Atypical Parkinsonian Disorders

CURRENT CLINICAL NEUROLOGY

Daniel Tarsy, MD, SERIES EDITOR

Atypical Parkinsonian Disorders
Clinical and Research Aspects

Edited by

Irene Litvan, MD

University of Louisville School of Medicine,
Louisville, KY

Foreword by

Yves Agid, MD, PhD

Hôpital de la Salpêtriere, Paris, France

HUMANA PRESS ✳ TOTOWA, NEW JERSEY

Due diligence has been taken by the publishers, editors, and authors of this book to assure the accuracy of the information published and to describe generally accepted practices. The contributors herein have carefully checked to ensure that the drug selections and dosages set forth in this text are accurate and in accord with the standards accepted at the time of publication. Notwithstanding, as new research, changes in government regulations, and knowledge from clinical experience relating to drug therapy and drug reactions constantly occurs, the reader is advised to check the product information provided by the manufacturer of each drug for any change in dosages or for additional warnings and contraindications. This is of utmost importance when the recommended drug herein is a new or infrequently used drug. It is the responsibility of the treating physician to determine dosages and treatment strategies for individual patients. Further it is the responsibility of the health care provider to ascertain the Food and Drug Administration status of each drug or device used in their clinical practice. The publisher, editors, and authors are not responsible for errors or omissions or for any consequences from the application of the information presented in this book and make no warranty, express or implied, with respect to the contents in this publication.

This publication is printed on acid-free paper. ∞
ANSI Z39.48-1984 (American Standards Institute) Permanence of Paper for Printed Library Materials.

Cover illustrations from Fig. 7B in Chapter 4, "Neuropathology of Atypical Parkinsonian Disorders," by Ian R. A. Mackenzie; Fig. 13A in Chapter 19, "Corticobasal Degeneration: *The Syndrome and the Disease*," by Bradley F. Boeve; Fig. 6 in Chapter 24, "Role of Electrophysiology in Diagnosis and Research in Atypical Parkinsonian Disorders," by Josep Valls-Solé; and Fig. 5D in Chapter 25, "Role of CT and MRI in Diagnosis and Research," by Mario Savoiardo and Marina Grisoli.

Cover design by Patricia F. Cleary

For additional copies, pricing for bulk purchases, and/or information about other Humana titles, contact Humana at the above address or at any of the following numbers: Tel.: 973-256-1699; Fax: 973-256-8314; E-mail: humana@humanapr.com, or visit our Website: http://humanapress.com

Printed in the United States of America. 10 9 8 7 6 5 4 3 2 1

eISBN: 1-59259-834-X

Library of Congress Cataloging in Publication Data

Atypical Parkinsonian disorders / edited by Irene Litvan.
      p. ; cm. -- (Current clinical neurology)
  Includes bibliographical references and index.
  ISBN 1-58829-331-9 (alk. paper)
  1. Parkinson's disease.
  [DNLM: 1. Parkinsonian Disorders. WL 359 A8874 2004] I. Litvan, Irene. II. Series.
  RC382.A89 2004
  616.8'33--dc22

                                                                                          2004008993

Series Editor's Introduction

Since the original classic description of Parkinson's disease, there have been swings in concept from a unitary disease with characteristic clinical features and unique neuropathologic changes to that of a more variable disorder with multiple etiologies owing to a spectrum of pathological processes. Originally, the terms *paralysis agitans* and Parkinson's disease first used in the 19th century implied a unitary disease. The concept of parkinsonism as a special disease entity was supported by the stereotyped features of akinesia, rigidity, tremor, and postural instability. The appearance of postencephalitic parkinsonism and later the recognition of "arteriosclerotic parkinsonism" led to the realization that there must be multiple forms of the disease. Idiopathic Parkinson's disease finally became anchored by identification of the Lewy body, which provided the necessary objective marker for what, at least temporarily, quite remarkably came to be called "Lewy body disease." However, the later discovery that parkinsonism and dementia arise from a more diffuse distribution of Lewy bodies led to the designation of dementia with Lewy bodies, one of the first of the new generation of atypical parkinsonian disorders to be recognized. Striatonigral degeneration, multiple system atrophy, progressive supranuclear palsy, and corticobasal degeneration soon followed and rapidly evolved from relatively exotic disorders to household words, at least among the rapidly growing community of movement disorder neurologists. Finally, more recently, even the unitary concept of idiopathic Parkinson's disease has been shaken by the discovery of multiple genetic types of Parkinson's disease that may occur with or without Lewy bodies!

Currently, patients are increasingly aware of the possibility of atypical parkinsonism. Many ask about it at early visits and understand their dismal prognosis and treatment prospects if they should have one of these disorders. Dr. Irene Litvan has been at the front line for many years in the effort to make sense of this bewildering array of atypical parkinsonian syndromes. In this volume she has brought together an impressive group of experts in the field. All aspects of these disorders are covered by highly knowledgeable and thoughtful investigators. Some of the clinical and scientific disciplines which are reviewed are clearly more mature than others, but it would be safe to say that our understanding of these disorders remains very much in its infancy. A particularly unique and very useful aspect of the book is that each chapter concludes with a section on future directions in research. As Dr. Litvan states in her preface, an important goal of this book is to enlist new researchers to further our knowledge about the cause and treatment of these devastating disorders. *Atypical Parkinsonian Disorders: Clinical and Research Aspects* will serve as the comprehensive reference to current state-of-the-art scientific developments in the field and will hopefully provide a launching pad for future fundamental discoveries in the pathophysiology and treatment of these currently hopeless disorders.

Daniel Tarsy, MD

Foreword

The term "atypical parkinsonian disorders" has the unavoidable connotation of neurodegeneration. Neurodegeneration can be defined as a loss of neurons that is both selective (i.e., several neuronal systems are affected, but not all), and slow (although faster than similar effects caused by aging). This definition excludes both sequelae of brain insults and diffuse lesions of the nervous system such as vascular parkinsonism and encephalopathies (Chapter 23).

What's in a name? A less depressing definition of parkinsonian disorders (or parkinsonism) might well be the following: an akinetic-rigid syndrome associated with the selective dysfunction of the nigrostriatal dopaminergic system. This definition is broad enough to include both typical and atypical neurodegenerative parkinsonian disorders. Parkinson's disease is what we call a "typical" parkinsonian disorder. Parkinson's disease is characterized by progressive akinesia and rigidity, usually unilateral at onset, with or without resting tremor, which responds significantly to levodopa treatment or other kinds of dopaminergic replacement therapy. However, the diagnosis of Parkinson's disease is difficult to establish for several reasons:

1. Akinesia and rigidity are heterogeneous symptoms that can differ from one patient to another. Plastic rigidity (associated with the classical cogwheel phenomenon and predominant in the extremities), is different from the diffuse rigidity of the Gegenhalten type (*rigidité oppositioniste*) observed in atypical parkinsonian disorders. Akinesia is a general term that is frequently used inappropriately, and does in fact include several symptoms: akinesia per se, which means delayed initiation of movement (increased reaction time); bradykinesia (slowness of movement); hypokinesia (easily observed when testing repetitive movements of the extremities); difficulty in performing consecutive or sequential gestures; and decreased motivation to move, whatever its origin.

2. Parkinson's disease is also difficult to diagnose because in most patients, other symptoms occur during the course of the disease, including cognitive decline (cortical and/or subcortical dysfunction) and axial symptoms such as dysarthria, swallowing difficulties, neck rigidity, postural abnormalities, urinary dysfunction, gait disorders, postural instability (all symptoms that represent a major component of atypical parkinsonian disorders), which respond poorly to Levodopa replacement therapy.

3. Before reaching a diagnosis of Parkinson's disease, it is indeed crucial to be sure that the patient shows a significant response to levodopa treatment (or related therapy) used at adequate doses. What we mean by "significant" is either (a) an objective 30% improvement in parkinsonian motor disability (as evaluated before and after the administration of Levodopa), or (b) a subjective 30% improvement in motor disability as assessed from the patient interview, either at the start of treatment (i.e., "What was the percentage improvement in your condition when you received levodopa treatment for the first time?") or later, during the course of the disease (i.e., "What was the percentage improvement in your condition when you took your first dose of levodopa?"). A clear-cut response to levodopa treatment (or dopamine agonists) is a prerequisite for a diagnosis of Parkinson's disease, as it indirectly reflects the existence of a dysfunction of dopaminergic neurons in the striatum of patients. A lack of response to levodopa treatment (using adequate doses of levodopa) does not mean that there is no nigrostriatal deficiency (inherent in the definition of parkinsonism), but rather indicates that the reestablishment of normal brain dopaminergic transmission is not followed by an improvement in motor disability owing to the presence of nondopaminergic lesions located downstream of the output of the basal ganglia.

4. Finally, Parkinson's disease is a heterogeneous disorder that includes several clinical phenotypes identified in recent years. The term "Parkinson's disease" should in fact be replaced by "Parkinson's diseases," as several phenotypes of this disorder have been described resulting from

different mutations within different genes in patients with familial and sporadic forms of the disease. This suggests that many, if not all, clinical phenotypes of sporadic Parkinson's disease have either a monogenic cause or at least involve a significant predisposition to develop the illness.

By deduction, atypical parkinsonian disorders can be defined as a mirror image of typical parkinsonism, i.e., an akinetic-rigid syndrome that is not improved by the reestablishment of normal dopaminergic transmission in the brain. Within the spectrum of diseases that constitute the syndrome of atypical parkinsonism, akinesia, and rigidity become rapidly severe and characteristically involve the axis of the body. Shortly after onset other signs become more prominent, leaving parkinsonism in the background: supranuclear gaze palsy, early falls and frontal lobe symptomatology will suggest progressive supranuclear palsy (Chapter 18); dysautonomia and cerebellar signs: multiple system atrophy (Chapter 20); unilateral apraxia, corticobasal degeneration (Chapters 13 and 19); dementia of the cortico-subcortical type with early visual hallucinations, Lewy body disease (Chapter 21). Additional symptoms may help to establish the diagnosis of atypical parkinsonism, including speech disorders (Chapter 14), various behavioral disorders (Chapters 12 and 13), dystonia, pyramidal signs and pseudo-bulbar palsy. A thorough physical examination (Chapter 10) will either allow a final diagnosis to be made or will suggest appropriate laboratory tests. Apart from electrophysiological investigations (Chapter 28), which are mostly interesting in terms of research, three investigations will provide decisive information as far as the diagnosis is concerned: a careful neuropsychological examination to evaluate the different cortical (and subcortical) components of cognitive disorders (Chapters 13, 16, and 24), ocular movement recording (Chapter 17), and neuroimaging, with particular reference to MRI (Chapter 25) (functional neuroimaging and positron emission tomography are mainly used for research purposes). Nevertheless, the diagnosis of atypical parkinsonian disorders is not easy to establish, and proves to be erroneous in about 10% of cases even in the hands of experts in the field of movement disorders.

The best definition of atypical parkinsonism is probably an anatomo-clinical one, since postmortem examination of the brains of patients does not always result in an accurate histological diagnosis. There is, indeed, an increasing number of postmortem cases in which histopathology does not entirely fulfill the diagnostic criteria for these disorders (Chapters 4 and 8), either because the distribution of the lesions is unusual or because atypical histopathological stigmata are associated with the characteristic hallmarks of the different diseases. Histopathological phenotypes have recently been identified, based on the presence of various abnormal tau proteins (Chapter 5) or synucleins (Chapter 6). These pathological classifications are of great interest in studying the pathogenesis of the disorders but, unfortunately, are of limited value to the patients and their caregivers. It is hoped that molecular and cellular research in these fields will help to delineate new clinical and pathological entities alongside those that have currently been identified in clinical practice.

During the past 5 years, aided by the unrelenting efforts of disease associations and lay groups, an enormous amount of research has been undertaken with two main aims. One is to find new symptomatic treatments. This implies understanding the neuronal substrate underlying each of the many and complex symptoms characteristic of each disorder, with a special focus on the anatomo-physiological organization of the neocortex and basal ganglia. The other is to cure the diseases, i.e., to understand the various mechanisms of nerve cell death that are directly related to the cause (or causes) of the diseases. The only way to define a disease is, indeed, to define it by its origin, whether the cause is genetic-monofactorial inheritance or multifactorial predisposition (Chapter 9), whether environmental factors play a predominant or contributive role (Chapter 3), or whether both of these causes are involved. The progress of research into the pathophysiology and pathogenesis of all these disorders is impressive, when one takes into account their relative recent description (Chapter 2).

An effort needs to be made by our institutions to develop research programs specifically dedicated to atypical parkinsonian disorders, from molecular and cellular biology to neurophysiology and behavioral sciences. The main objective, during the years ahead, must be to discover new drugs to improve the symptoms, to limit or stop the process of cell loss, and to repair the affected brain tissues. Yet, there has been a notable improvement in patient management during the last few years (Chapter 11). Though there is no available curative treatment (does one know of a neurodegenerative disease that can be cured?), there are numerous symptomatic treatments (Chapter 20) and rehabilitation approaches (Chapter 30) that will help to reduce disability and improve both the patients' well being and the quality of life for both patients and caregivers. This is perhaps the most important message of this book, *Atypical Parkinsonian Disorders: Clinical and Research Aspects*.

Irene Litvan, who has devoted the greater part of her clinical and research activities to these mysterious and distressing disorders, is to be applauded for having convinced so many leading experts in the field to contribute to this promising book.

Yves Agid, MD, PhD

Preface

The "atypical parkinsonian disorders," previously known as "Parkinson plus syndromes," are characterized by a rapidly evolving parkinsonism that usually has a poor or transient response to dopaminergic therapy and often associates with one or more atypical features. These disorders may be difficult to accurately diagnose, but an early and correct diagnosis is relevant for both patients and physicians, since it allows for appropriate management and prognosis, which in turn, improves patients and families quality of life. An accurate diagnosis also allows patients to participate in research and may increase survival.

This book, *Atypical Parkinsonian Disorders: Clinical and Research Aspects*, the first of its kind, provides an all-encompassing view of the current status of atypical parkinsonian disorders from both clinical and research viewpoints. Its goals are threefold: (1) to provide critical, state-of-the-art insight into both the clinical and research aspects of the atypical parkinsonian disorders; (2) to increase clinicians' index of suspicion by providing them with appropriate tools for an accurate diagnosis; and (3) to enlist new researchers who will further our knowledge on the etiopathogenesis of these devastating disorders and hopefully allow for the identification of new therapeutic paradigms.

The chapters have been written by world-leading experts in their fields, and their efforts have culminated in a truly unique compilation of what is currently known about the historic aspects, epidemiology, neuropathology, genetics, neuropsychological, neuropsychiatric, ophthalmologic, neurologic, and radiologic diagnostic evaluations and therapeutic approaches, as well as overall understanding of atypical parkinsonian disorders. We anticipate that the enclosed DVD, containing visual and auditory aids, will help clinicians, fellows, residents, students, and neuroscience researchers alike to characterize and differentiate the various atypical parkinsonian disorders. Audio segments will be helpful to characterize and distinguish the diverse speech disturbances found in these disorders. Current controversies and the role of genetics and neurological and pathological phenotypes in the nosologic classification of these disorders as well as each chapter author's view on where research should focus in the future are offered.

Movement disorder specialists, neurologists, neuro-ophthalmologists, neuropathologists, psychiatrists, neuropsychologists, geriatricians, and physical and occupational therapists alike may find these pages indispensable. Clinicians, residents, and students may find the chapters on epidemiology, medical and physical history techniques, neuropsychiatric and neuropsychological testing, praxis, visuospatial cognition, neuro-ophthalmology, and speech and language assessments invaluable tools for clinical diagnosis, while the disease-specific videos, tables, and figures may provide them with a visual handbook for frequent reference. Researchers and fellows will gain further insight into their own work, which will add to the progression of the knowledge presented in theses pages.

Atypical Parkinsonian Disorders would have not been possible without the hard work and dedication of friends and colleagues who graciously provided state-of-the-art chapters, excellent figures, and unique video and audio segments that we believe are crucial tools for learning, teaching, and research. I want particularly to thank Dr. Daniel Tarsy for encouraging me to edit this exciting book. I also want to acknowledge the help provided by Theresa Perry and Whitney Rogers in its preparation, and the support from Michael Gruenthal and the University of Louisville. Finally, I want to thank patients and caregivers for their time and dedication to our research and for their patience waiting for a therapeutic paradigm shift. It is hoped that their increasing participation in research and the knowledge summarized in this book will provide the needed enthusiasm to attract new researchers into this field who will further our understanding of these diseases so they can soon be eradicated from the face of the earth.

Carol Frattali, co-author of Chapter 16 on speech and language, passed away suddenly while this book was in press. Carol was a superb clinician, valued colleague, and was developing a new program of research at the National Institutes of Health when she was taken from us. Carol was not afraid to begin a new research project, no matter how difficult the challenge. I am sure that attitude kept her young at heart and permeated all facets of her life. She was inspirational to patients, colleagues and friends, and we all surely miss her.

Irene Litvan, MD

Contents

Contributors

DAG AARSLAND, PhD • Centre for Neuro and Geriatric Psychiatric Research, Rogaland Central Hospital, Stavanger, Norway

YVES AGID, MD, PhD • INSERM U-289, Hôpital de la Salpêtriere, Paris, France

CLIVE BALLARD, PhD • Wolfson Centre for Age-Related Diseases, Kings College London, London, UK

YOAV BEN-SHLOMO, MRCP, FFPHM • Department of Social Medicine, University of Bristol, Bristol, UK

BRADLEY F. BOEVE, MD • Division of Behavioral Neurology, Department of Neurology, Mayo Clinic College of Medicine, Rochester, MN

FRÉDÉRIC BOURDAIN • Department of Neurology, Saint-Antoine Hospital, and U289 Hôpital de la Salpêtrière, Paris, France

DAVID J. BROOKS, MD, DSC, FRCP • MRC Cyclotron Unit Department of Neurology, Faculty of Medicine, Hammersmith Hospital, Imperial College, London, UK

DAVID J. BURN, MD, FRCP • Institute for Aging and Health, Wolfson Research Centre, Regional Neurosciences Centre, Department of Neurology, Newcastle General Hospital and University of Newcastle-upon-Tyne, Newcastle-upon-Tyne, UK

LAURA BUYAN-DENT, MD, PhD • Department of Neurology, Boston University School of Medicine, Boston, MA

THOMAS N. CHASE, MD • Experimental Therapeutics Branch, National Institute of Neurological Disorders and Stroke, National Institutes of Health, Bethesda, MD

JOSÉ LUIS CONTRERAS-VIDAL, PhD • Department of Kinesiology and Graduate Program in Neuroscience and Cognitive Science (NACS), University of Maryland, College Park, MD

BRUNO DUBOIS, MD • Clinique de Neurologie et Neuropsychologie, INSERM U 610, Hôpital de la Salpêtriere, Paris, France

GÜNTHER DEUSCHL, MD • Department of Neurology, Christian-Albrechts-University, Kiel, Germany

JOSEPH R. DUFFY, PhD, BC-NCD • Department of Neurology, Division of Speech Pathology, Mayo Clinic and Medical School, Rochester, MN

CHARLES DUYCKAERTS, MD • Laboratoire de Neuropathologie Escourolle, Hôpital de la Salpêtrière, Paris, France

UWE EHRT, MD • Centre for Neuro and Geriatric Psychiatric Research, Rogaland Central Hospital, Stavanger, Norway

TERRY ELLIS, MSPT, NCS • Sargent College of Health and Rehabilitation Sciences, Boston University, Boston, MA

ELMYRA V. ENCARNACION, MD • Movement Disorders Section, Neurosciences Department, Wellspan Health, York, PA

VIRGILIO H. EVIDENTE, MD • Department of Neurology, Mayo Clinic, Scottsdale, AZ; Mayo Medical School, Rochester, MN

CAROL FRATTALI, PhD, BC-NCD • Rehabilitation Medicine Department, Speech-Language Pathology Section, W.G. Magnuson Clinical Center, National Institutes of Health, Bethesda, MD; Department of Hearing and Speech Sciences, University of Maryland at College Park, College Park, MD

THOMAS GASSER, MD • Department of Neurodegenerative Diseases, Hertie-Institute for Clinical Brain Research, University of Tübingen, Tübingen, Germany

ALEXANDER GERHARD, MD • MRC Clinical Sciences Centre and Division of Neuroscience, Faculty of Medicine, Hammersmith Hospital, Imperial College, London, UK

FELIX GESER, MD • Department of Neurology, University Hospital, Innsbruck, Austria

MICHEL GOEDERT, MD, PhD, FRS • MRC Laboratory of Molecular Biology, Cambridge, UK

CHRISTOPHER G. GOETZ, MD • Departments of Neurological Sciences and Pharmacology, Rush University/Rush University Medical Center, Chicago, IL

MARINA GRISOLI, MD • Department of Neuroradiology, Istituto Nazionale Neurologico "C. Besta," Milan, Italy

MICHAEL HUTTON, PhD • Department of Neuroscience, Mayo Clinic Jacksonville, Jacksonville, FL

JOSEPH JANKOVIC, MD • Parkinson's Disease Center and Movement Disorders Clinic, Department of Neurology, Baylor College of Medicine, Houston, TX

DOUGLAS I. KATZ, MD • Healthsouth Braintree Rehabilitation Hospital, Braintree, MA; Department of Neurology, Boston University School of Medicine, Boston, MA

ANDREW LEES, MD, FRCP • Reta Lila Weston Institute of Neurological Studies, Windeyer Medical Institute, University College London WC1 UK

R. JOHN LEIGH, MD • Departments of Neurology, Neurosciences, and Biomedical Engineering, Veterans Affairs Medical Center and Case Western Reserve University, Cleveland OH; Department of Neurology, University Hospitals, Cleveland, OH

RAMÓN LEIGUARDA, MD • Professor of Neurology, Raúl Correa Institute of Neurological Research, FLENI, Buenos Aires, Argentina

JADA LEWIS, PhD • Department of Neuroscience, Mayo Clinic Jacksonville, Jacksonville FL

IRENE LITVAN, MD • Raymond Lee Lebby Professor of Parkinson Disease Research, Director, Movement Disorder Program, Department of Neurology, University of Louisville School of Medicine, Louisville, KY

IAN R. A. MACKENZIE, MD, FRCPC • Department of Pathology and Laboratory Medicine, University of British Columbia, Vancouver, Canada

ANNA MAGHERINI, MD • Clinica Neurologica, Università di Modena e Reggio Emilia, Modena, Italy

IAN G. McKEITH, MD, FRCPSYCH • Institute for Aging and Health, Wolfson Research Centre, Newcastle General Hospital and University of Newcastle-upon-Tyne, Newcastle-upon-Tyne, UK

URS P. MOSIMANN, MD • Institute for Aging and Health, Wolfson Research Centre, Newcastle General Hospital and University of Newcastle-upon-Tyne, Newcastle-upon-Tyne, UK

PAOLO NICHELLI, MD • Clinica Neurologica, Università di Modena e Reggio Emilia, Modena, Italy

BERNARD PILLON, PhD • Clinique de Neurologie et Neuropsychologie, INSERM U 610, Hôpital de la Salpêtriere, Paris, France

MARIE H. SAINT-HILAIRE, MD, FRCAC • Healthsouth Braintree Rehabilitation Hospital, Braintree, MA; Department of Neurology, Boston University School of Medicine, Boston, MA

MARIO SAVOIARDO, MD • Department of Neuroradiology, Istituto Nazionale Neurologico "C. Besta," Milan, Italy

ANETTE SCHRAG, MD, PhD • University Department of Clinical Neurosciences, Royal Free and University College Medical School, London, UK

CAROLINE E. SELAI, PhD, CPSYCHOL • Department of Motor Neuroscience and Movement Disorders, Institute of Neurology, Queen Square, London UK

HARTWIG ROMAN SIEBNER, MD • Department of Neurology, Christian-Albrechts-University, Kiel, Germany

MARIA GRAZIA SPILLANTINI, PhD • Centre for Brain Repair, Department of Neurology, University of Cambridge, Cambridge, UK

MADHAVI THOMAS, MD • Experimental Therapeutics Branch, National Institutes of Neurologic Disorders and Stroke, National Institutes of Health, Bethesda, MD

JEAN-MARC TROCELLO • Department of Neurology, Saint-Antoine Hospital, and U289 Hôpital de la Salpêtrière, Paris, France

YOSHIO TSUBOI, MD • Department of Neurology, Mayo Clinic, Jacksonville, FL; (Currently at) Fifth Department of Internal Medicine, Fukuoka University School of Medicine, Fukuoka, Japan

JOSEP VALLS-SOLÉ, MD • Unitat d'EMG, Servei de Neurologia, Departament de Medicina, Hospital Clínic, Institut d'Investigacio Biomedica August Pi i Sunyer (IDIBAPS), Universitat de Barcelona, Barcelona, Spain

MARIE VIDAILHET, MD • Department of Neurology, Saint-Antoine hospital, and U289 Hôpital de la Salpêtrière, Paris, France

GREGOR K. WENNING, MD, PhD • Department of Neurology, University Hospital, Innsbruck, Austria

DANIEL K. WHITE, MSPT • Healthsouth Braintree Rehabilitation Hospital, Braintree, MA; Sargent College of Health and Rehabilitation Sciences, Boston University, Boston, MA

ZBIGNIEW K. WSZOLEK, MD • Department of Neurology, Mayo Clinic, Jacksonville, FL; Mayo Medical School, Rochester, MN

DAVID S. ZEE, MD • Departments of Neurology and Neurosciences, The Johns Hopkins University School of Medicine, Baltimore, MD

ADAM ZERMANSKY, MBCHB, MRCP • Regional Neurosciences Centre, University of Newcastle-upon-Tyne, Newcastle-upon-Tyne, UK

Companion DVD

To use this DVD-ROM, you will need a computer with a DVD drive. This DVD will not operate in a CD-ROM drive. To view the PDF files on this DVD-ROM, you will need Adobe Reader. To view the video clips, you will need an MPEG-1 compatible video player (Windows Media Player, Quicktime, Real Player, etc.). Most computers and operating systems will play these videos without further installation or modification.

What is an Atypical Parkinsonian Disorder?

Irene Litvan

INTRODUCTION

A parkinsonism is a syndrome defined by akinesia associated with rigidity or rest tremor. The akinesia can be expressed as motor slowness (bradykinesia) or as a paucity of movement (hypokinesia), i.e., difficulty in the initiation of or decreased amplitude of movements such as arm swing or facial expression. This syndrome is usually the result of a dysfunctional nigrostriatal pallidal pathway. Impairment of postural reflexes is not included as one of the features of the parkinsonian syndrome since abnormal postural reflexes are generally the consequence of dysfunction of other motor pathways. There are a variety of causes of parkinsonism, but Parkinson's disease (PD) is the most common (Fig. 1). Although there is extensive literature on PD, this is one of the few books dedicated to the remaining atypical parkinsonian disorders. To appropriately diagnose PD, one should be aware of when to suspect that a patient does not have PD and may be suffering from one of these atypical disorders.

The "atypical parkinsonian disorders" (previously known as "Parkinson plus syndromes") are characterized by a *rapidly evolving* parkinsonism that has a poor or transient response to dopaminergic therapy and often associates with one or more *atypical features* for PD. Some of these features include early presence of postural instability, early autonomic failure, vertical supranuclear gaze palsy, pyramidal or cerebellar signs, alien limb syndrome, and apraxia (Table 1; *see* corresponding video segments on accompanying DVD). Making the distinction between these two major groups of disorders is critical for both clinical practice and research because the prognosis and treatment of patients with an atypical parkinsonian disorder and those with PD differ *(1–4)*. In the clinical setting, although patients with PD may have an almost normal life-span if treated appropriately *(4–6)*, those with atypical parkinsonian disorders have a shorter survival time and more complications occur at early stages and are frequently more severe *(3,7–10)* (*see* Table 2 for an example). Moreover, indicated therapies (particularly surgical approaches) differ significantly since some may not be indicated to treat patients with atypical parkinsonian disorders. Until recently, clinicians would "lump" all the atypical parkinsonian disorders together and would only distinguish between this group and PD. However, the need for early identification of the different atypical parkinsonian disorders is becoming increasingly recognized *(11)*, as their prognosis, complications, and survival differ *(3,7,8,12–19)*.

For research, this distinction is crucial; homogenous groups are a necessity for studies that lead to firm conclusions. Genetic, analytical, epidemiological, and clinical trials require the inclusion of accurately diagnosed patients. However, diagnosis of the atypical parkinsonian disorders can be at times challenging *(20–25)* since these disorders may have similar presentations at early disease stages

From: *Current Clinical Neurology: Atypical Parkinsonian Disorders*
Edited by: I. Litvan © Humana Press Inc., Totowa, NJ

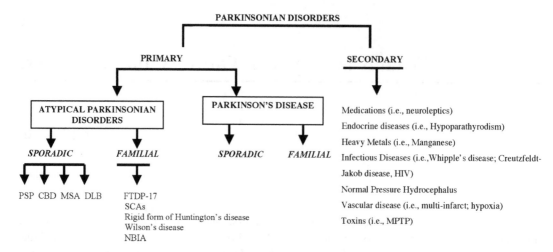

Fig. 1. PSP, progressive supranuclear palsy; CBD, corticobasal degeneration; MSA, multiple system atrophy; DLB, dementia with Lewy bodies; FTDP-17, frontotemporal dementia with parkinsonism linked to chromosome 17; SCAs, spinocerebellar atrophy; NBIA, Neurodegeneration With Brain Iron Accumulation, previously called Hallervorden–Spatz Syndrome; HIV, human immunodeficiency virus.

Table 1
When Should an Atypical Parkinsonian Disorder be Suspected?

Features suggestive of an atypical parkinsonian disorder

Motor
  Rapid disease progression
  Early instability and falls
  Absent, poor, or not maintained response to levodopa therapy
  Myoclonus
  Pyramidal signs
  Cerebellar signs
  Early dysarthria and/or dysphagia
  Early dystonia/contractures (unrelated to treatment)
Autonomic Features
  Impotence/decreased genital sensitivity in females
  Early orthostatic hypotension unrelated to treatment
  Early and/or severe urinary disturbances
Oculomotor
  Marked slowing of saccades
  Difficulty initiating saccades, gaze (oculomotor apraxia)
  Supranuclear gaze palsy
  Nystagmus
Cognitive and behavioral
  Early and severe frontal or cortical dementia
  Visual hallucinations not induced by treatment
  Ideomotor apraxia
  Sensory or visual neglect/cortical disturbances

Table 2
Progression of Various Parkinsonian Disorders

Disorder	Sample Size (N)	Median Age at Onset (yr)	Median HY II Latencies (mo)	Median HY III Latencies (mo)	Median HY IV Latencies (mo)	Median HY V Latencies (mo)	Median survival After HY V Onset (mo)
PD	18	60	36[*]	66[**]	166[**]	179[**]	12
CBD	13	64	25	42	55	62	43
DLB	11	65	12	43	45	59	12
MSA	15	56	0	3	56	73	10
PSP	24	65	—	0	38	56	9

Modified from Muller et al., with permission *(17)*.
[*]$p < 0.05$; [**]$p < 0.001$ Parkinson's disease (PD) vs atypical parkinsonian disorders (CBD, DLB, MSA, PSP), (Mann–Whitney U Test). PD patients had a significantly longer latency to each Hoehn and Yahr (HY) stage than those with atypical parkinsonian disorders, confirming the more rapid progression of motor disability in patients with atypical parkinsonian disorders. Most MSA and PSP patients developed postural instability with or without falls significantly earlier than those with CBD and DLB. Postural instability and falls are the most common initial symptoms in PSP, and almost all PSP patients developed an HY stage III within 1 yr of motor onset. The majority of MSA (67%), the majority of DLB (55%), and 38% of CBD patients also reached this stage early.

(i.e., progressive falls, parkinsonism not responsive to dopaminergic therapy). Tell-tale signs may take 2 to 4 yr after symptom onset to develop, or early features may be either disregarded or misdiagnosed by clinicians.

Misdiagnosis of these disorders is frequent, as patients exhibit a variety of symptoms that may lead them to be initially evaluated by internists or specialists (e.g., ophthalmologists, urologists, neurologists, psychiatrists, neurosurgeons). For example, it is not unusual for a patient with progressive supranuclear palsy (PSP) to be evaluated by several ophthalmologists (and have their glasses changed several times) or to have multiple unnecessary studies for evaluating the cause of their falls prior to being seen by a neurologist. Similarly, patients with corticobasal degeneration (CBD) may present after unsuccessful carpal tunnel surgery, or those with multiple system atrophy (MSA) may present only after failed prostate surgery; in both cases these types of surgery can worsen the patients' symptoms. Diagnostic accuracy would greatly improve, however, if clinicians from different disciplines would have a broader knowledge of the typical and atypical presentations of these disorders and use proposed clinical diagnostic criteria *(26)*.

In the absence of biological markers and known pathogenesis, current diagnosis requires the presence of certain clinical features that allow for clinical diagnosis and eventual pathologic verification. As a result, diagnostic accuracy requires that both clinical and pathological sets of diagnostic criteria be valid and reliable *(27,28)*. Neuropathologic diagnostic criteria for most parkinsonian disorders have been validated and standardized *(27,29)*; the exceptions are those for dementia with Lewy bodies (DLB) and PD with later onset dementia (PDD). Similarly, recently the clinical diagnostic criteria have undergone the same process of rigorous operationalization and validation for most of these disorders *(26,30–35)*.

Though consensus for the diagnosis of several of these disorders has been put forward *(30–33)*, and validation studies of diagnostic criteria have been performed for most of the atypical parkinsonian disorders *(36)*, refinement of the criteria is still needed *(36)*. In practice, clinicians are exposed to patients who exhibit different parkinsonian disorders, and so validation studies should compare the accuracy of several sets of criteria with neuropathology. The Scientific Issue Committee of the Movement Disorder Society created a task force to critically review the accuracy of different sets of diagnostic criteria for parkinsonian disorders *(36)*. The task force analyzed how well each set of diagnostic criteria identified all subjects with the disease as having the disease (i.e., sensitivity); identified sub-

Table 3
Validity of the Clinical Diagnostic Criteria for PSP, MSA, DLB, and VaD

Disorder	Criteria	Sensitivity (%)	Specificity (%)	Positive Predictive Value (%)	Author	n/n TOTAL
PSP	Blin et al. *(47)*				Litvan et al.	
	Probable/Possible	21/63	100/85	100/63	(29)	24/83
	Blin et al. *(47)*					
	Probable/Possible-1st visit	13/34	100/98	100/85	Litvan	
	Probable/Possible-last visit	55/89	94/74	73/50	(19)	24/105
	Clinician's own criteria					
	First visit	72	93	76	Litvan et al.	
	Last visit	80	92	76	(19)	24/105
	Collins et al. *(51)*				Litvan et al.	
	Probable/Possible	25/42	100/92	100/67	(29)	24/83
	Golbe et al. *(49)*					
	First visit	49	97	85	Litvan et al.	
	Last visit	67	94	76	(19)	24/105
	Golbe et al. *(49)*	50	98	92		24/83
	Lees (48)					
	First visit	53	95	77		
	Last visit	78	87	65		24/105
					Litvan	
	Lees *(48)*	58	95	82	(29)	24/83
	NINDS-SPSP				Litvan et al.	
	Probable/Possible	50/83	100/93	100/83	(29)	24/83
	NINDS-SPSP				Lopez	
	Probable/Possible	62/75	100/98.5	100/96	(25)	8/40
	Queen Square Movement Disorder neurologists				Hughes	
	diagnosis	84.2	96.8	80	(52)*	20/143
	Tolosa et al. *(50)*				Litvan	
	Probable/Possible	54/54	98/98	93/93	(19)	24/83
	Clinician's own criteria					
	First visit	56	96.6	75.5	Litvan et al.	
MSA	Last visit	69	97	80	(21)	16/105
	Clinician's prospective diagnosis in life					
	First visit	22		92	Oaski et al.	
	Last visit	100		86	(33)	51/59
	Consensus Criteria *(55)*					
	Probable/Possible	16/28		100/93		
	Consensus Criteria *(55)*					
	Probable/Possible	63/92		91/86		
	Queen Square movement disorder neurologist's				Hughes et al.	
	diagnosis	88		86	(52)*	34/143
	Quinn *(54)*					
	Probable/Possible	37/63		95/82		
	Quinn *(54)*					
	Probable/Possible	94/98		87/86		

(continued)

Table 3 *(continued)*
Validity of the Clinical Diagnostic Criteria for PSP, MSA, DLB, and VaD

Disorder	Criteria	Sensitivity (%)	Specificity (%)	Positive Predictive Value (%)	Author	n/n TOTAL
	Quinn *(54)*				Litvan et al.	
	Probable/Possible	44/53	97/79	68/30	*(53)*	16/105
	First visit					
DLB	CERAD	75	50		Mega *(56)*	4/24
	CDLB *(30)*	75	79	100	Mega *(56)*	4/24
	CDLB (30)					
	First visit	17.8		75		
	Last visit	28.6	NR	55.8	Litvan *(62)*	14/105
	CDLB*(30)*	22	100	100	Holmes *(57)*	9/80
	CDLB*(30)*	57	90	91	Luis *(58)*	35/56
	CDLB *(30)*				Verghese	
	Probable/Possible	61/89	84/23	48/23	*(59)*	18/94
	CDLB *(30)*					
	Probable/Possible	0/34	100/94	NA/55	Lopez *(25)*	8/40
	CDLB *(30)*				McKeith	
	Probable/Possible	83/83	95/91	96/92	*(64)*	29/50
	CDLB *(30)*					
	Probable/Possible	100/100	8/0	83/NA	Hohl *(60)*	5/10
	CDLB *(30)*	30.7	100		Lopez *(34)**	13/26
	Clinician's own criteria					
	First visit	17.8	99	75		
	Last visit	28.6	99	55.8	Litvan *(61)*	14/105
	Clinicians own criteria					
	First visit	35	99.6	80		
VaD	Last visit	48	99.6	100	Litvan *(62)*	10/105
	Queen Square movement disorder neurologists' diagnosis	25	98.6	33.3	Hughes et al. *(52)**	3/143

Revised from Litvan et al. *(36)*.

*Prospective studies. Note that all other studies are retrospective. CDLB, consensus criteria for dementia with Lewy bodies.

jects without the disease as not having the disease (i.e., specificity); and provided reasonable estimates of disease risk (i.e., positive predictive value or PPV). *See* summary table (Table 3) and refer to the actual publication *(36)* and specific disease-related chapters in this book for detailed comments. Overall, most of these criteria are specific but not very sensitive. It is worth noting that a validation of pathologic and clinical diagnostic criteria for PD is still needed. Standardization of diagnostic criteria, clinical scales, and identification of outcome measures *(37,38)* set the stage for conducting appropriate clinical trials.

CLASSIFICATION OF ATYPICAL PARKINSONIAN DISORDERS

Atypical parkinsonian disorders can be caused by primary or secondary diseases (*see* Fig. 1). The primary causes consist of neurodegenerative processes such as PSP, CBD, MSA, DLB, and PDD. Interestingly, one of the earlier historical cases thought to have the typical features of PSP was recently found to have a midbrain tumor through autopsy examination. As discussed in Chapter 23, secondary causes also include drugs, infections, toxins, or vascular disease *(21,23,39–44)*.

Table 4
Classification of Atypical Parkinsonian Disroders

Tauopathies	Synucleinopathies
Progressive supranuclear palsy	Parkinson's disease
Corticobasal degeneration	Multiple system atrophy
Lytico-bodig disease	Dementia with Lewy bodies
West-French Indies parkinsonian disorder	Parkinson disease and dementia
Frontotemporal dementias with parkinsonism linked to chromosome 17	Neurodegeneration with brain iron accumulation

An alternative classification (mostly helpful for research and future therapeutic approaches rather than for clinical use) considers the type of aggregated proteins in the brain lesions and classifies these disorders as tauopathies and synucleinopathies (Table 4; *see also* Chapters 4 and 8). Commonalities in clinical, biological, or genetic findings question the nosological classification of some of these disorders; for further information the reader is referred to Chapters 8 and 9.

PSP and DLB/PDD are the most frequent neurodegenerative primary cause of an atypical parkinsonian disorders *(31,45–47)*. A good history and physical examination will rule out drug-induced atypical parkinsonian disorders and supports the diagnosis of these specific disorders (Chapter 10). Each disorder is specifically covered in Chapters 18–23. The role of ancillary and laboratory tools to assist in the diagnosis of these disorders is discussed in Chapters 11–16 and 24–27. Ancillary tests (e.g., neuroradiologic or cerebrospinal studies) also help with the diagnosis of disorders caused by vascular diseases, tumors, or infection (e.g., Whipple's disease, Creutzfeldt–Jakob disease, human immunodeficiency virus). Specific therapeutic and rehabilitation approaches for all of these disorders are provided in each disease chapter and an overview of future biologic and rehabilitation approaches is provided in Chapters 28 and 29.

It is our expectation that this book will continue to improve the accuracy of the diagnosis of these disorders by raising awareness of their different presentations and by increasing diagnosticians' index of suspicion. An early and accurate diagnosis will allow better management of these patients and increase research potential.

There has been a tremendous increase in our knowledge concerning the proteins that characterize and aggregate in the brain in each of these disorders. Moreover, animal models are now available to help test potential new therapies (*see* Chapters 5 and 6). Hence, in addition to serving as a reference source, it is hoped that this book will stimulate new investigators to join us in the search for answers to the multiple questions raised throughout the book and in the battle against these disorders. It is anticipated that a better understanding of these diseases, their nosology, and etiopathogenesis (*see* Chapters 3–9) will lead to better management, quality of life (*see* Chapter 17), and treatment for patients who suffer them. We anticipate that the eradication of these devastating diseases from the face of the earth will occur in not such a remote future.

VIDEOTAPE

Postural Instability: Video segment shows a patient with a history of falls and an impaired postural reflex with the backward pull test. The patient would have fallen, unless aided by the examiner. The gait is stable but slightly wide-based.

Supranuclear gaze palsy: This patient shows a severe limitation in the range of ocular motor movements observed, which affects more upward than downward voluntary and pursuit gaze. As observed, the oculocephalic reflex is preserved when the the doll's head maneuver is performed.

Slowing of vertical saccades: Patient shows markedly slow vertical saccades and relatively preserved horizontal saccades.

Ocular motor apraxia: The patient shows difficulty initiating the voluntary gaze and saccades but exhibits a preserved pursuit and optokinetic nystagmus. Once the saccades are initiated their speed is normal.

Corticosensory deficits: This patient shows right sensory neglect and agraphesthesia. These lateralized cognitive features in conjunction with the progressive development of a right ideomotor apraxia, dystonia, and stimulus sensitive myoclonus led to the diagnosis of corticobasal degeneration (corticobasal syndrome).

Limb kinetic apraxia: The performance of this patient does not improve with imitation. Movements are coarse and do not represent the intended action.

Blepharospasm: Difficulty opening the eyes because of inhibition of eyelid opening, which is followed by blepharospasm.

REFERENCES

1. Litvan I. Parkinsonian features: when are they Parkinson disease? JAMA 1998;280:1654–1655.
2. Wenning GK, Ebersbach G, Verny M, et al. Progression of falls in postmortem-confirmed parkinsonian disorders. Mov Disord 1999;14:947–950.
3. Muller J, Wenning GK, Verny M, et al. Progression of dysarthria and dysphagia in postmortem-confirmed parkinsonian disorders. Arch Neurol 2001;58:259–264.
4. Elbaz A, Bower JH, Peterson BJ, et al. Survival study of Parkinson disease in Olmsted County, Minnesota. Arch Neurol 2003;60:91–96.
5. Mortality in DATATOP: a multicenter trial in early Parkinson's disease. Parkinson Study Group. Ann Neurol 1998;43:318–325.
6. Scigliano G, Musicco M, Soliveri P, et al. Mortality associated with early and late levodopa therapy initiation in Parkinson's disease. Neurology 1990;40:265–269.
7. Wenning GK, Ben-Shlomo Y, Magalhaes M, Daniel SE, Quinn NP. Clinicopathological study of 35 cases of multiple system atrophy. J Neurol Neurosurg Psychiatry 1995;58:160–166.
8. Wenning GK, Litvan I, Jankovic J, et al. Natural history and survival of 14 patients with corticobasal degeneration confirmed at postmortem examination. J Neurol Neurosurg Psychiatry 1998;64:184–189.
9. Ben-Shlomo Y, Wenning GK, Tison F, Quinn NP. Survival of patients with pathologically proven multiple system atrophy: a meta-analysis. Neurology 1997;48:384–3893.
10. Nath U, Ben-Shlomo Y, Thomson RG, Lees AJ, Burn DJ. Clinical features and natural history of progressive supranuclear palsy: A clinical cohort study. Neurology 2003;60:910–916.
11. Siderowf A, Quinn NP. Progressive supranuclear palsy: setting the scene for therapeutic trials. Neurology 2003;60:892–893.
12. Litvan I, Mangone CA, McKee A, et al. Natural history of progressive supranuclear palsy (Steele–Richardson–Olszewski syndrome) and clinical predictors of survival: a clinicopathological study. J Neurol Neurosurg Psychiatry 1996;60:615–6120.
13. Maher ER, Lees AJ. The clinical features and natural history of the Steele–Richardson–Olszewski syndrome (progressive supranuclear palsy). Neurology 1986;36:1005–1008.
14. Watanabe H, Saito Y, Terao S, et al. Progression and prognosis in multiple system atrophy: an analysis of 230 Japanese patients. Brain 2002;125:1070–1083.
15. Wenning GK, Geser F, Stampfer-Kountchev M, Tison F. Multiple system atrophy: an update. Mov Disord 2003;18(Suppl 6):S34–S42.
16. Wenning GK, Braune S. Multiple system atrophy: pathophysiology and management. CNS Drugs 2001;15:839–852.
17. Muller J, Wenning GK, Jellinger K, McKee A, Poewe W, Litvan I. Progression of Hoehn and Yahr stages in Parkinsonian disorders: a clinicopathologic study. Neurology 2000;55:888–891.
18. Wenning GK, Ben Shlomo Y, Magalhaes M, Daniel SE, Quinn NP. Clinical features and natural history of multiple system atrophy. An analysis of 100 cases. Brain 1994;117(Pt 4):835–845.
19. Golbe LI. The epidemiology of PSP. J Neural Transm Suppl 1994;42:263–273.
20. Litvan I, Agid Y, Jankovic J, et al. Accuracy of clinical criteria for the diagnosis of progressive supranuclear palsy (Steele–Richardson–Olszewski syndrome). Neurology 1996;46:922–930.
21. Litvan I, Agid Y, Goetz C, et al. Accuracy of the clinical diagnosis of corticobasal degeneration: a clinicopathologic study. Neurology 1997;48:119–125.
22. Litvan I, Goetz CG, Jankovic J, et al. What is the accuracy of the clinical diagnosis of multiple system atrophy? A clinicopathologic study. Arch Neurol 1997;54:937–944.

23. Boeve BF, Maraganore DM, Parisi JE, et al. Pathologic heterogeneity in clinically diagnosed corticobasal degeneration. Neurology 1999;53:795–800.

24. Wenning GK, Ben-Shlomo Y, Hughes A, Daniel SE, Lees A, Quinn NP. What clinical features are most useful to distinguish definite multiple system atrophy from Parkinson's disease? J Neurol Neurosurg Psychiatry 2000;68:434–440.

25. Bhatia KP, Lee MS, Rinne JO, et al. Corticobasal degeneration look-alikes. Adv Neurol 2000;82:169–182.

26. Lopez OL, Litvan I, Catt KE, et al. Accuracy of four clinical diagnostic criteria for the diagnosis of neurodegenerative dementias. Neurology 1999;53:1292–1299.

27. Litvan I, Hauw JJ, Bartko JJ, et al. Validity and reliability of the preliminary NINDS neuropathologic criteria for progressive supranuclear palsy and related disorders. J Neuropathol Exp Neurol 1996;55:97–105.

28. Litvan I. Methodological and research issues in the evaluation of biological diagnostic markers for Alzheimer's disease. Neurobiol Aging 1998;19:121–123.

29. Dickson DW, Bergeron C, Chin SS, et al. Office of Rare Diseases neuropathologic criteria for corticobasal degeneration. J Neuropathol Exp Neurol 2002;61:935–946.

30. Litvan I, Agid Y, Calne D, et al. Clinical research criteria for the diagnosis of progressive supranuclear palsy (Steele–Richardson–Olszewski syndrome): report of the NINDS-SPSP international workshop. Neurology 1996;47:1–9.

31. McKeith IG, Galasko D, Kosaka K, et al. Consensus guidelines for the clinical and pathologic diagnosis of dementia with Lewy bodies (DLB): report of the consortium on DLB international workshop. Neurology 1996;47:1113–1124.

32. McKeith IG, Perry EK, Perry RH. Report of the second dementia with Lewy body international workshop: diagnosis and treatment. Consortium on Dementia with Lewy Bodies. Neurology 1999;53:902–905.

33. Gilman S, Low P, Quinn N, et al. Consensus statement on the diagnosis of multiple system atrophy. American Autonomic Society and American Academy of Neurology. Clin Auton Res 1998;8:359–362.

34. Osaki Y, Wenning GK, Daniel SE, et al. Do published criteria improve clinical diagnostic accuracy in multiple system atrophy? Neurology 2002;59:1486–1491.

35. Lopez OL, Becker JT, Kaufer DI, et al. Research evaluation and prospective diagnosis of dementia with Lewy bodies. Arch Neurol 2002;59:43–46.

36. Litvan I, Bhatia KP, Burn DJ, et al. SIC Task Force appraisal of clinical diagnostic criteria for parkinsonian disorders. Mov Disord 2003;18:467–486.

37. Goetz CG, Leurgans S, Lang AE, Litvan I. Progression of gait, speech and swallowing deficits in progressive supranuclear palsy. Neurology 2003;60:917–922.

38. Tison F, Yekhlef F, Balestre E, et al. Application of the International Cooperative Ataxia Scale rating in multiple system atrophy. Mov Disord 2002;17:1248–1254.

39. Averbuch-Heller L, Paulson GW, Daroff RB, Leigh RJ. Whipple's disease mimicking progressive supranuclear palsy: the diagnostic value of eye movement recording. J Neurol Neurosurg Psychiatry 1999;66:532–535.

40. Siderowf AD, Galetta SL, Hurtig HI, Liu GT. Posey, Spiller and progressive supranuclear palsy: an incorrect attribution. Mov Disord 1998;13:170–174.

41. Berger JR, Arendt G. HIV dementia: the role of the basal ganglia and dopaminergic systems. J Psychopharmacol 2000;14:214–221.

42. Mirsattari SM, Power C, Nath A. Parkinsonism with HIV infection. Mov Disord 1998;13:684–689.

43. Wojcieszek J, Lang AE, Jankovic J, Greene P, Deck J. What is it? Case 1, 1994: rapidly progressive aphasia, apraxia, dementia, myoclonus, and parkinsonism. Mov Disord 1994;9:358–366.

44. Amarenco P, Roullet E, Hannoun L, Marteau R. Progressive supranuclear palsy as the sole manifestation of systemic Whipple's disease treated with pefloxacine. J Neurol Neurosurg Psychiatry 1991;54:1121–1122.

45. Nath U, Ben-Shlomo Y, Thomson RG, et al. The prevalence of progressive supranuclear palsy (Steele–Richardson–Olszewski syndrome) in the UK. Brain 2001;124:1438–1449.

46. Bower JH, Maraganore DM, McDonnell SK, Rocca WA. Incidence of progressive supranuclear palsy and multiple system atrophy in Olmsted County, Minnesota, 1976 to 1990. Neurology 1997;49:1284–1288.

47. Bower JH, Maraganore DM, McDonnell SK, Rocca WA. Incidence and distribution of parkinsonism in Olmsted County, Minnesota, 1976-1990. Neurology 1999;52:1214–1220.

48. Blin J, Baron JC, Dubois B, et al. Positron emission tomography study in progressive supranuclear palsy. Brain hypometabolic pattern and clinicometabolic correlations. Arch Neurol 1990;47:747–752.

49. Lees A. The Steele–Richardson–Olszewski sydrome (progressive supranuclear palsy). In: Marsden CD, Fahn S, eds. Movement Disorders 2. London: Butterworths, 1987;272–287.

50. Golbe LI. Progressive supranuclear palsy. In: Jankovic J, Tolosa E, eds. Parkinson's Disease and Movement Disorders. Baltimore: Williams & Wilkins, 1993;145–161.

51. Tolosa E, Valldeoriola F, Marti MJ. Clinical diagnosis and diagnostic criteria of progressive supranuclear palsy (Steele–Richardson–Olszewski syndrome). J Neural Transm Suppl 1994;42:15–31.

52. Collins SJ, Ahlskog JE, Parisi JE, Maraganore DM. Progressive supranuclear palsy: neuropathologically based diagnostic clinical criteria. J Neurol Neurosurg Psychiatry 1995;58:167–173.

53. Hughes AJ, Daniel SE, Ben-Shlomo Y, Lees AJ. The accuracy of diagnosis of parkinsonian syndromes in a specialist movement disorder service. Brain 2002;125:861–870.

54. Litvan I, Booth V, Wenning GK, et al. Retrospective application of a set of clinical diagnostic criteria for the diagnosis of multiple system atrophy. J Neural Transm 1998;105:217–227.

55. Quinn N. Multiple system atrophy. In: Marsden CD, Fahn S, eds. Movement Disorders 3. London: Butterworths, 1994:262–281.

56. Gilman S, Low PA, Quinn N, et al. Consensus statement on the diagnosis of multiple system atrophy. J Neurol Sci 1999;163:94–98.

57. Mega MS, Masterman DL, Benson DF, et al. Dementia with Lewy bodies: reliability and validity of clinical and pathologic criteria. Neurology 1996;47:1403–1409.

58. Ballard C, Holmes C, McKeith I, et al. Psychiatric morbidity in dementia with Lewy bodies: a prospective clinical and neuropathological comparative study with Alzheimer's disease. Am J Psychiatry 1999;156:1039–1045.

59. Duara R, Barker W, Luis CA. Frontotemporal dementia and Alzheimer's disease: differential diagnosis. Dement Geriatr Cogn Disord 1999;10:37–42.

60. Verghese J, Crystal HA, Dickson DW, Lipton RB. Validity of clinical criteria for the diagnosis of dementia with Lewy bodies. Neurology 1999;53:1974–1982.

61. Hohl U, Tiraboschi P, Hansen LA, Thal LJ, Corey-Bloom J. Diagnostic accuracy of dementia with Lewy bodies. Arch Neurol 2000;57:347–351.

62. Litvan I, MacIntyre A, Goetz CG, et al. Accuracy of the clinical diagnoses of Lewy body disease, Parkinson disease, and dementia with Lewy bodies: a clinicopathologic study. Arch Neurol 1998;55:969–978.

63. Litvan I, Agid Y, Goetz C, et al. Accuracy of the clinical diagnosis of corticobasal degeneration: a clinicopathological study. Neurology 1997;48:119–125.

64. McKeith IG, Ballard CG, Perry RH, et al. Prospective validation of consensus criteria for the diagnosis of dementia with Lewy bodies. Neurology 2005;54:1050–1058.

2

Historical Issues and Atypical Parkinsonian Disorders

Christopher G. Goetz

Studying archetypes is a fundamental task in nosography. Duchenne de Boulogne practiced it instinctively, and many others have done it before and after him: It is indispensable, and the only way to extract a specific pathological state from the chaos of imprecision. The history of medicine, which is long and grand, shows this truth well. But once the archetype is established, the second nosographic operation begins: dissect the archetype and analyze its parts. One must, in other words, learn how to recognize the imperfect cases, the *formes frustes*, or examples where only one feature occurs in isolation. Using this second method, the physician will see the archetypal illness in an entirely new light. One's scope enlarges, and the illness becomes much more important in the doctor's daily practice. To the patient's benefit, the doctor becomes attentive and sensitive to recognizing a disease, even when it is in its earliest developmental stages *(1)*.

INTRODUCTION

As shown in the above quotation from Jean-Martin Charcot's teaching of the late 19th century, the concept of *atypical Parkinsonian disorders* and *formes frustes* of the classic disease emerged in parallel with the definition of Parkinson's disease itself. In 1817, James Parkinson, a London general practitioner, described resting tremor and gait impairment in the small sample of subjects whose symptoms would later be coalesced into a disorder that would bear his name *(2)*. Nearly 50 yr later, Charcot returned to this early description and used his large patient population to study Parkinson's disease in full detail. With access to thousands of elderly patients who lived in the sprawling hospital-city of the Hôpital de la Salpêtrière in central Paris, Charcot studied the evolution of signs from very early disease through the most advanced stages *(3,4)*. Charcot used specialized recording equipment to distinguish the rest tremor of typical Parkinson's disease from the tremors typical of multiple sclerosis and other conditions where posture- or action-induced exacerbation occurred *(5)*. He was particularly adept in distinguishing bradykinesia as a cardinal feature of the illness and separating it from weakness. These studies led him to discourage the original designation of *paralysis agitans*, because patients did not develop clinically significant loss of muscle power until very late. Charcot further emphasized the distinctive elements of rigidity and delineated its distinction from spasticity or other forms of hypertonicity. Finally, he succinctly described the stance and gait of the subject with Parkinson's disease:

His head bends forward, he takes a few steps and they become quicker and quicker to the point that he can even bump into the wall and hurt himself. If I pull on his trousers from behind, he will retropulse in the same distinctive way *(4)*.

From: *Current Clinical Neurology: Atypical Parkinsonian Disorders*
Edited by: I. Litvan © Humana Press Inc., Totowa, NJ

Charcot's celebrated teaching courses and publications established these four features—rest tremor, bradykinesia, rigidity, and postural reflex impairment in balance and stance—as the cardinal features of typical Parkinson's disease. Charcot complemented these studies with documentation of trophic and arthritic features of the illness, with further studies of pain and autonomic nervous system alterations, and with pharmacological observations *(3)*. At the same time, however, as indicated in the introductory quotation of this chapter, he emphasized the importance of recognizing cases that he termed variants or *formes frustes*, cases that were similar to and yet distinct from the classic, archetypal form of the disease. These cases were termed *atypical Parkinson's disease*, at a time when the pathological substrate of Parkinson's disease itself remained unknown. As a historical introduction to the conditions that are the primary focus of this book and today collectively termed *atypical parkinsonian disorders*, these historical cases provide source material for the early study of conditions later to be separated from Parkinson's disease and defined in the mid- and late-20th century as progressive supranuclear palsy, multiple system atrophy, and corticobasal degeneration.

EARLY CONCEPTS OF ATYPICAL PARKINSON'S DISEASE

Nineteenth-century neurologists recognized three basic categories of parkinsonism that were suitably different from typical Parkinson's disease to merit designation: cases without typical tremor, those with atypical postures (extension rather than flexion), and those with marked asymmetry in the form of seeming hemiplegia. Within these categories, modern neurologists will find characteristics that typify progressive supranuclear palsy, multiple system atrophy, and corticobasal degeneration, though these latter diagnoses were not defined specifically until clinical-pathological studies distinguished them as distinct from Parkinson's disease itself. Each of these clinical categories is described from the perspective of 19th-century neurology and then followed by a specific discussion of the history of progressive supranuclear palsy, multiple system atrophy, and corticobasal degeneration.

Parkinsonism Without Prominent Rest Tremor

Early neurologists recognized resting tremor as the most distinctive feature of typical Parkinson's disease, and placed patients who had unusual, intermittent tremor patterns or no tremor into the clinical category termed "Parkinson's disease without tremor" *(3,4)*. Some of these cases actually had tremor, but the movements were mild in severity or intermittent and primarily induced with emotion or action *(3)*. It is possible that myoclonus, a feature frequently seen in corticobasal degeneration, and mild action tremor that can be seen in multiple system atrophy would have been categorized as one of these intermittent tremors. Myoclonus was appreciated in the 19th century, especially by Germanic and Austrian researchers *(6,7)*, but not specifically designated as an aspect of atypical Parkinson's disease. Charcot studied tremor extensively and drew attention to its typical features in Parkinson's disease. He conducted his tremor examination with patients at rest and during activity. In addition to clinical observation, he used tremor oscillometers (Fig. 1) and small portable lamps that he attached to the shaking extremities in order to record the trajectory movements on light-sensitive paper *(8)*. To accentuate an appreciation of very mild tremor, he attached feathers or other lightweight objects to the shaking body part to magnify the oscillations. He held strongly that titubation was not part of typical Parkinson's disease, but lip and tongue tremors could occur. Because parkinsonian cases without tremor were still considered as variants of the primary disease, Charcot advocated the use of the term Parkinson's disease, rather than "paralysis agitans," as coined by Parkinson himself *(3,4)*.

Parkinsonism With Atypical Postures

Charcot studied muscle tone extensively and established that most Parkinson's disease subjects showed a flexed posture with the shoulders hunched forward, neck bent down toward the chest, and the arms held in partial flexion at rest. In contrast, he found a small number of parkinsonian patients

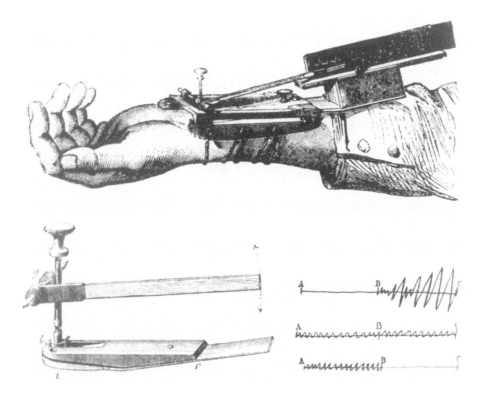

Fig. 1. Tremor recording machine used by Charcot to separate cases of typical rest tremor from those with postural tremor and action-induced tremor. Early studies focused on the differentiation by tremor type of multiple sclerosis and Parkinson's disease, but this apparatus was later used to study the various *formes frustes* of Parkinson's disease as well. In the insert, tremor recordings are shown for resting posture (AB) and action (BC) in patients with different tremor patterns. From *Dictionnaire Encyclopédique des Sciences Médicales*, 1883.

who were bradykinetic, unstable in their stance and gait, and yet showed a very different posture. These subjects, collectively termed "Parkinson's disease with extended posture," were of particular interest to Charcot, and he recognized several features of these cases that distinguished them from the archetypal cases of Parkinson's disease. These cases are further discussed later in the subheading on Progressive Supranuclear Palsy and shared several additional features of this diagnosis including the distinctive facial expression, swallowing difficulties, and frequent falls (Fig. 2).

Hemiplegic Parkinson's Disease

Early neurologists considered Parkinson's disease to be a bilateral condition, but often commented on the mild asymmetry of tremor, especially in the early years of disease. Within the context of this asymmetric but bilateral archetype, they distinguished another form of Parkinson's disease that was highly asymmetric with prominent disability in the involved upper extremity beyond that expected with bradykinesia alone *(3)*. Collectively termed *hemiplegic Parkinson's disease*, these cases form a large series in the French neurological literature of the late 19th century and include cases of abrupt strokelike onset as well as slowly progressive disability *(9)* (Fig. 3). They are discussed in the section on corticobasal degeneration, because they clinically fit best into this designation among the group of atypical parkinsonian disorders. Because infectious disease (abscess and hemorrhagic strokes especially from military tuberculosis) were frequent disorders in the 19th century, some of these cases may not have related to primary neurodegeneration. Furthermore, autopsy reports were not systematically recorded, so that analysis of cases as corticobasal degeneration remains only suggestive.

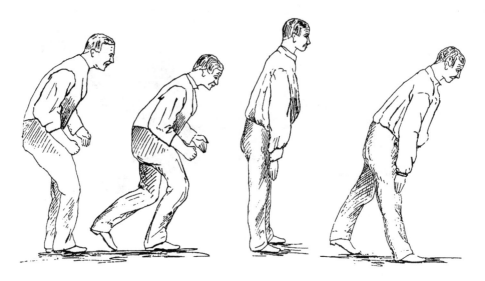

Fig. 2. Drawing by J-M Charcot comparing two patients: (left) typical Parkinson's disease with flexed posture and (right) another patient with an atypical variant of extended posture *(4)*.

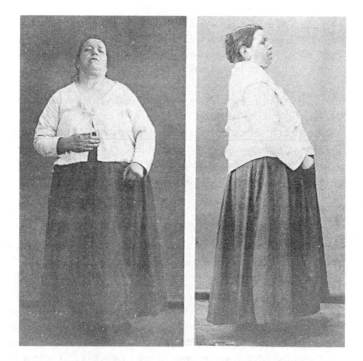

Fig. 3. Photograph from an article by Dutil *(17)* showing asymmetric parkinsonism suggestive of corticobasal degeneration but with an extended trunk and neck posture with gaze impairment suggestive of progressive supranuclear palsy.

HISTORICAL DESCRIPTIONS OF ATYPICAL PARKINSONIAN DISORDERS

Progressive Supranuclear Palsy

In 1963, Steele, Richardson, and Olszewski presented a report at the American Neurological Association of a new syndrome typified by parkinsonism, marked vertical gaze paresis, dementia, and axial rigidity *(10,11)*. Though they felt they were describing a new syndrome, they referred colleagues to similar cases from the recent past *(12–14)* (Fig. 4). H. Houston Merritt opened the discussion, commenting that he had not seen similar cases, that the involved areas all related to cell populations of similar phylogenetic age, and that dementia was of particular interest. F. McNaughton acclaimed: "I believe that the authors have described a clear-cut neurological syndrome and to judge from the pathological studies, it may, in fact, represent a new disease entity." D. Denny-Brown was less sure and ascribed the cases to variants of Jakob's "spastic pseudosclerosis" *(10)*.

Prior to these 20th-century descriptions, several cases of "Parkinson's disease with extended posture" can be identified with characteristics suggestive of progressive supranuclear palsy. Charcot presented a man, named Bachère, to his students on several occasions *(see* Fig. 2). Commenting on June 12, 1888, Charcot mentioned that Bachère did not have marked tremor and emphasized the issue of extension posture:

> There is something else unusual here worth noting. Look how he stands. I present him in profile so you can see the inclination of the head and trunk, well described by Parkinson. All this is typical. What is atypical, however, is that Bachère's forearms and legs are extended, making the extremities like rigid bars, whereas in the ordinary case, the same body parts are partly flexed. One can say then that in the typical case of Parkinson's disease, flexion is the predominant feature, whereas here, extension predominates and accounts fro this unusual presentation. The difference is even more evident when the patient walks *(3)*.

In addition to extended posture, this patient had particular facial bradykinesia and contracted forehead muscles *(15)*. Charcot commented that the patient had the perpetual look of surprise because the eyes remained widely opened and the forehead continually wrinkled (Fig. 5). In a modern setting, Jankovic has detailed similar facial morphology in Parkinsonism-plus patients, specifically those with progressive supranuclear palsy *(16)*. The extended truncal posture of this patient would be compatible with the posture of progressive supranuclear palsy, although Charcot did not comment on specific supranuclear eye movement abnormalities. Another Salpêtrière patient with "Parkinson's disease in extension" was described by Dutil in 1889 and eye movement abnormalities are mentioned, although a supranuclear lesion is not documented clinically *(17,18)* *(see* Fig. 3). This case also had highly asymmetric rigidity of the extremities, a feature more reminiscent of corticobasal degeneration than progressive supranuclear palsy (see next subheading). In this case, the extended neck posture was graphically emphasized:

> The face is masked, the forehead wrinkled, the eyebrows raised, the eyes immobile. This facies, associated with the extended posture of the head and trunk, gives the patient a singularly majestic air *(17,18)*.

With clinical features reminiscent of both progressive supranuclear palsy and corticobasal degeneration, this patient was mentioned in several articles from the Salpêtrière school, although no autopsy was apparently performed.

In their studies of tremor and Parkinson's disease, Charcot and contemporary colleagues described several other cases of parkinsonian patients who never suffered with either prominent resting or postural tremor. Although the descriptive details are often cursory, several of these cases may well represent cases of progressive supranuclear palsy. Bourneville published two cases in 1876 *(19)*, and later French students chose this subclass of patients for special clinical emphasis *(20)*. In his thesis on

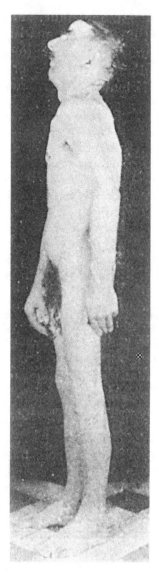

Fig. 4. Photograph from 1951 article by Chavany *(12)* showing a patient with extended posture suggestive of progressive supranuclear palsy prior to the definitive description by Steele and colleagues in 1964.

atypical forms of parkinsonism, Compin specifically noted that parkinsonian cases without tremor showed especially marked rigidity and often fall *(20)*. His first case history documented several additional features typical of the group of parkinsonism-plus syndromes, including early age of onset (age 45), prominent gait and balance difficulty within the first years of illness, and other midline dysfunction such as marked and early speech impairment.

Historical research on early medical diagnoses has occasionally benefited from nonmedical sources, especially literary descriptions. Because movement disorders are particularly visual in their character, it is reasonable to search the writings of celebrated authors known for their picturesque descriptive

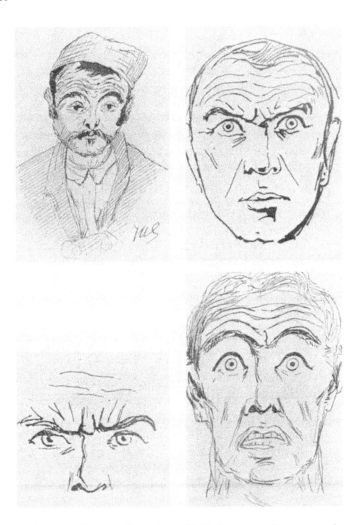

Fig. 5. Four pictures drawn by Charcot of a patient with likely progressive supranuclear palsy. The top two sketches emphasize the superior orbicularis contracture of the forehead, whereas the lower sketches capture the activation of the palpebral portion of the orbicularis (muscle of reflection, left) and the combined activation of the frontalis superior portion of the orbicularis and platysma, giving a frightened expression (right) *(4)*.

writings. In this context, Larner proposed that Charles Dickens captured the essential features of progressive supranuclear palsy in his description of a character in *The Lazy Tour of Two Idle Apprentices (21)*. Dickens wrote:

A chilled, slow, earthy, fixed old man. A cadaverous man of measured speech. An old man who seemed as unable to wink, as if his eyelids had been nailed to his forehead. An old man whose eyes—two spots of fire—had no more motion than if they had been connected with the back of his skull by screws driven through it and riveted and bolted outside, among his grey hair. He had come in and shut the door, and he now sat down. He did not bend himself to sit, as other people do, but seemed to sink bold upright, as if in water until the chair stopped him *(22)*.

For the medical reader with a knowledge of progressive supranuclear palsy, this description provides images compatible with the medical diagnosis. On the other hand, the passage falls short of the more convincing descriptions of sleep apnea in the *Pickwick Papers* or torticollis in *Little Dorrit*.

Corticobasal Degeneration

The clinical and pathological hallmarks of corticobasal degeneration were delineated in 1968 by Rebeiz *(23)*. Asymmetric parkinsonism in the context of a progressive dyspraxia, unilateral dystonia, and cortical sensory impairment are the major clinical findings found in association with corticodentatonigral degeneration with neuronal achromasia. In addition to the Dutil report cited earlier *(see* Fig. 3), a thesis by Béchet *(24)*, dated 1892, documents a patient (case VIII) with possible corticobasal degeneration. The patient's hallmarks were progressive tremor and contracture of the right upper extremity. Gradually, the trunk and neck developed extreme rigidity as well. The remarkable posture of the right upper extremity dominated the atypical picture:

> The right upper extremity is held along side the body, extended and stiff, the elbow held straight, the wrist flexed, the hand pronated and held in front of the thigh. The hand is markedly contorted . . . the fingers completely flexed, especially the last three digits to the point that the finger nails sometimes leave impressions on the palm. The flexion of the index finger is less marked and the adducted thumb is held over the palmer surface of the middle finger. This contracture of the flexor muscles, however is only one of appearance, for the examiner can (with a some effort, admittedly) extend the hand and fingers completely, and afterwards, they can hold this position briefly *(24)*.

Further discussing the functional impairment of the involved right upper extremity and the asymmetry of the case, he continued:

> Spontaneous movements of the upper extremity are practically impossible, very limited and extremely slow. The upper left extremity is only mildly flexed and the hand has no notable deformity *(24)*.

No photographs or medical drawings accompanied the report.

Nearly 30 yr later, in 1925, J. Lhermitte reported a case to the French Neurological Society that may also represent an early case of the same diagnosis *(25,26)*. A carpenter retired at age 67 because of progressive right-hand clumsiness. At age 72, he could no longer walk independently and ambulated with a wide-based, shuffling gait with the right arm flexed. In addition, his right arm moved involuntarily "like a foreign body." In spite of normal primary sensation, he could not recognize objects placed in his right hand. The patient did not have an autopsy (Fig. 6).

With the advent of cognitive neurology as a subspecialization of neurology, historical research efforts related to corticobasal degeneration have focused on descriptions of cases with signs of cortical dysfunction rather than motor. The clinical disorder of the celebrated composer, Maurice Ravel, has been retrospectively diagnosed as corticobasal degeneration, focal dementia, and progressive aphasia without dementia *(27,28)*. These analyses provide interesting reading, but, because the medical information is incomplete and no autopsy material has been identified, they do not substantially advance historical understanding of corticobasal degeneration.

Multiple System Atrophy

This diagnosis is particularly difficult to study historically, because the variety of symptoms and different phenotypes have been labeled with a wide vocabulary and nosology. In 1865, Sanders introduced the term "dystaxia or pseudo-paralysis agitans" to describe a patient with severe action tremor and gait impairment without sensory loss *(29)*. Dejerine and Thomas described olivopontocerebellar atrophy in 1900 and emphasized varying mixtures of parkinsonian, cerebellar, and autonomic dysfunction *(30)*. Critchley and Greenfield reviewed cases from the early 20th century, citing such names as Pierre Marie, Murri, Lhermitte, and Wilson, commenting on the changing terminology and nosographic confusion related to this disorder *(31)*. In 1925, Ley reported the same type of presentation as Dejerine and Thomas in a 50-yr-old man, and at autopsy, he noted not only olivopontocerebellar lesions, but also atrophic substantia nigra *(32,33)*.

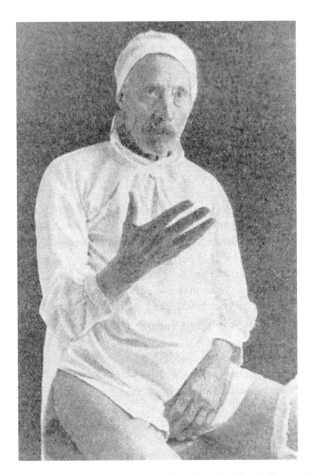

Fig. 6. Photograph from 1925 article by Lhermitte *(25)* and studied by Ballan and Tisson *(26)*, showing a patient with possible corticobasal degeneration. The picture captures his unusual posturing of the right arm and hand with marked dyspraxia.

In 1960, Shy and Drager described two patients with orthostatic hypotension and parkinsonism or pyramidal/cerebellar features, who showed highly distinctive autopsy features including vacuolation of the autonomic ganglia, shrunken, hyperchromatic cells in the intermediolateral column, and degenerative changes in the pons, substantia nigra, hypothalamus, locus ceruleus, and Purkinje layer of the cerebellum *(34)*. Striatonigral degeneration became widely known after Adams, van Bogaert, and van der Eecken published their series in 1961 *(35)*. The conditions were consolidated in the seminal article by Graham and Oppenheimer *(36)*.

Early reports of multiple system atrophy of the striatonigral phenotype were written by Lewy's student, Fleischhacker, in 1924 and Scherer in 1933, both analyzed by Wenning and colleagues *(37–39)*. Of these five subjects, three had severe parkinsonism and two had more prominent cerebellar features. All had neuropathological evidence of putaminal and pallidal degeneration as well as depigmentation and degeneration of the small cells of the substantia nigra. Those with cerebellar features had additional olivopontocerebellar lesions. Fleischhacker's case had been clinically diagnosed during life as paralysis agitans, but the author argued that both clinically and pathologically, the findings were atypical for Parkinson's disease. Clinically, he emphasized the atypical tremor (coarse and postural rather than resting), an early age of disease onset, and prominent rigidity. Berciano considers that Scherer's contribution was essential in establishing the striatal-nigral lesions that underlie parkinsonism in this phenotype. With his report, he definitively established that parkinsonism in olivopontocerebellar atrophies related to additional degenerative changes outside this system *(33)*.

FUTURE PERSPECTIVES

The study of early texts that describe Parkinson's disease and other forms of parkinsonism remains vital as the search for causes of these illnesses intensifies. Epidemiological and neurotoxicological research that will be reviewed in this text has focused increasingly on the putative role of environmental factors to parkinsonian syndromes, and many current industrial exposures did not exist in prior eras. It may not be by chance that the first medical description of Parkinson's disease emerged from the center of international industrialization in the midst of the Industrial Revolution. The identification of atypical parkinsonian disorders naturally followed the identification of the archetype of Parkinson's disease, but establishing exactly when such cases came to medical attention has not been precisely defined. In this light, readers of early medicine, literature, and other disciplines offer an important resource for research efforts in the 21st century. As readers examine the evidence for genetic and environmental causes of the atypical parkinsonian disorders discussed in this book, a vigilance to literature, artworks, and early medical descriptions will complement these data and may further the understanding of these collective entities.

REFERENCES

1. Charcot J-M. (March 20, 1888) Leçons du Mardi: Policlinique à la Salpêtrière. Paris: Bureaux du Progrès Médical, 1887–1888.
2. Parkinson J. The Shaking Palsy. London: Whittingham & Rowland, 1817.
3. Charcot J-M. De la paralysie agitante, Leçon 5. In: Oeuvres Complètes, vol 1. Paris: Bureaux du Progrès Médical, 1892:155–189 [In English: On paralysis agitans. In: Lectures on Diseases of the Nervous System, Sierson, G, trans. Philadelphia:HC Lea, 1879:105–127.
4. Charcot J-M. (Leçon 21: June 12, 1888) Leçons du Mardi: Policlinique à la Salpêtrière. Paris:Bureaux du Progrès Médical, 1888.
5. Goetz CG, Bonduelle M, Gelfand T. Charcot: Constructing Neurology. New York: Oxford University Press, 1995.
6. Friedreich N. Neuropathologische Beobachtung beim Paramyoklonus mutiplex. Virchow Arch Path Anat 1881; 86:421–434.
7. Unverricht H. Die Myoclonie. Leipsig:Franz Deuticke, 1891.
8. Goetz CG. Visual art in the neurological career of Jean-Martin Charcot. Arch Neurol 1991;48:421–425.
9. Marie P. Hémiplégie chez les parkinsoniens. In: Brouardel P, Gilbert JP, eds. Traité de Médecine et de Thérapeutique. Masson, 1911.
10. Transactions of the American Neurological Association. St. Paul MN: American Neurological Association, 1963.
11. Steele J, Richardson JC, Olszewski J. Progressive supranuclear palsy. A heterogeneous degeneration involving the brain stem, basal ganglia and cerebellum with verticle gaze and pseudobulbar palsy, nuchal dystonia and dementia. Arch Neurol 1964;10:333–359.
12. Chavany JA, van Bogaert L, Godlewski S. Sur un syndrome de rigidité, à prédominance axiale avec perturbation des automatismes oculo-palpébraux d'origine encéphalopatique. Presse Méd 1951;50:958–962.
13. Brusa A. Dégénérescence plurisystèmatisée du névraxe, de charactère sporadique. Rev Neurol 1961;104:412–429
14. Steele JC. Historical notes. J Neural Transm 1994(Suppl);42:3–14.
15. Goetz CG. Charcot, the Clinician: The Tuesday Lessons. New York: Raven, 1987.
16. Jankovic J. Progressive supranuclear palsy. Neurol Clin 1984;2:473–486.
17. Dutil A. Sur un cas de paralysie agitante à forme hemiplégique avec attitude anormale de la tête et du tronc (extension). Nouv Icon Salpêtrière 1889;2:165–169.
18. Goetz CG. Visual art in the neurological career of Jean-Martin Charcot. Arch Neurol 1991;48:421–425.
19. Bourneville D-M. Deux cas de la maladie de Parkinson sans tremblement. Prog Méd Sept. 17, 1876, Paris.
20. Compin P. Etude clinique des formes anormales de la maladie de Parkinson (Thèse de Médecine). Lyon: FA Rey, 1902.
21. Larner AJ. Did Charles Dickens described progressive supranuclear palsy in 1857? Mov Disorders 2002;17:832–833.
22. Dickens C. The lazy tour of two idle apprentices. Household Words 1857;3:44–46, 4:66–72; 5:72–89.
23. Rebeiz JL, Kolodny EW, Richardson EP. Corticodentatonigral degeneration with neuronal achromasia. Arch Neurol 1968;18:20–33.

24. Béchet A. Etude clinique des formes de la maladie de Parkinson (Thèse de Médecine). Paris: Bureaux du Progrès Médical, 1892.
25. Lhermitte J, Lévy G, Kyriaco N. Les perturbations de la representation spatial chez les apraxiques. Rev Neurolog (Paris) 1925;2:586–600.
26. Ballan G, Tison F. A historical case of probable corticobasal degeneration? Mov Disord 1997;12:1073–1074
27. Baeck E. Was Maurice Ravel's illness a corticobasal degeneration? Clin Neurol and Neurosurg 1996;98:57–61.
28. Cytowic RE. Aphasia in Maurice Ravel. Bull Los Angeles Neurol Soc 1976;41:109–114.
29. Sanders WR. Case of an unusual form of nervous disease, dystaxia or pseudo-paralysis agitans. Edinburgh Med J 1865;10:987–997.
30. Dejerine J, Thomas AA. L'atrophie olivo-ponto-cérébelleuse. Nouv Icon Salepêtrière 1900;13:330–370.
31. Critchley M, Greenfield JG. Olivo-ponto-cerebellar atrophy. Brain 1948;61:343–364.
32. Ley R. Forme atypique d'atrophie olivo-ponto-cérébelleuse. J Belge Neurol Psychiatr 1925;25:92–108.
33. Berciano J, Combarros O, Polo JM. An early description of striatonigral degeneration. J Neurol 1999;246:462–466.
34. Shy SM, Drager GA. A neurological syndrome associated with orthostatic hypotension. Arch Neurol 1963;2:511–517.
35. Adams RD, van Bogaert L, Vander Eecken H. Striato-nigral degeneration. J Neuropath Exper Neurol 1964;23:584–608.
36. Graham JG, Oppenheimer DR. Orthostatic hypotension and nicotine sensitivity in a case of multiple system atrophy. J Neurol Neurosurg Psychiat 1969;32:28–34.
37. Fleischhacker H. Afamiliäre chronisch-progressive Erkankung des mitteren Lebensalters vom Pseudosklerosetyp. Z ges Neurol Psyschiat 1924;91:1–22
38. Scherer HJ. Extrapyramidale Storungen bei der Olivopontocerebellarer Atrophie. Ein Beitrag zum Problem des lokalen vorzeitigen Alterns. Zbl ges Neurol Psychiat 1933;145:406–419.
39. Wenning GK, Jellinger KJ, Quinn NP, Werner HP. An early report of striatonigral degeneration. Mov Disord 2000;15(1):159–162.

3

Epidemiology of Progessive Supranuclear Palsy and Multiple System Atrophy

Adam Zermansky and Yoav Ben-Shlomo

INTRODUCTION

Epidemiology seeks to prevent disease by identifying risk factors, be they genetic and/or environmental, that are of etiological relevance through the use of descriptive studies, natural experiments, and very occasionally randomized trials. In addition, clinical epidemiology can examine the utility of diagnostic tests, determine predictors of disease prognosis, and test whether therapies can modify disease progression. This chapter will focus on descriptive studies that have either measured disease frequency (prevalence or incidence) or estimated the risk associated with environmental exposures. We have chosen to focus solely on progressive supranuclear palsy (PSP) and multiple system atrophy (MSA) as there is hardly any data for other atypical parkinsonian disorders such as corticobasal degeneration or dementia with Lewy bodies. For any uncommon disease, undertaking epidemiological studies presents several major challenges: case identification, representativeness of cases, and obtaining adequate sample sizes. For both PSP and MSA, there are additional problems as both these conditions can be difficult to diagnose. As there are no adequate tests that are both highly sensitive and specific, the gold standard remains the diagnostic expertise of a movement disorders specialist (1).

THE PREVALENCE AND INCIDENCE OF PSP AND MSA

Measuring the prevalence and incidence of disease serves several important functions. First, each measure enables health planners to estimate the number of existing cases (prevalence) and new cases (incidence) that one would expect to find in a community and hence provide the appropriate health staff required for their care. Second, by comparing age-standardized rates in different populations or over different time periods, one may observe differences, which if not artifactual or merely because of chance, that provide etiological clues and enable the formulation of hypotheses concerning risk factors. Marked changes over time, unless a result of increased disease awareness and hence a greater likelihood of diagnosis, strongly suggest an environmental factor or a genetic environmental interaction. Geographical variations are more complex as they may reflect differences in health services, variations in disease survival if only comparing prevalence rates, methodological differences in study design and/or diagnostic criteria, chance variations, or genuine population differences in genetic and/ or environmental factors.

Current consensus diagnostic criteria for PSP and MSA were only published in 1996 and 1999 respectively (2,3). Prevalence studies prior to these dates relied upon heterogeneous groups of published criteria and some used none (or did not state which were used) at all. This makes any interpre-

From: *Current Clinical Neurology: Atypical Parkinsonian Disorders*
Edited by: I. Litvan © Humana Press Inc., Totowa, NJ

tation of data from such studies even more complex as these different criteria would have had differing sensitivities and specificities *(4)*. Even the current consensus criteria, which at least enable a more standardized approach, have yet to be tested in large-scale representative prognostic cohorts with postmortem-validated diagnoses so their true diagnostic utility remains to be elucidated.

Despite these difficulties, such studies provide the empirical basis for suggesting or testing ideas concerning causal agents.

Prevalence of PSP and MSA

Measures of the prevalence of PSP vary from 0.97 to 6.54 per 100,000 (eight studies) and for MSA from 2.29 to 39.3 per 100,000 (five studies) (Table 1). A study from Sicily *(8)* reported one of the highest rates of 28.6 per 100,000 but this was for unspecified parkinsonism, so this category may have included cases other than MSA and PSP. The results presented in Table 1 are simple crude rates for the whole population rather than age-standardized rates. Though some studies do report such standardized rates, each study generally uses a different standard population and some studies fail to present age-specific rates making it impossible to restandardize the rates to a single population. The purpose of standardization is to remove any confounding effect owing to the age structure of the population. As all the studies except one from Libya *(7)* have been undertaken in a developed world population, it is likely that such confounding is not too large. In fact, differences between the crude and standardized rates are often small. For example, the crude rate for the New Jersey study is 1.38 per 100,000 and after standardization this increases to 1.39 per 100,000 *(6)*. In the London study, the crude PSP rate of 4.9 per 100,000 increased to 6.4 per 100,000 *(14)*. However, the incidence rate from Benghazi, Libya, is misleadingly small as a large proportion of this population will be under 55 yr of age and standardizing this rate to a European population will certainly increase this rate by a large degree.

Despite the various different diagnostic criteria, the rates for PSP and MSA across all studies are not too dissimilar. One obvious observation is that studies with very large populations, e.g., New Jersey *(6)* or United Kingdom *(15)*, produce lower prevalence estimates whereas very small populations produce high rates. The effect of varying population size and hence intensity of case finding is most elegantly demonstrated by the "Russian Doll Method" method employed by Nath and colleagues *(15)*. This general pattern is also well noted with prevalence studies for multiple sclerosis *(16)*. This is unsurprising because, although large populations give precise estimates, they are likely to be biased downward as it is easier to miss a proportion of cases. On the other hand, smaller populations will enable much more thorough case ascertainment and hence less biased but imprecise estimates. The highest prevalence rate (39.3 per 100,000) was observed in a study from rural Bavaria *(10)*. However being based on only three cases in a very small population, its lower 95% confidence interval is still 8.1 per 100,000, which will overlap with most of the other estimates. Almost all the studies except that from Nath and colleagues *(15)* estimate rates based on 11 or fewer cases, which demonstrates the problem with studying rare neurological disorders.

Some studies have specifically aimed to detect cases of PSP and/or MSA whereas others have been generic prevalence studies for parkinsonism. Interestingly, there is little difference between the estimates for these different studies. Perhaps more surprising is that studies that have screened a whole population *(9,10)* did not find higher rates than those using existing medical records or other databases. It is well recognized in the Parkinson's disease (PD) literature that a proportion of PD cases will be detected *de novo* by the screening procedure, though this varies across European centers *(17)*. It is possible that this "clinical iceberg" phenomenon is less important for PSP and MSA because their symptoms and disease progression make them less likely to be undetected. However, studies aimed at parkinsonism may underestimate rates of MSA since cases with predominantly cerebellar features may be undetected. Similarly, excluding patients who became demented before the onset of parkinsonism *(14)* will assist in the exclusion of dementia with Lewy bodies, in which a supranuclear gaze palsy may occur, but may also exclude cases of PSP.

Table 1
Prevalence Studies of PSP and MSA

Lead Author (Ref. No.)	Year of Publication	Generic (G) or Specific (S)	Location	Population Size (Total Estimated)	Case Ascertainment	Diagnostic Criteria	PSP Prevalence per 100,000 (No. of Cases)	MSA Prevalence per 100,000 (No. of Cases)
Golbe (6)	1988	S	New Jersey, USA	799,022	Neurologists, PD support group, nursing homes	Clinical diagnosis aimed at specificity	1.38* (11)	
Morgante (8)	1992	G	3 areas in Sicily	24,496	Two-phase screening	Validated screening tool but no specific criteria for PSP, MSA	28.6 (7) unspecified parkinsonism so covers both MSA and PSP as well as other conditions	
de Rijk (9)	1995	G	Suburb of Rotterdam Netherlands	6969 (≥ 55 yr) (34,845)* assuming 20% ≥ 55	Two phase screening	Clinical diagnosis	2.87* (1)	5.74* (2)
Trenkwalder (10)	1995	G	Rural villages in Bavaria, Germany	1190 (7628)	Two phase screening	Quinn criteria for MSA		39.3 (3)
Wermuth (12)	1997	G	Faroe Islands	43,709	Neurologists, GPs, nursing homes, pharmacies	Clinical diagnosis	4.58 (2)	2.29 (1)
Chio (13)	1998	G	Cosatto, Italy	61,830	Neurologists, GPs, hospital records, pharmacies	Clinical diagnosis	3.23 (2)	4.85 (3)
Schrag (14)	1999	S	London, UK	121,608	GP records	Quinn criteria for MSA & NINDS criteria for PSP	4.93 (6)	3.29 (4)
Nath (15)	2001	S	United Kingdom	59,236,500	Neurologist (BNSU), PSP support group	NINDS criteria for PSP	0.97 (577)	
Nath (15)	2001	S	North of England Region, UK	2,589,240	Neurologists, care of the elderly consultants, hospital records & databases	NINDS criteria for PSP	3.09 (80)	
Nath (15)	2001	S	Newcastle-upon-Tyne, UK	259,998	GP records	NINDS criteria for PSP	6.54 (17)	

*Estimated from paper

The study by Schrag and colleagues *(14)* had an additional important feature in that all subjects that were categorized as "unclassifiable parkinsonism," were reevaluated at 1 yr for signs of PSP or MSA. This approach is clearly helpful, as some patients who look like PSP or MSA may not fulfill diagnostic criteria at the time of screening but with further follow-up will develop these features.

Incidence of PSP and MSA

There are even fewer estimates of incidence and two of these are based in almost the same population *(5,11)* (Table 2). The relatively low rate from the first paper from Rochester, Minnesota *(5)*, may have reflected less recognition for PSP than in the later study *(11)*. The estimates by Schrag and colleagues *(14)* are remarkably similar to that by Bower and colleagues *(11)*, though the former are only indirect estimates based on prevalence data and dividing this by the median survival. This was probably a fortuitous coincidence but further studies are required to confirm these rates.

Implications From Prevalence and Incidence Data

Despite rather limited data, there are no clear signs that there are widespread geographical differences in PSP and MSA, however there are almost no data from developing countries and one cannot exclude that in other populations or ethnic groups there may be higher rates. Atypical parkinsonism has been reported with greater frequency in the Caribbean *(18)* and among South Asians and African Caribbeans *(19)* in the United Kingdom, though these latter observations remain controversial. Little obvious differences exist across Europe, as has been noted for PD *(17)*, or North America, yet more higher-quality studies are required especially to estimate incidence rates.

RISK FACTORS FOR PSP AND MSA

The epidemiology of PD has been greatly aided by two natural experiments that generated important hypotheses regarding its etiology. The first was the encephalitis lethargica epidemic, which suggested a role for an infective agent *(20)*. The second was the strange occurrence of MPTP-induced parkinsonism *(21)*, which suggested the role of a neurotoxic agent and led to studies examining the role of pesticides because of its similarity with paraquat *(22)*. The relevance of these models for the etiology of PSP and/or MSA is far more questionable. However, in the absence of any other clues, most researchers have simply used risk factors that have been suggested to be important for PD, e.g., smoking behavior, head injury, pesticides, well water, etc., and tested them out in PSP and MSA as essentially a hypothesis-generating exercise.

Risk Factors for PSP

One possible "natural experiment" has been the study of an atypical form of parkinsonism in Guadeloupe, clinically indistinguishable from PSP, which was prompted by the discovery that an unexpectedly high proportion of parkinsonian patients were unresponsive to levodopa *(23)*. Based upon the hypothesis that some of the herbal tea and tropical fruits consumed in Guadeloupe contain benzyltetrahydoisoquinolones, which are known to be neurotoxic, a case-control study was undertaken *(see* Table 3). During a 1-yr period, they compared herbal tea and tropical fruit consumption among 87 parkinsonism patients referred to the sole neurological center in Guadeloupe (22 had IPD [idiopathic Parkinson's disease], 31 PSP, 30 could not be classified, and 4 had atypical parkinsonism with motor neurone disease) with 65 hospital inpatients with non-neurodegenerative diseases. They demonstrated a higher consumption of herbal teas and tropical fruits in PSP patients and atypical parkinsonism. This was associated with a fourfold increased risk for both groups compared to controls. Although the confidence intervals for the odds ratios are wide and approach unity, further evidence supporting a causal role for these agents comes from the observation that two of the PSP patients and four of the atypical cases improved significantly after stopping their consumption of these substances, one patient being able to return to work. It remains unclear whether these atypical

Table 2
Incidence Studies of PSP and MSA

Lead Author (Ref. No.)	Year of Publication	Generic (G) or Specific (S)	Location	Population Size	Case Ascertainment	Diagnostic Criteria	PSP Incidence per 100,000 (No. of Cases)	MSA Incidence per 100,000 (No. of Cases)
Rajput (5)	1984	G	Rochester, USA	53,885*	Hospital medical records	Clinical diagnosis	0.29* (2)	0.71* (5)
Radhakrishnan (7)	1988	G	Benghazi, Libya	519,000	Polyclinics, hospitals, rehab centers, and neurology dept.	Clinical diagnosis	0.29 (6)	
Bower (11)	1997	S	Olmsted County, USA	94,965	Hospital medical records	MSA consensus 1996 & Collins 1995	1.12 (16)	0.63 (9)
Schrag (14)	1999	S	London, UK	121,608	GP records	Quinn criteria for MSA &NINDS criteria for PSP	1.41**	0.46**

*Estimated from paper.
**Indirect estimates based on prevalence and median survival.

Table 3
Case control studies of PSP and MSA

Lead Author (Ref. No.)	Year of Publication	Design	Location	Cases	Controls	Results - Odds Ratios (95% CI)
PSP						
Davis (24)	1988	Case-control study	New Jersey, USA	50 cases from neurologists and tertiary center	100 hospital controls	Finished high school 3.1, finished college 2.9, rural residence 2.4
Golbe (25)	1996	Case-control study	New Jersey, USA	75 cases from tertiary center (91 unmatched)	75 neurology outpatients excluding neurodegenrative diseases (106 unmatched)	At least 12 years education 0.35 (0.12 to 0.96); no difference by rurality
Caparros-Lefebvre (23)	1999	Case-control study	French West Indies	31 PSP and 30 atypical parkinsonism from neurology dept.	65 hospital controls	Fruit or herbal tea 4.35, (1.25 to 15.2) for PSP, 4.27, (1.22 to 14.9), for atypical parkinsonism
Vanacore (26)	2000	Case-control study	Mainly Italy but also Austria and Germany	55 cases from tertiary centers	134 relatives of patients with non-neurological controls	Smoking OR 0.91 (0.42–1.98); no dose-response
MSA						
Nee (27)	1991	Case-control study	USA	60 cases from NINDS, newsletters, or private doctors	60 controls from spouses, friends, and volunteers	College education 0.39 (0.16–0.90); significant associations with metal dust and fumes 14.8, pesticides 5.8, plastic monomers and addditives 5.3
Vanacore (26)	2000	Case-control study	Mainly Italy but also Austria and Germany	75 cases from tertiary centers	134 relatives of patients with non-neurological controls	Smoking 0.56 (0.29–1.06); dose-response effect

cases represent PSP or not. Only one patient in their study had a neuropathological examination, which showed changes seen in amyotrophic lateral sclerosis (ALS). It is not clear whether this was one of the PSP, PSP and ALS, or unclassifiable patients. Circumstantial evidence that the PSP-like syndrome may be PSP comes from a neuropathological study of five PSP patients from Guadeloupe, all of whom consumed large amounts of either tropical fruits or herbal teas. All these cases had neuropathologically confirmed PSP, with four-repeat tau deposition.

Although this study provides a model for the role of dietary factors or a neurotoxin, the specific dietary components are fairly unique to this population and can provide clues to other substances only by analogy. Two case-control studies in New Jersey, conducted by the same research group 8 yr apart tried to identify a wide range of possible factors. The first *(24)*, in 1988, compared 50 PSP patients (Golbe diagnostic criteria) in a tertiary-referral center with 100 age- and sex-matched inpatients with non-neurological disorders. It examined 85 potential factors including educational attainment, family history, and toxin exposures. In an attempt to improve the quality of information and possibly reduce recall bias between control and patient groups, questionnaires were administered to surrogate respondents only (the patient's spouse or offspring or sibling). This may have led to reducing any true association as relatives may not have been aware of all occupational exposures resulting in nondifferential misclassification toward the null. The only significant finding was that PSP patients were more likely to have completed high school, completed 4 yr at college, and live in an area with a population of less than 10,000 as an adult. It is unsurprising that out of 85 hypothesis tests, 3–4 tests were significant by chance at the 5% level (type I error). These findings could also be explained, as discussed in the paper, by selection bias; patients identified from tertiary referral centers are more likely to have a higher educational level and come from a wider catchment area than inpatients with acute medical problems from the local community. These findings failed to replicate in the follow-up study in 1996 *(25)*. On this occasion, to avoid selection bias, non-neurodegenerative controls were drawn from the same pool of neurology outpatient referrals as the patients. Using a self-completed postal questionnaire, the study examined factors that neared statistical significance in the previous study. Now, PSP patients were less likely to have completed 12 yr at school, but no other factors were significant. The authors hypothesized that this may be a proxy for either lower nutritional status, somehow leading to a propensity to develop PSP, or possibly exposure to an unknown neurotoxin in early life. However, it is unclear how representative was the sample of controls. Given the severity of PSP, it is likely that all cases will eventually be referred for a neurological opinion, though not always to a tertiary specialist center. However, other neurological conditions, e.g., headaches, sciatica, etc., may be referred to a wide variety of other clinicians. Those reaching a tertiary center may be biased toward a higher educational level.

Since smoking shows a negative association with Parkinson's disease, Vanacore and colleagues examined this factor among PSP patients *(26)*. The study recruited 55 PSP and 134 control subjects. The control subjects were healthy relatives of patients with non-neurodegenerative diseases. Any further information about control selection was not given nor were the response rates reported. Since smokers are likely to be overrepresented in any randomly selected patient cohort, there is the possibility that controls were more likely to be relatives of patients who smoked. This bias would tend to show an inverse association with PSP but in fact there was little evidence of any association, though the wide 95% confidence intervals mean it is not possible to exclude even a halving of risk as seen with PD.

Risk Factors for MSA

Only two case-control studies have been reported for MSA. The first examined family history and specific occupational exposures. This noted significant odds ratios for organic solvents (2.4), metallic dusts (14.8), pesticides (5.8), and plastic monomers and additives (5.3) *(27)*. Anecdotal case reports have also suggested pesticides *(28)*, heavy metals *(28)*, and organic solvents *(28,29)*.

Logistic regression analysis uncovered an increased risk of MSA with a positive family history of any neurological disease. No response rates were reported for cases and controls and the use of spouse, friends, and volunteer controls may have introduced substantial selection bias. In particular, as more male cases were ascertained, the use of female spouses will artifactually increase the risk of any occupationally related exposure found in male jobs. The increased odds ratio of having a family history of neurological disorders may have been spurious, since only 33 of the 60 MSA subjects' family members participated, and attempts to recruit MSA-subject family members were made only if the MSA patients thought their relatives would be interested.

Vanacore and colleagues in the same study mentioned earlier did find an inverse association between smoking and MSA. Although the odds rations for smoking were not significant at the 5% level, they did observe a dose–response effect with decreasing odds as the number of pack-years increased. This may have been biased, owing to the control selection, however their results for PD are consistent with other studies suggesting that this may not have been a real problem.

Implications From Case-Control Studies of PSP and MSA

Summarizing the current published data, it appears that there is no evidence identifying any clear environmental risk factor for PSP, other than tropical fruit and herbal tea consumption for the PSP-like disorder in Guadeloupe. Evidence for environmental factors in MSA is mainly anecdotal, although the study by Nee and colleagues implicates various nonspecific occupational exposures. This does not, however, exclude the possibility of the role for an environmental factor in the etiology of either disorder. Furthermore, none of these studies recruited more than 100 cases. This means they are limited in statistical power with a high likelihood of a type II error, accepting the null hypothesis when the alternative hypothesis is true. Even with a study recruiting 100 cases and 200 controls, at a 5% level of significance and 90% power, one could only detect an odds ratio of 2.3 for a common exposure with 50% prevalence in the control group. For a rarer exposure with only 10% prevalence, this further deteriorates to an odds ratio of 3.0.

CONCLUSIONS

Remarkably little good-quality evidence exists on the epidemiology of PSP and MSA. Basic descriptive data on the variations of both diseases in time, place, and person are sparse. There is at this stage little evidence of widespread geographical variations, but many areas of the world have yet to report prevalence and incidence rates. Other than the possible rare exposure of benzyl-tetrahydoisoquinolones, we have little to go on for specific environmental clues. Positive findings with occupational exposures may reflect publication bias and negative studies may simply be under-powered to detect modest increased risks. Single centers are unlikely to be able to undertake sufficiently large and powerful studies so future research must either use a multicenter approach or use standardized methods to enable future meta-analysis of results. The challenges of undertaking high-quality epidemiology of PSP and MSA are likely to remain well into the 21st century.

FUTURE DIRECTIONS

The future direction for PSP and MSA epidemiology will depend on various factors. Firstly, clinical anecdotes or natural experiments as occurred with MPTP and parkinsonism, will generate new hypotheses. Whilst many of these will be red herrings, true etiological insights can be gained by methodological sound exploration of such reports. Secondly, new developments in laboratory-based research may highlight etiological factors that have an analogous lifestyle exposure. This in turn can be tested using either questionnaires or, better still, with some plausible biomarker. Finally, well undertaken large case control studies will be necessary to refute or support plausible hypotheses.

REFERENCES

1. Hughes AJ, Daniel SE, Ben-Shlomo Y, Lees AJ. The accuracy of diagnosis of parkinsonian syndromes in a specialist movement disorder service. Brain 2002;125:861–870

2. Gilman S, Low P, Quinn N, et al. Consensus statement on the diagnosis of multiple system atrophy. J Neurol Sci 1999;163(1):94–98.

3. Litvan I, Agid Y, Calne D, et al. Clinical research criteria for the diagnosis of progressive supranuclear palsy (Steele–Richardson–Olszewski syndrome): report of the NINDS-SPSP international workshop. Neurology 1996;47(1):1–9.

4. Litvan I, Bhatia KV, Burn DJ, et al. Movement Disorders Society Scientific Issues Committee report: SIC Task Force appraisal of clinical diagnostic criteria for Parkinsonian disorders. Mov Disord 2003;18(5):467–486.

5. Rajput AH, Offord KP, Beard M, Kurland LT. Epidemiology of parkinsonism: incidence, classification and mortality. Ann Neurol 1984;16:278–282.

6. Golbe LI, Davis PH, Schoenberg, et al. Prevalence and Natural History of Progressive Supranuclear Palsy. Neurology 1988;38:1031–1034.

7. Radhakrishnan K, Thacker AK, Maloo JC, et al Descriptive epidemiology of some rare neurological diseases in Benghazi, Libya. Neuroepidemiology 1988;7(3):159–164.

8. Morgante L, Rocca WA, Di Rosa AE, et al. Prevalence of Parkinson's disease and other types of Parkinsonism: a door-to-door survey in three Sicillian municipalities. Neurology 1992;42:1901–1907.

9. de Rijk MC, Breteler MMB, Graveland GA, et al. Prevalence of Parkinson's disease in the elderly: the Rotterdam Study. Neurology, 1995;45(12):2143–2146.

10. Trenkwalder C, Schwarz J, Gebhard J, et al. Starnberg trial on epidemiology of Parkinsonism and hypertension in the elderly. Prevalence of Parkinson's disease and related disorders assessed by a door-to-door survey of inhabitants older than 65 years. Arch Neurol 1995;52(10):1017–1022.

11. Bower JH, Maranganore DM, McDonnell SK, Rocca W. Incidence of progressive supranuclear palsy and multiple system atrophy in Olmsted County, Minnesota, 1976 to 1990. Neurology 1997;49(5):1284–1288.

12. Wermuth, L, Joensen P, Bunger N, Jeune B. High prevalence of Parkinson's disease in the Faroe Islands. Neurology 1997;49(2):426–432.

13. Chio A, Magnani C, Schiffer D. Prevalence of Parkinson's disease in Northwestern Italy: comparison of tracer methodology and clinical ascertainment of cases. Mov Disord 1998;13(3):400–405.

14. Schrag A., Ben-Shlomo Y, Quinn NP. Prevalence of progressive supranuclear palsy and multiple system atrophy: a cross-sectional study. Lancet 1999;354:1771–1775.

15. Nath U, Ben-Shlomo Y, Thomson RG, et al. The Prevalence of progressive supranuclear palsy (Steele–Richardson–Olszewski syndrome) in the UK. Brain 2001;124:1438–1449.

16. Matthews WB, Compston A, Allen IV, Martyn CN. McAlpine's Mmultiple sclerosis, 2 ed. Edinburgh: Churchill Livingstone, 1990.

17. de Rijk MC, Tzourio C, Breteler MM, et al. Prevalence of parkinsonism and Parkinson's disease in Europe: the EUROPARKINSON Collaborative Study. European Community Concerted Action on the Epidemiology of Parkinson's disease. J Neurol Neurosurg Psychiatry 1997;62:10–15.

18. Steele JC, Caparros-Lefebvre D, Lees AJ, Sacks OW. Progressive supranuclear palsy and its relation to pacific foci of the parkinsonism-dementia complex and Guadeloupean parkinsonism. Parkinsonism Relat Disord 2003;9:39–54.

19. Chaudhuri KR, Hu MT, Brooks DJ. Atypical parkinsonism in Afro-Caribbean and Indian origin immigrants to the UK. Mov Disord 2000;15(1):18–23.

20. Duvoisin RC, Yahr MD, Schweitzer MD, Merritt HH. Parkinsonism before and since the epidemic of Encephalitis Lethargic. Arch Neurol 1963;9:232–236.

21. Langston JW, Ballard P, Tetrud JW, Irwin I. Chronic parkinsonism in humans due to a product of meperidine-analog synthesis. Science 1983;219:970–980.

22. Sanchez-Ramos JR, Hefti F, Weiner WJ. Paraquat and Parkinson's disease. Neurology 1987;37:728.

23. Caparros-Lefebvre D, Elbaz A, and the Caribbean Parkinsonism Study Group. Possible relation of atypical parkinsonism in the French West Indies with consumption of tropical plants: a case-control study. Lancet 1999;354:281–286.

24. Davis PH, Golbe LI, Duvoisin RC, Schoenberg BS. Risk factors for progressive supranuclear palsy. Neurology 1988;38(10):1546–1552.

25. Golbe LI, Rubin RS, Cody RP et al. Follow-up study of risk factors in progressive supranuclear palsy. Neurology 1996;47(1):148–54.

26. Nee LE, Gomez MR, Dambrosia J, Bale S, Eldridge R, Polinsky RJ. Environmental-occupational risk factors and familial associations in multiple system atrophy: a preliminary investigation. Clin Auton Res 1991;1(1):9–13.

27. Vanacore, N., et al., Smoking habits in multiple system atrophy and progressive supranuclear palsy. European Study Group on Atypical Parkinsonisms. Neurology 2000;54(1):114–119.

28. Hanna PA, Jankovic J, Kirkpatrick JB. Multiple system atrophy: the putative causative role of environmental toxins. Arch Neurol 1999;56(1):90–94.

29. McCrank E. PSP risk factors. Neurology 1990; 40:1637.

4

Neuropathology of Atypical Parkinsonian Disorders

Ian R. A. Mackenzie

INTRODUCTION

Although the clinical syndrome of parkinsonism (rigidity, bradykinesia, and tremor) is most often owing to idiopathic Parkinson's disease (PD), it may also be associated with a variety of other underlying pathologies (Table 1) *(1–3)*. Each of these other pathological conditions tends to have a characteristic clinical phenotype, however atypical cases are increasingly recognized *(4–8)*. Moreover, some patients with PD have additional clinical features such as dementia, autonomic dysfunction, or gastrointestinal dysmotility *(9–13)*. As a result, the accurate diagnosis of a patient with parkinsonism, and especially those with atypical or additional clinical features, ultimately depends on neuropathological examination. This chapter will review the pathological changes that characterize those conditions that may present with or have parkinsonism as a major feature, either in isolation or combined with other clinical manifestations. Although the focus of this text and chapter are the *atypical* causes of parkinsonism, a description of the pathological features of typical PD is included for comparison.

Most of the conditions that cause parkinsonism have damage of the striatonigral system as the common anatomicopathological substrate. Some have additional neuropathology, which is more disease specific, such as the presence of characteristic cellular inclusions in many of the idiopathic neurodegenerative disorders (Table 2). Others, such as many toxic and metabolic conditions, show only nonspecific chronic degeneration with neuronal loss and reactive gliosis. In this chapter, greater discussion will be devoted to those disease entities that more commonly cause parkinsonism and have distinctive pathology, whereas conditions that rarely cause parkinsonism and those with nonspecific pathology will receive less attention.

IDIOPATHIC PARKINSON'S DISEASE

Although there is some controversy as to the most appropriate use of the term *(14)*, *Parkinson's disease* is most often used to denote idiopathic parkinsonism associated with the pathological finding of neuronal loss and Lewy bodies in the substantia nigra.

External examination of the brain is generally unremarkable, although PD patients who develop dementia may have mild to moderate cerebral atrophy. On cut sections, there is usually loss of pigment from the substantia nigra and locus ceruleus (Fig. 1A). The caudate, putamen, globus pallidus, thalamus, and other brainstem structures appear normal.

The histopathological hallmark of PD is the loss of dopaminergic neurons from the substantia nigra associated with the presence of intraneuronal inclusions called Lewy bodies (LBs). Cell loss in the substantia nigra occurs in a region-specific manner, with the lateral ventral tier of the pars compacta being most affected *(15)*. It is estimated that at least 50% of the nigral neurons must degenerate

From: *Current Clinical Neurology: Atypical Parkinsonian Disorders*
Edited by: I. Litvan © Humana Press Inc., Totowa, NJ

Table 1
Causes of Parkinsonism

1. Neurodegenerative disease:
   synucleinopathies
   - Lewy body disorders
     - idiopathic Parkinson's disease
     - dementia with Lewy bodies
   - multiple system atrophy
   - Hallervorden–Spatz syndrome
   tauopathies
   - corticobasal degeneration
   - progressive supranuclear palsy
   - FTDP-17
   - parkinsonism/dementia complex of Guam
   other:
   - Alzheimer's disease
   - motor neuron disease and frontotemporal dementia with MND-type inclusions
   - Huntington's disease
   - spinocerebellar ataxia
2. Infectious disease:
   - postencephalitic parkinsonism
   - HIV
   - other (bacteria, viruses, parasites, fungi)
3. Vascular disease
4. Trauma
5. Toxins:
   - MPTP
   - others
6. Dugs:
   - neuroleptics (phenothiazines)
7. Metabolic disease:
   - Wilson's disease
   - aceruloplasminemia
8. Space-occupying lesions
9. Hydrocephalus

Note: It has recently become popular to classify some neurodegenerative diseases based on the protein abnormality (molecular pathology) that is believed to be central to the pathogenesis. This interpretation is often supported by genetic analysis of familial cases. Although this type of classification may help to organize discussion of the comparative pathology and biochemistry between conditions, it may be an oversimplification, which will require revision in the future. For instance, it is increasingly recognized that many of the "tauopathies" often have some accumulation of α-synuclein and vice versa.

to produce symptoms and, at autopsy, most cases show more than 80% reduction *(15)*. Significant neuronal loss also occurs in the locus ceruleus, dorsal motor nucleus of the vagus, raphe nuclei, and nucleus basalis. LBs may be found in all of these locations as well as numerous other subcortical structures. Neurodegeneration is accompanied by reactive changes including astrogliosis and microglial cell activation. In pigmented nuclei, neuromelanin is released from dying neurons and may lie free within the neuropil or be taken up by macrophages.

In 1912, Frederich H. Lewy first described intraneuronal inclusions in the substantia innominata and dorsal motor nucleus of the vagus, in patients with paralysis agitans *(16)*. Seven years later, Tretiakoff recognized similar inclusions in the substantia nigra and called them *corps de Lewy (17)*. Since then, LBs have been considered the pathological hallmark of idiopathic PD and most

Table 2
Comparative Neuropathology of Major Causes of Parkinsonism

Disease	Most Diagnostic Pathology	Other Characteristic Pathology
idiopathic Parkinson's disease	• subcortical LBs[a]	• cortical LBs[a] • pale bodies[a] • Lewy neurites[a]
dementia with Lewy bodies	• cortical LBs[a]	• subcortical LBs[a] • Lewy neurites[a]
multiple system atrophy	• glial cytoplasmic inclusions[a]	• glial intranuclear inclusions[a] • neuronal cytoplasmic and intranuclear inclusions[a]
corticobasal degeneration	• achromatic neurons • astrocytic plaques[b] • threads[b]	• cortical neuronal cytoplasmic inclusions[b] • corticobasal bodies[b] • thorn-shaped astrocytes[b] • coiled bodies[b]
progressive supranuclear palsy	• subcortical NFTs[b] • tufted astrocytes[b]	• cortical NFTs[b] • thorn-shaped astrocytes[b] • coiled bodies[b] • threads[b] • grumose degeneration
FTDP-17T	• various neuronal cytoplasmic inclusions[b] • various glial cytoplasmic inclusions[b]	• achromatic neurons
ALS/parkinsonism/ dementia complex of Guam	•cortical and subcortical NFTs[b]	• glial cytoplasmic inclusions[b]
Alzheimer's disease	• cortical SPs • cortical NFTs[b]	• subcortical SPs (subcortical NFTs[b]
postencephalitic parkinsonism	• cortical and subcortical NFTs[b]	• glial cytoplasmic inclusions[b]
vascular parkinsonism	• cerebral infarcts	
posttraumatic parkinsonism	• NFTs[b] • SPs	

LB, Lewy body; NFT, neurofibrillary tangle
[a]α-synuclein immunoreactive
[b]tau-immunoreactive

neuropathologists are reluctant to make the diagnosis in their absence. Classical LBs are spherical intracytoplasmic neuronal inclusions, measuring 8–30 μm in diameter, with an eosinophilic hyaline core and a pale-staining peripheral halo (Fig. 1B). They occasionally have a more complex, multilobar shape and more than one LBs may occur in a single cell. Following neuronal death, LBs may remain as an extracellular deposit in the neuropil. Ultrastructurally they are composed of radially arranged 7- to 20-nm filaments associated with granular electron-dense material.

An additional finding in most cases of PD is the presence of *pale* bodies: ill-defined rounded areas of granular pale-staining eosinophilic material that also occur in pigmented neurons of the substantia nigra and locus ceruleus (Fig. 1C). Although they are distinguished from LBs histologically, their similar immunocytochemical profile suggests they likely represent precursors to LBs *(18,19)*.

LBs are difficult to isolate and purify and so most of our understanding of their chemical composition is based on immunohistochemical studies. Until recently, the two main components were

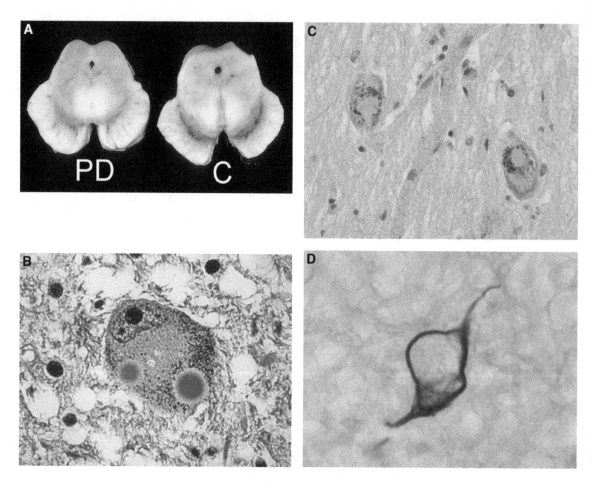

Fig. 1. Idiopathic Parkinson's disease (PD). (**A**) Gross photograph of the midbrain showing loss of pigmentation of the substantia nigra in PD compared with normal control (C). (**B**) Classical Lewy body in pigmented neuron of the substantia nigra (H&E stain). (**C**) Pale bodies in pigmented neurons of the substantia nigra (H&E stain). (**D**) Filamentous cytoplasmic inclusion in glial cell (Gallyas silver stain).

thought to be neurofilament proteins and ubiquitin, although many other protein and non-proteinaceous elements are also recognized *(20–22)*. The biochemistry of LBs was clarified following the discovery of mutations in the gene for α-synuclein in some families with autosomal dominant PD *(23)*. α-Synuclein is a presynaptic nerve terminal protein and immunohistochemistry of normal brain tissue shows punctate staining around neuronal perikarya. Direct involvement of α-synuclein in the pathogenesis of all LB disorders (sporadic as well as familial PD and dementia with LB) is supported by immunohistochemical studies confirming α-synuclein as a major component of both brainstem and cortical LB, as well as pale bodies and Lewy-related neurites *(19,24)*. In addition to these neuronal pathologies, recent reports have described the presence of argyrophilic, α-synuclein-positive cytoplasmic inclusions in both astrocytes and oligodendrocytes in PD (Fig. 1D) *(25,26)*. The consistency and significance of this glial pathology awaits clarification.

DEMENTIA WITH LEWY BODIES

Although it has long been recognized that a significant proportion of PD patients develop dementia *(12)*, the pathological substrate for this cognitive dysfunction remained uncertain. In 1961, Okazaki reported finding LBs in the cerebral cortex of two patients with PD and atypical dementia *(27)*.

Although subsequent cases of *diffuse Lewy body disease* (DLBD) were published, the condition was initially considered rare. In the late 1980s, with greater awareness of cortical LBs and the development of more sensitive staining methods, several groups reported finding cortical LBs in 15–25% of elderly demented patients, both with and without parkinsonism *(28,29)*. It has recently been proposed that dementia associated with Lewy bodies (DLB) represents a recognizable clinicopathological syndrome that may be distinguishable during life from other causes of dementia *(30)*. The proposed diagnostic criteria are purely clinical however, and recommendations as to how to quantitate LBs are only designed to assess the hypothesis that dementia is more likely to occur when LBs are numerous and widespread (i.e., DLB = DLBD) *(30)*. Although numerous cortical LBs are most characteristic of DLB, smaller numbers are found in most (if not all) patients with idiopathic PD, even in the absence of dementia *(31)*. As a result, the clinical and pathological relationship between PD and DLB and the appropriate terminology remains an ongoing source of controversy.

Some cases of DLB show microvacuolation of the superficial neocortex, particularly in the temporal lobe. Cortical LBs occur primarily in small and medium-size pyramidal neurons of the deeper cortical layers and are most abundant in the transentorhinal and cingulate cortex, less numerous in neocortex, and generally spare the hippocampus. They tend to be less well defined and are more difficult to recognize than classical brainstem LBs, using conventional staining methods (Fig. 2A). It is largely the advent of more sensitive immunohistochemical methods of detection (especially for ubiquitin and α-synuclein) that has allowed the extent of cortical LB pathology to be fully appreciated (Fig. 2B).

A distinctive neuritic degeneration was first reported in cases of DLB *(32)* but has subsequently been found in many cases of PD, as well *(33)*. These abnormally swollen neuronal processes are not seen using hematoxylin and eosin (H&E) or conventional silver stains but are well demonstrated using ubiquitin and α-synuclein immunohistochemistry (Fig. 2C) *(19)*. Often referred to as *Lewy neurites*, they are most concentrated in the CA2/3 region of the hippocampus but are also found in the amygdala, nucleus basalis, and various brainstem nuclei. In addition to accumulating in neuronal cell bodies and processes, α-synuclein-positive glial inclusions have also been reported in DLB *(25,34)*.

Most, but not all, cases of DLB have some degree of Alzheimer's disease (AD)-like pathology *(28,35)*. Senile plaques (SPs) are the most common finding with the majority being of the "diffuse" type. When neuritic plaques are present, most contain only tau-negative, ubiquitin-positive neurites. Neurofibrillary tangles (NFTs) and neuropil threads, containing paired helical filaments, may be found in the limbic structures and mesial temporal lobe but are uncommon in the neocortex. This pattern of pathology may be sufficient to fulfil pathological criteria for AD that are based on SP numbers (such as CERAD) *(36)* but not those that stress the importance of NFTs (such as Braak staging) *(37)*. This overlap between DLB and AD pathology, combined with the lack of universally accepted pathological diagnostic criteria for either disorder, has resulted in confusion over the relationship between the conditions and the appropriate terminology. It also raises questions as to the pathological substrate for dementia in DLB patients. Although some studies have shown a correlation between the numbers of cortical LBs and cognitive dysfunction *(38–41)*, others have not *(29)*. This suggests that coexisting AD pathology, Lewy neurites, and/or degeneration of specific neuronal populations could all contribute to dementia, possibly in an additive fashion *(42,43)*.

THE SPECTRUM OF LB DISORDERS

There is striking clinical and pathological overlap between PD and DLB. Up to one-third of patients with a clinical diagnosis of PD will develop dementia *(9,12,42)* and most (but not all) patients with DLB display some degree of parkinsonism *(30)*. LBs are the defining histopathological feature of both conditions. In PD, LBs are most numerous in subcortical nuclei and it is the associated loss of dopaminergic neurons that is largely responsible for the characteristic extrapyramidal features. However, small numbers of cortical LBs may be found in virtually all cases of PD, even in the absence of dementia *(31)*. In DLB, cortical LBs are usually more numerous and some studies have shown a

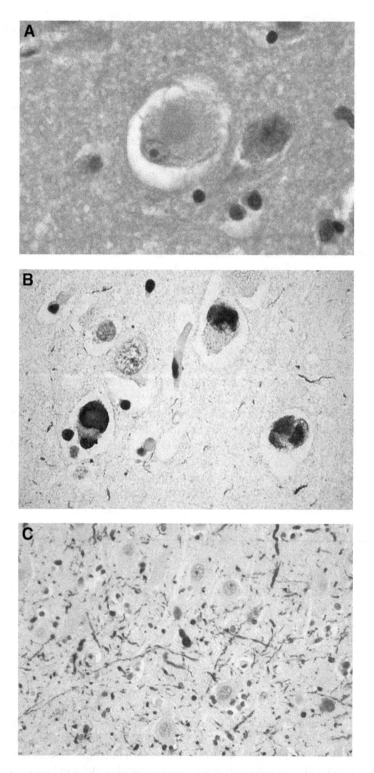

Fig. 2. Dementia with Lewy bodies. (**A**) Cortical Lewy body (LB) (H&E stain). (**B**) Three neurons in deep layers of neocortex containing LBs (α-synuclein immunohistochemistry). (**C**) Lewy neurites in CA2 region of hippocampus (ubiquitin immunohistochemistry).

correlation between their number and the degree of dementia *(38–41)*. Even in the absence of parkinsonism, however, the vast majority of DLB cases display some brainstem LB. Recognition of this overlap has led to the concept of a spectrum of LB disorders with different clinical features, depending on the severity and anatomic distribution of LB involvement *(44–46)*. Other less common clinical manifestations may be associated with involvement of other neuroanatomic regions, autonomic dysfunction with involvement of sympathetic ganglia, dysphagia when the dorsal motor nucleus of the vagus is damaged, and gastrointestinal dysmotility with LBs in enteric plexi *(10,11)*. Each condition may occur in isolation or in various combinations. Although this concept is attractive, at least one recent study failed to demonstrate the degree of clinical-anatomic correlation predicted *(38)*.

FAMILIAL PARKINSON'S DISEASE

At the time this manuscript was being prepared, at least 11 different genetic loci had been linked to familial PD, including mutations in four specific genes *(47,48)*. The pattern of inheritance includes both autosomal dominant and recessive and the clinical phenotypes vary from typical PD to families with juvenile or early onset and others with atypical clinical features. For most of these, information about the pathological findings is not yet available. Families with autosomal dominant PD and mutation of the gene for α-synuclein have changes similar to sporadic PD, with nigral degeneration and LBs *(23)*. Cases of autosomal recessive, juvenile-onset PD and *parkin* mutations have neuronal loss in the substantia nigra and locus ceruleus, but only one report has described finding LBs *(49)*. A single family has been identified with a mutation in the gene for ubiquitin C-terminal hydrolase L1 (UCH-L1) *(50)*. No pathological information is available from this family but mice with intronic deletion of this gene develop axonal degeneration *(51)*.

MULTIPLE SYSTEM ATROPHY

Although the term *multiple system atrophy* (MSA) has been used rather indiscriminately in the past, recent advances in our understanding of the genetic, biochemical, and pathological basis of a number of neurodegenerative diseases has resulted in some reclassification and refinement of the definition. On the basis of a common pathological substrate, the diagnosis of MSA is currently restricted to include cases formerly designated as striatonigral degeneration (SND), olivopontocerebellar atrophy (OPCA), and some (but not all) cases of Shy–Drager syndrome. Because of the high degree of clinical and pathological overlap between these conditions, a recent Consensus Conference recommended using the terms MSA-P for cases with prominent parkinsonism and MSA-C for those with mainly cerebellar features *(52)*. A review of 100 cases of the clinical course of MSA found that almost all eventually developed parkinsonism and autonomic dysfunction whereas cerebellar features occurred in less than half *(53)*.

Several excellent reviews of the neuropathology of MSA have recently been published *(54,55)*. Macroscopically, there is atrophy of specific cortical and subcortical regions, which reflects the anatomic distribution of degenerative change. In cases previously designated as SND (most probably corresponding to MSA-P), there tends to be severe atrophy and discoloration of the putamen and loss of pigmentation of the substantia nigra and locus ceruleus (Fig. 3A), whereas in OPCA (MSA-C) the cerebellum, middle cerebellar peduncles, and basis pontis are most affected (Fig. 3B).

Microscopically, the involved gray matter structures show neuronal loss and reactive gliosis whereas associated white matter tracts demonstrate loss of myelin. The degree and pattern of degeneration vary from case to case but the putamen, substantia nigra, locus ceruleus, inferior olives, pontine nuclei, Purkinje cell layer, and intermediolateral columns are most often affected in some combination *(56)*. Nerve biopsy may show a reduction in the number of unmyelinated fibres *(57)*.

The specific histopathological changes that characterize MSA, and which are now considered mandatory for the diagnosis *(58)*, were first described in a series of articles by Papp and Lantos *(59–61)*. The most characteristic change is the presence of small flame or sickle-shaped structures in the

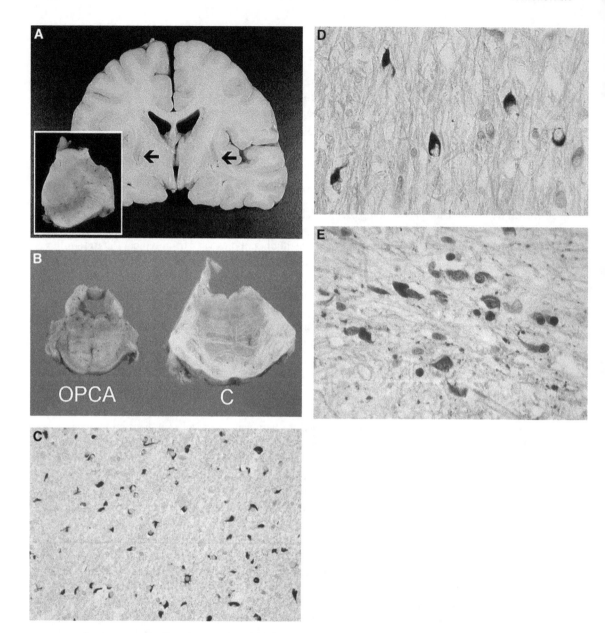

Fig. 3. Multiple system atrophy. (**A**) Gross photographs of a case of striatonigral degeneration showing atrophy and discoloration of the putamen (arrows) and loss of pigmentation of the substantia nigra (inset). (**B**) Gross photograph showing atrophy of the pons in a case of olivopontocerebellar atrophy (OPCA) compared with normal control (C). (**C,D**) Numerous glial cytoplasmic inclusions (GCIs) in oligodendrocytes (Gallyas silver stain). (**E**) GCIs immunoreactive for α-synuclein.

cytoplasm of oligodendrocytes, referred to as *glial cytoplasmic inclusions* (GCIs). They are difficult to detect in routine H&E-stained sections but are well demonstrated with a variety of silver stains, particularly the Gallyas method (Fig. 3C,D). Although GCIs show variable immunoreactivity for a variety of proteins including tau, ubiquitin, tubulins, and B-crystallin *(59,62–64)*, they are most strongly immunoreactive for α-synuclein (Fig. 3E) *(65,66)*. The ultrastructural composition includes tubules and straight and twisted filaments associated with granular material *(59,60,62–65)*. GCIs tend to be widely distributed throughout the brain, beyond the areas showing obvious degeneration. They are found in motor cortex, putamen, globus pallidus, subthalamic nucleus, pontine nuclei, various cranial nerve nuclei, and several white matter tracts in the cerebrum, brainstem, and spinal cord. In addition to GCI, argyrophilic, ubiquitin-, and α-synuclein immunoreactive fibrillar or filamentous inclusions are also found in the cytoplasm of neurons and the nuclei of both neurons and glia in MSA *(60,63,67)*. These other types of inclusions tend to be less numerous and have a more restricted anatomical distribution, found primarily in the putamen and basis pontis, and their presence is not required for diagnosis.

CORTICOBASAL DEGENERATION

This clinicopathological entity was first described under the name *corticodentonigral degeneration with neuronal achromasia (68)* and early reports stressed the characteristic movement abnormalities, which often include akinetic rigidity *(69)*. More recently, however, a number of postmortem studies have found abnormalities of higher mental function, such as language disturbance and dementia, to be a common and sometimes predominant feature in patients with corticobasal degeneration (CBD) pathology *(6,8,70–74)*.

Cortical atrophy is often focal and asymmetric with parasagittal, peri-Rolandic, or peri-Sylvian regions most often involved (Fig. 4A). Macroscopic degeneration of subcortical structures is variable with depigmentation of the substantia nigra being most consistent. Microscopically, degenerative changes are more widespread but the severity and anatomical distribution vary between cases. In addition to neuronal loss and gliosis, the affected cortical regions may show superficial laminar or transcortical microvacuolation. Of subcortical structures, the substantia nigra tends to be the most severely and consistently affected whereas involvement of globus pallidus, striatum, subthalamic, thalamic nuclei, and brainstem regions is more variable.

The original description identified numerous swollen achromatic neurons (ANs) as the characteristic histopathological feature of CBD *(68)*. ANs are most numerous in limbic cortex and amygdala in CBD, however this finding is not disease specific *(75,76)*. Of greater diagnostic significance is the presence of neocortical ANs, which are most common in layers III, V, and VI of posterior frontal and parietal lobes. They may also be present in small numbers in subcortical regions. ANs resemble cells undergoing central chromatolysis; the perikaryon is swollen and often rounded, the Nissl substance is inconspicuous, and the nucleus is often in an eccentric position (Fig. 4B). They occasionally show cytoplasmic vacuolation. Although easy to recognize with standard H&E stain, ANs are best demonstrated by their strong cytoplasmic immunoreactivity for phosphorylated neurofilament and αB-crystallin (Fig. 4C) *(75,77)*. Argyrophilia, tau-, and ubiquitin-immunoreactivity are more variable *(72,78)*.

The other change visible with H&E stain is the presence of ill-defined faintly basophilic filamentous cytoplasmic inclusions in surviving neurons of the substantia nigra and some other subcortical structures (Fig. 4D). These were originally termed *corticobasal bodies (79)* but appear to have the same immunophenotype and ultrastructure as the NFTs found in broader distribution in progressive supranuclear palsy (PSP) *(80,81)*.

The major recent advance in understanding the pathology of CBD has been the demonstration of widespread accumulation of abnormal phosphorylated tau protein in both glia and neurons *(72,80,82–84)*. Tau is a microtubule-associated protein (MAP) whose primary function is to promote the assembly and stabilization of microtubules. It is constitutively expressed and is normally found in axons

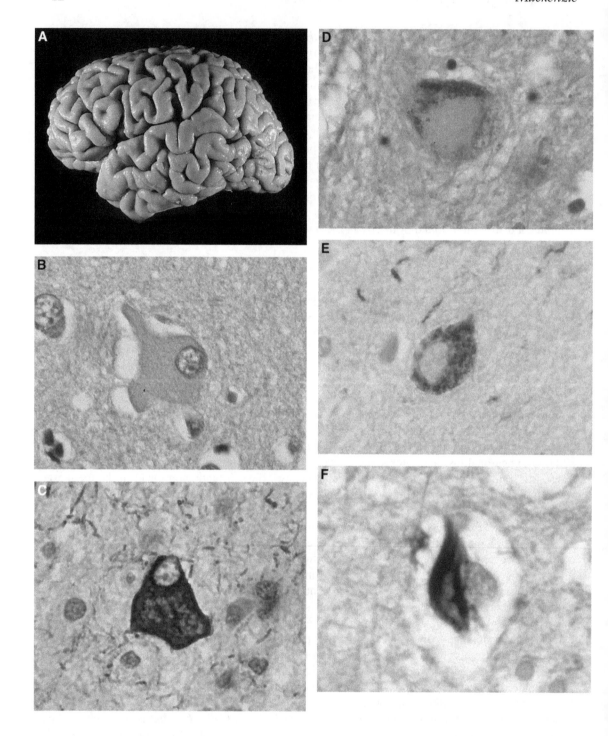

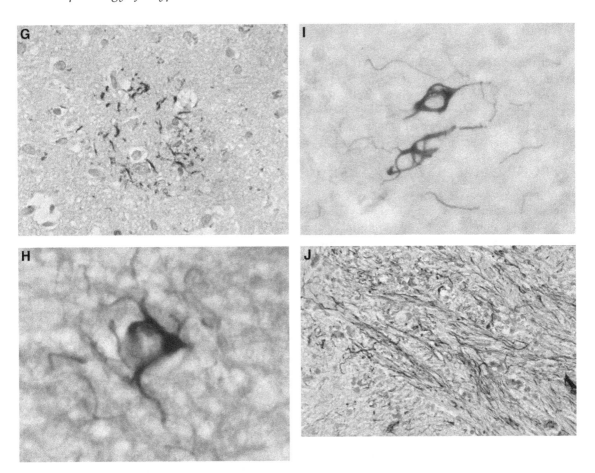

Fig. 4. Corticobasal degeneration. (**A**) Gross photograph showing mild peri-Rolandic cortical atrophy. (**B**) Achromatic neuron (AN) in neocortex (H&E stain). (**C**) AN showing cytoplasmic immunoreactivity for phosphorylated neurofilament. (**D**) Corticobasal body in pigmented neuron of substantia nigra (H&E stain). (**E,F**) Neuronal inclusions in neocortex. Diffuse cytoplasmic immunoreactivity for phosphorylated tau (E) and argyrophilic neurofibrillary tangle (F) (Gallyas silver stain). (**G–J**) Glial inclusions. (G) Astrocytic plaque (tau immunohistochemistry). (H) Thorn-shaped astrocyte (Gallyas silver stain). (I) Coiled bodies in oligodendrocytes (Gallyas silver stain). (J) Thread-like processes in cerebral white matter (tau-immunohistochemistry).

and mature neurons. Most of the tau-positive inclusions of CBD are also well demonstrated with silver stains such as Gallyas method but tend to react poorly with antibodies against ubiquitin protein. Neurons in the cerebral cortex may show diffuse granular cytoplasmic staining or contain denser inclusions, resembling either Pick's bodies or small NFTs (Fig. 4E,F) *(72,80,85)*. Filamentous or fibrillar cytoplasmic inclusions are also found in some subcortical neurons, especially in the substantia nigra, where they correspond to the corticobasal bodies *(80,81)*.

Several types of tau-immunoreactive, argyrophilic inclusions are found in the cytoplasm of glial cells. The most specific is the *astrocytic plaque*, which consists of a circular arrangement of short cell processes in the cortical or subcortical gray matter (Fig. 4G) *(72,82,83,86,87)*. Although vaguely resembling the neuritic plaques of AD, these structures are not associated with extracellular amyloid and double-immunolabeling has confirmed they represent tau accumulation in the most distal portion of astrocytic processes *(72)*. More numerous but less disease specific are *thorn-shaped astrocytes* and *coiled bodies (83,88,89)*. Thorn-shaped astrocytes result from the accumulation of tau in the cell body and most proximal portion of astrocytic processes, producing short, sharp processes (Fig. 4H).

These are seen in cortical and subcortical gray matter and white matter. Coiled bodies occur in oligodendrocytes and appear as delicate bundles of fibrils that wrap around the nucleus and extend into the proximal cell process (Fig. 4I). They are located primarily in the subcortical white matter. One of the most striking changes in CBD is the presence of numerous tau-immunoreactive, silver-positive threadlike processes in affected gray and white matter (Fig. 4J) *(72,80,82,83,85,90)*. In contrast with the neuropil threads of AD, which are exclusively neuronal in origin, the threads of CBD are primarily glial *(72,90)*. Although similar threads are found in some other conditions such as PSP, their extreme number in CBD is diagnostically helpful.

PROGRESSIVE SUPRANUCLEAR PALSY

In the original description of this disease entity, patients with supranuclear ophthalmoplegia, pseudobulbar palsy, dysarthria, rigidity, and mild cognitive deficits were found to have abundant NFTs in subcortical nuclei *(91)*. The clinical phenotype is now recognized to be much more variable and includes both pure parkinsonism and frontotemporal dementia with no movement abnormality *(1,2,4,5,71)*.

The macroscopic changes are quite variable. The cerebral cortex often appears normal but may show significant frontotemporal atrophy that may be quite circumscribed (Fig. 5A). The midbrain and pontine tegmentum are often atrophic whereas the globus pallidus is the most commonly affected part of the basal ganglia (Fig. 5B). Microscopic degeneration with neuronal loss and gliosis also tends to be more widespread and severe in PSP than CBD, with substantia nigra, locus ceruleus, globus pallidus, subthalamic nucleus, midbrain tegmentum, cerebellar dentate nucleus, and pontine nuclei usually involved.

As with CBD, the histopathology of PSP is characterized by the abnormal accumulation of tau protein, in both neurons and glia, which can be demonstrated with immunohistochemistry or silver methods such as Gallyas *(82,83,86,88,90,92)*. The most characteristic feature is widespread NFT formation (Fig. 5C) *(91)*. Current diagnostic criteria require the presence of numerous NFTs in at least three of the following sites: pallidum, subthalamic nucleus, substantia nigra, or pons, and at least some tangles in three of striatum, oculomotor nucleus, medulla, or dentate *(93,94)*. The tangles in these subcortical regions often have a rounded or *globose* shape (Fig. 5D) and ultrastructural studies show they are composed predominantly of 12–20 nm straight filaments. NFTs may also be found in cerebral cortex where their morphology more closely resemble those seen in AD, being flame-shaped and composed of paired helical filaments *(95–97)*. Although the number and distribution of cortical NFTs in PSP is usually more restricted than in AD, some studies have shown a correlation with cognitive dysfunction *(98)*. ANs (more characteristic of CBD) may be found in some cases of PSP but tend to be limited to limbic cortex *(76)*.

Several types of argyrophilic, tau-positive glial inclusions occur consistently in PSP. Many of these, such as thorn-shaped astrocytes, coiled bodies, and threadlike lesions, are nonspecific, also being seen in other *tauopathies* such as CBD and Pick's disease *(82,83,88–90)*. The most diagnostic glial pathology in PSP is the presence of *tufted* astrocytes, which are most numerous in striatum but that are also found in other subcortical regions and frontal cortex *(86,88)*. Although immunoreactive for tau, the morphology is best appreciated with Gallyas silver method, which shows the filamentous inclusion material surrounding the astrocyte nucleus and extending into a complex collection of long delicate processes, producing a *shrublike* appearance (Fig. 5E). This is different from thorn-shaped astrocytes where the inclusion material is restricted to more proximal processes (Fig. 4G) and astrocytic plaques in which only the most distal parts of processes are involved (Fig. 4F).

Finally, a unique pathology, which may be seen in the cerebellar dentate nucleus in PSP, is *grumose degeneration* in which granular eosinophilic material surrounds neurons, some of which are achromatic (Fig. 5F). Ultrastructural studies have shown the granular material to be degenerating axon terminals of Purkinje cells *(99)*.

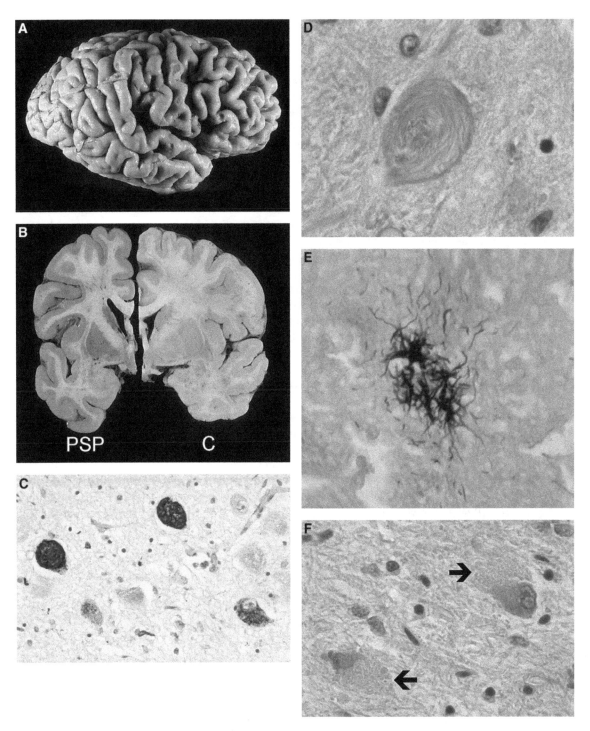

Fig. 5. Progressive supranuclear palsy. Gross photographs showing (**A**) lobar frontal atrophy and (**B**) atrophy and discoloration of basal ganglia. (**C**) Multiple neurofibrillary tangles (NFTs) and pretangles in midbrain (tau-immunohistochemistry). (**D**) Globose NFT (H&E stain). (**E**) Tufted-astrocyte (Gallyas silver stain). (**F**) Grumose degeneration (arrows) of neurons in cerebellar dentate nucleus (H&E stain).

FTDP-17*T*

The term *frontotemporal dementia and parkinsonism linked to chromosome 17* (FTDP-17) was recommended at a consensus conference in 1997 to denote a growing number of families recognized, in which frontotemporal dementia (FTD), behavioral disturbances, language abnormalities, and/or parkinsonism are inherited in an autosomal dominant fashion and genetic analysis shows linkage to chromosome 17 *(100)*. The following year, a number of reports were published, describing mutations in the tau gene in some of these families *(101–104)*. It is now common for a "*T*" to be added to the end of the acronym to distinguish these cases from other chromosome 17-linked FTD in which the tau gene is normal and there is no tau accumulation in the brain *(105,106)*. At the present time, more than 80 FTDP-17*T* kindreds have been identified, with more than 30 different tau mutations *(107)*. The types of genetic abnormality include missense, deletion, and silent transition mutations in the coding region of the tau gene and intronic mutations near the splice site of the intron following exon 10 *(108)*. Sufficient material is just now becoming available to allow for detailed examination of how different genetic abnormalities correlate with the clinical and pathological phenotypes *(108,109)*.

FTDP-17*T* shows significant heterogeneity in both the clinical manifestations and the underlying neuropathology *(100,108–110)*. In some families, FTD predominates and parkinsonism is variable, mild, or of late onset, whereas other pedigrees have parkinsonism as the major feature. A limited amount of postmortem information is available on FTDP-17*T* families. Most cases show frontotemporal atrophy with varying degeneration of subcortical nuclei and tracts *(100,110)*. Loss of pigmentation of the substantia nigra is common. The histopathology of all cases described to date is characterized by the accumulation of abnormal hyperphosphorylated tau in neurons and/or glial cells *(108,110)*. Neuronal changes may include ballooned neurons, pretangles, NFTs, Pick's-like bodies, and/or neuropil threads. A variety of tau-positive inclusions may be seen in both astrocytes and oligodendrocytes. In some cases, the pattern of pathology closely resembles one of the sporadic tauopathies such as AD *(111)*, CBD *(112,113)*, PSP *(114)*, or Pick's disease *(115,116)*, whereas others show some novel combination of findings *(117)*. Although a detailed description of each of the different patterns of pathology in FTDP-17*T* is not possible in this review, two specific conditions are worth mentioning because of the prominence of parkinsonism and availability of detailed neuropathology.

Parkinsonism is the dominant feature of several families with the N279K mutation in the alternatively spliced exon 10; this includes the American kindred designated as having *pallido-ponto-nigral degeneration* (PPND), for which there is detailed pathological information *(118)*. Most patients show mild frontotemporal atrophy with grossly obvious degeneration of the globus pallidus and substantia nigra. The histopathologic and immunohistochemical findings include ballooned neocortical neurons and tau-positive subcortical threadlike structures, globose NFTs (corticobasal bodies), and oligodendroglial inclusions resembling coiled bodies. Astrocytic inclusions are uncommon and tufted astrocytes and astrocytic plaques are not a feature. Although these findings most closely resemble sporadic CBD, the anatomic distribution is more similar to that seen in PSP.

Parkinsonism is also a major feature in the Irish-American kindred with *disinhibition-dementia-parkinsonism-amyotrophy-complex* (DDPAC). This was the first family to be linked to chromosome 17 and has subsequently been show to be owing to an intronic mutation of the exon 10 5' slice site *(119)*. There is gross atrophy of temporal lobes, prefrontal cortex, cingulum, basal ganglia, and substantia nigra *(120)*. Affected cortical regions show gliosis, occasional ballooned neurons, and tau-positive NFTs and spheroids. The hippocampus is relatively spared. Subcortical regions affected include the amygdala, substantia nigra, globus pallidus, striatum, midbrain tegmentum, and hypothalamus. In these areas, neuronal loss and gliosis are accompanied by small numbers of ballooned neurons, argyrophilic neuronal inclusions, and spheroids. Some neuronal inclusions resembled AD-type NFTs and are immunoreactive for tau whereas other have a more spiculated appearance and are positive for neurofilament and ubiquitin but are tau negative. Argyrophilic, tau-positive tanglelike inclusions are also present in oligodendrocytes in various white matter tracts.

ALS/PARKINSONISM DEMENTIA COMPLEX OF GUAM

A high incidence of neurodegenerative disease is found within the Chamorro population of the Western Pacific island of Guam, and includes parkinsonism, dementia, and amyotrophic lateral sclerosis (ALS), each of which may occur in isolation but are more commonly combined *(121)*. The cause is unknown but a toxic or viral etiology has been postulated *(122–124)*. The histopathology is dominated by the presence of numerous NFTs *(125,126)*, with similar immunohistochemical, biochemical, and ultrastructural features as those seen in AD *(127,128)*, but usually in the absence of SP (Fig. 6A,B). The anatomical distribution of NFTs is different from AD *(129)* and more similar to that seen in PSP and postencephalitic parkinsonism (PEP) *(130,131)*. Chronic degenerative changes including neuronal loss and gliosis are found in regions where NFTs are numerous, including the frontotemporal neocortex, hippocampus, entorhinal cortex, nucleus basalis, basal ganglia, thalamus, subthalamus, substantia nigra, locus ceruleus, and periaqueductal gray *(125,126,129)*. Glial pathology has recently been described and includes argyrophilic, tau-positive coiled bodies in oligodendroglia and granular inclusions in astrocytes *(132)*. There tends to be large numbers of Hirano bodies and abundant granulovacuolar degeneration in the hippocampus *(133)*. Cases with clinical features of ALS have pathologic changes in the pyramidal motor system, similar to sporadic ALS *(134)*.

OTHER NEURODEGENERATIVE CONDITIONS

Many other common idiopathic neurodegenerative conditions have parkinsonism as an inconsistent or minor clinical feature. Extrapyramidal symptoms are very common in AD and may take the form of true parkinsonism *(135–137)*. Many patients with a clinical diagnosis of AD and parkinsonism are found to have coexisting LB pathology at autopsy, either restricted to subcortical structures or also involving the cerebral cortex *(35,136,138)*. The correct terminology for these cases is uncertain, because of the lack of universally accepted neuropathological diagnostic criteria for both AD and DLB (*see* subheading Dementia with Lewy Bodies). Interpretation is further complicated by recent reports of LBs as a common incidental finding in AD patients, even in the absence of extrapyramidal features *(139)*. However, parkinsonism also occurs in some AD patients who have only SP and NFT pathology *(136,138,140)*. SPs are a consistent finding in the striatum and are occasionally seen in the substantia nigra in AD, however most are the *diffuse* type of SP, which lack amyloid and are thought not to be injurious to neurons *(137,141,142)*. Numerous NFTs in the substantia nigra is also a consistent feature of AD *(137,141–143)*. Whereas some studies have reported loss of pigmented neurons in the nigra in AD *(143)*, others have found the difference not to be significantly different from age-matched controls *(141)*. It is not clear which, if any, of these changes is the substrate for parkinsonism in AD. Though several studies have found that extrapyramidal features in AD correlate with pathology in the substantia nigra (and not the striatum), there is disagreement as to whether the association is a result of neuronal loss or the number of NFTs *(140,144)*.

Motor neuron disease (MND) may be complicated by dementia and/or akinetic-rigidity *(145)*. In addition to the characteristic changes in the pyramidal motor system, cases of MND with dementia have a unique pathology in the extramotor cortex; ubiquitin-immunoreactive neuronal cytoplasmic inclusions and dystrophic neurites ae present in the neocortex and the hippocampal dentate granule layer *(146)*. Degeneration of various subcortical structures, including substantia nigra and basal ganglia, is well recognized in MND *(145)*. Recently, several studies have described various types of ubiquitin-positive neuronal inclusions and dystrophic neurites in a wide range of these subcortical locations (Fig. 7A,B) *(147–149)*. Although detailed clinicopathological correlation is still lacking, we have recently reported that MND-dementia patients with extrapyramidal features have a greater burden of ubiquitin pathology in the substantia nigra and striatum (Fig. 6) *(150)*.

Although the movement abnormality in most cases of Huntington's disease (HD) is chorea, juvenile or early-onset cases may have akinetic-rigidity. The most characteristic pathological feature of HD is severe atrophy of the caudate nucleus and putamen, with neuronal loss and gliosis (Fig. 8A).

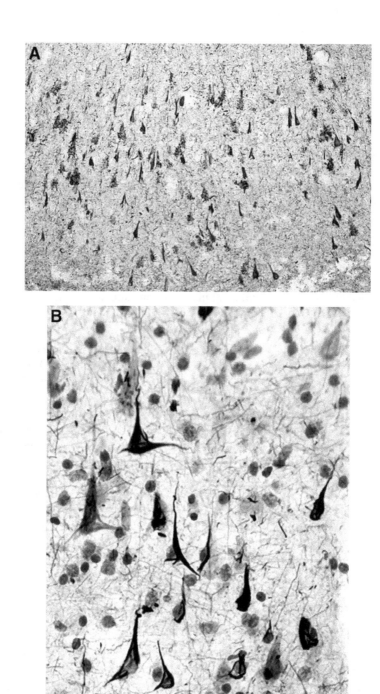

Fig. 6. ALS/parkinsonism/dementia complex of Guam. (**A,B**) Numerous neurofibrillary tangles in CA1 region of hippocampus (A, tau-immunohistochemistry) and temporal neocortex (B, Bielschowsky silver stain). Photographs courtesy of C. Schwab.

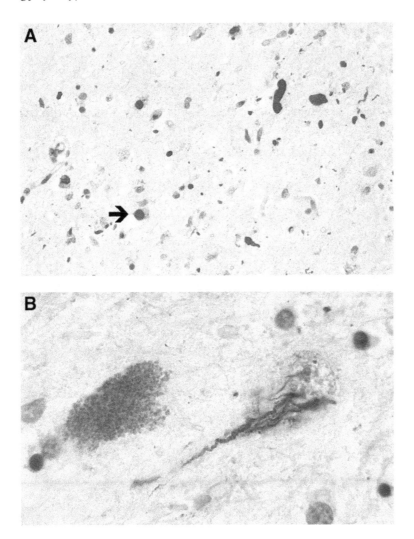

Fig. 7. Case of motor neuron disease with dementia and parkinsonism. (**A**) Dystrophic neurites and neuronal cytoplasmic inclusions (arrow) in striatum (ubiquitin-immunohistochemistry). (**B**) Filamentous *skeinlike* cytoplasmic inclusion in substantia nigra neuron (ubiquitin-immunohistochemistry).

The globus pallidus, thalamus, and cerebral cortex may also be affected and loss of pigmented neurons has been reported in the substantia nigra *(151)*. A recent finding in HD is the presence of intranuclear neuronal inclusions and dystrophic neurites that are immunoreactive for *huntingtin*, ubiquitin, and polyglutamine repeats, in the striatum, allocotex, and neocortex (Fig. 8B) *(152,153)*.

Parkinsonism may be a presenting or prominent feature in some types of autosomal dominant spinocerebellar ataxia (SCA) *(154)*, particularly those caused by trinucleotide repeat expansions. Degenerative changes are most severe in the cerebellum and its connections but are also found in the substantia nigra and basal ganglia *(155,156)*. Many of these conditions have neuronal intranuclear inclusions that are immunoreactive for ubiquitin, polyglutamine repeats, and/or the disease-specific mutant protein *(157,158)*.

Hallervorden–Spatz disease (HSD), recently renamed *neurodegenertion with brain iron accumulation type I* (NBIA-1), is a rare neurodegenerative disorder in which various abnormalities of movement are associated with cognitive decline. Some cases are familial, usually with an autosomal

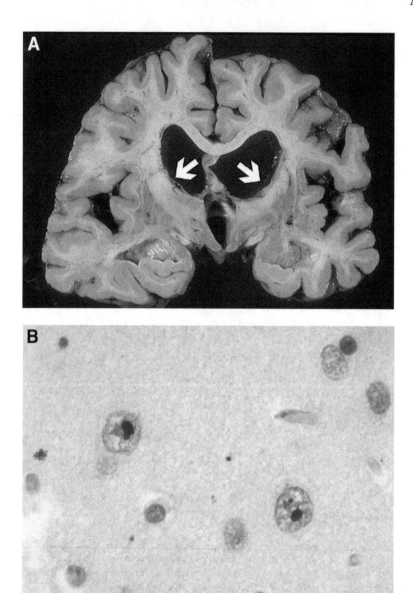

Fig. 8. Huntington's disease. (**A**) Gross photograph showing severe atrophy of caudate nuclei (arrows). (**B**) Intranuclear neuronal inclusions (ubiquitin-immunohistochemistry).

recessive inheritance pattern. Extrapyramidal features are more often a presenting feature in adult-onset cases *(159)*. The neuropathology is characterized by axonal dystrophy (spheroids) and the intra- and extracellular accumulation of iron in the globus pallidus, substantia nigra, and other locations (Fig. 9A,B). It has been recognized for some time that some cases of HSD have LBs *(160)*. Recent reports of α-synuclein immunoreactivity in LBs, axonal spheroids, and neuronal and glial inclusions *(161–163)* has resulted in HSD being classified as a *synucleinopathy*, along with more classical LB disorders (PD and DLB).

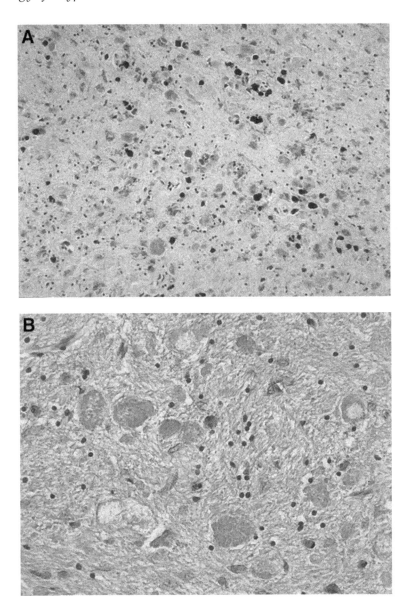

Fig. 9. Hallervorden–Spatz disease. (**A**) Iron deposition (black) and numerous axonal spheroids in globus pallidus (H&E stain). (**B**) Numerous axonal spheroids in globus pallidus (H&E stain).

POSTENCEPHALITIC PARKINSONISM

Following the pandemic of encephalitis lethargica (von Economo's disease), in the early part of the 20th century, a large proportion of individuals who survived the acute encephalitic phase developed parkinsonism, after a latency of several years or decades. PEP was therefore common in the 1940s and 1950s but is now rarely encountered. Although a viral etiology (possibly influenza A) has long been suspected, this remains to be proven *(164,165)*.

Most detailed accounts of the neuropathology of PEP were published several decades ago *(166,167)*. There may be mild cerebral atrophy and the substantia nigra and locus ceruleus show loss of pigmentation (Fig. 10A). There is severe chronic degeneration of substantia nigra with neuronal loss and gliosis. The histopathology is characterized by the presence of numerous NFTs (Fig. 10B). The tangles may be either flame-shaped or globose *(164)* and have the same immunohistochemical and ultrastructural features as those seen in AD *(168,169)*. NFTs are most numerous in the substantia nigra, locus ceruleus, hippocampus, and nucleus basalis, but are also found in many other cortical and subcortical regions *(130)*. This distribution is different from that seen in AD *(170)* and more similar to other causes of parkinsonism with numerous NFTs, such as PSP and parkinsonism-dementia complex of Guam *(94,130,131)*. Tau-positive glial inclusions include tufted astrocytes, thorn-shaped astrocytes, and astrocytic plaques *(164,171,172)*.

VASCULAR PARKINSONISM

Patients with cerebrovascular disease may develop features of parkinsonism *(173–175)* and a small but significant fraction of those with a clinical diagnosis of idiopathic PD will turn out to have vascular lesions demonstrated by neuroimaging or at autopsy *(2,176)*. This "vascular pseudoparkinsonism" is most often seen in patients with cerebral arteriolosclerosis and multiple small lacunar infarcts affecting the basal ganglia or deep cerebral white matter *(173–177)* but has also been reported with isolated lesions of the substantia nigra *(178,179)*.

POSTTRAUMATIC PARKINSONISM

Parkinsomism immediately following a single episode of acute head injury is rare *(180)* but has been reported with direct penetrating lesions of the midbrain *(181)* and with subdural hematoma *(182)*. Epidemiologic studies have shown a history of remote head trauma to be a risk factor for PD, however the mechanism is unclear *(183–184)*. Repeated head injury may result in a syndrome that includes psychiatric symptoms, memory loss, and/or parkinsonism (dementia pugilistica, punch-drunk syndrome). This most often occurs in professional and amateur boxers, with the onset of symptoms occurring several years after the end of their athletic career. Pathological studies have shown loss of pigmented neurons in the substantia nigra and the presence of widespread AD-like pathology, with numerous tau-immunoreactive NFTs and amyloid β (Aβ) containing SPs *(185,186)*. A direct link between these pathological changes and preceding trauma is supported by studies showing Aβ deposits in the brains of individuals dying a few weeks following severe head injury *(187)* and evidence that both Aβ and phosphorylated tau accumulate following brain injury in experimental animals *(188,189)*. Anatomical-pathologic correlation for movement disorder in some of these patients is supported by in vivo neuroimaging, showing damage or dysfunction of the nigrostriatal system *(190–192)*.

MPTP INTOXICATION

Some intravenous drug addicts who use a synthetic heroin-like drug (meperidine) develop chronic parkinsonism as a result of contamination by 1-methyl-4-phenyl-1,2,3,6-tetrahydropyridine (MPTP) *(193)*. MPTP is metabolized in the brain to 1-methyl-4-phenylpyridinium (MPP+) *(194)* and is selectively transported into dopaminergic cells, which it kills by inhibiting mitochondrial function *(195)*. Human postmortem studies reveal severe depletion of pigmented neurons in the substantia nigra without LBs *(196)*. The presence of active gliosis and microglial activity has been interpreted as indicating ongoing neurodegeneration, years after the initial exposure. MPTP-induced parkinsonism in experimental nonhuman primates has become a valuable model for studying idiopathic PD *(197)*. In addition to nerve cell degeneration in both the substantia nigra and the locus ceruleus, these animals develop eosinophilic neuronal inclusions that show both similarities and differences compared with LBs in human disease *(198)*.

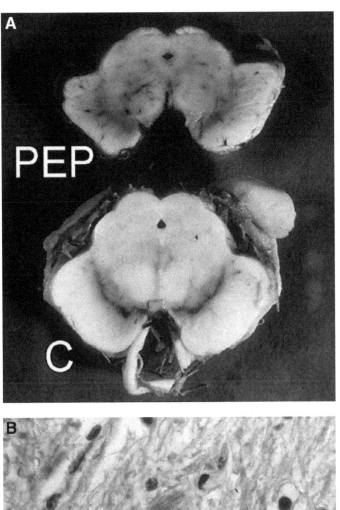

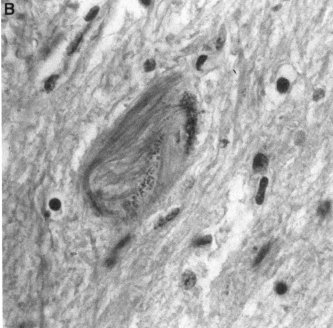

Fig. 10. Postencephalitic parkinsonism (PEP). (**A**) Gross photograph showing atrophy of the midbrain with degeneration of the substantia nigra in PEP compared with normal control (C). (**B**) Globose neurofibrillary tangle (H&E stain).

WILSON'S DISEASE

Wilson's disease is an autosomal recessively inherited disorder of copper metabolism in which the metal deposits in a number of organs including brain. Neurologic findings vary but often include extrapyramidal features. The neuropathology also varies depending on the rate of disease progression. There is degeneration of the basal ganglia, which may appear shrunken or even cavitated and often has a brown discoloration (Fig. 11A). The putamen tends to be more severely affected than the caudate, globus pallidus, and substantia nigra. Other areas that may be involved include the pons, thalamus, cerebellum, and subcortical white matter. There is neuronal loss, extensive fibrillary gliosis, and macrophages containing lipid and hemosiderin pigment. There may be visible accumulation of copper around capillaries. A number of more disease-specific cellular changes may be present. Alzheimer type II astrocytes are commonly seen in cases of chronic hepatic failure with neurological dysfunction and are numerous in most cases of Wilson's disease. They have swollen pale nuclei with little chromatin, prominent nucleoli, and sometimes contain small dots of glycogen (Fig. 11B). Large multinucleate Alzheimer type I cells are rare and not seen in every case *(199)*. Most disease specific is the presence of cells with small nuclei, abundant granular or foamy cytoplasm, and no obvious processes *(200)*. These "Opalski" cells are of uncertain origin, possible derived from astrocytes, macrophages, or degenerating neurons (Fig. 11C). They are most numerous in the thalamus, globus pallidus, and substantia nigra and rare in the striatum.

CONCLUSION

Parkinsonism may be associated with a wide range of underlying pathologies, in which the common feature is damage to the striatonigral system. In addition to the diseases discussed, virtually any pathological process that affects the striatonigral system has the potential to produce parkinsonism; these include various toxins *(201–206)*, infections *(207–212)*, mass lesions *(213)*, and other conditions. As a result, neuropathological examination is essential for accurate diagnosis in an individual with clinical parkinsonism.

FUTURE RESEARCH

It was the recognition of a unique pattern of histopathology that originally allowed most of the conditions described in this chapter to be designated as specific disease entities. Over the past few decades, greater understanding of the biochemical and genetic basis of these conditions has helped to clarify the disease pathogenesis and has shed light on the relationship between diseases (e.g., tauopathies, synucleinopathies, etc.). Although it is anticipated that future advances will occur primarily in the field of molecular genetics, the role of tissue pathology should not be overlooked. Defining the cellular localization and anatomical distribution of abnormal protein accumulations in postmortem tissue will continue to illuminate mechanisms of disease and help to confirm the relevance of new molecular findings. It will be the combination of genetic, biochemical, and histopathological research, matched with appropriate clinical correlative studies, that will further our understanding of these fascinating conditions.

MAJOR POINTS

- Parkinsonism may be associated with a variety of underlying pathologies.
- Most of the conditions that cause parkinsonism have damage of the striatonigral system as the anatomicopathological substrate.
- The most common causes of parkinsonism are neurodegenerative diseases, each of which has a defining pattern of neuropathology, often characterized by the abnormal accumulation of protein in the form of a cellular inclusion.
- For many of these conditions, recent molecular genetic findings have helped to define disease pathogenesis and have clarified the relationship between disease entities.

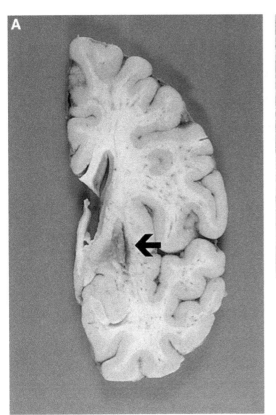

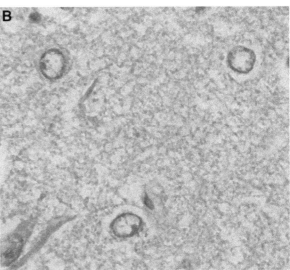

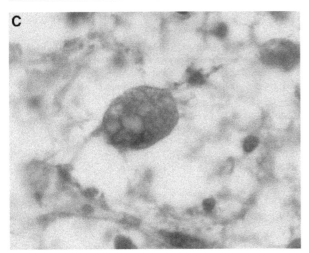

Fig. 11. Wilson's disease. (**A**) Gross photograph showing cystic degeneration of putamen. (**B**) Alzheimer type II astrocytes with swollen pale nuclei (H&E stain). (**C**) Opalski cell (H&E stain).

REFERENCES

1. Hughes AJ, Daniel SE, Ben-Shlomo Y, et al. The accuracy of diagnosis of parkinsonism syndromes in a specialist movement disorder service. Brain 2002;125:861–870.
2. Hughes AJ, Daniel SE, Kilford L, Lees AG. Accuracy of clinical diagnosis of idiopathic Parkinson's disease: a clinico-pathological study of 100 cases. J Neurol Neurosurg Psych 1992;55:181–184.
3. Rajput AH, Rozdilsky B, Rajput A. Accuracy of clinical diagnosis of parkinsonism—a prospective study. Can J Neurol Sci 1991;18:275–278.
4. Daniel SE, Bruin VMS, Lees AJ. The clinical and pathological spectrum of Steele–Richardson–Olszewski syndrome (progressive supranuclear palsy): a reappraisal. Brain 1995;118:759–770.
5. Gearing M, Olson DA, Watts RL, Mirra SS. Progressive supranuclear palsy: neuropathologic and clinical heterogeneity. Neurology 1994;44:1015–1024.
6. Litvan I, Agid Y, Goetz C, et al. Accuracy of the clinical diagnosis of corticobasal degeneration: a clinicopathologic study. Neurology 1997;48:119–125.
7. Litvan I, Goetz CG, Jankovic J, et al. What is the accuracy of the clinical diagnosis of multiple system atrophy? A clinicopathological study. Arch Neurol 1997;54:937–944.
8. Schneider JA, Watts RL, Gearing M, Brewer RP, Mirra SS. Corticobasal degeneration: neuropathological and clinical heterogeneity. Neurology 1997;48:959–969.
9. Aarsland D, Landberg E, Larsen JP, Cummings J. Frequency of dementia in Parkinson's disease. Arch Neurol 1996;53:538–542.
10. Edwards LL, Quigley EM, Harned RD, Hofman R, Pfeiffer RF. Characterization of swallowing and defecation in Parkinson's disease. Am J Gastroenterol 1994;89:15–25.
11. Edwards LL, Quigley EM, Pfeiffer RF. Gastrointestinal dysfunction in Parkinson's disease: frequency and pathophysiology. Neurology 1992;32:726–732.
12. Mayeux R, Stern Y, Rosenstein, et al. An estimate of the prevalence of dementia in idiopathic Parkinson's disease. Arch Neurol 1988;45:260–262.
13. Olanow CW. Tatton WG. Etiology and pathogenesis of Parkinson's disease. Ann Rev Neurosci 1999;22:123–144.
14. Calne DB. Parkinson's disease is not one disease. Parkinsonism Rel Dis 2000;17:3–7.
15. Fearnley JM, Lees AJ. Ageing and Parkinson's disease: substantia nigra regional selectivity. Brain 1991;114:2283–2301.
16. Lewy FH. Paralysis agitans. Pathologische anatomie. In: Lewandowsky M, eds. Handbuch der Neurologie. New York: Springer, 1912: 920–933.
17. Tretiakoff MC. Contribution a l'etude de l'anatomie pathologique de Locus Niger de Soemmerling. Paris: Universite de Paris, 1919.
18. Dale GE, Probst A, Luthert P, Martin J, Anderton BH, Leigh PN. Relationship between Lewy bodies and pale bodies in Parkinson's disease. Acta Neuropathol 1992;83:525–529,
19. Irizarry MC, Growdon W, Gomez-Isla T, et al. Nigral and cortical Lewy bodies and dystrophic nigral neurites in Parkinson's disease and cortical Lewy body disease contain α-synuclein immunoreactivity. J Neuropathol Exp Neurol 1998;57:334–337.
20. Bancher C, Lassmann H, Budka H, et al. An antigenic profile of Lewy bodies: immunocytochemical indication for protein phosphorylation and ubiquitination. J Neuropathol Exp Neurol 1989;48:81–93.
21. Goldman J, Yen SH, Chui F, et al. Lewy bodies in Parkinson's disease contain neurofilament antigens. Science 1983;221:4.
22. Kuzuhara S, Mori H, Izumiyama N, Yoshirmura M, Ihara Y. Lewy bodies are ubiquitinated. A light and electron microscopic immunocytochemical study. Acta Neuropathol 1988;75:345–353.
23. Polymeropoulos MHC, Leroy E, Ide SE, et al. Mutation in the alpha-synuclein gene identified in families with Parkinson's disease. Science 1997;276:2045–2047.
24. Spillantini MG, Schmidt ML, Lee VM, Trojanowski JQ, Jakes R, Goedert M. Alpha-synuclein in Lewy bodies. Nature 1997;388:839–840.
25. Arai T, Ueda K, Ikeda K, et al. Argyrophilic glial inclusions in the midbrain of patients with Parkinson's disease and diffuse Lewy body disease are immunopositive for NACP/alpha-synuclein. Neurosci Lett 1999;259:83–86.
26. Wakabayashi K, Hayashi S, Yoshimoto M, Kudo H, Takahashi H. NACP/alpha-synuclein-positive filamentous inclusions in astrocytes and oligodendrocytes of Parkinson's disease brains. Acta Neuropathol 2000;99:14–20.
27. Okazaki H, Lipkin LS, Aronson SM. Diffuse intracytoplasmic ganglionic inclusions (Lewy type) associated with progressive dementia and quadraparesis in flexion. J Neuropathol Exp Neurol 1961;20:237–244.
28. Hansen L, Salmon D, Galasko D, et al. The Lewy body variant of Alzheimer's disease: a clinical and pathological entity. Neurology 1990;40:1–8.
29. Perry RH, Irving D, Blessed G, Fairbairn A, Perry EK. Senile dementia of Lewy body type: a clinically and pathologically distinct form of Lewy body dementia in the elderly. J Neurol Sci 1990;95:119–139.
30. McKeith IG, Galasko D, Kosaka K, et al. Consensus guidelines for the clinical and pathological diagnosis of dementia with Lewy bodies (DLB): report of the consortium on DLB International Workshop. Neurology 1996;47:1113–1124.

31. Hughes AJ, Daniel SE, Blankson S, et al. A clinicopathological study of 100 cases of Parkinson's disease. Arch Neurol 1993;50:140–148.
32. Dickson DW, Ruan D, Crystal H, et al. Hippocampal degeneration differentiates diffuse Lewy body disease (DLBD) from Alzheimer's disease. Neurology 1991;41:1402–1409.
33. De Vos RA, Jansen EN, Stam FC, et al. Lewy body disease: clinicopathological correlations in 18 consecutive cases of Parkinson's disease with and without dementia. Clin Neurol Neurosurg 1995;97:13–22.
34. Piao YS, Wakabayashi K, Hayashi S, yoshimoto M, Takahashi H. Aggregation of α-synuclein/NACP in the neuronal and glial cells in diffuse Lewy body disease: a survey of six patients. Clin Neuropathol 2000;19:163–169.
35. Hansen LA, Masliah E, Galasko D, Terry RD. Plaque-only Alzheimer disease is usually the Lewy body variant and vice versa. J Neuropathol Exp Neurol 1993;52:648–654.
36. Mirra SS, Heyman A, McKeel D, et al. The consortium to establish a registry for Alzheimer's disease (CERAD). Part II. Standardisation of the neuropathologic assessment for Alzheimer's disease. Neurology 1991; 41:479–486.
37. Braak H, Braak E. Neuropathological staging of Alzheimer related changes. Acta Neuropathol 1991;82:239–259.
38. Gomez-Tortosa E, Newell K, Irizarry MC, Albert M, Growdon JH, Hyman BT. Clinical and quantitative pathologic correlates of dementia with Lewy bodies. Neurology 1999;53:1284–1291.
39. Lennox G, Lowe J, Landon M, Bryne EJ, Mayer RJ, Godwin-Austen RB. Diffuse Lewy body disease: correlative neuropathology using anti-ubiquitin immunohistochemistry. J Neurol Neurosurg Psychiatry 1989;52:1236–1247.
40. Mattila PM, Roytta M, Torikka H, Dickson DW, Rinne JO. Cortical Lewy bodies and Alzheimer-type changes in patients with Parkinson's disease. Acta Neuropathol 1998;95:576–582.
41. Samuel W, Galasko D, Masliah E, Hansen LA. Neocortical Lewy body counts correlate with dementia in Lewy body variant of Alzheimer's disease. J Neuropathol Exp Neurol 1996;55:44–52.
42. Jellinger KA. Morphological substrates of dementia in parkinsonism. A critical update. J Nerual Trans (Suppl) 1997;51:57–82.
43. Samuel W, Alford M, Hofstetter R, Hansen L. Dementia with Lewy bodies versus pure Alzheimer disease: differences in cognition, neuropathology, cholinergic dysfunction, and synapse density. J Neuropathol Exp Neurol 1997;56:499–508.
44. Ince PG, Perry EK, Morris CM. Dementia with Lewy bodies. A distinct non-Alzheimer dementia syndrome. Brain Pathol 1998;8:299–324.
45. Kosaka K, Iseki E. Diffuse Lewy body disease within the spectrum of Lewy body disease. In: Perry R, McKeith I, Perry E, eds. Dementia with Lewy Bodies. New York: Cambridge University Press, 1996:238–247.
46. Kosaka K, Tsuchiya K, Yoshimura M. Lewy body disease with and without dementia: a clinicopathological study of 35 cases. Clin Neuropathol 1989;7:299–305.
47. Bonifati V, Rizzu P, van Baren MJ, et al. Mutations in the DJ-1 gene associated with autosomal recessive early-onset parkinsonism. Science 2003;299:256–259.
48. Mouradian MM. Recent advances in the genetics and pathogenesis of Parkinson disease. Neurology 2002;58:179–185.
49. Farrer M, Chan P, Chen R, et al. Lewy bodies and parkinsonism in families with parkin mutation. Ann Neurol 2001;50:293–300.
50. Wintermeyer P, Kruger R, Kuhn W, et al. Mutation analysis and association studies of the UCHL1 gene in German Parkinson's disease patients. Neuroreport 2000;11:2079–2082.
51. Saigoh K, Wang YL, Suh JG, et al. Intragenic deletion in the gene encoding ubiquitin carboxy-terminal hydrolase in gad mice. Nat Genet 1999;23:47–51.
52. Gilman S, Low PA, Quinn N, et al. Consensus statement on the diagnosis of multiple system atrophy. J Neurol Sci 1999;163:94–98.
53. Wenning GK, Ben Shlomo Y, Magalhaes M, Daniel SF, Quinn NP. Clinical features and natural history of multiple system atrophy. An analysis of 100 cases. Brain 1994;117:835–845.
54. Lantos PL. The definition of multiple system atrophy: a review of recent developments. J Neuropathol Exp Neurol 1998;57:1099–1111.
55. Dickson DW, Lin WL, Liw WK, yen SH. Multiple system atrophy: a sporadic synucleinopathy. Brain Pathol 1999.9:721–732.
56. Wenning GK, Tison F, Ben Shlomo Y, Daniel SE, Quinn NP. Multiple system atrophy: a review of 203 pathologically proven cases. Mov Disord 1997;12:133–147.
57. Kanada T, Tsukagoshi H, Oda M, et al. Changes of unmyelinated nerve fibres in sural nerve in amyotrophic lateral sclerosis, Parkinson's disease, and multiple system atrophy. Acta Neuropathol 1996;91:145–154.
58. Lantos PL. Neuropathological diagnostic criteria of multiple system atrophy: a review. In Cruz-Sanchez FF, Ravid R, Cuzner ML, eds. Neuropathological Diagnostic Criteria for Brain Banking, Amsterdam: IOS Press, 1995:116–121.
59. Papp MI, Kahn JE, Lantos PL. Glial cytoplasmic inclusions in the CNS of patients with multiple system atrophy (striatonigral degeneration, olivopontocerebellar atrophy and Shy–Drager syndrome). J Neurol Sci 1989;94:79–100.
60. Papp MI, Lantos PL. Accumulation of tubular structures in oligodendroglial and neuronal cells as the basic alteration in multiple system atrophy. J Neurol Sci 1992;107:172–182.
61. Papp MI, Lantos PL. The distribution of oligodendroglial inclusions in multiple system atrophy and its relevance to clinical symptomatology. Brain 1994;117:235–243.

62. Abe H, Yagishita S, Amano N, et al. Argyrophilic glial intracytoplasmic inclusions in multiple system atrophy: immunocytochemical and ultrastructural study. Acta Neuropathol 1992 84:273–277.

63. Arima K, Murayama S, Mukoyama M, Inose T. Immunocytochemical and ultrastructural studies of neuronal and oligodendroglial cytoplasmic inclusions in multiple system atrophy. 1. Neuronal cytoplasmic inclusions. Acta Neuropathol 1992;83:453–460.

64. Murayama S, Arima K, Nakazato Y, Satoh J, Oda M, Inose T. Immunocytochemical and ultrastructural studies of neuronal and oligodendroglial cytoplasmic inclusions in multiple system atrophy. 2. Oligodendroglial cytoplasmic inclusions. Acta Neuropathol 1992;84:32–38.

65. Spillantini MG, Crowther RA, Jakes R, Cairus NJ, Lantos PL, Goedert M. Filamentous α-synuclein inclusions link multiple system atrophy with Parkinson's disease and dementia with Lewy Bodies. Neurosci Lett 1998;251:205–208.

66. Wakabayashi K, Yoshimoto M, Tsuji S, takahashi H. α-synuclein immunoreactivity in glial cytoplasmic inclusions in multiple system atrophy. Neruosci Lett 1998;249:180–182.

67. Kato S, Nakamura H. Cytoplasmic argyrophilic inclusions in neurons of pontine nuclei in patients with olivopontocerebellar atrophy: immunohistochemical and ultrastructural studies. Acta Neuropathol 1990;79:584–594.

68. Rebeiz JJ, Kolodny EH, Richardson EP. Corticodentonigral degeneration with neuronal achromasia. Arch Neurol 1968;18:20–33.

69. Rinne JO, Lee MS, Thompson PD, Marsden CD. Corticobasal degeneration. A clinical study of 36 cases. Brain 1994;117:1183–1196.

70. Arima K, Uesugi H, Fujita I, et al. Corticonigral degeneration with neuronal achromasia presenting with primary progressive aphasia: ultrastructural and immunocytochemical studies. J Neurol Sci 1994;127:186–197.

71. Bergeron C, Davis A, Lang AE. Corticobasal ganglionic degeneration and progressive supranuclear palsy presenting with cognitive decline. Brain Pathol 1998;8:355–365.

72. Feany MB, Dickson DW. Widespread cytoskeletal pathology characterizes corticobasal degeneration. Am J Pathol 1995;146:1388–1396.

73. Kertesz A, Hudson L, Mackezie IRA, et al. The pathology and nosology of primary progressive aphasia. Neurology 1994;44:2065–2072.

74. Kertesz A, Martinez-Lage P, Davidson W, Munoz DG. The corticobasal degeneration syndrome overlaps progressive aphasia and frontotemporal dementia. Neurology 2000;55:1368–1375.

75. Dickson DW, Yen SH, Suzuki KI, Davies P, Garcia JH, Hiraqno A. Ballooned neurons in select neurodegenerative diseases contain phosphorylated neurofilament epitopes. Acta Neuropathol 1986;71:216–223.

76. Mackenzie IRA, Hudson LP. Achromatic neurons in the cortex of progressive supranuclear palsy. Acta Neuropathol 1995;90:615–619.

77. Lowe J, Errington DR, Lennox G, et al. Ballooned neurons in several neurodegenerative diseases and stroke contain alpha B crystallin. Neruopathol Appl Neurobiol 1992;18:515–516.

78. Smith TW, Lippa CF, de Girolami U. Immunocytochemical study of ballooned neurons in cortical degeneration with neuronal achromasia. Clin Neuropathol 1992;11:28–35.

79. Gibb WR, Luthert PJ, Marsden CD. Corticobasal degeneration. Brain 1989;112:1171–1192.

80. Mori H, Nishimura M, Namba Y, Oda M. Corticobasal degeneration: a disease with widespread appearance of abnormal tau and neurofibrillary tangles and its relation to progressive supranuclear palsy. Acta Neuropathol 1994;88:113–121.

81. Paulus W, Selim M. Corticonigral degeneration with neuronal achromasia and basal neurofibrillary tangles. Acta Neuropathol 1990;81:89–94.

82. Feany MB, Dickson DW. Neurodegenerative disorders with extensive tau pathology: a comparative study and review. Ann Neurol 1996;40:139–148.

83. Feany MB, Mattiace LA, Dickson DW. Neuropathologic overlap of progressive supranuclear palsy, Pick's disease and corticobasal degeneration. J Neuropathol Exp Neurol 1996;55:53–67.

84. Wakabayashi K, Oyamagi K, Makifuchi T, et al. Corticobasal degeneration: etiopathological significance of the cytoskeletal alterations. Acta Neuropathol 1994;87:545–553.

85. Dickson DW, Bergeron C, Chin WW, et al. Office of rare diseases. Neuropathologic criteria for corticobasal degeneration. J Neuropathol Exp Neurol 2002; 61:935–946.

86. Komori T, Arai N, Oda M, et al. Astrocytic plaques and tufts of abnormal fibres do not coexist in corticobasal degeneration and progressive supranuclear palsy. Acta Neuropathol 1998;96:401–408.

87. Mattice LA, Wu E, Aronson M, Dickson D. A new type of neuritic plaque without amyloid in corticonigral degeneration with neuronal achromasia. J Neuropathol Exp Neurol 1991;50:310.

88. Chin SSM, Goldman JE. Glial inclusions in CNS degenerative diseases. J Neuropathol Exp Neurol 1996;55:499–508.

89. Ikeda K, Akiyama H, Kondo H, et al. Thorn-shaped astrocytes: possibly secondarily induced tau-positive glial fibrillary tangles. Acta Neuropathol 1995;90:620–625.

90. Ikeda K, Akiyama H, Haga C, Kondo H, Arima K, Oda T. Argyrophilic thread-like structure in corticobasal degeneration and supranuclear palsy. Neurosci Lett 1994;174:157–159.

91. Steele JC, Richardson JC, Olszewski J. Progressive supranuclear palsy. Arch Neurol 1964;10:333–359.

92. Dickson DW. Neuropathologic differentiation of progressive supranuclear palsy and corticobasal degeneration. J Neurol 1999;246(Suppl 2):II6–II15.
93. Hauw JJ, Daniel SE, Dickson D, et al. Preliminary NINDS neuropathologic criteria for Steele–Richardson–Olszewski syndrome (progressive supranuclear palsy). Neurology 1994;44:2015–2019.
94. Litvan I, Hauw JJ, Bartko JJ, et al. Validity and reliability of the preliminary NINDS neuropathologic criteria for progressive supranuclear palsy and related disorders. J Neuropathol Exp Neurol 1996;55:97–105.
95. Braak H, Jellinger K, Braak E, et al. Allocortical neurofibrillary changes in progressive supranuclear palsy. Acta Neuropathol 1992;84:478–483.
96. Hauw JJ, Verny M, Delaere P, Cervera P, He Y, Duyckaerts C. Constant neurofibrillary changes in the neocortex in progressive supranuclear palsy. Basic differences with Alzheimer's disease and aging. Neurosci Lett 1990;119:182–186.
97. Hof PR, Delacourte A, Bouras C. Distribution of cortical neurofibrillary tangles in progressive supranuclear palsy: a quantitative analysis of six cases. Acta Neruoapathol 1992;84:45–51.
98. Bigio EH, Brown DF, White CL. Progressive supranuclear palsy with dementia: cortical pathology. J Neuroapthol Exp Neurol 1999;58:359–364.
99. Arai N. "Grumose degeneration" of the dentate nucleus. A light and electron microscopic study in progressive supranuclear palsy and dentatorubropallidoluysial atrophy. J Neurol Sci 1989;90:131–145.
100. Foster NL, Wilhelmsen K, Sima AA, Jones MZ, D'Amato CJ, Gilman S. Frontotemporal dementia and parkinsonism linked to chromosome 17: a consensus conference. Conference Participants. Ann Neurol 1997;41:706–715.
101. Clark LN, Poorkaj P, Wszolek Z, et al. Pathogenic implications of mutations in the tau gene in pallido-ponto-nigral degeneration and related neurodegenerative disorders linked to chromosome 17. Proc Natl Acad Sci USA 1998;95: 13103–13107.
102. Dumanchin C, Camuzat A, Campion D, et al. Segregation of a missense mutation in the microtubule-associated protein tau gene with familial frontotemporal dementia and parkinsonism. Hum Mol Genet 1998;7:1825–1829.
103. Hutton M, Lendon CL, Rizzu P, et al. Association of missense and 5' splice-site mutations in tau with the inherited dementia FTDP-17. Nature 1998;393:702–705.
104. Spillantini MG, Murrell JR, Goedert M, et al. Mutation in the tau gene in a familial multiple system tauopathy with presenile dementia. Proc Natl Acad Sci USA 1998;95:7737–7741.
105. Kertesz A, Kawarai T, Rogaeva E, et al. Familial frontotemporal dementia with ubiquitin-positive, tau-negative inclusions. Neurology 2000;54:818–827,
106. Rosso SM, Kamphorst W, de Graaf B, et al. Familial frontotemporal dementia with ubiquitin-positive inclusions is linked to chromosome 17q21-22. Brain 124;1948–1957.
107. Ghetti B, Hutton ML, Wszolek ZK. Frontotemporal dementia and parkinsonism linked to chromosome 17 associated with tau gene mutations (FTDP-17T). In: Dickson D, ed. Neurodegeneration: The Molecular Pathology of Dementia and Movement Disorders. Los Angeles: ISN Neuropath Press, 2003:86–102.
108. Reed LA, Wszolek ZK, Hutton M. Phenotypic correlations in FTDP-17. Neurbiol Aging 2001;22:89–107.
109. van Swieten JC, Stevens M, Rosso SM, et al. Phenotypic variation in hereditary frontotemporal dementia with tau mutations. Ann Neurol 1999;46:617–626.
110. Spillantini MG, Bird TD, Ghetti B. Frontotemporal dementia and parkinsonism linked to chromosome 17; a new group of tauopathies. Brain Pathol 1998;8:386–402.
111. Sumi SM, Bird TD, Nochlin D, raskind MA. Familial presenile dementia with psychosis associated with corticoal neurofibrillary tangles and degeneration of the amygdala. Neurology 1992;42:120–127.
112. Mirra SS, Murrell JR, Gearing M, et al. Tau pathology in a family with dementia and P301L mutation in tau. J Neuropathol Exp Neurol 1999;58:335–345.
113. Spillantini MG, Yoshida H, Rizzini C, et al. A novel tau mutation (N296N) in familial dementia with swollen achromatic neurons and corticobasal inclusion bodies. Ann Neurol 2000;48:939–943.
114. Stanford PM, Halliday GM, Brooks WS, et al. Progressive supranuclear palsy pathology caused by a novel silent mutation in exon 10 of the tau gene: expansion of the disease phenotype caused by tau gene mutations. Brain 2000;123:880–893.
115. Murrell Jr, Spillantini MG, Zolo P, et al. Tau gene mutation G389R causes a tauopathy with abundant pick body-like inclusions and axonal deposits. J Neuropathol Expo Neurol 1999;58:1207–1226.
116. Rizzini C, Goedert M, Hodges JR, et al. Tau gene mutation K257T causes a tauopathy similar to Pick's disease. J Neuropathol Exp Neurol 2000;59:990–1001.
117. Spillantini MG, Goedert M, Crowther RA, Smith MJ, Jakes R, Hills R. Familial multiple system tauopathy: a new neurodegenerative disease of the brain with tau neurofibrillary pathology. Proc Natl Acad Sci USA 1997;95:4113–4118.
118. Reed LA, Schmidt ML, Wszolek ZK, et al. The neuropathology of a chromosome 17-linked autosomal dominant parkinsonism and dementia ("pallido-ponto-nigral degeneration"). J Neuropathol Exp Neurol 1998;57:588–601.
119. Wilhelmsen KC, Lynch T, Pavlou E, et al. Localization of disinhibition-parkinsonism-amyotrophy complex to 17q21-22. Am J Hum Genet 1994;55:1159–1165.

120. Sima AA, Defendini R, Keohane C, et al. The neuropathology of chromosome 17–linked dementia. Annals of Neurology 1996;39:734–743.

121. Hirano A, Kurland LT, Krooth RS, lessell S. Parkinsonism-dementia complex, an endemic disease on the island of Guam. I. Clinical features. Brain 1961;84:642–661.

122. Gibbs CJ, Gajdusek DC. An update on long-term in vivo and in vitro studies designed to identify a virus as the cause of amyotrophic lateral sclerosis, parkinsonism dementia and Parkinson's disease. Adv Neurol 1982;36:343–353.

123. Hudson AJ, Rice GP. Similarities of guamanian ALS/PD to post-encephalitic parkinsonism/ALS: possible viral cause. Can J Neurol Sci 1990;17:427–433.

124. Spencer PS, Nunn PB, Hugon J, et al. Guam amyotrophic lateral sclerosis-parkinsonism-dementia linked to a plant excitant neurotoxin. Science 1987;237:517–522.

125. Hirano A, Malamjud N, Kurland LT. Parkinsonism-dementia complex, an endemic disease on the island of Guam. II. Pathological features. Brain 1961;84:662–679.

126. Malamud N, Hirano A, Kurland LT. Pathoanatomic changes in amyotrophic lateral sclerosis on Guam. Neurology 1961;5:401–414.

127. Buee-Scherrer V, Buee L, Hof PR, et al. Neurofibrillary degeneration in amyotrophic lateral sclerosis/parkinsonism-dementia complex of Guam. Immunochemical characterization of tau proteins. Am J Pathol 1995;146:924–932,

128. Shankar SK, Yanagihara R, Garruto RM, Grundke-Iqbal I, Kosik KS, Gajdusek DC. Immunocytochemical characterization of neurofibrillary tangles in amyotrophic lateral sclerosis and parkinsonism-complex of Guam. Ann Neurol 1989;25:146–151.

129. Hof PR, Nimchinsky EA, Buee-Scherrer V, et al. Amyotrophic lateral sclerosis/parkinsonism dementia-complex from Guam: quantitative neuropathology, immunohistochemical analysis of neuronal vulnerability and comparison with related neurodegenerative disorders. Acta Neuropathol 1994;88:397–404.

130. Geddes JF, Hughes AJ, Lees AJ, Daniel SE. Pathological overlap in cases of parkinsonism associated with neurofibrillary tangles. A study of recent cases of postencephalitic parkinsonism and comparison with progressive supranuclear palsy and Guamanian parkinsonism-dementia complex. Brain 1993;116:281–302.

131. Hudson AJ. Amyotrophic lateral sclerosis/parkinsonism/dementia: clinico-pathological correlations relevant to Guamanian ALS/PD. Can J Neurol Sci 1991;19:458–461.

132. Oyanagi K, Makifuchi T, Ohtoh T, Chen KM, Gajdusek DC, Chase TN. Distinct pathological features of the Gallyas- and tau-positive glia in the Parkinsonism-dementia complex and amyotrophic lateral sclerosis of Guam. J Neuropathol Exp Neurol 1997;56:308–316.

133. Hirano A, Dembitzer HM, Kurland.LT. The fine structure of some intraganglionic alterations. Neurofibrillary tangles, granulovacuolar bodies and "rod-like" structures as seen in Guam amyotrophic lateral sclerosis and parkinsonism-dementia complex. J Neuropathol Exp Neurol 1968;27:167–182.

134. Oyanagi K, Makifuchi T, Ohtoh T, et al. Amyotrophic lateral sclerosis of Guam: the nature of the neuropathological findings. Acta Neuropathol 1994;88:405–412.

135. Merello M, Sabe L, Teson A, et al. Extrapyramidalism in Alzheimer's disease: prevalence, psychiatric and neuropsychological correlates. J Neurol Neurosurg Psychiatry 1994;57:1503–1509.

136. Morris JC, Drazner M, Fulling K, Grant EA, Goldring J. Clinical and pathological aspects of parkinsonism in Alzheimer's disease. A role for extranigral factors? Arch Neurol 1989;46:651–657.

137. Tsolaki M, Kokarida K, Iakovidou V, et al. Extrapyramidal symptoms and signs in Alzheimer's disease: prevalence and correlation with the first symptom. Am J Alz Dis 2001;16:268–278.

138. Hulette C, Mirra S, Wilkinson W, et al. The consortium to establish a registry for Alzheimer's disease (CERAD). Part IX. A prospective cliniconeuropathologic study of Parkinson's features in Alzheimer's disease. Neurology 1995;45:1991–1995.

139. Stern Y, Jacobs D, Goldman J, et al. An investigation of clinical correlates of Lewy bodies in autopsy-proven Alzheimer's disease. Arch Neurol 2001;58:460–465.

140. Lui Y, Stern Y, Chun MR, Jacobs DM, Yan P, Goldman JR. Pathological correlates of extrapyramidal signs in Alzheimer's disease. Ann Neurol 1997;41:368–374.

141. Love S, Wilcock GK, Matthews SM. No correlation between nigral degeneration and striatal plaques in Alzheimer's disease. Acta Neuropathol 1996;91:432–436.

142. Uchihara T, Kondo H, Ikeda K, et al. Alzheimer-type pathology in melanin-bleached sections of substantia nigra. J Neurol 1995;242:485–489.

143. Uchihara T, Kondo H, Kosaka K, Tsukagoshi H. Selective loss of nigral neurons in Alzheimer's disease: a morphometric study. Acta Neuropathol 1992;83:271–276.

144. Kazee AM, Cox C, Richfield EK. Substantia nigra lesions in Alzheimer's disease and normal aging. Alz Dis Assoc Disord 1995;9:61–67.

145. Hudson AJ. Amyotrophic lateral sclerosis and its association with dementia, parkinsonism and other neurological disorders: a review. Brain 1981;104:217–247.

146. Okamoto K, Murakami N, Kusaka H, et al. Ubiquitin-positive intraneuronal inclusions in the extramotor cortices of presenile dementia patients with motor neuron disease. J Neurol 1992;239:426–430.

147. Kawashima T, Kikuchi H, Takita M, et al. Skein-like inclusions in the neostriatum from a case of amyotrophic lateral sclerosis with dementia. Acta Neuropathol 1998;96:541–545.

148. Su M, Yoshida Y, Ishiguro H, et al. Nigral degeneration in a case of amyotrophic lateral sclerosis: evidence of Lewy-like and skein-like inclusions in the pigmented neurons. Clin Neuropathol 1999;18:293–300.

149. Wakabayashi K, Piao YS, Hayashi S, et al. Ubiquitinated neuronal inclusions in the neostriatum in patients with amyotrophic lateral sclerosis with and without dementia—a study of 60 patients 31 to 87 years of age. Clin Neuropathol 2001;20:47–52.

150. Mackenzie IR, Feldman H. Extrapyramidal features in patients with motor neuron disease and dementia; a clinico-pathological correlative study. Acta Neuropathol 2004;107:336–340.

151. Oyanagi K, Takeda S, Takahashi H, Ohama E, Ikuta F. A quantitative investigation of the substantia nigra in Huntington's disease. Ann Neurol 1989;26:13–19.

152. DiFiglia M, Sapp E, Chase KO, et al. Aggregation of huntingtin in neuronal intranuclear inclusions and dystrophic neurites in brain. Science 1997;227:1990–1993.

153. Maat-Schieman MLC, Dorsman JC, Smoor MA, et al. Distribution of inclusions in neuronal nuclei and dystrophic neurites in Huntington Disease brain. J Neuropathol Exp Neurol 1999;58:129–137.

154. Harding A. The clinical features and classification of the late onset autosomal dominant cerebellar ataxias: a study of eleven families including descendants of the "Drew family of Walworth." Brain 1982;105:1–28.

155. Estrada R, Galarraga J, Orozco G, Nodarse A, Auburger G. Spinocerebellar ataxia 2 (SCA2): morphometric analyses in 11 autopsies. Acta Neuropathol 1999;97:306–310.

156. Martin JJ, van Regemorter N, Krols L, et al. On an autosomal dominant form of retinal-cerebellar degeneration: an autopsy study of five patients in one family. Acta Neuropathol 1994;88:277–286.

157. Fujigasaki H, Uchihara T, Koyano S, et al. Ataxin-3 is translocated into the nucleus for the formation of intranuclear inclusions in normal and Macado-Joseph disease brains. Exp Neurol 2000;165:248–256.

158. Koyano S, Uchihara T, Fujigasaki H, Nakamura A, Yagishita S, Iwabuchi K. Neuronal intanuclear inclusions in spinocerebellar ataxia type 2: triple-labelling immunofluorescent study. Neuro Sci Lett 1999;273:117–120.

159. Jankovic J, Kirkpatrick JB, Blomquist KA, et al. Late-onset Hallervorden-Spatz disease presenting as familial parkinsonism. Neurology 1985;35:227–234.

160. Antoine JC, Tommasi M, Chalumeau A. Hallervorden–Spatz disease with Lewy bodies. Rev Neurol Paris 1985;141:806–809.

161. Arawaka S, Saito Y, Murayama S, Mori H. Lewy body in neurodegeneration with brain iron accumulation type I is immunoreactive for alpha-synuclein. Neurology 1998;51:887–889.

162. Galvin JE, Giasson B, Hurtig HI, lee V, Trojanowski JQ. Neurodegeneration with brain iron accumulation, type 1 is characterized by alpha-, beta-, and gamma-synuclein neuropathology. Am J Pathol 2000;157:361–368.

163. Wakabayashi K, Yoshimoto M, Fikushima T, et al. Widespread occurrence of alpha-synuclein/NACP-immunoreactive neuronal inclusions in juvenile and adult-onset Hallervorden-Spatz disease with Lewy bodies. Neuropathol Exp Neurol 1999;25:363–368.

164. McCall S, Henry JM, Reid AH, Taubenberger JK. Influenza RNA not detected in archival brain tissues from acute encephalitis lethargica cases or in postencephalitic Parkinson cases. J Neuropathol Exp Neurol 2001;60:696–704.

165. Reid AH, McCall S, Henry JM, Taubenberger JK. Experimenting on the past: the enigma of von Economo's encephalitis lethargica. J Neuropathol Exp Neurol 2001;663–670.

166. Hallervorden J. Anatomische untersuchungen zur pathologenese des postencephaliticshen Parkinsonismus. Dtsch Z Nervenheilkunde 1935;136:68–77.

167. Torvik A, Meen D. Distribution of the brainstem lesions in postencephalitic parkinsonism. Acta Neurol Scand 1966;42:415–425.

168. Buee-Scherrer V, Buee L, Leveugle B, et al. Pathological tau proteins in postencephalitic parkinsonism: comparison with Alzheimer's disease and other neurodegenerative disorders. Ann Neurol 1997;42:924–932.

169. Ishii T, Nakamura Y. Distribution and ultrastructure of Alzheimer's neurofibrillary tangles in postencephalitic parkinsonism of Economo type. Acta Neuropathol 1981;55:59–62.

170. Hof PR, Charpiot A, Delacourte A, Purohit D, Perl DP, Bouras C. Distribution of neurofibrillary tangles and senile plaques in the cerebral cortex in postencephalitic parkinsonism. Neurosci Lett 1992;139:10–14.

171. Haraguchi T, Ishizu H, Terada S, et al. An autopsy case of postencephalitic parkinsonism of von Economo type: some new observations concerning neurofibrillary tangles and astrocytic tangles. Neuropathology 2000;20:143–148.

172. Ikeda K, Akiyama H, Kondo H, Ikeda K. Anti-tau-positive glial fibrillary tangles in the brain of postencephalitic parkinsonism of Economo type. Neurosci Lett 1993;162:176–178.

173. Reider-Groswasser I, Bornstein NM, Korczyn AD. Parkinsonism in patients with lacunar infarcts of the basal ganglia. Eur Neurol 1996;36:248–249.

174. Tomonaga M, Yamanouchi H, Tohgi H, Kameyama M. Clinicopathologic study of progressive subcortical vascular encephalopathy (Binswanger type) in the elderly. J Am Geriatr Soc 1982;30:524–529.

175. Van Zagten M, Lodder J, Kessels F. Gait disorder and parkinsonian signs in patients with stroke related to small deep infarcts and white matter lesions. Mov Disord 1998;13:89–95.

176. Chang CM, Yu YL, Ng HK, et al. Vascular pseudoparkinsonism. Acta Neurol Sci 1992;86;588–592.

177. Murrow RW. Schweiger GD, Kepes et al. Parkinsonism due to basal ganglia lacunar state: clinicopathologic correlation. Neurology 1990;40:897–900.

178. De Reuck J, Sieben G, de Coster W, et al. Parkinsonism in patients with cerebral infarcts. Clin Neurol Neurosurg 1980;82:177–218.

179. Hunter R, Smith J, Thomson T, et al. Hemiparkinsonism with infarction of the ipsilateral substantia nigra. Neuropathol Appl Neurobiol 1978;4:297–301.

180. Krauss JK, Jankovic J. Head injury and posttraumatic movement disorders. Neurosurgery 2002;50:927–940.

181. Rondot P, Bathien N, De Recondo J, et al. Dystonia-parkinsonism syndrome from a bullet injury in the midbrain. J Neurol Neurosurg Psychiatry 1994;57:658.

182. Wiest RG, Burgunder JM, Krauss JK. Chronic subdural haematomas and Parkinsonian syndromes. Acta Neurochir 1999;141:753–758.

183. Taylor CA, Saint-Hilaire MH, Cupples LA, et al. Environmental, medical and family history risk factors for Parkinson's disease: a New England-based case control study. Am J Med Genet 1999;88:742–749.

184. Tsai CH, Lo SK, See LC, et al. Environmental risk factors of young onset Parkinson's disease: a case-control study. Clin Neurol Neurosurg 2002;104:328–333.

185. Clinton J, Ambler MW, Roberts GW. Post-traumatic Alzheimer's disease: preponderance of a single plaque type. Neuropathol Appl Neurobiol 1991;17:69–74.

186. Tokuda T, Ikeda S, Yanagisawa N, Ihara Y, Glenner GG. Re-examination of ex-boxers' brains using immunohistochemistry with antibodies to amyloid beta-protein and tau protein. Acta Neuropathol 1991;82:280–285.

187. Roberts GW, Gentleman SM, Lynch A, Graham DI. βA4-amyloid protein deposition in the brain after head injury. Lancet 1991;338:1422–1423.

188. Hoshino S, Tamaoka A, Takahashi M, et al. Emergence of immunoreactivities for phosphorylated tau and amyloid-beta protein in chronic stage of fluid percussion in rat brain. Neuroreport 1998;9:1879–1893.

189. Smith DH, Chen XH, Nonaka M, et al. Accumulation of amyloid β and tau and the formation of neurofilament inclusions following diffuse brain injury in the pig. J Neuropathol Exp Neurol 1999;58:982–992.

190. Bhatt M, Desai J, Mankodi A, Elias M, Wadia N. Posttraumatic akinetic-rigid syndrome resembling Parkinson's disease: a report on three patients. Mov Disord 2000;15:313–317.

191. Nayernouri T. Posttraumatic parkinsonism. Surg Neurol 1985;24:263–264.

192. Turjanski N, Lees AJ, Brooks DJ. Dopaminergic function in patients with posttraumatic parkinsonism: an 18F-dopa PET study. Neurology 1997;49:183–189.

193. Langston JW, Ballard P, Tetrud JW, Irwin I. Chronic parkinsonism in humans due to a product of meperidine-analogue synthesis. Science 1983;219:979–980.

194. Langston JW, Irwin I, Langston EB, et al. 1-methyl-4-phenylpyridinium (MPP+): identification of a metabolite of MPTP, a toxin selective to the substantia nigra. Neurosci Lett 1984;48:87–92.

195. Singer TP, Ramsay RR. Mechanism of the neurotoxicity of MPTP. An update. FEBS Lett 1990;274:1–8.

196. Langston JW, Forno LS, Tetrud J, Reeves AG, Kaplan JA, Karluk D. Evidence of active nerve cell degeneration in the substantia nigra of humans years after 1-methyl-4-phenyl-1,2,3,6-tetrahydropyridine exposure. Ann Neurol 1999;46:598–605.

197. Tetrud JW, Langston JW. MPTP-induced parkinsonism as a model for Parkinson's disease. Acta Neurol Scand 1989;126:35–40.

198. Forno LS, DeLanney LE, Irwin I, Langston JW. Similarities and differences between MPTP-induced parkinsonism and Parkinson's disease. Neuropathologic considerations. Adv Neurol 1993;60:600–608.

199. Lapham LW. Cytologic and cytochemical studies of neuroglia. I. A study of the problem of amitosis in reactive astrocytes. Am J Pathol 1962;41:1–21.

200. Opalski A. Uber eine besondere Art von Gliazellen bei der Wilson-Pseudosklerosegruppe. Z Ges Neurol Psychiat 1930;124:420–425.

201. Huang CC, Chu NS, Lu CS, et al. Chronic manganese intoxication. Arch Neurol 1989;46:1104–1106.

202. Klawans HL, Stein RW, Tanner CM, Goetz CG. A pure parkinsonian syndrome following acute carbon monoxide intoxication. Arch Neurol 1983;39:302–304.

203. McLean DR, Jacobs H, Mielke BW. Methanol poisoning: a clinical and pathological study. Ann Neurol 1980;8:161–167.

204. Okuda B, Iwamoto Y, Tachibana H, et al. Parkinsonism after acute cadmium poisoning. Clin Neurol Neurosurg 1997;99:263–265.

205. Peters HA, Levine RL, Matthew CG, Chapman LJ. Extrapyramidal and other neurologic manifestations associated with carbon disulfide fumigant exposure. Arch Neurol 1998;45:537–540.

206. Uitti RJ, Rajput AH, Ashenhurst EM, Rozdilsky B. Cyanide-induced parkinsonism: a clinicopathologic report. Neurology 1985;35:921–925.

207. Kim JS, Choi IS, Lee MC. Reversible parkinsonism and dystonia following probable mycoplasma pneumoniae infection. Mov Disord 1995;10:510–512.

208. Mirsattari SM, Power C, Nath A. Parkinsonism with HIV infection. Mov Disord 2000;15:1032–1033.
209. Murakami T, Nakajima M, Nakamura T, et al. Parkinsonian symptoms as an initial manifestation in a Japanese patient with acquired immunodeficiency syndrome and Toxoplasma infection. Intern Med 2000;39:1006–1007.
210. Viader F, Poncelet AM, Chapon F, et al. Neurologic forms of Lyme disease. Rev Neurol 1989;145:362–368.
211. Wszolek Z, Monsour H, Smith P, et al. Cryptococcal meningoencephalitis with parkinsonian features. Mov Disord 1988;3:271–273.
212. Yazaki M, Yamazaki M, Urasawa N, et al. Successful treatment with alpha-interferon of a patient with chronic measles infection of the brain and parkinsonism. Eur Neurol 2000;44:184–186.
213. Lhermitte F, Agid Y, Serdaru M, Guimaraes J. Parkinson syndrome, frontal tumor and L-dopa. Rev Neurol 1984;140:138–139.

5

Animal Models of Tauopathies

Jada Lewis and Michael Hutton

INTRODUCTION

The discovery of mutations in the tau gene in frontotemporal dementia and parkinsonism linked to chromosome 17 (FTDP-17) *(1–4)* has demonstrated that tau dysfunction can result in neurodegeneration and has allowed researchers to generate transgenic models of the human tauopathies *(5)* (*see* Table 1 for summary). Transgenic models permit studies on the mechanisms of formation of filamentous tau lesions in neurons and glia as well as their role in neurodegeneration. They also serve as models to develop treatments for tauopathies.

The tau gene is subject to alternative splicing of three exons, which generates six tau isoforms *(6,7)* (Fig. 1). Additional heterogeneity is derived from posttranslational modifications of tau. Two exons in the amino half of the molecule (exon 2 and exon 3) and one exon in the microtubule-binding domain (exon 10) are alternatively spliced *(8)*. Exon 2 is included (1N) or excluded (0N), whereas exon 3 is always coexpressed with exon 2 (2N). Exon 10 contains a conserved repeat domain that is also present in exons 9, 11, and 12. Inclusion of exon 10 generates tau with 4 repeats (4R), whereas exclusion generates tau with 3 repeats (3R). The various splice combinations of tau are thus abbreviated as follows: 0N3R, 0N4R, 1N3R, 1N4R, 2N3R, and 2N4R. Adult brain has all six isoforms, whereas fetal tau is composed of 3R tau *(9)*.

MICE EXPRESSING TRANSGENES THAT ALTER TAU KINASE OR PHOSPHATASE ACTIVITY

The filamentous tau lesions observed in human neurodegenerative disease invariably contain tau that is hyperphosphorylated at specific residues *(10)*. As a result, there has been much speculation about the role of abnormal tau phosphorylation in the development of neurofibrillary pathology in Alzheimer's disease (AD) and the tauopathies. To examine this question, several groups have generated mice that overexpress transgenes designed to upregulate tau phosphorylation.

Transgenic mice were generated using a tetracycline-regulated system for conditional gene expression to express glycogen synthase 3 β (GSK3β) in adult animals thus avoiding possible deleterious effects of expression during development *(11)*. Strong somatodendritic immunostaining of hyperphosphorylated tau was detected in cortex and hippocampus, but no thioflavin-S fluorescence was detected. Western blotting with the phospho-tau antibodies (e.g., PHF-1 and AD2) in cortex, striatum, hippocampus, and cerebellum revealed increased levels of tau phosphorylation in the hippocampus. Increased TUNEL staining and astrogliosis further suggested that increased GSK3β activity was initiating neurodegenerative changes in the mice; however, these changes occurred in the absence

From: *Current Clinical Neurology: Atypical Parkinsonian Disorders*
Edited by: I. Litvan © Humana Press Inc., Totowa, NJ

Table 1
Summary of Tau Transgenic Mouse Models

Reference	Promoter	Isoform	Mutation	Mouse Strain	Tau Immunoreactivity Observed
19,20	mouse prion	0N3R	Wild-type	B6/D2	12E8, AT8, AT270, PHF1, PHF6, T3P
23	2α Ta1-tubulin	(0N,1N,2N)3R	Wild-type	B6/SJL	AT8, AT270, PHF1, PHF6, T3P
21	PAC (tau)	(0N,1N,2N)3R > (0N,1N,2N)4R	Wild-type	B6/D2/SW	MC-1
22	PAC (tau)/murine tau KO	(0N,1N,2N)3R > (0N,1N,2N)4R	Wild-type	B6/D2/SW	CP13, MC-1, PHF1
16	mouse thy-1	2N4R	Wild-type	B6/D2	AT8, AT180, PHF1
17	mouse thy-1	2N4R	Wild-type	FVB/N	ALZ50, AT8, AT180, AT270, MC1, PHF1
24	mouse prion	0N4R	P301L	B6/D2/SW	ALZ50, AT8, AT100, AT180, CP3, CP9, CP13, MC1, PHF1
31	mouse thy-1	2N4R	P301L	B6/D2	AD199, AT8, AT180, MC1, TG3
41	mouse thy-1	0N4R	P301S	B6/CBA	12E8, ALZ50, AT8, AT100, AT180, AP422, CP3, PG5, PHF1
40	mouse prion-tTA/ tetOp-tau	2N4R	G272V	B6/D2	12E8, AD2, AT8,TG3
37,38	PDGFβ	2N4R	V337M	B6/SJL	ALZ50, AT8, PS199
39	CamKII	2N4R	R406W	B6/SJL	ALZ50, AT180, PS199, PS404
36	mouse thy-1	2N4R	G272V, P301L, R406W	B6/CBA	AT8, AT180

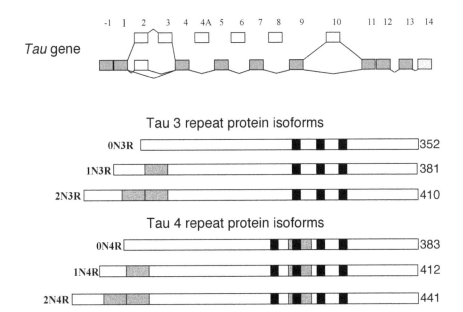

Fig. 1. Tau Isoforms. A. The tau gene is encoded on chromosome 17q21. Alternatively spliced exons 2, 3, and 10 are shown above the constitutive exons. Exons 4A, 6, and 8 are generally excluded from human tau mRNA. Most tau transcripts include the intron between exons 13 and 14. B. Exons 2, 3, and 10 (shaded boxes) are alternatively spliced to yield six tau isoforms (3R0N, 3R1N, 3R2N, 4R0N, 4R1N, 4R2N). *The microtubules binding domains (black boxes) are encoded by exons 9–12.*

of neurofibrillary pathology *(11)*. In a separate study, Ahlijanian and coworkers *(12)* overexpressed p25, a calpain cleavage product of p35, the endogenous regulator of another potential tau kinase, cdk5 *(13)*. P25 lacks the regulatory region of p35 and thus causes constitutive activation of cdk5. P25 production has been suggested to underlie tau hyperphosphorylation in AD *(13)*. Mice expressing p25 developed hyperphosphorylated tau and silver-positive inclusions that also had neurofilament immunoreactivity, but again neurofibrillary pathology was not observed *(12)*. Bian and colleagues *(14)* recently generated another transgenic mouse line, which overexpressed p25 in neurons. Despite the elevated cdk5 activity observed in these animals, axonal degeneration resulted in the absence of neurofibrillary tau pathology.

Kins and colleagues *(15)* addressed the role of tau hyperphosphorylation by generating mice that expressed a dominant negative mutant of the catalytic subunit of protein phosphatase 2A transgene in neurons. Abnormal tau phosphorylation (AT8 immunoreactivity) was observed in Purkinje cells of these transgenic mice. Ubiquitin immunoreactivity colocalized with the AT8 immunopositive aggregates; however, neurofibrillary lesions were not identified.

Transgenesis that resulted in altered tau kinase or phosphatase activity has produced some of the initial features of the tau pathology seen in human disease; however, the absence of neurofibrillary pathology or pronounced cell loss suggests that these enzymes may not initiate mature tau pathology. These models have now been bred with various tau transgenic models to further define the role that altered kinase or phosphatase activity has in the presence of early and late tau pathology.

TRANSGENIC MICE EXPRESSING WILD-TYPE TAU TRANSGENES

Two tau transgenic models have been reported that overexpress the longest isoform of wild-type 4R tau (2N4R). These mice expressed the transgene up to 10-fold over the level of endogenous tau and displayed somatodendritic localization of tau in neurons reminiscent of the "pre-tangle" state observed in human tauopathies including AD *(16,17)*. The 2N4R animals also showed motor distur-bances in tasks involving balancing on a rod and clinging from an inverted grid. This observation was consistent with the presence of prominent axonopathy characterized by swollen axons with neurofilament, tubulin, mitochondria, and vesicles in the brains and spinal cords of these mice. Dys-trophic neurites that stained with antibodies recognizing hyperphosphorylated and conformational tau epitopes (e.g., Alz50) were also identified. Astrogliosis, demonstrated by glial fibrillary acidic protein (GFAP) immunoreactivity, was also observed in the cortex and spinal cord. Wild-type 4R tau transgenic mice did not, however, develop filamentous tau inclusions characteristic of neurofibrillary tangles (NFTs) and neuronal loss was not observed.

To examine the role of tau hyperphosphorylation in disease pathogenesis, 2N4R wild-type tau animals were crossed with mice overexpressing GSK3β, a possible tau protein kinase *(18)*. These mice displayed a twofold increase in GSK3β activity and tau phosphorylation that surprisingly did not lead to NFTs, but instead resulted in rescue of axonopathy and motor deficits observed in the wild-type tau 2N4R transgenic mice. This observation indicates that tau hyperphosphorylation does not inevitably result in abnormal tau aggregation, although clearly GSK3β and tau hyperphosphorylation could still play a role in the pathogenesis of tauopathies.

The adult mouse brain predominantly expresses 4R tau isoforms. Therefore, Ishihara and co-workers generated transgenic mice that overexpress the shortest tau isoform (0N3R) to test the hy-pothesis that absence of 3R tau inhibits the development of neurofibrillary pathology *(19)*. Five- to 10-fold overexpression of the 0N3R wild-type transgene resulted in axonal spheroids in the spinal cord from 1 mo of age that were immunopositive for multiple phospho-dependent tau antibodies. The spheroids also stained for neurofilament. The spinal cord inclusions in the 3R mice were argy-rophilic with the Gallyas stain, but negative for thioflavin S. Binding of thioflavin S and other "congophilic" dyes to the neurofibrillary pathology in AD and other tauopathies is consistent with the presence of tau filaments with a β-sheet structure. It was therefore interesting that after 2 yr of age, occasional (1–2 NFTs per mouse brain section) NFTs were observed in the hippocampus of these mice. These inclusions consisted of straight tau filaments of 10- to 20-nm diameter that did not stain with neurofilament antibodies. Additionally, insoluble tau accumulated in the brains and spi-nal cords of these tau mice with age. Because the NFTs were sparse and required up to 2 yr to develop, it has been suggested that these mice represent a model of normal aging *(20)*. It will be interesting to determine whether modifying factors can be identified that accelerate the development of neurofibrillary pathology in these mice.

Duff and coworkers *(21)* created mice that expressed a P1-derived artificial chromosome (PAC) transgene containing the entire human tau gene to drive expression of all six human tau isoforms. Despite the almost fourfold overexpression of transgenic tau, robust tau pathology and behavioral changes were absent. These mice produce all six human tau isoforms with a 3.7-fold increase in total tau levels. Interestingly, in the mouse brain, splicing of the human genomic tau transgene is altered to favor the production of exon 10-negative mRNA and 3R tau. In these mice neuronal processes and synaptic terminals were positive for human tau. With the exception of immunoreactivity with certain conformation-specific tau antibodies (e.g., MC-1), these mice lacked evidence of abnormal tau pathol-ogy or behavioral changes up to 8 mo of age. It is uncertain why these mice, despite relatively high tau expression levels, develop little overt pathology; however, subsequent breeding of these mice onto a background lacking endogenous tau suggests that the presence of the mouse tau, which is largely 4R, may have inhibited the development of robust pathology.

Andorfer et al. subsequently bred the wild-type genomic tau mice to mice lacking the endogenous murine tau *(22)*. At early ages, the axons of these animals (Htau) are immunopositive for phospho-tau (CP13); however, this pathologic tau redistributes into the cells bodies with age, similarly to that observed in human tauopathies. Significantly, neurons in the hippocampus and cortex of Htau mice stained with PHF-1, MC1, and CP13. Similarly to the parental genomic tau line, these Htau preferen-tially produce 3R human tau isoforms. Sarkosyl-insoluble tau accumulated as early as 2 mo of age and was immunopositive for phosphotau epitopes as well as an antibody for 3R tau. Soluble, but not insoluble, tau fractions from these Htau mice stained with 4R tau antibody. Ultrastructural analysis showed remarkable similarity between human AD and the Htau isolated filaments. The extent to which the tauopathy matures in these animals is still somewhat unclear. Staining with Thioflavin S, Congo Red, and a variety of silver stains may be able to clarify the stage to which the animals progress. Also, there are currently no published reports of neurodegeneration or behavior deficits in association with the tau pathology in these mice. Despite this, these mice are currently the most impressive model employing wild-type tau to mimic human tauopathy and will be useful in testing therapeutic strategies. Additionally, these mice may prove valuable in determining the role of 3R and 4R tau in human tauopathies.

Higuchi and coworkers generated transgenic mice using the T1 α-tubulin promoter to obtain 3R tau expression *(23)*, but instead of a cDNA with 0N3R tau, they used a minigene construct that permitted expression of three human tau isoforms (0N3R, 1N3R, and 2N3R). Hyperphosphoryated tau accumulated in glia and insoluble tau, extracted in formic acid, accumulated in spinal cord and cerebellum by 12 mo. At 24 mo of age the glial inclusions were argyrophilic and immunoelectron microscopy showed tau immunoreactive fibrils within oligodendrocyte inclusions. There was also an age-related decrease in oligodendrocytes in spinal cord.

TRANSGENIC MICE EXPRESSING FTDP-17-ASSOCIATED P301L MUTANT TAU TRANSGENES

Overexpression of wild-type tau transgenes has had only limited success in modeling the pathology observed in the human tauopathies. As a result, several groups have generated mice that express human tau containing FTDP-17-associated mutations in an attempt to accelerate the development of neurofibrillary inclusions and other tau-related pathology.

Lewis and coworkers *(24)* reported a tau (P301L) transgenic mouse that expresses at about one- to twofold above endogenous levels the shortest 4R tau isoform (0N4R) with the P301L mutation in exon 10. Hemizygous and homozygous animals developed motor and behavioral deficits, as shown in the accompanying video, initially presenting with hind-limb dysfunction starting at 7 and 4.5 mo, respectively. Dystonic posturing and immobility developed within 1–2 mo of the initial symptoms. Additional features of the phenotype included docility, reduced weight, decreased vocalization, and eye irritations.

The P301L tau mice developed NFTs composed of 15- to 20-nm diameter straight and wavy tau filaments that were concentrated in the spinal cord, brainstem, and basal telencephalon. Occasional NFTs (one to two per section) were observed in the cortex and hippocampus. Pretangles had a much wider brain distribution. The NFTs contained hyperphosphorylated tau, were congophilic, and were positive with silver stains. Additionally, NFTs were negative for neurofilament and some were positive for ubiquitin. In addition to NFT, argyrophilic oligodendroglial inclusions were also detected in the spinal cord, and the glial inclusions were composed of tau-immunoreactive fibrils with electron microscopy *(25)*. Tau-immunoreactive astrocytes were also detected, but they did not have argyrophilia and ultrastructural studies showed dispersed tau fibrils *(25)*. Consistent with the neuropathology, the mice accumulated hyperphosphorylated tau that was insoluble after sarkosyl extraction of brain tissue including a prominent hyperphosphorylated 64kD species that comigrated with pathologic tau from FTDP-17 and AD patients *(24,26)*. Associated with the neurofibrillary pathology, the P301L animals demonstrated almost 50% neuronal loss in the spinal cord (neuronal counts in other brain regions were not reported), which likely explains much of the motor dysfunction in these mice.

Subsequent studies with these animals have evaluated the interaction of tau with APP/Aβ and the kinases GSK3 and cdk5. Breeding of these P301L mice with a transgenic model for amyloid deposition (Tg2576) *(27)* resulted in enhanced neurofibrillary tau pathology in the limbic system and olfactory cortex of double transgenic animals (TAPP), supporting an interaction between amyloid precursor protein (APP) or amyloid β (Aβ) and tau pathology in human AD *(28)*. Additionally, neurons containing tangle, but not pretangle, pathology from the P301L mice showed the abnormal accumulation of tyrosine-phosphorylated GSK3 *(29)*. Consistent with the enhanced neurofibrillary pathology, TAPP mice contained larger numbers of neurons that were immunopositive for this abnormal GSK3 sequestration. Noble and colleagues *(30)* investigated the interaction of tau with cdk5 by breeding mice that overexpressed the constitutive activator of cdk5 (p25) *(12)* onto the P301L tau background. In these double transgenic mice, increased cdk5 activity, either alone or in conjunction with GSK3, increased tau hyperphosphorylation and enhanced the degree of tau neurofibrillary pathology. The evidence that GSK3 and cdk5 may play a role in the tauopathy in these mice suggests that therapeutics aimed at reducing kinase activity may be beneficial in human tauopathies.

A second P301L tau transgenic mouse expressing the longest 4R tau isoform (2N4R) under the mouse Thy-1 promoter was described by Götz and coworkers *(31)*. Pretangles and some thioflavin-S-positive neurofibrillary-like structures were identified in the cortex, brainstem, and spinal cord of 8-mo-old P301L animals. Tau filaments with straight and twisted ribbon morphologies were observed in brain extracts. Additionally, astrocytosis and neuronal apoptosis, as demonstrated with terminal deoxyribonucleotide transferase-mediated dUTP nick end labeling (TUNEL), accompanied the tau pathology. Direct injection of Aβ42 fibrils into the brains of this P301L model resulted in a significant enhancement (5X) in the degree of neurofibrillary tau pathology in the amygdala *(32)*. These results demonstrated that Aβ42 can accelerate tau pathology in this mouse model, supporting the role of Aβ peptide in the development of tauopathy in humans.

Recently, Oddo et al. generated a mouse model expressing both a P301L tau transgene and an APP transgene with the Swedish mutation on a gene-targeted mutant presenilin 1 (M146V) background *(33)*. These animals deposit extracellular Aβ in the cortex and hippocampus followed by the development of tau pathology, initially in the CA1. This is a model of both tau and amyloid pathology in regions directly relevant to AD; however, most interesting is the initial pathological appearance of intraneuronal Aβ in this model. This accumulation of intracellular Aβ appeared to be responsible for the synaptic dysfunction and long-term potentiation deficits reported in this model. Ultrastructural analysis of the tau pathology and sarkosyl-insoluble tau analysis have not been published in these mice; therefore, the filamentous nature of the tau pathology has not been fully defined. Additionally, the impact of both intracellular and extracellular amyloid as well as the tau pathology on the behavioral features of these mice should prove interesting.

To determine if α-synuclein could promote the fibrillization of tau, Giasson and colleagues generated single transgenic lines expressing wild-type α-synuclein protein or mutant (P301L) tau protein under the direction of the murine 2',3'-cyclic nucleotide 3'-phosphodiesterase promoter *(34)*. Mice expressing just one of the two transgenes failed to develop synuclein or tau inclusions; however, bigenic tau/synuclein mice developed inclusions for both proteins at 12 mo of age that were positive for thioflavin S. Data from these bigenic mice suggests that α-synuclein and tau may interact, resulting in fibrillization, and therefore promote the hypothesis that future therapeutic strategies for synucleinopathies may also prove effective for tauopathies.

Models expressing the P301L human tau protein have been utilized in three novel ways to support the role of amyloid in the development of human AD. Additionally, results from one P301L model suggests that tau and synuclein pathology may be linked, supporting a role for tau in Parkinson's disease (PD). It is possible that the inclusion of the P301L mutation in these mice, which has not been identified in human AD or PD, may complicate these results; however, attempts to reproduce these findings using wild-type tau may be unsuccessful given the abbreviated life-span of the model organism. Nonetheless, the pathology of many of these P301L models at the cellular level closely recapitulates the tau pathological features of human AD and other tauopathies.

TRANSGENIC MICE EXPRESSING OTHER FTDP-17-ASSOCIATED MUTANT TAU TRANSGENES

Similar to Christi and colleagues' approach to modeling accelerated amyloid pathology in transgenic mice *(35)*, Lim and coworkers generated transgenic mice expressing 4R2N human tau containing three different FTDP-17 mutations under the mouse Thy-1 promoter *(36)*. These mice were termed VLW because of inclusion of the G272V, P301L, and R406W mutations in the transgenic tau. Dystrophic neurites and hyperphosphorylated tau were detected in cortex and hippocampus. The lesions resembled pretangles in their lack of immunoreactivity with phospho-tau antibodies that recognize NFTs (phosphoserine 396/404). Electron microscopy revealed tau immunoreactive filamentous structures 2- to 8-nm in diameter that were negative for neurofilament. Presence of tau-positive filaments was confirmed with ultrastructural analysis of sarkosyl-insoluble tau; however, immunogold labeling with phosphoepitopes of tau filaments was not reported *in situ* or in extracts. Increased lysosomal bodies were identified in the VLW animals, particularly in the neurons that were immunopositive for tau, as early as 1 mo of age.

Tanemura and coworkers *(37,38)* generated transgenic mice expressing V337M in 2N4R tau under the PDGFβ promoter. The construct contained myc and FLAG epitope tags at the amino- and carboxyl-terminal ends. Hippocampal neurons from 14-mo transgenic mice displayed myc and phospho-tau immunoreactivity, which was lacking in nontransgenic littermates. The immunoreactive neurons were irregularly shaped and darkly stained with a variety of staining methods, and ultrastructural studies showed organelles, lipofuscin pigment, and cytoskeletal elements, but no definitive evidence of NFTs. Using a similar strategy, Tatebayashi and coworkers *(39)* generated transgenic mice expressing R406W mutation under the calcium calmodulin kinase-II promoter, again with myc and FLAG tags on amino and carboxyl terminal ends. Mutant tau was expressed from 7- to 18-fold over endogenous tau, and mutant tau was detected predominantly in forebrain neurons. In animals more than 18 mo of age there was abnormal tau immunoreactivity in neurons, and some of the neurons had argyrophilia or weak Congo red birefringence. Ultrastructural studies showed cytoplasmic bundles of thin filaments that were different from thicker tubular fibrils that characterize human tauopathies. Transgenic animals also showed impairment in tests for contextual and cued fear conditioning.

Götz and coworkers generated transgenic mice with tetracycline-inducible expression of G272V tau under the mouse prion promotor *(40)*. The expression was above endogenous levels and expressed in both neurons and glia. By 6 mo of age thioflavin-S-positive oligodendroglial inclusions were detected in the spinal cord. The oligodendroglial inclusions were not argyrophilic with Gallyas stain, but at the electron microscopic level contained tubulofilamentous aggregates, with individual fibrils measuring 17–20 nm in width. Neurons formed tau-positive pretangles, but were not filamentous lesions and there was only a small amount of insoluble tau in formic acid extractable fractions.

Most recently, Allen and colleagues *(41)* utilized the mouse thy-1 promoter to drive expression of 0N4R human tau with the P301S mutation at approximately twofold the endogenous levels. Homozygous and hemizygous P301S mice developed paraparesis at approx 6 and 12 mo of age, respectively. Insoluble, hyperphosphorylated tau accumulated in the brains and spinal cords of the P301S animals that showed identical mobility to aggregated tau from human patients. Abnormally phosphorylated tau largely accumulated in nerve cells of the brainstem and spinal cords of the P301S animals with reduced immunoreactivity in the regions of the forebrain. Argyrophilic, thioflavin S neurons were also reported in the regions of concentrated tau pathology. Ultrastructurally, the lesions predominantly consisted of "half-twisted" ribbons that almost exclusively stained for human tau and lacked murine tau. Apoptosis did not appear to cause the neuronal loss (49%) that was reported in the ventral horn of the P301S mice. Interestingly, these mice shared many characteristics with the P301L 0N4R mice generated by Lewis et al. *(24)* including the development of frequent eye irritations.

OTHER ANIMAL MODELS OF TAU DYSFUNCTION

In addition to the range of mouse models now available, there have been attempts to use nonmammalian systems to model the tau dysfunction observed in human tauopathies. Although often ignored by many mouse-based researchers, these systems have proven useful in modeling some aspects of the disease while providing relatively simple screening systems for potential therapeutics before trials in mammals.

One such system is a lamprey model for tau dysfunction developed by Hall and colleagues *(42)*. By expressing wild-type human tau in the large anterior bulbar cells (ABCs) of the lamprey, Hall et al. *(42)* succeeded in producing a fish model of tau dysfunction. Tau within these ABCs became hyperphosphorylated and filamentous, and the neurons degenerated, resulting in a lamprey tauopathy that can be staged similarly to human tauopathies. The ease of therapeutic trials using this lamprey system allows the model to be a valuable link between cellular models and the in vivo mammalian models detailed earlier. Hall et al. *(43)* has recently utilized this system to screen a novel proprietary compound aimed at blocking tau filament formation. Limitations of this model system include differences of central nervous system and the inability to perform cognitive and motor tests that accompany the tauopathies that occur in complex organisms.

Kraemer et al. recently generated a *Caenorhabditis elegans* model of tau pathology *(44)*. Expression of tau with either the P301L or V377M mutation resulted in worms with locomotor deficits, accumulation of insoluble tau protein, and increased tau phosphorylation. Axonal degeneration and neuronal loss were also reported in this mold. The simplicity of this model makes it an attractive system with which to screen potential therapeutic compounds before trials in mammals.

A *Drosophila* model of tauopathy expressing the human tau containing the R406W mutation also mimicked many aspects of tauopathy without the development of NFTs *(45)*. Aged flies showed progressive neurodegeneration, accumulation of abnormally phosphorylated tau, but lacked the large neurofibrillary accumulations of tau that characterize human tauopathies. This model system suggested that mature tau pathology may not be necessary to result in the neurodegenerative process. Additionally, this model has now been used to examine the gene expression changes that occur as the result of tau-related neurodegeneration *(46)*. Evidence of these expression changes such as those in lysosomal and cellular stress response genes in the *Drosophila* model will now allow us to more closely investigate similar changes in both mouse models and human tauopathies.

CONCLUSION

A range of different in vivo model systems is now available that can be used to investigate both the development and progression of tauopathies (*see* Table 2 for future directions). These models mimic many of the basic cellular changes that accompany development of tauopathy. Additionally, some of the models share clinical features and distribution of tau pathology that could be compared to human 4R tauopathies such as progressive supranuclear palsy (PSP). PSP is a rare parkinsonian movement disorder that is associated with early postural instability and supranuclear vertical gaze palsy *(47)*. The brains of PSP patients display neurofibrillary tangles that are primarily localized to the basal ganglia, diencephalon, and the brainstem *(48,49)*. Brainstem regions that are usually affected in PSP included the locus ceruleus, pontine nuclei, and pontine tegmentum. Additionally, the cerebellar dentate nuclei and spinal cord are frequently affected in PSP patients *(48,49)*. The distribution of the neurofibrillary tau pathology in the JNPL3 mice overlaps many of the same regions affected in PSP, including the pontine nucleus, the dentate nucleus, and the spinal cord. 0N4R P301S mice *(41)* also showed a similar distribution of pathology. Additionally, the reduced vocalization and progressive

Table 2
Future Directions in Animal Modeling of Tauopathies

- Determine gene expression changes that accompany tauopathies.
- Isolate loci or specific alleles that modify the progression of tauopathy based on comparison of different mouse models and different strains and based on simple models of tauopathy.
- Develop and utilize inducible mouse models of tauopathy to determine at which stages tauopathies are targets for therapeutic efforts.
- Design, develop,a nd screen therapeutic strategies using the current and future transgenic tau models.
- Utilize current models to understand the interaction of tau with other disease-related processes.
- Understand how and at which stage tau leads to neurodegeneration.

movement disorder, including rigidity, observed in the JNPL3 model is similar to that observed in PSP patients. In addition, the selective distribution of 4R tau in both neurons and glia is a feature observed in both PSP and these mouse models.

The neuronal response to tauopathy, including of gene expression and protein (level and modification) changes, can now be investigated at various pathological stages in these models and compared with observations from end-stage human tissue. Additionally, multiple disease modifiers may now be identified in the more simple systems such as in the fly or worm, which may lead to a greater understanding of the mechanisms that result in tau-induced neurodegeneration and perhaps identify additional therapeutic targets. It is important however to recognize the limitations of these simple "genetic" animal models and follow-up studies in mouse models will be required to verify the relevance of the findings in these systems.

The development of multiple animal models of tauopathy has also enabled the field to investigate the relationship between tau dysfunction and other proteins previously implicated in neurodegenerative disease including Aβ, α-synuclein, and various tau kinases/phosphatases. Given the similarities between the various protein aggregation disorders, these interactions may provide essential clues for understanding the basic process of tau-associated neurodegeneration and for developing therapeutic strategies (Fig. 2).

Comparisons of various tau transgenic mice on different mouse strain backgrounds should further our understanding of how genetic or environmental factors modify the progression of tauopathy. Novel inducible models of tauopathy should also help determine which aspects of the disease process are reversible and which stages are associated with functional deficits. Overall the rapid development of animal models of tauopathy in the last 4 yr will inevitably accelerate progress in understanding the pathogenesis of tauopathy and should also identify potential therapeutic approaches that can be used to treat these diseases in human patients.

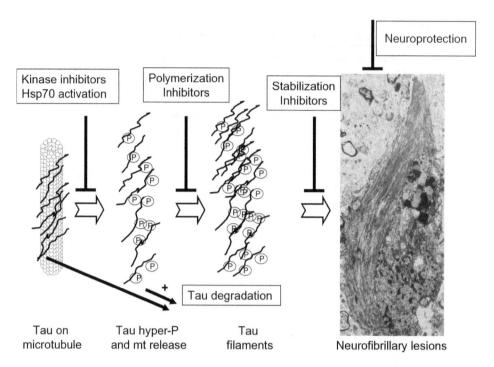

Fig. 2. Tau therapeutic targets. Therapeutic targets may be aimed at different stages of tau dysfunction. Kinase inhibitors could be tested to prevent hyperphosphorylation of tau and dissociation from microtubules (mt). Compounds that prevent or dissociate the polymerization of tau into lesions might also be effective therapies. Additionally, it may be possible to target therapies to decrease the stabilization of tau lesions or to increase the turnover of abnormal tau. Finally, neuroprotective agents may be effective in maintaining or recovering functional neurons.

REFERENCES

1. D'Souza, I, Poorkaj P, Hong M, et al. Missense and silent tau gene mutations cause frontotemporal dementia with parkinsonism-chromosome 17 type, by affecting multiple alternative RNA splicing regulatory elements. Proc Natl Acad Sci USA 1999;96:5598–5603.
2. Hutton M, Lendon CL, Rizzu P, et al. Association of missense and 5'-splice site mutations in tau with the inherited dementia FTDP-17. Nature 1998;393:702–705.
3. Poorkaj P, Bird TD, Wijsman E, et al. Tau is a candidate gene for chromosome 17 frontotemporal dementia. Ann Neurol 1998;43:815–825.
4. Spillantini MG, Murrell JR, Goedert M, Farlow MR, Klug A, Ghetti B. Mutation in the tau gene in familial multiple system tauopathy with presenile dementia. Proc Natl Acad Sci USA 1998;95:7737–7741.
5. Spillantini MG, Bird TD, Ghetti B. Frontotemporal dementia and parkinsonism linked to chromosome 17: a new group of tauopathies. Brain Pathol 1998;8:387–402.
6. Goedert M, Spillantini MG, Potier MC, Ulrich J, Crowther RA. Cloning and sequencing of the cDNA encoding an isoform of microtubule-associated protein tau containing four tandem repeats: differential expression of tau protein mRNAs in human brain. EMBO J 1989;8:393–399.
7. Goedert M, Spillantini MG, Jakes R, Rutherford D, Crowther RA. Multiple isoforms of human microtubule-associated protein tau: sequences and localization in neurofibrillary tangles of Alzheimer's disease. Neuron 1989;3:519–526.
8. Lee G, Neve RL, Kosik KS. The microtubule binding domain of tau protein. Neuron 1989;2:1625–1624.
9. Kosik KS, Orecchio LD, Bakalis S, Neve RL. Developmentally regulated expression of specific tau sequences. Neuron 1989;2:1389–1397.
10. Spillantini MG, Goedert M. Tau protein pathology in neurodegenerative diseases. Trends Neurosci 1998;21:428–433.
11. Lucas JJ, Hernandez F, Gomez-Ramos P, Moran M, Hen R, Avila J. Decreased nuclear α-catenin, tau hyperphosphorylation and neurodegeneration in GSK-3beta conditional transgenic mice. EMBO J 2001;20:27–39.

12. Ahlijanian MK, Barrezueta NX, Williams RD, et al. Hyperphosphorylated tau and neurofilament and cytoskeletal disruptions in mice overexpressing human p25, an activator of Cdk5. Proc Natl Acad Sci USA 2000;97:2910–2915.

13. Patrick GN, Zukerberg L, Nikolic M, de la Monte S, Dikkes P, Tsai LH. Conversion of p35 to p25 deregulates Cdk5 activity and promotes neurodegeneration. Nature 1999;402:615–622.

14. Bian F, Nath R, Sobocinski G, et al. Axonopathy, tau abnormalities, and dyskinesia, but no neurofibrillary tangles in p25-transgenic mice. J Comp Neurol 2002;446:257–266.

15. Kins S, Crameri A, Evans DRH, Hemmings BA, Nitsch R, Gotz J. Reduced PP2A activity induces tau hyperphosphorylation and altered compartmentalization of tau in transgenic mice. J Biol Chem 2001;276:38193–38200.

16. Probst A, Götz J, Wiederhold KH, et al. Axonopathy and amyotrophy in mice transgenic for human four-repeat tau protein. Acta Neuropathol 2000;99:469–481.

17. Spittaels K, Van den Haute C, Van Dorpe J, et al. Prominent axonopathy in the brain and spinal cord of transgenic mice overexpressing four-repeat human tau protein. Am J Pathol 1999;155:2153–2165.

18. Spittaels K, Van den Haute C, Van Dorpe J, et al. Glycogen synthase kinase-3β phosphorylates protein tau and rescues the axonopathy in the central nervous system of human four-repeat tau transgenic mice. J Biol Chem 2000;275:41340–41349.

19. Ishihara T, Hong M, Zhang B, et al. Age-dependent emergence and progression of a tauopathy in transgenic mice overexpressing the shortest human tau isoform. Neuron 19999;24:751–762.

20. Ishihara T, Zhang B, Higuchi M, Yoshiyama Y, Trojanowski JQ, Lee VM. Age-dependent induction of congophilic neurofibrillary tau inclusions in tau transgenic mice. Am J Pathol 2001;158:555–562.

21. Duff K, Knight H, Refolo LM, et al. Characterization of pathology in transgenic mice over-expressing human genomic and cDNA tau transgenes. Neurobiol Dis 2000;7:87–98.

22. Andorfer C, Kress Y, de Silva R, et al. Hyperphosphorylation and aggregation of tau in mice expressing normal human tau isoforms. J Neurochem 2003;86:582–590.

23. Higuchi M, Ishihara T, Zhang B, et al. Transgenic mouse model of tauopathies with glial pathology and nervous system degeneration. Neuron 2002;35:433–446.

24. Lewis J, McGowan E, Rockwood J, et al. Neurofibrillary tangles, amyotrophy and progressive motor disturbance in mice expressing mutant (P301L) tau protein. Nat Genet 2000;25:402-–405.

25. Lin W-L, Lewis J, Yen S-H, Hutton M, Dickson DW. Filamentous tau in oligodendrocytes and astrocytes of transgenic mice expressing the human tau isoform with the P301L mutation. Am J Pathol 2003;162:213–218.

26. Sahara N, Lewis J, DeTure M, et al. Assembly of tau in transgenic animals expressing P301L tau: alterations of phosphorylation and solubility. J Neurochem 2002;83:1498–1508.

27. Hsiao K, Chapman P, Nilsen S, et al. Correlative memory deficits, Abeta elevation, and amyloid plaques in transgenic mice. Science 1996;274:99–102.

28. Lewis J, Dickson DW, Lin WL, et al. Enhanced neurofibrillary degeneration in transgenic mice expressing mutant tau and APP. Science 2001;293:1487–1491.

29. Ishizawa T, Sahara N, Ishiguro K, et al. Co-localization of glycogen synthase kinase-3 with neurofibrillary tangles and granulovacular degeneration in transgenic mice. Am J Pathol 2003;163:1057–1067.

30. Noble W, Olm V, Takata K, et al. Cdk5 is a key factor in tau aggregation and tangle formation in vivo. Neuron 2003;38:555–565.

31. Götz J, Chen F, Barmettler R, Nitsch RM. Tau filament formation in transgenic mice expressing P301L tau. J Biol Chem 2001;276:529–534.

32. Gotz J, Chen F, van Dorpe J, Nitsch RM. Formation of neurofibrillary tangles in P301L tau transgenic mice induced by Abeta fibrils. Science 2001;293:1491–1495.

33. Oddo S, Caccamo A, Shepherd JD, et al. Triple-transgenic model of Alzheimer's Disease with plaques and tangles: intracellular Ab and synaptic dysfunction. Neuron 2003; 39:409–421.

34. Giasson BI, Forman MS, Higuchi M, et al. Initiation and synergistic fibrillization of tau and alpha-synuclein. Science 2003;300:636–640.

35. Chrishti MA, Yang DS, Janus C, et al. Early-onset amyloid deposition and cognitive deficits in transgenic mice expressing a double mutant form of amyloid precursor protein 695. J Biol Chem 2001;276:21562–21570.

36. Lim F, Hernandez F, Lucas JJ, Gomez-Ramos P, Moran MA, Avila J. FTDP-17 Mutations in tau transgenic mice provoke lysosomal abnormalities and tau filaments in forebrain. Mol Cell Neurosci 2001;18:702–714.

37. Tanemura K, Akagi T, Murayama M, et al. Formation of filamentous tau aggregates in transgenic mice expressing V337M human tau. Neurobiol Disease 2001;8:1036–1045.

38. Tanemura K, Murayama M, Akagi T, et al. Neurodegeneration with tau accumulation in a transgenic mouse expressing V337M human tau. J Neurosci 2002;22:133–141.

39. Tatebayashi Y, Miyasaka T, Chui D-H, et al. Tau filament formation and associative memory deficit in aged mice expressing mutant (R406W) human tau. Proc Natl Acad Sci USA 2002;99:13896–13901.

40. Götz J, Tolnay M, Barmettler R, Chen F, Probst A, Nitsch RM. Oligodendroglial tau filament formation in transgenic mice expressing G272V tau. Eur J Neurosci 2001;13:2131–2140.

41. Allen B, Ingram E, Takao M, et al. Abundant tau filaments and nonapoptotic neurodegeneration in transgenic mice expressing human P301S tau protein. J Neurosci 2002;22:9340–9351.

42. Hall GF, Lee VM, Lee G, Yao J. Staging of neurofibrillary degeneration caused by human tau overexpression in a unique cellular model of human tauopathy. Am J Pathol 2001;158:235–246.

43. Hall GF, Lee S, Yao J. Neurofibrillary degeneration can be arrested in an in vivo cellular model of human tauopathy by application of a compound which inhibits tau filament formation in vitro. J Mol Neurosci 2002;19:253–260.

44. Kraemer BC, Zhang B, Leverenz JB, Thomas JH, Trojanowski JQ, Schellenberg G. Neurodegeneration and defective neurotransmission in a *Caenorhabditis elegans* model of tauopathy. Proc Natl Acad Sci USA 2003;100:9980–9985.

45. Whitmann CW, Wszolek MF, Shulman JM, et al. Tauopathy in Drosophila: neurodegeneration without neurofibrillary tangles. Science 2001;293:711–714.

46. Scherzer CR, Jensen RV, Gullans SR, Feany MB. Gene expression changes presage neurodegeneration in a Drosophila model of Parkinson's disease. Hum Mol Genet 2003;12:2457–2466.

47. Litvan I, Hutton M. Clinical and genetic aspects of progressive supranuclear palsy. J Geriatr Psychiatry Neurol 1998;11:107–114.

48. Dickson DW. Neuropathologic differentiation of progressive supranuclear palsy and corticobasal degeneration. J Neurol 1999;246(Suppl 2):II/6–II/15.

49. Ishizawa K, Dickson DW. Microglial activation parellels system degeneration in progression supranuclear palsy and corticobasal degeneration. J Neuropathol Exp Neurol 2001;60:647–657.

6

Neurodegenerative α-Synucleinopathies

Michel Goedert and Maria Grazia Spillantini

INTRODUCTION

Parkinson's disease (PD) is the most common movement disorder *(1)*. Neuropathologically, it is defined by nerve cell loss in the substantia nigra and the presence there of Lewy bodies and Lewy neurites. Nerve cell loss and Lewy body pathology are also found in a number of other brain regions, such as the dorsal motor nucleus of the vagus, the nucleus basalis of Meynert, and some autonomic ganglia. Lewy bodies and Lewy neurites also constitute the defining neuropathological characteristics of dementia with Lewy bodies (DLB), a common late-life dementia that exists in a pure form or overlaps with the neuropathological characteristics of Alzheimer's disease (AD) *(2)*. Unlike PD, DLB is characterized by large numbers of Lewy bodies in cortical brain areas. Ultrastructurally, Lewy bodies and Lewy neurites consist of abnormal filamentous material. Despite the fact that the Lewy body was first described in 1912 *(3)*, its molecular composition remained unknown until 1997.

The two developments that imparted a new direction to research on the aetiology and pathogenesis of PD and DLB were the twin discoveries that a missense mutation in the α-synuclein gene is a rare genetic cause of PD *(4)* and that α-synuclein is the main component of Lewy bodies and Lewy neurites in idiopathic PD, DLB, and several other diseases *(5)*. Subsequently, the filamentous glial and neuronal inclusions of multiple system atrophy (MSA) were also found to be made of α-synuclein, revealing an unexpected molecular link with Lewy body diseases *(6–8)*. These findings have placed the dysfunction of α-synuclein at the center of PD and several atypical parkinsonian disorders (Table 1).

THE SYNUCLEIN FAMILY

Synucleins are abundant brain proteins whose physiological functions are only poorly understood. The human synuclein family consists of three members—α-synuclein, β-synuclein, and γ-synuclein—which range from 127 to 140 amino acids in length and are 55–62% identical in sequence, with a similar domain organization (Fig. 1) *(9–11)*. The amino-terminal half of each protein is taken up by imperfect 11-amino acid repeats that bear the consensus sequence KTKEGV. Individual repeats are separated by an interrepeat region of five to eight amino acids. The repeats are followed by a hydrophobic intermediate region and a negatively charged carboxy-terminal domain; α- and β-synuclein have identical carboxy-termini. By immunohistochemistry, α- and β-synuclein are concentrated in nerve terminals, with little staining of somata and dendrites. Ultrastructurally, they are found in close proximity to synaptic vesicles *(12)*. In contrast, γ-synuclein is present throughout nerve cells in many brain regions. In rat, α-synuclein is most abundant throughout telencephalon and diencephalon, with lower levels in more caudal regions *(13)*. β-Synuclein is distributed fairly evenly throughout the central nervous system, whereas γ-synuclein is most abundant in midbrain, pons, and spinal cord,

From: *Current Clinical Neurology: Atypical Parkinsonian Disorders*
Edited by: I. Litvan © Humana Press Inc., Totowa, NJ

Table 1
α-Synuclein diseases

Lewy body diseases
    Idiopathic Parkinson's disease
    Dementia with Lewy bodies
    Pure autonomic failure
    Lewy body dysphagia
    Inherited Lewy body diseases

Multiple system atrophy
    Olivopontocerebellar atrophy
    Striatonigral degeneration
    Shy–Drager syndrome

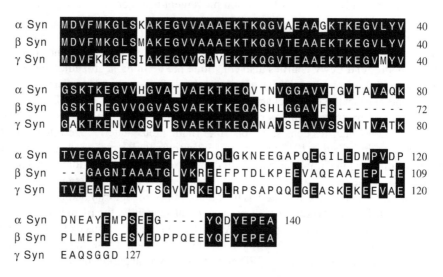

Fig. 1. Sequence comparison of human α-synuclein (α Syn), β-synuclein (β Syn), and γ-synuclein (γ Syn). Amino acid identities between at least two of the three sequences are indicated by black bars. As a result of a common polymorphism, residue 110 of γ-synuclein is either E or G.

with much lower levels in forebrain areas. At the level of neurotransmitter systems, α-synuclein is particularly abundant in central catecholaminergic regions, β-synuclein in somatic cholinergic neurons, whereas γ-synuclein is present in both catecholaminergic and cholinergic systems.

Synucleins are natively unfolded proteins with little ordered secondary structure that have only been identified in vertebrates *(14)*. Experimental studies have shown that α-synuclein can bind to lipid membranes through its amino-terminal repeats, indicating that it may be a lipid-binding protein *(15,16)*. It adopts structures rich in α-helical character upon binding to synthetic lipid membranes containing acidic phospholipids. This conformation is taken up by amino acids 1–98 and consists of two α-helical regions (residues 1–42 and 45–98) that are interrupted by a break of two amino acids (residues 43 and 44) *(17,18)*. Residues 99–140 are unstructured. In cell lines and primary neurons treated with high fatty acid concentrations, α-synuclein was found to accumulate on phospholipid monolayers surrounding triglyceride-rich droplets *(19)*. β-Synuclein bound in a similar way, but γ-synuclein failed to bind to lipid droplets and remained cytosolic. Accordingly, α-synuclein has been shown to bind fatty acids in vitro, albeit with a lower affinity than physiological fatty acid-binding proteins *(20,21)*. Both α- and β-synucleins have been shown to inhibit phospholipase D2 *(22)*. This isoform of phospholipase D localizes to the plasma membrane, where it might be involved in signal-induced cytoskeletal regulation and endocytosis. It is therefore possible that α- and β-synucleins regulate vesicular transport processes.

Little is known about posttranslational modifications of synucleins in the brain. In transfected cells, α-synuclein is constitutively phosphorylated at residues 87 and 129, with residue 129 being the predominant site *(23)*. However, in normal brain, only a small fraction of α-synuclein is phosphorylated at S129 *(24)*. Casein kinase-1 and casein kinase-2 phosphorylate S129 of α-synuclein in vitro, as do several G protein-coupled receptor kinases *(23–25)*. Phosphorylation at S129 has been reported to result in a reduced ability of α-synuclein to interact with phospholipids and phospholipase D2 in one study, whereas another study found no effect of phosphorylation on lipid binding *(25,26)*. α-Synuclein contains four tyrosine residues, three of which are located in the carboxy-terminal region. Tyrosine kinases of the Src family phosphorylate Y125 in vitro and in transfected cells *(27,28)*. The same site also becomes phosphorylated following exposure of cells to osmotic stress *(29)*, suggesting that tyrosine phosphorylation of α-synuclein may be regulated. However, it remains to be seen whether synucleins are phosphorylated on tyrosines in brain. Like some other natively unfolded proteins, α-synuclein can be degraded by the proteasome in the absence of polyubiquitination *(30)*.

Inactivation of the α-synuclein gene by homologous recombination does not lead to a neurological phenotype, with the mice being largely normal *(31–35)*. So, a loss of function of α-synuclein is unlikely to account for its role in neurodegeneration. Analysis of mice lacking γ-synuclein has similarly failed to reveal any gross abnormalities *(34)*. Mice lacking β-synuclein have not yet been reported. Ultimately, mice lacking all three synucleins may be needed for an understanding of the physiological functions of these abundant brain proteins. One study has reported that targeted disruption of the α-synuclein gene confers specific resistance of dopamine neurons to the toxic effects of 1-methyl-4-phenyl-1,2,3,6-tetrahydropyridine (MPTP) *(35)*. The resistance to neurodegeneration appeared to be mediated through the inability of MPTP to inhibit the complex I activity of the mitochondrial respiratory chain. A second study on two additional lines of mice without α-synuclein has reported partial resistance to MPTP in one line and normal sensitivity to the toxin in the other *(36)*. It thus appears that α-synuclein is not obligatorily coupled to sensitivity to MPTP, but that it can influence MPTP toxicity on some genetic backgrounds.

LEWY BODY DISEASES

The PARK1 Locus

In 1990, Golbe, Duvoisin, and colleagues described an autosomal-dominantly inherited form of PD in an Italian-American family (Contursi kindred; *see* ref. *37*). It was the first familial form of disease in which Lewy bodies had been shown to be present. Subsequently, several more families with autopsy-confirmed Lewy body disease were identified. In 1996, Polymeropoulos and colleagues mapped the genetic defect responsible for disease in the Contursi kindred to chromosome 4q21-23 (PARK1) *(38)*. One year later, they reported a missense mutation (A53T) in the α-synuclein gene as the cause of familial PD in this kindred and several PD families of Greek origin (Fig. 2) *(4)*. A founder effect probably accounts for the relatively frequent occurrence of the A53T mutation in southern Italy and Greece. In 1998, a second mutation (A30P) in the α-synuclein gene was identified in a German pedigree with early-onset PD (Fig. 2) *(39)*. In 2003, the genetic defect responsible for a familial form of PD dementia in a large family (the Iowa kindred; *see* ref. *40*) was shown to be a triplication of a 1.6–2.0 Mb region on the long arm of chromosome 4 *(41)*. One of an estimated 17 genes located in this region is the α-synuclein gene. These findings thus suggest that that the simple overproduction of wild-type α-synuclein may be sufficient to cause PD dementia. Moreover, polymorphic variations in the 5' noncoding region of the α-synuclein gene have been found to be associated with idiopathic PD in some, but not all, studies *(42–45)*. They probably influence the level of α-synuclein expression *(46)*.

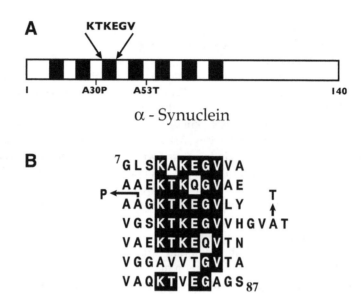

Fig. 2. Mutations in the α-synuclein gene in familial Parkinson's disease. (**A**) Schematic diagram of human α-synuclein. The seven repeats with the consensus sequence KTKEGV are shown as black bars. The two known missense mutations are indicated. Triplication of a region on chromosome 4 that comprises the α-synuclein gene causes familial PD dementia. Therefore, it appears likely that the overexpression of wild-type α-synuclein can also cause disease (**B**) Repeats in human α-synuclein. Residues 7–87 of the 140-residue protein are shown. Amino acid identities between at least five of the seven repeats are indicated by black bars. The A to P mutation at residue 30 between repeats two and three and the A to T mutation at residue 53 between repeats four and five are shown.

α-Synuclein and Sporadic Lewy Body Diseases

Shortly after the identification of the genetic defect responsible for PD in the Contursi kindred, Lewy bodies and Lewy neurites in the substantia nigra from patients with sporadic PD were shown to be strongly immunoreactive for α-synuclein (Fig. 3) *(5)*. Subsequently, Lewy bodies and isolated Lewy body filaments from PD brain were found to be decorated by antibodies directed against α-synuclein *(47,48)*. In addition to PD, Lewy bodies and Lewy neurites also constitute the defining neuropathological characteristics of DLB. Unlike PD, DLB is characterized by large numbers of Lewy bodies and Lewy neurites in cortical brain areas. But like PD, DLB is also characterized by Lewy body pathology in the substantia nigra, and the Lewy bodies and neurites associated with DLB are strongly immunoreactive for α-synuclein (Fig. 4) *(5)*. Filaments from Lewy bodies in DLB are decorated by α-synuclein antibodies, and their morphology closely resembles that of filaments extracted from the substantia nigra of PD brains *(49,50)*.

The α-synuclein filaments associated with PD and DLB are unbranched, with a length of 200–600 nm and a width of 5–10 nm. Full-length α-synuclein is present, with its amino- and carboxy-termini being exposed on the filament surface. Protease digestion and site-directed spin labeling studies have shown that the core of the α-synuclein filaments extends over a stretch of about 70 amino acids, from residues 34–101 *(51,52)*. This sequence overlaps almost entirely with the lipid-binding region of α-synuclein. Biochemically, the presence of α-synuclein inclusions has been found to correlate with the accumulation of α-synuclein. Of the three human synucleins, only α-synuclein is associated with the filamentous inclusions of Lewy body diseases. Using specific antibodies, β- and γ-synucleins are absent from these inclusions *(5,50)*.

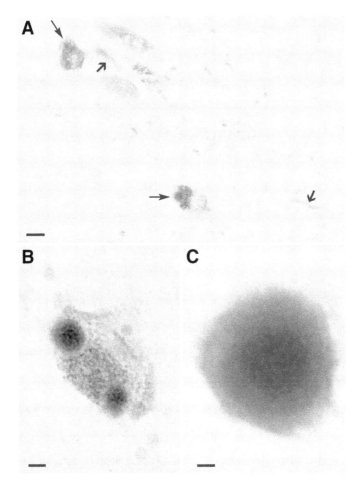

Fig. 3. Substantia nigra from patients with Parkinson's disease immunostained for α-synuclein. (**A**) Two pigmented nerve cells, each containing an α-synuclein-positive Lewy body. Lewy neurites (small arrows) are also immunopositive. Scale bar, 20 μm. (**B**) Pigmented nerve cell with two α-synuclein-positive Lewy bodies. Scale bar 8 μm. (**C**) α-Synuclein-positive extracellular Lewy body. Scale bar, 4 μm.

Prior to this work, ubiquitin staining had been the preferred immunohistochemical marker of Lewy body pathology *(53)*. By double-labeling immunohistochemistry, the number of α-synuclein-positive structures was greater than that stained for ubiquitin, suggesting that the ubiquitination of α-synuclein occurs after its assembly into filaments *(50,54,55)*. In DLB brain, α-synuclein is mostly mono- or diubiquitinated *(54–56)*. Phosphorylation and nitration are two additional posttranslational modifications of filamentous α-synuclein. Phosphorylation at S129 has been documented in Lewy bodies and Lewy neurites by mass spectrometry and phosphorylation-dependent antibodies *(24)*. It has been suggested that phosphorylation of α-synuclein at S129 may trigger filament assembly. However, it remains to be determined whether it occurs before or after filament assembly in human brain. Nitration of tyrosine residues in proteins is the result of the action of oxygen, nitric oxide, and their products, such as peroxynitrite. Nitration of filamentous α-synuclein was found using antibodies specific for nitrated tyrosine residues *(57)*. As for ubiquitin, staining for nitrotyrosine was less extensive than staining for α-synuclein, suggesting that nitration of α-synuclein occurs after its assembly into filaments.

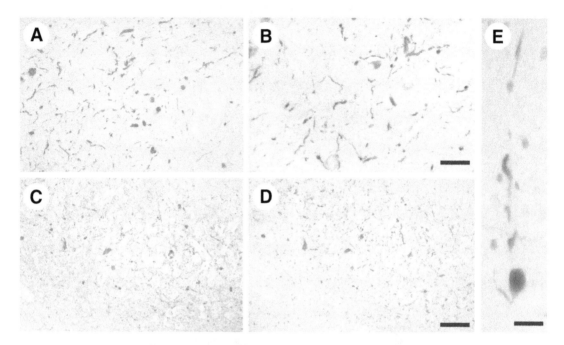

Fig. 4. Brain tissue from patients with dementia with Lewy bodies immunostained for α-synuclein. (**A,B**) α-Synuclein-positive Lewy bodies and Lewy neurites in substantia nigra stained with antibodies recognizing the amino-terminal (A) or the carboxy-terminal (B) region of α-synuclein. Scale bar, 100 μm (in B, for A,B). (**C,D**) α-Synuclein-positive Lewy neurites in serial sections of hippocampus stained with antibodies recognizing the amino-terminal (C) or the carboxy-terminal (D) region of α-synuclein. Scale bar, 80 μm (in D, for C,D). (**E**), α-Synuclein-positive intraneuritic Lewy body in a Lewy neurite in substantia nigra. Scale bar, 40 μm.

Lewy body pathology is also the defining feature of several other, rarer diseases. Cases in which α-synuclein immunoreactivity has been examined have shown its presence. Thus, pure autonomic failure is characterized by α-synuclein-positive Lewy body pathology in sympathetic ganglia *(58,59)*. Incidental Lewy body disease describes the presence of small numbers of Lewy bodies and Lewy neurites in the absence of clinical symptoms. It is observed in 5–10% of the general population over the age of 60, and is believed to represent a preclinical form of Lewy body disease *(60,61)*. In cases with incidental Lewy body disease, the first pathological α-synuclein-immunoreactive structures do not form in dopaminergic nerve cells of the substantia nigra, but in non-catecholaminergic neurons of the dorsal glossopharyngeus-vagus complex, projection neurons of the reticular zone, and in the locus coeruleus, raphe nuclei, and the olfactory system *(62)*. Incidental Lewy body disease may be at one end of the spectrum of Lewy body diseases, with DLB at the other end and PD somewhere in between. The Lewy body pathology that is sometimes associated with other neurodegenerative diseases, such as Alzheimer's disease, the parkinsonism-dementia complex of Guam, and neurodegeneration with brain iron accumulation type I has also been shown to be immunoreactive for α-synuclein *(7,63,64)*. However, it is not an invariant feature of these diseases. Nevertheless, understanding why α-synuclein pathology develops in a proportion of cases in these apparently unrelated conditions may shed light on the mechanisms operating in the diseases defined by the presence of Lewy body pathology.

α-*Synuclein and Inherited Lewy Body Diseases*

The discovery that α-synuclein is the major component of Lewy bodies and Lewy neurites in idiopathic PD raised the question of the neuropathological picture in cases of familial PD with mutations in the α-synuclein gene. Widespread Lewy bodies and Lewy neurites immunoreactive for α-synuclein were described in the brainstem pigmented nuclei, hippocampus, and temporal cortex in two individuals from an Australian family of Greek origin with the A53T mutation *(65)*. Lewy neurites accounted for much of the pathology, underscoring their relevance for the neurodegenerative process. As in other Lewy body diseases, the α-synuclein pathology was neuronal. However, it was much more widespread than in idiopathic PD. Similarly extensive deposits of α-synuclein have been found in a case of the Contursi kindred *(66)*. In addition, substantial tau pathology was reported in this case, suggesting that a missense mutation in the α-synuclein gene can somehow also lead to tau deposition. This is in line with recent studies that have reported that tau staining is frequently associated with Lewy bodies and that α-synuclein assemblies can induce tau filament formation in vitro *(67,68)*. Work so far has been on cases with the A53T mutation. Nothing is known about the neuropathology in cases of familial PD with the A30P mutation in α-synuclein.

In the Iowa kindred with a triplication of the region of chromosome 4 that encompasses the α-synuclein gene, abundant and widespread α-synuclein-immunoreactive Lewy bodies and Lewy neurites have been described *(69)*. The pathological picture resembled that of DLB. In addition, α-synuclein-positive glial inclusions were also present, suggesting that overproduction of wild-type α-synuclein may be a mechanism leading to the formation of glial cytoplasmic inclusions.

A genetic locus (PARK3) that is linked to autosomal-dominantly inherited PD has been mapped to chromosome 2p13 *(70)*. Although the underlying genetic defect is not yet known, neuropathological analysis has shown the presence of α-synuclein-immunoreactive Lewy bodies and Lewy neurites, with a distribution resembling PD *(71)*. It appears likely that the defective PARK3 gene product functions in the pathway that leads from soluble to filamentous α-synuclein.

Subsequent to the identification of the A53T mutation in the α-synuclein gene, a missense mutation (I93M) in the ubiquitin carboxy-terminal hydrolase L1 (UCHL1) gene was reported in a patient with familial PD (PARK5) *(72)*. UCHL1 is an abundant neuron-specific deubiquitinating enzyme. This mutation resulted in a partial loss of the catalytic activity of the thiol protease, which could, in principle, lead to protein aggregation. However, no information is available about neuropathology in this family, and the presence of Lewy body pathology with the accumulation of α-synuclein remains a possibility. In 1998, mutations in the gene *parkin* (PARK2) were identified as the genetic cause of a form of autosomal-recessive juvenile parkinsonism (AR-JP) *(73)*. These mutations constitute a common cause of parkinsonism, especially when the age of onset is relatively early in life. Parkin functions as a ubiquitin ligase, and the known mutations are believed to lead to a loss of its function *(74)*. It is possible that one or more proteins accumulate as a result, and that this causes nerve cell degeneration. Parkin has been reported to be present in Lewy bodies and to ubiquitinate a minor, O-glycosylated form of α-synuclein *(75–77)*. However, with one exception, mutations in parkin have, so far, not been found to lead to the development of Lewy body pathology *(78–80)*. Furthermore, a more rigorous study using well-characterized anti-parkin antibodies failed to confirm colocalization with α-synuclein *(81)*. In 2002, mutations in the gene *DJ-1* were found to cause another form of AR-JP (PARK7), presumably through a loss of function mechanism *(21)*. The physiological function of DJ-1 remains to be identified. To date, there is no information about the neuropathological features of cases with mutations in DJ-1. DJ-1-immunoreactivity does not colocalize with Lewy bodies or Lewy neurites *(83)*. It will be interesting to see whether there are links between the mechanisms that lead to Lewy body diseases and AR-JP, or whether they constitute distinct disease entities.

MULTIPLE SYSTEM ATROPHY

After the discovery of α-synuclein in the filamentous lesions of Lewy body diseases, multiple system atrophy (MSA) was also shown to be characterized by filamentous α-synuclein deposits (Fig. 5) *(6–8)*. Lewy body pathology is not generally observed in MSA. Instead, glial cytoplasmic inclusions,

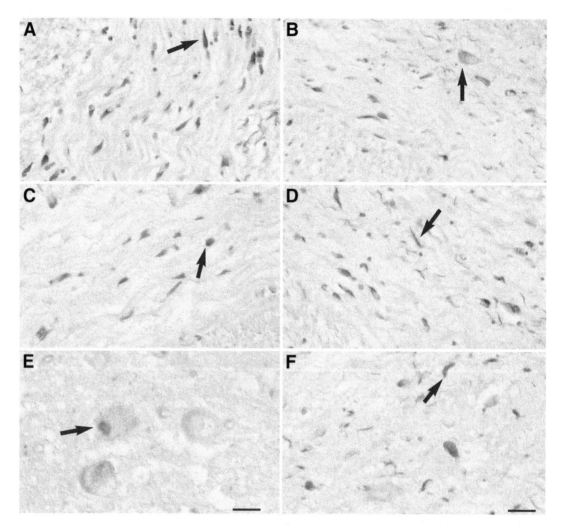

Fig. 5. Brain tissue from patients with multiple system atrophy immunostained for α-synuclein. (**A–D**) α-Synuclein-immunoreactive oligodendrocytes and nerve cells in white matter of pons (A,B,D) and cerebellum (C) identified with antibodies recognizing the amino-terminal (A,C) or the carboxy-terminal (B,D) region of α-synuclein. (**E,F**) α-Synuclein-immunoreactive oligodendrocytes and nerve cells in gray matter of pons (E) and frontal cortex (F) identified with antibodies recognizing the amino-terminal (E) or the carboxy-terminal (F) region of α-synuclein. Arrows identify representative examples of each of the characteristic lesions stained for α-synuclein: cytoplasmic oligodendroglial inclusions (A,F), cytoplasmic nerve cell inclusions (B), nuclear oligodendroglial inclusion (C), neuropil threads (D), and nuclear nerve cell inclusion (E). Scale bars, 33 μm (in E); 50 μm (in F, for A–D,F).

which consist of filamentous aggregates, are the defining neuropathological feature of MSA *(84)*. They are found mostly in the cytoplasm and, to a lesser extent, in the nucleus of oligodendrocytes. Inclusions are also observed in the cytoplasm and nucleus of some nerve cells, and in neuropil threads. The principal brain regions affected are the substantia nigra, striatum, locus coeruleus, pontine nuclei, inferior olives, cerebellum, and spinal cord. Typically, nerve cell loss and gliosis are observed. The formation of glial cytoplasmic inclusions might be the primary lesion that will eventually compromise nerve cell function and viability. Nerve cell loss and clinical symptoms of MSA in the presence of only glial cytoplasmic inclusions have been described *(85)*.

Glial cytoplasmic inclusions are strongly immunoreactive for α-synuclein, and filaments isolated from the brains of patients with MSA are labeled by α-synuclein antibodies *(6–8)*. No staining is obtained with antibodies specific for β- or γ-synuclein. As in DLB, assembled α-synuclein is nitrated and phosphorylated at S129, and the number of α-synuclein-positive structures exceeds that stained by anti-ubiquitin antibodies, indicating again that the accumulation of α-synuclein precedes ubiquitination. The filament morphologies and their staining characteristics were found to be similar to those of filaments extracted from the brains of patients with PD and DLB *(8)*. Two distinct morphologies were observed. Some filaments showed a distinctly twisted appearance, alternating in width between 5 and 18 nm, with a period of 70–90 nm. The other class of filaments had a more uniform width of approx 10 nm. The formation of inclusions was shown to correlate with decreased solubility of α-synuclein. However, the reduction in solubility was less marked than in PD and DLB *(86)*.

This work has revealed an unexpected molecular link between MSA and Lewy body diseases. The main difference is that in MSA most of the α-synuclein pathology is found in glial cells, whereas in Lewy body diseases most of the pathology is present in nerve cells.

SYNTHETIC α-SYNUCLEIN FILAMENTS

Recombinant α-synuclein assembles into filaments that share many of the morphological and ultrastructural characteristics of filaments present in humans (Fig. 6) *(87–89)*. Assembly is a nucleation-dependent process and occurs through the repeats in the amino-terminal half *(90,91)*. The carboxy-terminal region, in contrast, inhibits assembly *(87,92,93)*. It has been reported that the structural transformation involves a partially folded intermediate *(94)*. The A53T mutation increases the rate of filament assembly, indicating that this might be its primary effect *(88,89,92,95)*. The effect of the A30P mutation on the assembly of α-synuclein is less clear. One study reported an increase in filament assembly *(95)*, another study found no change *(92)*, and a third found an inhibitory effect on assembly *(96)*. The third study showed that the A30P monomer was consumed at a similar rate to wild-type α-synuclein, leading to the suggestion that oligomeric, nonfibrillar α-synuclein species might be detrimental to nerve cells. The A30P mutation has also been shown to produce reduced binding of α-synuclein to rat brain vesicles in vitro *(16,97)*, indicating that this might lead to its accumulation over time, resulting in filament assembly. Consistent with this, it has been shown that the α-helical conformation that is induced and stabilized by the interaction between α-synuclein and acidic phospholipids prevents its assembly into filaments *(98)*. Thus, lipid binding and self-assembly of α-synuclein appear to be mutually exclusive.

The assembly of α-synuclein is accompanied by the transition from random coil to a β-pleated sheet *(92,99)*. By electron diffraction, α-synuclein filaments have been found to show a conformation characteristic of amyloid fibers. Under the conditions of these experiments, β- and γ-synuclein failed to assemble into filaments, and remained in a random coil conformation *(92,100)*. This behavior is consistent with their absence from the filamentous lesions of the α-synuclein diseases. When incubated together with α-synuclein, β- and γ-synuclein markedly inhibit the fibrillation of α-synuclein, suggesting that they could indirectly influence the pathogenesis of Lewy body diseases and MSA *(101–103)*.

The sequence requirements for the assembly of α-synuclein are only incompletely understood. One difference between α- and β-synuclein is the presence of a stretch of 11 amino acids (residues 73–83) in α-synuclein that is missing from β-synuclein. It has been suggested that this sequence is both necessary and sufficient for the assembly of α-synuclein and that its absence explains why β-synuclein does not form filaments *(101,104)*. A similar sequence is present in γ-synuclein, but it differs at four positions from residues 73–83 of α-synuclein. Other studies have suggested that residues 71–84 *(105)*, 68–76 *(106)*, or 66–74 *(107)* of α-synuclein are essential for its ability to form filaments.

Many studies have identified factors that influence the rate and/or extent of α-synuclein assembly in vitro. Methionine-oxidized and nitrated α-synucleins were found to be poor at assembling into

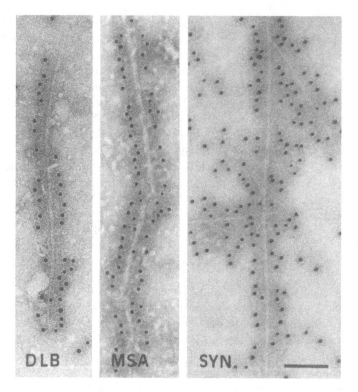

Fig. 6. Filaments extracted from the brains of patients with dementia with Lewy bodies (DLB) and multiple system atrophy (MSA) or assembled from bacterially expressed human α-synuclein (SYN) were decorated by an anti-α-synuclein antibody. The gold particles conjugated to the second antibody appear as black dots. Scale bar, 100 nm.

filaments compared with the unmodified proteins *(108,109)*. For the nitrated protein, stable oligomeric intermediates formed that were reminiscent of protofibrils. A similar inhibition of the protofibril to fibril conversion of α-synuclein has been reported for a number of catecholamines, including oxidized dopamine *(110)*. This has led to the suggestion that nonvesicular, cytoplasmic dopamine may be harmful by sustaining the accumulation of potentially toxic protofibrils. Factors that have been reported to accelerate the fibrillation of α-synuclein include cytochrome C *(111)*, some pesticides *(112)*, several di- and trivalent metal ions *(113)*, sulphated glycosaminoglycans *(114)*, polyamines *(115)*, and oxidized glutathione *(116)*.

The aforementioned substances were used largely because they had previously been implicated in the pathogenesis of PD. These findings in vitro are consistent with many of these hypotheses. However, the true relevance of these factors for the transition from soluble to filamentous α-synuclein in nerve cells in the brain remains to be established.

ANIMAL MODELS

Transgenic Mice

Experimental animal models of α-synucleinopathies are being produced by a number of laboratories (Table 2). They are essential for studying disease pathogenesis and for identifying ways to interfere with the disease process. Several transgenic mouse lines that express wild-type or mutant human

Table 2
Animal Models of α-Synucleinopathies

	Toxin Model	Genetic Models				
	Rotenone	Worm	Fly	Mouse	Rat	Marmoset
Dopaminergic nerve cell loss	+	+	+	–	+	+
Filamentous α-synuclein inclusions	+	–	+	+	u	u
Motor deficits	+	–	+	+	u	u
Complex I inhibition	+	u	u	u	u	u

The rotenone model is in the rat. The genetic models in worm, fly, and mouse are based on the transgenic expression of human α-synuclein (wild-type and mutant), whereas the rat and marmoset models are based on viral vector-mediated transfer of human α-synuclein (wild-type and mutant). u = unknown.

α-synuclein in nerve cells have been described. One study has reported on the effects of α-synuclein overexpression in glial cells. In all published studies, mice developed numerous α-synuclein-immunoreactive cell bodies and processes.

The first study to be published described the expression of wild-type human α-synuclein driven by the human platelet-derived growth factor-β promoter *(117)*. The mice developed cytoplasmic and nuclear intraneuronal inclusions in neocortex, hippocampus, olfactory bulb, and substantia nigra. These inclusions were α-synuclein-immunoreactive, with some being ubiquitin-positive as well. By electron microscopy, they consisted of amorphous, nonfilamentous material. The mice showed a reduction in dopaminergic nerve terminals in the striatum and signs of impaired motor function, but they failed to exhibit nerve cell loss in the substantia nigra. Two studies have reported the expression of wild-type and A53T or A30P mutant human α-synuclein driven by the murine Thy-1 promoter. In one study *(118)*, mice expressing wild-type or A53T mutant α-synuclein developed an early-onset motor impairment that was associated with axonal degeneration in the ventral roots and signs of muscle atrophy. Some α-synuclein inclusions were argyrophilic and ubiquitin-immunoreactive, but they lacked the filaments characteristic of the human diseases. In the second study *(119,120)*, mice expressing A30P mutant α-synuclein developed a neurodegenerative phenotype consisting of the accumulation of protease-resistant human α-synuclein phosphorylated at S129. Occasional inclusions were also ubiquitin-positive. By electron microscopy, filamentous structures were observed, although they were not shown to be made of α-synuclein. The transgenic mice showed a progressive deterioration of motor function. It remains to be seen whether the accumulation of mutant α-synuclein was accompanied by nerve cell loss.

Three studies have described the expression of wild-type and A53T or A30P mutant human α-synuclein under the control of the murine prion protein promoter *(121–123)*. A severe movement disorder was observed that was accompanied by the accumulation of α-synuclein in nerve cells and their processes. One study documented the presence of abundant α-synuclein filaments in brain and spinal cord of mice transgenic for A53T α-synuclein *(121)*. The formation of filamentous inclusions closely correlated with the appearance of clinical symptoms, suggesting a possible cause-and-effect relationship. A minority of inclusions was ubiquitin-immunoreactive. Signs of Wallerian degeneration were much in evidence in ventral roots, but nerve cell numbers in the ventral horn of the spinal cord were unchanged. A major difference with PD was the absence of significant pathology in dopaminergic nerve cells of the substantia nigra. In mice, these neurons appear to be relatively resistant to the effects of α-synuclein expression. This is further supported by reports showing that the expression of wild-type and mutant human α-synuclein under the control of the tyrosine hydroxylase promoter did not lead to the formation of inclusions or neurodegeneration *(124,125)*.

Mouse lines transgenic for wild-type human α-synuclein under the control of a proteolipid protein promoter were generated to give high levels of expression in oligodendroglia *(126)*. Expression of human α-synuclein phosphorylated at S129 was obtained, but there was no sign of argyrophilic glial cytoplasmic inclusions or abnormal filaments. Behavioral changes were also not observed.

Transgenic Flies and Worms

One of the first reports describing the overexpression of α-synuclein made use of *Drosophila melanogaster*, an organism without synucleins *(127)*. Expression of wild-type and A30P or A53T mutant human α-synuclein in nerve cells of *D. melanogaster* resulted in the formation of filamentous Lewy body–like inclusions and an age-dependent loss of some dopaminergic nerve cells (Table 2). The inclusions were α-synuclein- and ubiquitin-immunoreactive. An age-dependent locomotor defect was observed that could be reversed by the administration of L-DOPA or several dopamine agonists, underscoring the validity of this model for PD *(128)*. Overexpression of wild-type and A53T mutant human α-synuclein in nerve cells of *Caenorhabditis elegans* resulted in a loss of dopaminergic nerve cells and motor deficits, in the apparent absence of filamentous α-synuclein inclusions (Table 2) *(129)*.

Disease models in *D. melanogaster* and *C. elegans* offer some advantages over mouse models, in particular with regard to the speed and relative ease with which genetic modifiers of disease phenotype can be discovered and pharmacological modifiers can be screened. Coexpression of human heat-shock protein 70 alleviated the toxicity of α-synuclein in transgenic flies *(130)*. Conversely, a reduction in the fly chaperone system exacerbated nerve cell loss. Increasing chaperone activity through the administration of geldanamycin delayed neurodegeneration in transgenic flies *(131)*. It thus appears that chaperones can modulate the neurotoxicity resulting from the overexpression of human α-synuclein.

Viral Vector-Mediated Gene Transfer

Viral vector-mediated gene transfer differs from standard transgenic approaches by being targeted to a defined region of the central nervous system and by being inducible at any point during the life of the animal. Recombinant adeno-associated virus and recombinant lentivirus vector systems have been used to express wild-type and mutant α-synuclein in the substantia nigra of rat and marmoset (Table 2).

In the rat, expression of α-synuclein was maximal 2–3 wk after virus injection *(132–134)*. At 8–10 wk, numerous swollen, dystrophic axons and dendrites were observed in conjunction with α-synuclein inclusions. Nerve cell bodies contained Lewy body–like inclusions and substantial nerve cell loss (30–80%) was present in the substantia nigra. The inclusions were α-synuclein-positive and ubiquitin-negative, but it remains to be determined whether they were also filamentous. Behaviorally, about a quarter of animals were impaired in spontaneous and drug-induced motor behaviors. Similar findings were reported for wild-type and A30P or A53T mutant human α-synuclein. One study has reported that degeneration of transduced nigral cells was seen upon expression of human, but not rat, α-synuclein *(134)*. In the marmoset, dopaminergic nerve cells of the substantia nigra were transduced with high efficiency and human α-synuclein was expressed *(135)*. Similar to the rat, α-synuclein-positive inclusions were observed, together with a loss of 40–75% of tyrosine hydroxylase-positive neurons. Overexpression of disease-causing gene products by using recombinant viral vectors constitutes a promising way forward for modeling human neurodegenerative diseases in a number of species, including primates.

Rotenone Neurotoxicity

A model of α-synuclein pathology has been developed in the rat by using the chronic administration of the pesticide rotenone, a high-affinity inhibitor of complex I, one of the five enzyme complexes of the inner mitochondrial membrane involved in oxidative phosphorylation *(136,137)*. The rats developed a progressive degeneration of nigrostriatal neurons and Lewy body-like inclusions that were immunoreactive for α-synuclein and ubiquitin (Table 2). Behaviorally, they showed bradykinesia, postural instability, and some evidence of resting tremor. Using this regime of rotenone administration, the inhibition of complex I was only partial, indicating that a bioenergetic defect with ATP (adenosine 5'-triphosphate) depletion was probably not involved. Instead, oxidative damage might have contributed to this condition, as partial inhibition of complex I by rotenone is known to stimulate the production of reactive oxygen species. It would therefore seem that oxidative stress can lead to the assembly of α-synuclein into filaments. Although it remains to be seen how robust a model rotenone administration is, it appears clear that it can lead to the degeneration of nigrostriatal dopaminergic nerve cells in association with α-synuclein-positive inclusions. This has so far not been achieved following the administration of either 6-hydroxydopamine or MPTP, the two most widely used toxin models of PD. It has been reported that the systemic administration of rotenone leads to the specific degeneration of dopaminergic nerve cells in the substantia nigra. However, a subsequent study has described additional nerve cell loss in the striatum *(138)*, raising the question of how valid a model rotenone intoxication is for PD.

CONCLUSION

The relevance of α-synuclein for the neurodegenerative process in Lewy body diseases and MSA is now well established. The development of experimental models of α-synucleinopathies has opened the way to the identification of the detailed mechanisms by which the formation of inclusions causes disease. These model systems have also made it possible to identify disease modifiers (enhancers and suppressors) that may well lead to the development of the first mechanism-based therapies for these diseases. At a conceptual level, it will be important to understand whether α-synuclein has a role to play in disorders, such as the autosomal-recessive juvenile forms of parkinsonism caused by mutations in the parkin and DJ-1 genes, or whether there are entirely separate mechanisms by which the dopaminergic nerve cells of the substantia nigra degenerate in PD and in inherited disorders with parkinsonism.

MAJOR RESEARCH ISSUES

The new work has established that a neurodegenerative pathway leading from soluble to insoluble, filamentous α-synuclein is central to Lewy body diseases and multiple system atrophy. The study of familial forms of diseases with filamentous α-synuclein inclusions has revealed that missense mutations in the α-synuclein gene or overexpression of wild-type protein are sufficient to cause neurodegeneration. It appears likely that these genetic defects induce the assembly of α-synuclein into filaments. What causes assembly of α-synuclein in the much more common cases of sporadic disease remains to be discovered. In normal brain, the biophysically driven propensity of α-synuclein to undergo ordered self-assembly is probably counterbalanced by a number of factors, including the ability of cells to dispose of the protein prior to assembly. Other factors may include the binding of α-synuclein to lipid membranes and its interactions with β- and γ-synucleins. Identification of the detailed mechanisms at work constitutes an important area for future research. In particular, we need to know more about the factors that regulate the production of α-synuclein and the mechanisms that ensure its degradation. We need to understand what the toxic α-synuclein species are and how they exert their effects. It appears probable that all familial forms of Lewy body disease are caused by genetic defects that act at the level of the neurodegenerative α-synuclein pathway. It remains to be seen whether they are mechanistically linked to familial forms of parkinsonism that lead to nerve cell loss in the substantia nigra, without formation of Lewy body pathology. The availability of ever better animal models of the α-synucleinopathies opens the way to the identification of genetic and pharmacological modifiers (enhancers and suppressors) of the disease process. This will be essential for a better understanding of the pathogenesis of Lewy body diseases and multiple system atrophy and for the discovery of novel therapeutic avenues.

REFERENCES

1. Jellinger KA, Mizuno Y. Parkinson's disease. In: Dickson D, ed. Neurodegeneration: The Molecular Pathology of Dementia and Movement Disorders. Basel: ISN Neuropath Press, 2003: 159–187.
2. Ince PG, McKeith IG. Dementia with Lewy bodies. In: Dickson D, ed. Neurodegeneration: The Molecular Pathology of Dementia and Movement Disorders. Basel: ISN Neuropath Press, 2003:188–199.
3. Lewy F. *Paralysis agitans*. In: Lewandowski M, Abelsdorff G, eds. Handbuch der Neurologie. Berlin: Springer Verlag, 1912: 920–933.
4. Polymeropoulos MH, Lavedan C, Leroy E, et al. Mutation in the α-synuclein gene identified in families with Parkinson's disease. Science 1997;276:2045–2047.
5. Spillantini MG, Schmidt ML, Lee VMY, Trojanowski JQ, Jakes R, Goedert M. α-Synuclein in Lewy bodies. Nature 1997;388:839–840.
6. Wakabayashi K, Yoshimoto M, Tsuji S, Takahashi H. α-Synuclein immunoreactivity in glial cytoplasmic inclusions in multiple system atrophy. Neurosci Lett 1998;249:180–182.
7. Tu PH, Galvin JE, Baba M, et al. Glial cytoplasmic inclusions in white matter oligodendrocytes of multiple system atrophy brains contain insoluble α-synuclein. Ann Neurol 1998;44:415–422.
8. Spillantini MG, Crowther RA, Jakes R, Cairns NJ, Lantos PL, Goedert M. Filamentous α-synuclein inclusions link multiple system atrophy with Parkinson's disease and dementia with Lewy bodies. Neurosci Lett 1998;251:205–208.
9. Ueda K, Fukushima H, Masliah E, et al. Molecular cloning of cDNA encoding an unrecognized component of amyloid in Alzheimer disease. Proc Natl Acad Sci USA 1993;90:11282–11286.
10. Jakes R, Spillantini MG, Goedert M. Identification of two distinct synucleins from human brain. FEBS Lett 1994;345:27–32.
11. Ji H, Liu YE, Jia T, et al. Identification of a breast cancer-specific gene, BCSG1, by direct differential cDNA sequencing. Cancer Res 1997;57:759–764.
12. Clayton DF, George JM. Synucleins in synaptic plasticity and neurodegenerative disorders. J Neurosci Res 1999;58:120–129.
13. Li JY, Jensen PH, Dahlström A. Differential localization of α-, β- and γ-synucleins in the rat CNS. Neuroscience 2002;113:463–478.
14. Weinreb PH, Zhen W, Poon AW, Conway KA, Lansbury PT. NACP, a protein implicated in Alzheimer's disease and learning, is natively unfolded. Biochemistry 1996;35:13709–13715.
15. Davidson WS, Jonas A, Clayton DF, George, JM. Stabilization of α-synuclein secondary structure upon binding to synthetic membranes. J Biol Chem 1998;273:9443–9449.
16. Jensen PH, Nielsen MH, Jakes R, Dotti CG, Goedert M. Binding of α-synuclein to rat brain vesicles is abolished by familial Parkinson's disease mutation. J Biol Chem 1998;273:26292–26294.
17. Chandra S, Cheng X, Rizo J, Jahn R, Südhof TC. A broken α-helix in folded α-synuclein. J Biol Chem 2003;278:15313–15318.
18. Bussell R, Eliezer D. A structural and functional role for 11-mer repeats in α-synuclein and other exchangeable lipid binding proteins. J Mol Biol 2003;329:763–778.
19. Cole NB, Murphy DD, Grider T, Rueter S, Brasaemle D, Nussbaum RL. Lipid droplet binding and oligomerization properties of the Parkinson's disease protein α-synuclein. J Biol Chem 2002;277:6344–6352.
20. Sharon R, Goldberg MS, Bar-Joseph I, Betensky RA, Shen J, Selkoe DJ. α-Synuclein occurs in lipid-rich high molecular weight complexes, binds fatty acids, and shows homology to the fatty acid-binding proteins. Proc Natl Acad Sci USA 2002;98:9110–9115.
21. Sharon R, Bar-Joseph I, Frosch MP, Walsh DM, Hamilton JA, Selkoe DJ. The formation of highly soluble oligomers of α-synuclein is regulated by fatty acids and enhanced in Parkinson's disease. Neuron 2003;37:583–595.
22. Jenco RM, Rawlingson A, Daniels B, Morris AJ. Regulation of phospholipase D2: selective inhibition of mammalian phospholipase D isoenzymes by α- and β-synucleins. Biochemistry 1998;37:4901–4909.
23. Okochi M, Walter J, Koyama A, et al. Constitutive phosphorylation of the Parkinson's disease–associated α-synuclein. J Biol Chem 2000;275:390–397.
24. Fujiwara H, Hasegawa M, Dohmae N, et al. α-Synuclein is phosphorylated in synucleinopathy lesions. Nature Cell Biol 2002;4:160–164.

25. Pronin AN, Morris AJ, Surguchov A, Benovic JL. Synucleins are a novel class of substrates for G protein–coupled receptor kinases. J Biol Chem 2000;275:26515–26522.
26. Ahn BH, Rhim H, Kim SY, et al. α-Synuclein interacts with phospholipase D isozymes and inhibits pervanadate-induced phospholipase D activation in human embryonic kidney-293 cells. J Biol Chem 2002;277:12334–12342.
27. Nakamura T, Yamashita H, Takahashi T, Nakamura S. Activated Fyn phosphorylates α-synuclein at tyrosine residue 125. Biochem Biophys Res Commun 2001;280:1085–1092.
28. Ellis CE, Schwartzberg PL, Grider TL, Fink DW, Nussbaum RL. α-Synuclein is phosphorylated by members of the Src family of protein tyrosine kinases. J Biol Chem 2001;276:3879–3884.
29. Nakamura T, Yamshita H, Nagano Y, et al. Activation of Pyk2/RAFTK induces tyrosine phosphorylation of α-synuclein via Src-family kinases. FEBS Lett 2002;521:190–194.
30. Tofaris GK, Layfield R, Spillantini MG. α-Synuclein metabolism and aggregation is linked to ubiquitin-independent degradation by the proteasome. FEBS Lett 2001;509:22–26.
31. Abeliovich A, Schmitz Y, Farinas I, et al. Mice lacking α-synuclein display functional deficits in the nigrostriatal dopamine system. Neuron 2000;25:239–252.
32. Cabin DE, Shimazu K, Murphy D, et al. Synaptic vesicle depletion correlates with attenuated synaptic responses to prolonged repetitive stimulation in mice lacking α-synuclein. J Neurosci 2002;22:8797–8807.
33. Specht CG, Schoepfer R. Deletion of the α-synuclein locus in a subpopulation of C57BL/6J inbred mice. BMC Neurosci 2001;2:11.
34. Ninkina N, Papachroni K, Robertson DC, et al. Neurons expressing the highest levels of γ-synuclein are unaffected by targeted inactivation of the gene. Mol Cell Biol 2003;23:8233–8245.
35. Dauer W, Kholodilov N, Vila M, et al. Resistance of α-synuclein null mice to the parkinsonian neurotoxin MPTP. Proc Natl Acad Sci USA 2002;99:14254–14259.
36. Schlüter OM, Fornai F, Alessandri MG, et al. Role of α-synuclein in 1-methyl-4-phenyl-1,2,3,6-tetrahydropyridine-induced parkinsonism in mice. Neuroscience 2003;118:985–1002.
37. Golbe LI, Di Iorio G, Sanges G, et al. Clinical genetic analysis of Parkinson's disease in the Contursi kindred. Ann Neurol 1990;27:276–282.
38. Polymeropoulos MH, Higgins JJ, Golbe LI, et al. Mapping of a gene for Parkinson's disease to chromosome 4q21-q23. Science 1996;274:1197–1199.
39. Krüger T, Kuhn W, Müller T, et al. Ala30Pro mutation in the gene encoding α-synuclein in Parkinson's disease. Nature Genet 1998;18:106–108.
40. Muenter MD, Forno LS, Hornykiewicz O, et al. Hereditary form of Parkinsonism-dementia. Ann Neurol 1998;43:768–781.
41. Singleton AB, Farrer M, Johnson J, et al. α-Synuclein locus triplication causes Parkinson's disease. Science 2003;302:841.
42. Krüger R, Vieira-Saecker AMM, Kuhn W, et al. Increased susceptibility to sporadic Parkinson's disease by a certain combined α-synuclein/apolipoprotein E genotype. Ann Neurol 1998;45:611–617.
43. Tan EK, Matsuura T, Nagamitsu S, Khajavi M, Jankovic J, Ashizawa T. Polymorphism of NACP-Rep1 in Parkinson's disease: an etiologic link with essential tremor? Neurology 2000;54:1195–1198.
44. Khan N, Graham E, Dixon P, et al. Parkinson's disease is not associated with the combined α-synuclein/apolipoprotein E susceptibility genotype. Ann Neurol 2001;49:665–668.
45. Farrer M, Maraganore DM, Lockhart P, et al. α-Synuclein gene haplotypes are associated with Parkinson's disease. Hum Mol Genet 2001;10:1847–1851.
46. Chiba-Falek O, Nussbaum RL. Effect of allelic variation at the NACP-Rep1 repeat upstream of the α-synuclein gene (SNCA) on transcription in a cell culture luciferase reporter system. Hum Mol Genet 2001;10:3101–3109.
47. Arima K, Ueda K, Sunohara N, et al. Immunoelectron microscopic demonstration of NACP/α-synuclein epitopes on the filamentous component of Lewy bodies in Parkinson's disease and in dementia with Lewy bodies. Brain Res 1998;808:93–100.
48. Crowther RA, Daniel SE, Goedert M. Characterisation of isolated α-synuclein filaments from substantia nigra of Parkinson's disease brain. Neurosci Lett 2000;292:128–130.
49. Spillantini MG, Crowther RA, Jakes R, Hasegawa M, Goedert M. α-Synuclein in filamentous inclusions of Lewy bodies from Parkinson's disease and dementia with Lewy bodies. Proc Natl Acad Sci USA 1998;95:6469–6473.
50. Baba M, Nakajo S, Tu PS, et al. Aggregation of α-synuclein in Lewy bodies of sporadic Parkinson's disease and dementia with Lewy bodies. Am J Pathol 1998;152:879–884.
51. Miake H, Mizusawa H, Iwatsubo T, Hasegawa M. Biochemical characterization of the core structure of α-synuclein filaments. J Biol Chem 2002;277:19213–19219.
52. Der-Sarkissian A, Jao CC, Chen J, Langen R. Structural organization of α-synuclein fibrils studied by site-directed spin labeling. J Biol Chem 2003;278:37530–37535.
53. Kuzuhara S, Mori H, Izumiyama N, Yoshimura M, Ihara Y. Lewy bodies are ubiquitinated: a light and electron microscopic immunocytochemical study. Acta Neuropathol 1988;75:345–353.
54. Sampathu DM, Giasson BI, Pawlyk AC, Trojanowski JQ, Lee VMY. Ubiquitination of α-synuclein is not required for formation of pathological inclusions in α-synucleinopathies. Am J Pathol 2003;163:91–100.

55. Tofaris GK, Razzaq A, Ghetti B, Lilley K, Spillantini MG. Ubiquitination of α-synuclein in Lewy bodies is a pathological event not associated with impairment of proteasome function. J Biol Chem 2003;278:44405–44411.

56. Hasegawa M, Fujiwara H, Nonaka T, et al. Phosphorylated α-synuclein is ubiquitinated in α-synucleinopathy lesions. J Biol Chem 2002;277:49071–49076.

57. Giasson BI, Duda JE, Murray IV, et al. Oxidative damage linked to neurodegeneration by selective α-synuclein nitration in synucleinopathy lesions. Science 2000;290:985–989.

58. Arai K, Kato N, Kashiwado K, Hattori T. Pure autonomic failure in association with human α-synucleinopathy. Neurosci Lett 2000;296:171–173.

59. Kaufmann H, Hague K, Perl D. Accumulation of alpha-synuclein in autonomic nerves in pure autonomic failure. Neurology 2001;56: 980–981.

60. Perry RH, Irving D, Tomlinson BE. Lewy body prevalence in the aging brain: relationship to neuropsychiatric disorders, Alzheimer-type pathology and catecholaminergic nuclei. J Neurol Sci 1990;100:223–233.

61. Saito Y, Kawashima A, Ruberu NN, et al. Accumulation of phosphorylated α-synuclein in aging human brain. J Neuropathol Exp Neurol 2003;62:644–654.

62. Del Tredici K, Rüb U, De Vos RAI, Bohl JRE, Braak H. Where does Parkinson disease pathology begin in the brain? J Neuropathol Exp Neurol 2002;61:413–426.

63. Lippa CF, Fujiwara H, Mann DM, et al. Lewy bodies contain altered α-synuclein in brains of many familial Alzheimer's disease patients with mutations in presenilin and amyloid precursor protein genes. Am J Pathol 1998;153:1365–1370.

64. Yamazaki M, Arai Y, Baba M, et al. α-Synuclein inclusions in amygdala in the brains of patients with the parkinsonism-dementia complex of Guam. J Neuropathol Exp Neurol 2000;59:585–591.

65. Spira PJ, Sharpe DM, Halliday G, Cavanagh J, Nicholson GA. Clinical and pathological features of a parkinsonian syndrome in a family with an Ala53Thr α-synuclein mutation. Ann Neurol 2001;49:313–319.

66. Duda JE, Giasson BI, Mahon ME, et al. Concurrence of α-synuclein and tau brain pathology in the Contursi kindred. Acta Neuropathol 2002;104:7–11.

67. Ishizawa T, Mattila P, Davies P, Wang D, Dickson DW. Colocalization of tau and alpha-synuclein epitopes in Lewy bodies. J Neuropathol Exp Neurol 2003;62:389–397.

68. Giasson BI, Forman MS, Higuchi M, et al. Initiation and synergistic fibrillization of tau and alpha-synuclein. Science 2003;300:636–640.

69. Gwinn-Hardy K, Mehta ND, Farrer M, et al. Distinctive neuropathology revealed by α-synuclein antibodies in hereditary parkinsonism and dementia linked to chromosome 4p. Acta Neuropathol 2000;99:663–672.

70. Gasser T, Müller-Myhsok B, Wszolek ZK, et al. A susceptiibility locus for Parkinson's disease maps to chromosome 2p13. Nature Genet 1998;18:262–265.

71. Wszolek ZK, Gwinn-Hardy K, Wszolek EK, et al. Neuropathology of two members of a German-American kindred (Family C) with late onset parkinsonism. Acta Neuropathol 2002;103:344–350.

72. Leroy E, Boyer R, Auburger G, et al. The ubiquitin pathway in Parkinson's disease. Nature 1998;395:451–452.

73. Kitada T, Asakawa S, Hattori N, et al. Mutations in the parkin gene cause autosomal recessive juvenile parkinsonism. Nature 1998;392:605–608.

74. Shimura H, Hattori N, Kubo S, et al. Familial Parkinson's disease gene product, parkin, is a ubiquitin-protein ligase. Nature Genet 2000;25:302–305.

75. Choi P, Golts N, Snyder H, et al. Co-association of parkin and alpha-synuclein. Neuroreport 2001;12:2839–2843.

76. Schlossmacher MG, Frosch MP, Gai WP, et al. Parkin localizes to the Lewy bodies of Parkinson disease and dementia with Lewy bodies. Am J Pathol 2002;160:1655–1667.

77. Shimura H, Schlossmacher MG, Hattori N, et al. Ubiquitination of a new form of alpha-synuclein by parkin from human brain: implications for Parkinson's disease. Science 2001;293:263–269.

78. Takahashi H, Ohama E, Suzuki S, et al. Familial juvenile parkinsonism: clinical and pathologic study in a family. Neurology 1994;44:437–441.

79. Mori H, Kondo T, Yokochi M, et al. Pathologic and biochemical studies of juvenile parkinsonism linked to chromosome 6q. Neurology 1998;51:890–892.

80. Farrer M, Chan P, Chen R, et al. Lewy bodies and parkinsonism in families with parkin mutations. Neurology 2001;50:293–300.

81. Pawlyk AC, Giasson BI, Sampathu DM, et al. Novel monoclonal antibodies demonstrate biochemical variation of brain parkin with age. J Biol Chem 2003;278:48,120–48,128.

82. Bonifati V, Rizzu P, van Baren MJ, et al. Mutations in the DJ-1 gene associated with autosomal recessive early-onset parkinsonism. Science 2003;299:256–259.

83. Takao M, Ghetti B, Yoshida H, et al. Early-onset dementia with Lewy bodies. Brain Pathol 2004;14:137–147.

84. Lantos PL, Quinn N. Multiple system atrophy. In: Dickson D, ed. Neurodegeneration: The Molecular Pathology of Dementia and Movement Disorders. Basel: ISN Neuropath Press, 2003: 203–214.

85. Wenning GK, Quinn N, Magalhaes M, Mathias C, Daniel SE. "Minimal change" multiple system atrophy. Mov Disord 1994;9:161–166.

86. Campbell BC, McLean CA, Culvenor JG, et al. The solubility of alpha-synuclein in multiple system atrophy differs from that of dementia with Lewy bodies and Parkinson's disease. J Neurochem 2001;76:87–96.

87. Crowther RA, Jakes R, Spillantini MG, Goedert M. Synthetic filaments assembled from C-terminally truncated α-synuclein. FEBS Lett 1998;436:309–312.

88. Conway KA, Harper DJ, Lansbury PT. Accelerated in vitro fibril formation by a mutant α-synuclein linked to early-onset Parkinson's disease. Nature Med 1998;4:1318–1320.

89. El-Agnaf IMA, Jakes R, Curran MD, Wallace A. Effects of the mutations Ala30 to Pro and Ala53 to Thr on the physical and morphological properties of α-synuclein implicated in Parkinson's disease. FEBS Lett 1998;440:67–70.

90. Giasson BI, Uryu K, Trojanowski JQ, Lee VMY. Mutant and wild-type human α-synuclein assemble into elongated filaments with distinct morphologies in vitro. J Biol Chem 1999;274:7619–7622.

91. Wood SJ, Wypych J, Steavenson S, Louis JC, Citron M, Biere AL. α-Synuclein fibrillogenesis is nucleation-dependent. J Biol Chem 1999;274:19509–19512.

92. Serpell LC, Berriman J, Jakes R, Goedert M, Crowther RA. Fiber diffraction of synthetic alpha-synuclein filaments shows amyloid-like cross-beta conformation. Proc Natl Acad Sci USA 2000;97:4897–4902.

93. Murray IVJ, Giasson BI, Quinn SM, et al. Role of α-synuclein carboxy-terminus on fibril formation in vitro. Biochemistry 2003;42:8530–8540.

94. Uversky VN, Li J, Fink AL. Evidence for a partially folded intermediate in α-synuclein fibril formation. J Biol Chem 2001;276:10737–10744.

95. Narhi L, Wood SJ, Steavenson S, et al. Both familial Parkinson's disease mutations accelerate α-synuclein aggregation. J Biol Chem 1999;274:9843–9846.

96. Conway KA, Lee SJ, Rochet JC, Ding TT, Williamson RE, Lansbury PT. Acceleration of oligomerization, not fibrillization, is a shared property of both alpha-synuclein mutations linked to early-onset Parkinson's disease: implications for pathogenesis and therapy. Proc Natl Acad Sci USA 2000;97:571–576.

97. Jo E, Fuller N, Rand PR, St George-Hyslop P, Fraser PE. Defective membrane interactions of familial Parkinson's disease mutant A30P α-synuclein. J Mol Biol 2002;315:799–807.

98. Zhu M, Fink AL. Lipid binding inhibits α-synuclein filament formation. J Biol Chem 2003;278:16873–16877.

99. Conway KA, Harper JD, Lansbury PT. Fibrils formed in vitro from alpha-synuclein and two mutant forms linked to Parkinson's disease are typical amyloid. Biochemistry 2000;39:2552–2563.

100. Biere AL, Wood SJ, Wypych J, et al. Parkinson's disease-associated α-synuclein is more fibrillogenic than β- and γ-synuclein and cannot cross-seed its homologs. J Biol Chem 2000;275:34574–34579.

101. Hashimoto M, Rockenstein E, Mante, Mallory M, Masliah E. β-Synuclein inhibits α-synuclein aggregation: a possible role as an antiparkinsonian factor. Neuron 2001;32:213–223.

102. Uversky VN, Li J, Souillac P, et al. Biophysical properties of the synucleins and their propensities to fibrillate: inhibition of α-synuclein assembly by β- and γ-synucleins. J Biol Chem 2002;277:11970–11978.

103. Park JY, Lansbury PT. β-Synuclein inhibits formation of α-synuclein protofibrils: a possible therapeutic strategy against Parkinson's disease. Biochemistry 2003;42:3696–3700.

104. Kahle PJ, Neumann M, Ozmen L, et al. Selective insolubility of α-synuclein in human Lewy body diseases is recapitulated in a transgenic mouse model. Am J Pathol 2001;159:2215–2225.

105. Giasson BI, Murray IVJ, Trojanowski JQ, Lee VMY. A hydrophobic stretch of 12 amino acid residues in the middle of α-synuclein is essential for filament assembly. J Biol Chem 2001;276:2380–2386.

106. Bodles AM, Guthrie DJS, Greer B, Irvine GB. Identification of the region of non-Aβ component (NAC) of Alzheimer's disease amyloid responsible for its aggregation and toxicity. J Neurochem 2001;78:384–395.

107. Du HN, Tang L, Luo XY, et al. A peptide motif consisting of glycine, alanine, and valine is required for the fibrillation and cytotoxicity of human α-synuclein. Biochemistry 2003;42:8870–8878.

108. Uversky VN, Yamin G, Souillac PO, Goers J, Glaser CB, Fink AL. Methionine oxidation inhibits fibrillation of human α-synuclein in vitro. FEBS Lett 2002;517:239–244.

109. Yamin G, Uversky VN, Fink AL. Nitration inhibits fibrillation of human α-synuclein in vitro by formation of soluble oligomers. FEBS Lett 2003;542:147–152.

110. Conway KA, Rochet JC, Bieganski RM, Lansbury PT. Kinetic stabilization of the α-synuclein protofibril by a dopamine-α-synuclein adduct. Science 2001;294:1346–1349.

111. Hashimoto M, Takeda A, Hsu LJ, Takenouchi T, Masliah E. Role of cytochrome C as a stimulator of α-synuclein aggregation in Lewy body disease. J Biol Chem 1999;274:28849–28852.

112. Uversky VN, Li J, Fink AL. Pesticides directly accelerate the rate of α-synuclein fibril formation: a possible factor in Parkinson's disease. FEBS Lett 2001;500:105–108.

113. Uversky VN, Li J, Fink AL. Metal-triggered structural transformations, aggregation and fibril formation of human α-synuclein. A possible molecular link between Parkinson's disease and heavy metal exposure. J Biol Chem 2001;276:44284–44296.

114. Cohlberg JA, Li J, Uversky VN, Fink AL. Heparin and other glycosaminoglycans stimulate the formation of amyloid fibrils from α-synuclein in vitro. J Biol Chem 2002;41:1502–1511.

115. Antony T, Hoyer W, Cherny D, Heim G, Jovin TM, Subramaniam V. Cellular polyamines promote the aggregation of α-synuclein. J Biol Chem 2003;278:3235–3240.

116. Paik SR, Lee D, Cho HJ, Lee EN, Chang CS. Oxidized glutathione stimulated the amyloid formation of α-synuclein. FEBS Lett 2003;537:63–67.

117. Masliah E, Rockenstein E, Veinbergs I, et al. Dopaminergic loss and inclusion body formation in α-synuclein mice: implications for neurodegenerative disorders. Science 2000;287:1265–1269.

118. Van der Putten H, Wiederhold KH, Probst A, et al. Neuropathology in mice expressing human α-synuclein. J Neurosci 2000;20:6021–6029.

119. Kahle PJ, Neumann N, Ozmen L, et al. Subcellular localization of wild-type and Parkinson's disease–associated mutant α-synuclein in human and transgenic mouse brain. J Neurosci 2000;20:6365–6373.

120. Neumann M, Kahle PJ, Giasson BI, et al. Misfolded proteinase K–resistant hyperphosphorylated α-synuclein in aged transgenic mice with locomotor deterioration and in human α-synucleinopathies. J Clin Invest 2002;110:1429–1439.

121. Giasson BI, Duda JE, Quinn SM, Zhang B, Trojanowski JQ, Lee VMY. Neuronal α-synucleinopathy with severe movement disorder in mice expressing A53T human α-synuclein. Neuron 2002;34:521–533.

122. Lee MK, Stirling W, Xu Y et al. Human α-synuclein-harboring familial Parkinson's disease–linked Ala53 to Thr mutation causes neurodegenerative disease with α-synuclein aggregation in transgenic mice. Proc Natl Acad Sci USA 2002;99:8968–8973

123. Gomez-Isla T, Irizarry MC, Mariash A, et al. Motor dysfunction and gliosis with preserved dopaminergic markers in human α-synuclein A30P transgenic mice. Neurobiol Aging 2003;24:245–258.

124. Matsuoka Y, Vila M, Lincoln S, et al. Lack of nigral pathology in transgenic mice expressing human α-synuclein driven by the tyrosine hydroxylase promoter. Neurobiol Dis 2001;8:535–539.

125. Richfield EK, Thiruchelvam MJ, Cory-Schlechta DA, et al. Behavioral and neurochemical effects of wild-type and mutated human α-synuclein in transgenic mice. Exp Neurol 2002;175:35–48.

126. Kahle PJ, Neumann M, Ozmen L, et al. Hyperphosphorylation and insolubility of α-synuclein in transgenic mouse oligodendrocytes. EMBO Rep 2002;3:583–588.

127. Feany MB, Bender WW. A *Drosophila* model of Parkinson's disease. Nature 2000;404:394–398.

128. Pendleton RG, Parvez F, Sayed M, Hillman R. Effects of pharmacological agents upon a transgenic model of Parkinson's disease in *Drosophila melanogaster*. J Pharmacol Exp Ther 2002;300:91–96.

129. Lakso M, Vartiainen S, Moilanen AM, et al. Dopaminergic neuronal loss and motor deficits in Caenorhabditis elegans overexpressing human α-synuclein. J Neurochem 2003;86:165–172.

130. Auluck PK, Chan E, Trojanowski JQ, Lee VMY, Bonini NM. Chaperone suppression of α-synuclein toxicity in a *Drosophila* model for Parkinson's disease. Science 2002;295:865–868.

131. Auluck PK, Bonini NM. Pharmacologic prevention of Parkinson's disease in *Drosophila*. Nature Med 2002;8:1185–1186.

132. Klein RL, King MA, Hamby ME, Meyer EM. Dopaminergic cell loss induced by human A30P α-synuclein gene transfer to the rat substantia nigra. Hum Gene Ther 2002;13:605–612.

133. Kirik D, Rosenblad C, Burger C, et al. Parkinson-like neurodegeneration induced by targeted overexpression of α-synuclein in the nigrostriatal system. J Neurosci 2002;22:2780–2791.

134. Lo Bianco C, Ridet JL, Schneider BL, Déglon N, Aebischer P. α-Synucleinopathy and selective dopaminergic neuron loss in a rat lentiviral-based model of Parkinson's disease. Proc Natl Acad Sci USA 2002;99:10813–10818.

135. Kirik D, Annett LE, Burger C, Muzyczka N, Mandel RJ, Björklund A. Nigrostriatal α-synucleinopathy induced by viral vector–mediated overexpression of human α-synuclein: a new primate model of Parkinson's disease. Proc Natl Acad Sci USA 2003;100:2884–2889.

136. Betarbet R, Sherer TB, MacKenzie G, Garcia-Osuna M, Panov AV, Greenamyre JT. Chronic systemic pesticide exposure reproduces features of Parkinson's disease. Nature Neurosci 2000;3:1301–1306.

137. Sherer TB, Kim JH, Betarbet R, Greenamyre JT. Subcutaneous rotenone exposure causes highly selective dopaminergic degeneration and α-synuclein aggregation. Exp Neurol 2003;179:9–16.

138. Höglinger GU, Féger J, Prigent A, et al. Chronic systemic complex I inhibition induces a hypokinetic multisystem degeneration in rats. J Neurochem 2003;84:491–502.

7

Computer Modeling in Basal Ganglia Disorders

José Luis Contreras-Vidal

1. INTRODUCTION

The last two decades have witnessed an increasing interest in the use of computational modeling and mathematical analysis as tools to unravel the complex neural mechanisms and computational algorithms underlying the function of the basal ganglia and related structures under normal and neurological conditions *(1–3)*. Computational modeling of basal ganglia disorders has until recently been focused on Parkinson's disease (PD), and to a smaller scale, Huntington's disease (HD) *(4–6)*. However, with the advent of large-scale neural network models of frontal, parietal, basal ganglia, and cerebellar network dynamics *(7–9)*, it is now possible to use these models as a window to study neurological disorders that involve more distributed pathology such as in atypical parkinsonian disorders (APDs). Importantly, computational models may also be used for bridging data across scales to reduce the gap between electrophysiology and human brain imaging *(10)*, to integrate data in all areas of neurobiology and across modalities *(11)*, and to guide the design of novel experiments and intervention programs (e.g., optimization of pharmacotherapy in PD) *(12)*.

This chapter aims to present the paradigm of computational modeling as applied to the study of PD and APDs so that it can be understood for those approaching it for the first time. Therefore, mathematical details are kept to a minimum; however, references to detailed mathematical treatments are given. The brain, in its intact state, is a very complex dynamical system both structurally and functionally, and many questions remain unanswered. However, theoretical and computational neuroscience approaches may prove to be a very valuable tool for the neuroscientist and the neurologist in understanding how the brain works in health and disease.

The Modeling Paradigm

Computational models of brain and neurological disorders vary widely in the focus and scale of the modeling, their degrees of simulated biological realism, and the mathematical approach used *(13)*. A combination of "top-down" and "bottom-up" approaches to computational modeling in neuroscience is depicted in Fig. 1, which shows the series of steps that need to be taken to study brain disorders computationally. One first has to measure the behavioral operating characteristics (BOCs), such as movement kinematics, average firing rates of homogenous cell populations, or neurotransmitter levels under intact conditions. The next step is to construct a mathematical model based on the behavioral, anatomical, neurophysiological, and pharmacological data concerned with the production of the BOCs. The specified model should be capable of reproducing the measured behavior. The modeled output is compared with the initial BOCs, leading to model refinement and further computer simulations until a reasonable match between the measured and the modeled BOC can be achieved.

From: *Current Clinical Neurology: Atypical Parkinsonian Disorders*
Edited by: I. Litvan © Humana Press Inc., Totowa, NJ

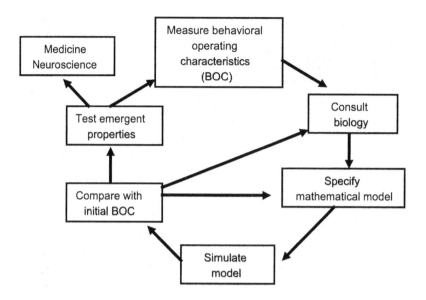

Fig. 1. The paradigm of neural network modeling.

Although models are usually developed to demonstrate the biological plausibility of a particular preexisting hypothesis, or to show how computational algorithms may be implemented in neural networks, the same models can be used to generate and test new ideas by analyzing the emergent properties of the model—model properties that cannot be explained by the operation or the wiring of individual model components alone. Moreover, by lesioning the intact structural components of the model, manipulating its dynamic mechanisms, or altering its inputs, it is possible to characterize the neuropathology of the disease and the associated changes in the behavior. It is then also possible to test the effect of surgical or pharmacological interventions to counteract the effects of lesions or disease *(2,12)*. Thus, computational modeling of neurological disorders involves a succession of modeling cycles to first account for neural mechanisms underlying the normative data, followed by the characterization and simulation of diseased mechanisms and abnormal behavior.

Modeling PD and APDs

Although a comprehensive review of the literature on modeling of basal ganglia function in health and disease is not possible because of space limitations, the reader is referred to the reviews of Beiser et al. *(1)*, Ruppin et al. *(2)*, and Gillies and Arbuthnott *(3)* for a detailed account. These efforts have focused on explaining the roles of the basal ganglia in procedural learning *(14–17)*, action selection *(18–20)*, serial order *(21–23)*, and movement planning and control *(24–27)*. Unfortunately, although these models have provided insights on the abnormal mechanisms underlying PD, few efforts have been put forward on modeling APDs. Thus, one goal of this chapter is to describe how existing models of cortical, basal ganglia, and cerebellar dynamics can be used to model and simulate APDs. In the next section, we briefly review the neuropathology in APDs. The reader is referred to Chapters 1, 4, 8, and 18–20 of this book for detailed reviews and discussion of the underlying neuropathology.

Neuropathology of the APDs

It is widely recognized that the differential diagnosis of APDs presents some difficult problems. First, clinical diagnostic criteria are often suboptimal or partially validated *(28)*; and second, the usefulness of routine brain-imaging techniques, such as magnetic resonance imaging (MRI), is still debatable because of issues such as specificity, sensitivity, variations in technical parameters, and the experience of radiologists and neurologists *(29)*. Nevertheless, modern MRI methodologies are useful to differentiate PD from APDs, as brain MRI in PD is grossly normal. Moreover, MRI studies suggest specific regional brain markers associated with the underlying pathology in APDs, such as multiple system atrophy (MSA), progressive supranuclear palsy (PSP), and corticobasal degeneration (CBD). Importantly, as these data can be used as a starting point for modeling purposes (Fig. 1), we briefly summarize the MRI findings.

Multiple system atrophy of the parkinsonian type (MSA-P) appears to be characterized by putaminal atrophy, T2-hypointensity, and "slit-like" marginal hyperintensity *(29–32)*, whereas MSA of the cerebellar type (MSA-C) usually is accompanied by atrophy of the lower brainstem, pons, middle cerebellar peduncles, and vermis, as well as signal abnormalities in the pontine and the middle cerebellar peduncles *(30,31,33,34)*. Mild-to-moderate cortical atrophy is also common to both MSA-P and MSA-C *(29,35)*.

PSP is usually characterized by widespread cell loss and gliosis in the globus pallidus, subthalamic nucleus, red nucleus, substantia nigra, dentate nucleus, and brainstem, and often cortical atrophy and lateral ventricle dilatation *(29)*. These patients also show decreased 18F-flurodopa in both anterior and posterior putamen and caudate nucleus, and an anterior–posterior hypometabolic gradient *(36)*. On the other hand, CBD may be differentiated by the presence of asymmetric frontoparietal and midbrain atrophy *(29)*.

Interestingly, cortical atrophy in APDs, particularly in cases involving damage of frontoparietal networks, is consistent with reports of ideomotor apraxia, which can also be seen in PD patients when their pathology is coincident with cortical atrophy *(36–39)*. In particular, patients with PD and PSP, who showed ideomotor apraxia, had the greatest deficits in movement accuracy, spatial and temporal coupling, and multijoint coordination *(38)*. However, as has been noted elsewhere, it remains to be seen if the kinematic deficits observed in this patients are characteristic of apraxia or are caused by elementary motor deficits *(40)*. Given the pathological heterogeneity seen in patients with APDs, and even in PD, it seems that computer modeling would be a useful tool to study how damage to frontoparietal networks and their interaction with a dysfunctional basal ganglia and/or cerebellar systems may increase the kinematic abnormalities beyond some threshold that would result in the genesis of limb apraxia.

MODELING STUDIES

In this section we present two examples of computational models of basal ganglia disorders. The first example presents a model formulated as a control problem to investigate akinesia and bradykinesia in PD, whereas the second example, formulated as a large-scale, dynamic neural network model involving frontoparietal, basal ganglia, and cerebellar networks, investigates the effects of PD and PSP on limb apraxia.

Modeling Hypokinetic Disorders in PD

Contreras-Vidal and Stelmach proposed a neural network model of the sensorimotor cortico-striato-pallido-thalamo-cortical system to explain some movement deficits (the "BOCs" in the modeling cycle) seen in PD patients *(24)*. This model, originally specified as a set of nonlinear differential equations, proposed the concept of basal ganglia gating of thalamo-cortical pathways involved in movement preparation (or priming), movement initiation and execution, and movement termination (Fig. 2A). In this model, three routes for cortical control of the basal ganglia output exist: activation of the "direct pathway" opens the gate by disinhibition of the thalamic neurons (route 1), whereas activation of both a slower indirect (through GPe, route 2) pathway and a faster direct cortical (route 3) pathway closes the gate through inhibition of thalamo-cortical neurons.

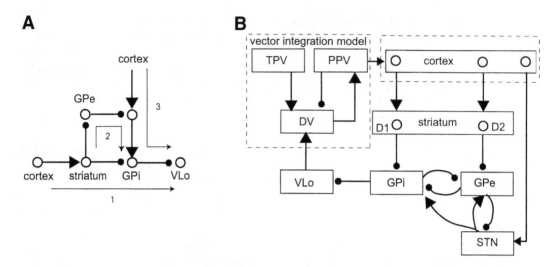

Fig. 2. (**A**) Three pathways for control of pallidal output by cortical areas. B) Block diagram of the cortico-basal ganglia-thalamo-cortical network of Contreras-Vidal and Stelmach *(24)*. The basal ganglia output (GPi) gates activity at the ventro-lateral thalamus (VLo), thus modulating cortico-cortical communication in the "vector integration model" that progressively moves the endeffector (PPV) to the target location (TPV). The basal ganglia gating allows priming and controls the speed of change from limb present position (PPV) to target position (TPV). Filled circles imply inhibitory connections, whereas arrows imply excitatory connections.

In this theoretical framework, activation of pathway 1 would result in activation of thalamo-cortical motor circuits leading to initiation and modulation of movement, whereas activation of pathway 2 would lead to breaking of ongoing movement. Activation of pathway 3 would facilitate rapid movement switching, or prevent the release of movement. The model postulated a role of the pallidal output for generating an analog gating signal (at the thalamus) that modulated a (hypothesized) cortical system that vectorially computed the difference between a target position vector and the present limb position vector, the so-called Vector-Integration-To-Endpoint (VITE) model (Fig. 2B) *(41)*.

In this computational model, the basal ganglia output had the role of gating the onset, timing, and the rate of change of the difference vector (DV), therefore controlling movement parameters such as movement initiation, speed, and size. Moreover, the proposed basal ganglia gating function allows three control modes: preparation for action or priming (gate is closed), initiation of action (gate starts to open), and termination of action (gate starts to close). Simulations of this model demonstrated a single mechanism for akinesia, bradykinesia, and hypometria, and a correlation between degree of striatal dopamine depletion and the severity of the PD signs.

In the terminology of control theory, it can been shown that the sensorimotor cortico-basal ganglia network of Contreras-Vidal and Stelmach *(24)* can be approximated as a proportional + derivative controller (Equation 1) with time-varying position (G_p; Equation 2) and velocity (G_v; Equation 3) gains. The system described by the second-order differential equation (1) represents the motion of the endpoint (P) toward the target (T) under the initial position and velocity conditions $P = P_0$ and $dP_0/dt = 0$, respectively.

$$\frac{d^2}{dt^2} P = G_v \frac{d}{dt} P - G_p (P - T) \qquad (1)$$

$$G_p = \alpha G_0 \frac{t}{1+t} \qquad (2)$$

$$G_v = \frac{1+t}{(1+t)^2} - \alpha \qquad (3)$$

where α represents an integration rate and G_0 is a scaling constant and t is the time in sec. The system given by Equations 1–3 is based on the experimentally testable assumption that pallidal signals modulate the ventro-lateral thalamus (VL_o) such that the pattern of thalamic output has a sigmoidal shape or is gradually increasing as a function of time as in Equation 4. This assumption implies that either a compact set of pallidal neurons progressively decrease their firing rate as a function of time before movement onset, therefore gradually disinhibiting the motor thalamus, or an increasing number of (inhibitory) pallidal cells, controlling the prime movers, are depressed as the movement unfolds.

$$VL_o = G_0 \frac{t}{1+t} \qquad (4)$$

Figure 3 shows the mean cumulative distributions of onsets (decreases and increases) for GPi neurons prior to movement onset obtained from a set of neurophysiological studies published between 1978 and 1998 (Table 1) in which information about the timing of internal globus pallidus (GPi) neurons was available. The plot shows a gradual buildup or decrease of the mean cumulative distribution of neurons whose activations were either enhanced or depressed prior to movement onset. Overall, increases in GPi activity were predominant (48% and 26% for increases and decreases, respectively). It is likely that the small percentage of GPi depressions prior to movement onset reflects the focused activation of prime mover muscles required to produce an arm movement. Interestingly, the mean cumulative distribution shows an increasing number of GPi neurons that are depressed, which supports the foregoing model's assumption.

Computer simulations of the set of equations (1–4) show that smaller-than-normal position and velocity gains can lead to bradykinesia (Fig. 4). Therefore, it is hypothesized that a function of basal ganglia networks is to compute these time-varying position and velocity gains. Low gains would prevent appropriate opening of the pallidal gate leading to poor activation of thalamo-cortical pathways involved in movement, whereas high gains may lead to excess or unstable movement. Interestingly, Suri and colleagues also used a dynamical linear model to model basal ganglia function and their simulations suggested that low gains in the direct and indirect pathways resulted in PD motor deficits *(26)*.

In addition, reduced movement amplitudes may be caused by premature resetting of these gains that prevent movement completion. Indeed, we have shown that smaller-than-normal (in duration and size) pallido-thalamic signals produced by dopamine depletion in the basal ganglia can reproduce micrographic handwriting *(12)*.

Modeling Abnormal Kinematics During Pointing Movement and Errors in Praxis in PD and APDs

To study the kinematic aspects of movement in basal ganglia disorders, we have performed computer simulations of the finger-to-nose task and a "bread-slicing gestural task"; the latter task is used commonly in testing for ideomotor apraxia *(38)*. These two tasks require the integration and transformation of sensory information into motor commands for movement, and therefore successful task completion depends on accurate spatial and temporal organization of movement.

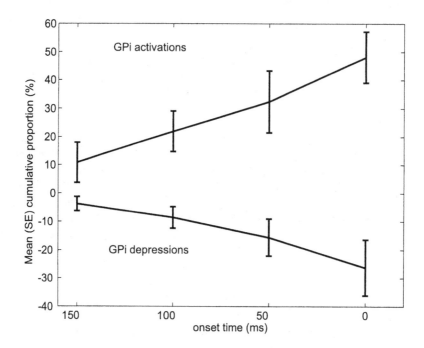

Fig. 3. Mean cumulative (SE) distributions of activations and depressions of GPi activity obtained from set of studies in Table 1.

Table 1
Cumulative Distribution of Onsets for GPi Cells

| | | Initial Timing of Discharge (%) Prior to: | | | | | | | | | cells |
| | | −150 ms | | −100 ms | | −50 ms | | 0 ms | | EMG | | |
Ref	Location	↑	↓	↑	↓	↑	↓	↑	↓	↑	↓	#
42[a]	C (m. N)	7	0	27	0	40	7	53	13	20	0	15
43[b]	NA[c]	—	—	—	—	2	2	—	—	7	7	35
44[d]	DL EP	22	14	45	29	48	31	53	34	37	24	114
45	NA	—	—	—	—	—	—	38	26	11	14	36
46[e]	VL	—	—	10[f]	4	—	—	29	12	2	1	41
47[g]	VL (m. 2)	—	—	19	3	81	14	84	15	37	7	68
48[h]	DL EP	57	16	57	16	63	18	66	19	NA	NA	28
49[i]	DL/VL	—	—	17	17	25	53	62	91	NA	NA	18
	Mean %	10.8	3.8	21.9	8.6	32.4	15.6	48.1	26.3	14.3	6.63	—
	Total											355

↑, increase; ↓, decrease; C, centered; DL, dorsolateral; EMG, onset of first muscle activity in prime movers; EP, entopenduncular nucleus (GPi-like structure in felines); GPi, internal globus pallidus; m., monkey; NA, data not available; VL, ventrolateral. All times with respect to movement onset, except EMG data. Notes: [a] biphasic stimulation trains (from Fig. 8), [b] EMG recordings were made at separate times from the single-cell recordings; [c] recording was done from "full extent of GP" and percentages of discharges were divided equally in increases and decreases; [d] estimated from Fig. 9 (61%: ↑, 39%: ↓); [e] for *VisStep* task (71% [29%] GPi increased [decreased] their discharge overall); [f] estimated from Fig. 5, by counting number of samples during time interval and dividing by the maximum number of conditions (four); [g] data estimated from Fig. 6C (85%: ↑, 15%: ↓); [h] estimated from Fig. 4 (assumes uniform distributions of 78% activations in EP); [i] data estimated from Fig. 3B.

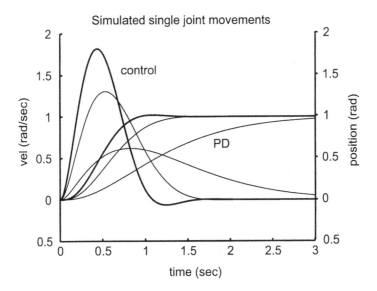

Fig. 4. Simulations of normal (thick lines) and Parkinson's disease (thin lines) movement control. Joint position (ramp trajectories) and velocity (bell-shaped trajectories) for three different position and velocity gain settings are shown ($\alpha = 10$; $G_0 = 10$; normal: *Gp = Gv = 1.0*; PD1: *Gp = Gv = 0.6*; PD2: *Gp = Gv = 0.2*). Reducing the gain resulted in slower movement (bradykinesia).

Figure 5 depicts a schematic diagram of frontal, parietal, basal ganglia, and cerebellar networks postulated to be engaged in the learning and updating of sensorimotor transformations for reaching to visual or proprioceptive targets. The model is based on an extension of the computational models of Bullock et al. *(9)* and Burnod et al. *(8)*, and recent imaging and behavioral experiments *(50–53)* that suggest distinct roles for fronto-parietal, basal ganglia, and cerebellar networks. In the model, visual and/or proprioceptive signals about target location and end-effector position are used to code an internal representation for target (T) and arm (Eff), presumably in posterior parietal cortex (PPC). These internal representations are compared to compute a spatial difference vector (DVs) as in the cortical "vector integration model" depicted in Fig. 2B. The DV's outflow must be transformed into a joint rotation vector (DVm) in order to guide the end-effector to the target. This spatial direction-to-joint rotation transformation is an inverse kinematic transformation and computationally, it can be learned through certain amount of simultaneous exposure to patterned proprioceptive and visual stimulation under conditions of self-produced movement—referred to as "motor babbling" *(8,9)*.

The cortical network just described is complemented by two subcortical networks connected in two distinct, parallel, lateral loops, namely, a frontostriatal network and a parieto-cerebellar system. The former provides a learned bias term that rotates the frame of reference for movement, whereas the latter provides a correction term that is added to the direction vector whenever the actual direction of movement deviates from the desired one. The frontostriatal network is modeled as an adaptive search element that performs search and action selection using reinforcement learning *(15)*. This system uses an explicit error (dopamine) signal to drive the selection and the reinforcement/punishment mechanisms used for learning new procedural skills. It searches and evaluates candidate visuomotor actions that would lead to acquisition of a spatial target. The cerebellar component is modeled as an adaptive error-correcting module that continuously provides a compensatory signal to drive the visuomotor error (provided by the climbing fibers) to zero *(7)*.

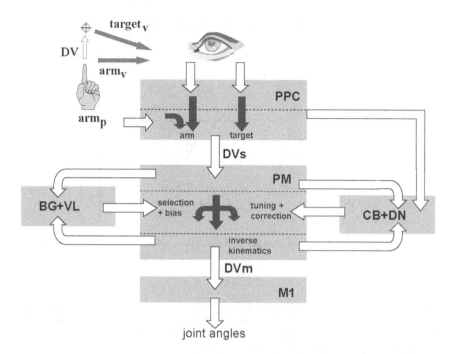

Fig. 5. Diagram of hypothesized networks involved in sensorimotor transformation for reaching. See text for description.

Simulating the Finger-to-Nose Test in Control, PD, and APD

The model summarized in the previous discussion was implemented in Matlab Simulink (following the mathematical equations in refs. *8* and *9*) to investigate the effects of PD and APDs in the spatial and temporal characteristics of repetitive pointing movement to the nose (a kinesthetic target). Figure 6 depicts the movement trajectories and the joint angles for a simulated arm with three joints (shoulder, elbow, wrist). The simulation assumed horizontal movements at the nose level, and therefore the paths are shown as two-dimensional plots. As expected, in the virtual control subject, the finger-to-nose trajectories were slightly curved and showed high spatial and temporal accuracy. The joint excursions reflected the repetitive nature of the task with most of the movement performed by elbow flexion/extension followed by the shoulder and to a lesser degree by the wrist.

To simulate PD, the gain of the basal ganglia gating signal was decreased by 30% with respect to that in the intact system. In addition, Gaussian noise ($N(0,1)*30$) was added to the internal representation of the hand to account for kinesthetic deficits reported in PD patients (degradation of the kinesthetic representation of the spatial location of the nose would have had the same effect) *(54)*. Computer simulations of the PD network showed decreased movement smoothness and increased spatial and temporal movement variability. Moreover, the joint rotations were slower and progressively decreased in amplitude. Thus, the simulation is consistent with reports of deficits in the production of multiarticulated repetitive movement in PD.

Following the observations of cortical atrophy in frontal and parietal areas in APD summarized in subheading Neuropathology of the APDs, we modeled this disease in two steps: First, we added noise (uniform distribution between 0 and 1.5) to the adaptive synaptic weights of the frontoparietal network in the intact ("control") system; second, we pruned the synaptic weights by randomly setting 50% of the weights to zero; and third, the gain of the basal ganglia gating signal was reduced to 50% of the control value. Simulation of the APD network model showed that the movement trajectories

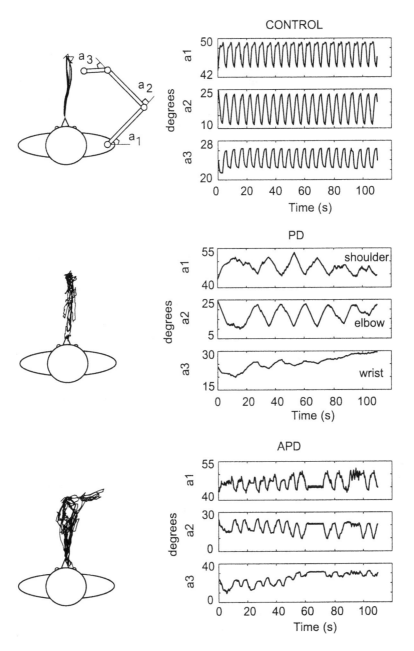

Fig. 6. Simulations of the finger-to-nose test in normal, PD, and APD models. Movement trajectories and joint angles are shown. See videoclip for real-time simulation.

were severely affected. The virtual subject showed misreaching to the nose and produced movement paths that varied widely in space. This was reflected in the joint excursions, which were characterized by noisy and asymmetrical flexion and extension ranges, as well as some periods of joint immobility. Thus, simulation of APD had the largest effect on the spatial and temporal aspects of movement coordination.

Simulating the Bread-Slicing Gesture in Control, PD, and APD

Recent clinical studies suggest that apraxia may be explained in terms of damage to a fronto-parietal network involved in reaching and prehension *(38)*. According to Rothi, ideomotor apraxia is characterized by "impairment in the timing, sequencing, and spatial organization of gestural movements" *(55)*. Studies involving patients with PD and APDs, including PSP and CBD, indicate that combined involvement of basal ganglia and cortical networks may underlie the presence of apraxia in these patients *(37,38)*. Moreover, in a group of studies by Leiguarda and colleagues, they found that patients with PD, PSP, and CBD, who tested positive for apraxia in the clinical test, showed larger kinematic abnormalities than those patients who do not show apraxia on clinical examination. However, as discussed initially by Roy, it is still a matter of debate whether these kinematic abnormalities are a result of an apraxia-like impairment or to basic motor control deficits *(40)*. For example, do the basic motor control deficits seen in these clinical populations explain the abnormal kinematic deficits seen in patients with ideomotor apraxia?

In the computer simulations that follow we focus on production errors, which are associated with deficits in the programming and execution of gestural movements, like the bread-slicing task. Simulations of higher-order content errors would require modeling of frontal areas related to ideational or conceptual processing, which are not included in the current model. In the model simulations, it is assumed that the planning and control components are disturbed because of the pathology in fronto-parietal networks.

Figure 7 shows the performance in the 'bread slicing' task in a normal virtual subject (Control), and after simulated PD and APD. Both diseases were simulated as in subheading Modeling Hypokinetic Disorders in PD. In the control simulation the slicing gesture, depicted as a continuous dark line, reflected a tight, curvilinear trajectory, which was primarily a result of the repetitive, periodic, shoulder rotations. Elbow and wrist joint angles also showed sustained, periodic patterns albeit of smaller amplitude. Simulation of the parkinsonian network resulted in reduced spatial and temporal accuracy of the slicing movement. This was accompanied by slower and asymmetrical joint oscillations that were maximal for the shoulder joint, but considerably reduced for the wrist joint. In fact, as the slicing gesture was generated, the wrist joint was progressively rotated from ~18° to ~38° (see geometry of the arm in top panel of Fig. 7). Simulation of PSP resulted in large production errors as evidenced by distorted spatial trajectories, some of which left the spatial area for the simulated bread surface. The profiles of the joint angles also resemble those reported in recent studies *(see* e.g., Fig. 5 in ref. *38)*. For example, the angular changes of virtual patients with PD and APDs are smaller, irregular, and distorted compared to the simulated control subject.

CONCLUSIONS

Models of basal ganglia disorders have been advanced in the last two decades. These models have mostly focused on PD, in part because of the computational burden of simulating large-scale models that include multiple brain areas. However, recent computational work on frontal, parietal, cerebellar, and basal ganglia dynamics involved in sensorimotor transformations for reaching provide a window to study widespread pathologies as those seen in APDs. These models can inform the experimentalist about the various potential sources of movement variability in various types of tasks (simple vs sequential, pantomime vs real tool use, kinesthetic vs visual cueing, etc.). Moreover, simulated lesions and interventions can be used to test hypotheses and guide new experiments.

For example, we modeled the pharmacokinetics and the pharmacodynamics using a neural network model parameterized by the measurements of the handwriting kinematics of PD patients *(12)*. Other mathematical treatments of the dose–effect relationship of levodopa and motor behavior treat the motor control system as a black-box system and do not provide insights on the mechanisms, although they may still be useful for therapy optimization purposes *(56)*. On the other hand, a biologically inspired, albeit highly simplified neural network model of cortico-basal ganglia dynamics

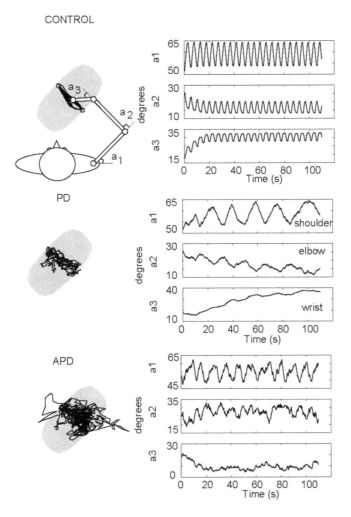

Fig. 7. Simulations of the bread-slicing gesture commonly used to test ideomotor apraxia in basal ganglia disorders. Simulations show movement trajectories and joint angles (shoulder, elbow, and wrist) for normal, PD, and APD simulations. See videoclip on accompanying DVD for real-time simulation.

during normal and neurological conditions would be valuable to assess which parameters might be most amenable to therapeutic intervention, including individual optimization of pharmacological therapy, while at the same time informing about abnormal mechanisms.

Limitations of Current Models of Basal Ganglia Disorders

APDs are caused by various diseases, therefore involving a complex neuropathophysiology and a wide spectrum of abnormal behavioral signs. Currently, there is no mathematical or conceptual model that can explain all the symptoms based on abnormal mechanisms within the basal ganglia, cerebellum, and/or cortical areas. This limitation is partially because of the necessary simplification of the neurobiology required to make the model computationally or mathematically tractable for formal investigation. Thus, it is likely that some aspect of any proposed model may be wrong; however, the likelihood of this happening can be minimized by developing a step-by-step reconstruction of the system under study, with each step required to account for additional sources of neural or motor variability. Moreover, manipulations of model components, such as simulated lesions or deep brain stimulation paradigms, are also oversimplifications of the processes occurring in the brain in response to such events.

We hope that computational models of basal ganglia disorders will be developed further to help elucidate and account for the complexity of the clinical symptoms seen in PD and APDs, in such a way that these models can guide further theoretical and applied research and foster interactions between clinicians, modelers, and neuroscientists.

FUTURE DIRECTIONS

A controversial question in apraxia research is the relevance of ideomotor apraxia for real-life action *(57)*. Earlier reports suggested that patients with apraxia may use single objects appropriately even when they are unable to pantomime their use *(58,59)*, whereas other have found the same types of spatiotemporal errors in both object pantomime and during tool use *(58)* or reported that subjects with ideomotor apraxia, assessed by gesture pantomime, had more errors with tools while eating than matched controls *(61)*. The large-scale neural network presented in this chapter may help to elucidate any potential relationship of ideomotor apraxia to skilled tool use in naturalistic situations. Extension of the large-scale neural network model to include visual and tactile signals produced by the sight and on-line interaction with the object would be critical to answer this question. Another important direction for future work relates to the integration of stored movement primitives (so-called gesture engrams) and dynamic movement features required to produce and distinguish a given gesture from others. Although the simulations of the "slicing" gesture in anapraxic neural network model presented in this chapter were based on degraded sensorimotor transformations for movement, it should also be possible to evaluate the effects of disruptions in the on-line sequential (dynamic) processes underlying the repetitive nature of the slicing task, which were intact in the present simulations. Finally, the hypothetical effects of neuromotor noise in different model components could also be assessed through neural network simulations.

ACKNOWLEDGMENTS

The author thanks Shihua Wen, University of Maryland's Department of Mathematics, for running the simulations shown in Figs. 6 and 7. The author's computational work summarized herein has been supported in part by INSERM and the National Institutes of Health.

FIGURES

Figures were generated in Matlab and filtered using Abobe Illustrator.

MEDIA

Procedure Used to Generate the MPEG Files:

In the CD disk, there are six mpeg files, the file names represent the simulated tasks, which are described below. The frames in format .avi were generated by the computational model written in MatLab's Simulink. The .avi files are generated by a shareware named "HyperCam" produced by Hypererionics Technology (www.hperionics.com). The mpeg files were obtained using the freeward softward "avi2meg" written by USH (www.ush.de). All the movies are recorded at a rate of 30 frames per second.

Description of Movies:

Finger-to-nose Control (duration: 1:48): Simulation shows the end-pont trajectories during the finger-to-nose task. A three segments arm is shown. These segments are linked by the shoulder, elbow, and wrist joints. This simulation of an intact (Control) network shows almost linear trajectories.

Finger-to-nose PD: This movie shows the performance of the computer model after simulating severe PD. In this simulation, the movement becomes slower, discrete, and noisy. Moreover, some of the targeted movements do not reach the nose.

Finger-to-nose APD: This movie shows the finger-to-nose simulations after damage to the fronto-parietal network involved in sensorimotor trnsformations for reaching, which simulated APD. The end-point trajectories become irregular, coarse, fragmented, and dyscoordinated.

Slicing Control: This clip shows a simulation of the "bread slicing" gesture as seen from directly above. The rectangle represents the loaf of bread. Note that there were not constrains on the way the virtual arm was supposed to produce the gesture. Note that during the repetitive movement the wrist joint was initially slightly flexed, but gradually became extended. This illustrates the fact that in a redundant arm there are many possible arm configurations that can be used to move the end point to a spatial target or along a given spatial trajectory.

Slicing PD: The PD simulation shows reduced range of motion for all joints, discontinuous movements, and a difficulty in generating the repetitive slicing gesture. In this particular simulation, the wrist is in the extended position from the onset of the movement.

Slicing APD: This video shows the slicing gesture task after simulated APD. This simulation shows production errors as the arm fails to move the end point along the desired slicing trajectory. This resulted in highly disrupted spatial and temporal organization.

REFERENCES

1. Beiser DG, Hua SE, Houk JC. Network models of the basal ganglia. Curr Opin Neurobiol 1997;7:185–190.
2. Ruppin E, Reggia JA, Glanzman D. Understanding brain and cognitive disorders: the computational perspective. Prog Brain Res 1999;121:ix–xv.
3. Gillies A, Arbuthnott G. Computational models of the basal ganglia. Mov Disord 2000;15:762–770.
4. Amos A. A computational model of information processing in the frontal cortex and basal ganglia. J Cogn Neurosci 2000;12:505–519.
5. Lorincz A. Static and dynamic state feedback control model of basal ganglia-thalamocortical loops. Int J Neural Syst 1997;8:339–357.
6. Wickens JR, Kotter R, Alexander ME. Effects of local connectivity on striatal function: stimulation and analysis of a model. Synapse 1995;20:281–298.
7. Contreras-Vidal JL, Grossberg S, Bullock D. A neural model of cerebellar learning for arm movement control: cortico-spino-cerebellar dynamics. Learn Mem 1997;3:475–502.
8. Burnod Y, Grandguillaume P, Otto I, Ferraina S, Johnson PB, Caminiti R. Visuomotor transformations underlying arm movements toward visual targets: a neural network model of cerebral cortical operations. J Neurosci 1992;12:1435–1453.
9. Bullock D, Grossberg S, Guenther FH. A self-organizing neural model of motor equivalent reaching and tool use by a multijoint arm. J Cogn Neurosci 1993;5:408–435.
10. Tagamets MA, Horwitz B. Interpreting PET and fMRI measures of functional neural activity: the effects of synaptic inhibition on cortical activation in human imaging studies. Brain Res Bull 2001;54:267–273.
11. Horwitz B, Poeppel D. How can EEG/MEG and fMRI/PET data be combined? Hum Brain Mapp 2002;17:1–3.
12. Contreras-Vidal JL, Poluha P, Teulings HL, Stelmach GE. Neural dynamics of short and medium-term motor control effects of levodopa therapy in Parkinson's disease. Artif Int Med 1998;13:57–79.
13. Bower JM. Modeling the nervous system. TINS 1992;15:411–412.
14. Schultz W, Dayan P, Montague R. A neural substrate of prediction and reward. Science 1997;275:1593–1599.
15. Contreras-Vidal JL, Schultz W. A predictive reinforcement model of dopamine neurons for learning approach behavior. J Comput Neurosci 1999;6:191–214.
16. Nakahara H, Doya K, Hikosaka O. Parallel cortico-basal ganglia mechanisms for acquisition and execution of visuomotor sequences—A computational approach. J Cogn Neurosci 2001;13:626–647.
17. Suri R, Schultz W. Learning of sequential movements by neural network model with dopamine-like reinforcement signal. Exp Brain Res 1998;121:350–354.
18. Contreras-Vidal, JL. The gating functions of the basal ganglia in movement control. In: JA Reggia, E Ruppin, DL Glanzman (eds.). Progress in Brain Research. Disorders of Brain, Behavior and Cognition: the Neurocomputational Perspective. Amsterdam: Elsevier, 1999:261–276.
19. Humphries MD, Gurney KN. The role of intra-thalamic and thalamocortical circuits in action selection. Network 2002;13:131–156.

20. Gurney K, Prescott TJ, Redgrave P. A computational model of action selection in the basal ganglia. II. Analysis and simulation of behaviour. Biol Cybern 2001;84:411–423.

21. Beiser D, Houk J. Model of cortical-basal ganglia ganglionic processing: encoding the serial order of sensory events. J Neurophysiol 1998;79:3168–3188.

22. Fukai T. Sequence generation in arbitrary temporal patterns from theta-nested gamma oscillations: a model of the basal ganglia-thalamo-cortical loops. Neural Netw 1999;12:975–987.

23. Berns GS, Sejnowski TJ. A computational model of how the basal ganglia produce sequences. J Cogn Neurosci 1998;10:108–121.

24. Contreras-Vidal JL, Stelmach GE. A neural model of basal ganglia–thalamocortical relations in normal and Parkinsonian movement. Biol Cybern 1995;73:467–476.

25. Connolly CI, Burns JB, Jog MS. A dynamical-systems model for Parkinson's disease. Biol Cybern 2000;83:47–59.

26. Suri RE, Albani C, Glattfelder AH. A dynamic model of motor basal ganglia functions. Biol Cybern 1997;76:451–458.

27. Borrett DS, Yeap TH, Kwan HC. Neural networks and Parkinson's disease. Can J Neurol Sci 1993;20:107–113.

28. Litvan I. Recent advances in atypical parkinsonian disorders. Curr Opin Neurol 1999;12:441–446.

29. Yekhlef F, Ballan G, Macia F, Delmer O, Sourgen C, Tison F. Routine MRI for the differential diagnosis of Parkinson's disease, MSA, PSP, and CBD. J Neural Transm 2003;110:151–169.

30. Schrag A, Kingsley D, Phatouros C, et al. Clinical usefulness of magnetic resonance imaging in multiple system atrophy. J Neurol Neurosurg Psychiatry 1998;65:65–71.

31. Schrag A, Good CD, Miszkiel K, et al. Differentiation of atypical parkinsonian syndromes with routine MRI. Neurology 2000;54:697–702.

32. Kraft E, Schwarz J, Trenkwalder C, Vogl T, Pfluger T, Oertel WH. The combination of hypointense and hyperintense signal changes on T2-weighted magnetic resonance maging sequences: a specific marker of multiple system atrophy? Arch Neurol 1999;56:225–228.

33. Savoiardo M, Strada L, Girotti F, Zimmerman RA, Grisoli M, Testa D, Petrillo R. Olivopontocerebellar atrophy: MR diagnosis and relationship to multisystem atrophy. Radiology 1990;174:693–669.

34. Savoiardo M, Grisoli M, Girotti F, Testa D, Caraceni T. MRI in sporadic olivopontocerebellar atrophy and striatonigral degeneration. Neurology 1997;48:790–792.

35. Horimoto Y, Aiba I, Yasuda T, et al.Cerebral atrophy in multiple system atrophy by MRI. J Neurol Sci 2000;173:109–112.

36. Fahn S, Green PE, Ford B, Bressman SB. Handbook of Movement Disorders. London: Blackwell Science, 1997.

37. Leiguarda RC, Marsden CD. Limb apraxias: higher-order disorders of sensorimotor integration. Brain 2000;123:860–79.

38. Leiguarda R, Merello M, Balej J, Starkstein S, Nogues M, Marsden CD. Disruption of spatial organization and interjoint coordination in Parkinson's disease, progressive supranuclear palsy, and multiple system atrophy. Mov Disord 2000;15:627–640.

39. Litvan I. Progressive supranuclear palsy and corticobasal degeneration. Baillieres Clin Neurol 1997;6:167–185.

40. Roy EA. Apraxia in diseases of the basal ganglia. Mov Disord 2000;15:598–600.

41. Bullock D, Grossberg S. Neural dynamics of planned arm movements: emergent invariants and speed-accuracy properties during trajectory formation. Psychol Rev 1988;95:49–90.

42. Anderson ME, Horak FB. Influence of the globus pallidus on arm movements in monkeys. III. Timing of movement-related information. J Neurophysiol 1985;54:433–448.

43. Brotchie P, Iansek R, Horne MK. Motor function of the monkey globus pallidus. 1. Neuronal discharge and parameters of movement. Brain. 1991;114:1667–1683.

44. Cheruel F, Dormont JF, Amalric M, Schmied A, Farin D. The role of putamen and pallidum in motor initiation in the cat. I. Timing of movement-related single-unit activity. Exp Brain Res 1994;100:250–266.

45. Georgopoulos AP, DeLong MR, Crutcher MD. Relations between parameters of step-tracking movements and single cell discharge in the globus pallidus and subthalamic nucleus of the behaving monkey. J Neurosci 1983;3:1586–1598.

46. Mink JW, Thach WT. Basal ganglia motor control. I. Nonexclusive relation of pallidal discharge to five movement modes. J Neurophysiol 1991;65:273–300.

47. Nambu A, Yoshida S, Jinnai K. Movement-related activity of thalamic neurons with input from the globus pallidus and projection to the motor cortex in the monkey. Exp Brain Res 1991;84:279–284.

48. Neafsey EJ, Hull CD, Buchwald NA. Preparation for movement in the cat. II. Unit activity in the basal ganglia and thalamus. Electroencephalogr Clin Neurophysiol 1978;44:714–723.

49. Turner RS, Anderson ME. Pallidal discharge related to the kinematics of reaching movements in two dimensions. J Neurophysiol 1997;77:1051–1074.

50. Contreras-Vidal JL, Buch ER. Effects of Parkinson's disease on visuomotor adaptation. Exp Brain Res 2003;150:25–32.

51. Buch ER, Young S, Contreras-Vidal JL. Visuomotor adaptation in normal aging. Learn Mem 2003;10:55–63.

52. Inoue K, Kawashima R, Satoh K, et al. A PET study of visuomotor learning under optical rotation. Neuroimage 2000;11:505–516.

53. Balslev D, Nielsen FA, Frutiger SA, et al. Cluster analysis of activity-time series in motor learning. Hum Brain Mapp 2002;15:135–45.

54. Klockgether T, Borutta M, Rapp H, Spieker S, Dichgans J. A defect of kinesthesia in Parkinson's disease. Mov Disord 1995;10:460–465.
55. Rothi LJG, Ochipa C, Heilman KM. A cognitive neuropsychological model of limb praxis. Cogn Neuropsychol 1991;8:443–458.
56. Hacisalihzade SS, Mansour M, Albani C. Optimization of symptomatic therapy in Parkinson's disease. IEEE Trans Biomed Eng 1989;36:363–372.
57. Buxbaum LJ. Ideomotor apraxia: A call to Action. Neurocase 2001;7:445–458.
58. Poizner H, Mack L, Verfaellie M, Rothi LJ, Heilman KM. Three-dimensional computer graphic analysis of apraxia. Neural representations of learned movement. Brain 1990;113:85–101.
59. Liepmann H. The left hemisphere and action. London, Ontario: University of Western Ontario, 1905.
60. De Rensi E, Motti F, Nichelli P. Imitating gestures. A quantitative approach to ideomotor apraxia. Arch Neurol 1980;37:6–10.
61. Foundas AL, Macauley BL, Raymer AM, Maher LM, Heilman KM, Gonzalez Rothi, LJ. Ecological implications of limb apraxia: evidence from mealtime behavior. J Int Neuropsychol Soc 1995;1:62–66.

8

Atypical Parkinsonian Disorders

Neuropathology and Nosology

Charles Duyckaerts

INTRODUCTION

In many neurological diseases the topography of the lesion, whatever its nature, determines the clinical signs, whereas the nature of the lesion (vascular, inflammatory, degenerative, etc.) whatever its topography, determines the time course. According to J. P. Martin *(1)*, this general principle cannot be simply applied to diseases of the basal ganglia since the nature of the lesions directly influence the clinical signs. Chorea, for instance, is associated with atrophy of the caudate nucleus but infarct of the caudate nucleus does not generally cause chorea.

What is the localizing value of parkinsonism? Parkinsonism is the clinical syndrome that is fully developed in idiopathic Parkinson's disease (IPD). Hypokinesia or bradykinesia, rigidity, and resting tremor are characteristic of IPD. In general, these features are eventually bilateral, but usually largely predominate on one side of the body *(2)*. In parkinsonian disorders not resulting from IPD, resting tremor is usually absent.

The Topography of the Lesions Causing Parkinsonism

When Lewy described the cerebral lesions found in patients with IPD, he correctly identified the cellular inclusions that are now known under his name. He also acknowledged the diffuse nature of the disease. Numerous figures in his monograph *(3)* show inclusions in the brainstem next to those in the basal nuclei. He mentioned the fact that Tretiakoff "and the French authors" had emphasized the importance of the alteration of the substantia nigra (which was macroscopically visible as a pallor) but he failed to appreciate the importance of this topography. In his view, the tonus was modulated by two antagonist structures, the cerebellum—the destruction of which caused hypotonia—and basal ganglia, the lesions of which caused hypertonia (rigidity). The equilibrium between both was regulated by a hypothetical mesencephalic tonus center that was not clearly identified and certainly not recognized as the substantia nigra (Fig. 1). It may seem surprising that Lewy, who had so many deep insights into the pathogenesis of IPD, did not appreciate the importance of the lesions of the substantia nigra. The reason is, probably, the knowledge of the anatomy at that time. The reading of old neuroanatomy books, such as the various editions of the classical Carpenter's *Neuroanatomy*, makes it clear that the connections of the substantia nigra with the striatum escaped the scrutiny of the anatomists until the development of the histofluorescence technique by Falck and Hillarp *(4)* *(see* Fig. 2). This method, which was able to reveal the thin catecholaminergic fibers, finally established that, indeed, the substantia nigra was connected with the striatum and truly belonged to the basal nuclei. The idea that the substantia nigra was the producer of dopamine that flowed into the striatum and that IPD was just caused by the mere interruption of this flow was put forward at that time.

From: *Current Clinical Neurology: Atypical Parkinsonian Disorders*
Edited by: I. Litvan © Humana Press Inc., Totowa, NJ

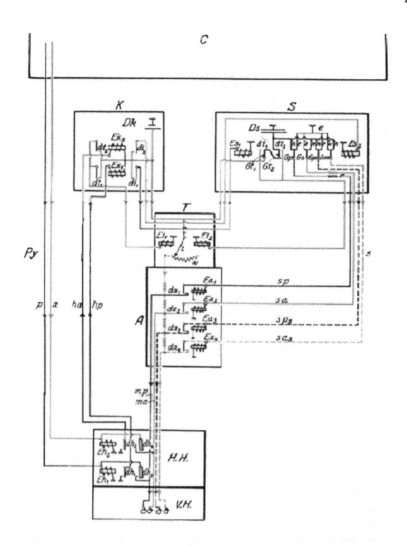

Fig. 1. A precursor of today's models: Lewy diagram explaining the motor symptoms of Parkinson disease. Reproduction in black and white of the color picture 546b of "Die Lehre vom Tonus und der Bewegung" by F. Lewy (Berlin, 1923). C is the cortex. K stands for Kleinhirn (cerebellum), and S for striatum. T is the Tonusregulationszentrum, located in A "Nucleus Associatorius motorius tegmenti" (defined in the text as a set of mesencephalic tegmental nuclei not identified as substantia nigra). Py is the pyramidal tract. H.H. is Hinterhornschaltzelle (the cells of the posterior horn [of the spinal cord]) and V.H. is the Vorderhorn (ventral horn).

Fig. 2. (*opposite page*) Stages in the understanding of the connections of substantia nigra as seen from anatomy book diagrams. Panel A is part of a diagram, which dates back to 1935 *(222)*. S. nigra , substantia nigra. Neorubr. , red nucleus - neoruber, i.e., parvocellular part of the nucleus. Paleorubr. = red nucleus - paleoruber i.e. magnocellular part of the nucleus. Corp quadr., colliculi. Tegm mes., Tegmentum of the mesencephalon. In 1935, the efferent fibers of the substantia nigra were thought to stop in the reticular formation of the mesencephalon, in or close to the red nucleus. Panel B is a diagram published in 1969 *(223)*. SN, substantia nigra. GPM, globus pallidus, pars medialis. VLM, medial part of the ventrolateral nucleus of the thalamus. Refer to the original drawing for other abbreviations. In 1969, the connections of the substantia nigra with the striatum were not yet illustrated. Panel C comes from the seventh edition of the book: on the diagram, the efferent fibers from the substantia nigra are indicated as reaching the striatum (putamen) *(224)*.

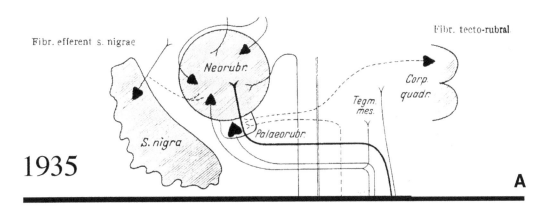

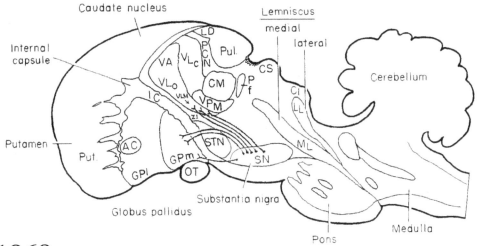

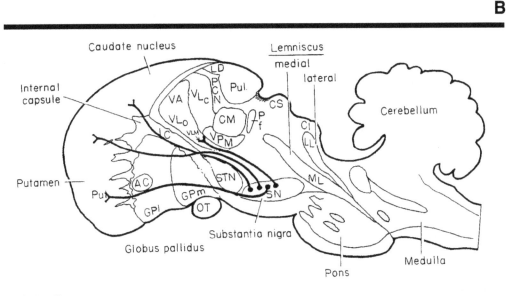

We now know that IPD cannot be reduced to a pure dopaminergic deficit *(5–7)*. α-Synuclein, which makes up the Lewy bodies, accumulates in many more nuclei or brain structures than just the substantia nigra. However, it remains true that the substantia nigra is involved in most disorders with parkinsonism, and that parkinsonism, as a clinical syndrome, points to a lesion of the substantia nigra. The substantia nigra is indeed, clearly involved in IPD, progressive supranuclear palsy (PSP), corticobasal degeneration (CBD), and multiple system atrophy (MSA), i.e., striatonigral degeneration, although most often in association with other structures. Infarction of the substantia nigra, rarely encountered, has been incriminated in unilateral parkinsonism *(8)*. Lymphoma invading the substantia nigra has been reported to cause parkinsonism *(9)*; postencephalitic parkinsonism, although causing diffuse alterations, massively affects the substantia nigra. It is also the substantia nigra that is involved in 1-methyl-4-phenyl-1,2,3,6-tetrahydropyridine (MPTP) intoxication, which is responsible for a severe parkinsonian syndrome.

The rule of a nigral involvement in parkinsonism suffers many exceptions, the most noticeable being patients with lacunes of the basal ganglia who frequently develop a shuffling gait, akinesia, and rigidity reminiscent of IPD. Vascular lesions of the basal ganglia can also cause a clinical syndrome of supranuclear palsy *(10)*. How lesions of the basal ganglia cause these symptoms is not clear. Large destructions of the lenticular nucleus in animals (already mentioned by Kinnear Wilson, ref. *11*) or in humans *(12)* do not cause a movement disorder that may be described as parkinsonism.

There are other lesions outside the basal ganglia nuclei accompanied by parkinsonism, usually without tremor; bradykinesia, rigidity, and gait disturbances have been associated with frontal-lobe infarcts and with periventricular and deep subcortical white matter lesions *(13)*. Bilateral frontal tumors such as meningioma *(14)* may also cause rigidity and bradykinesia reminiscent of IPD.

In brief, a lesion involving the substantia nigra, whatever its type, regularly causes parkinsonism, whereas only some types of alterations in the lenticular nucleus, or more rarely in other parts of the brain, may be held responsible for similar symptoms.

The Degenerative Processes Affecting the Basal Ganglia and Their Markers

As already briefly outlined, parkinsonism is a syndrome of many causes. The degenerative processes commonly involved are difficult to disentangle since the mechanisms leading to neuronal dysfunction or death are not understood. The topography of the neuronal loss could help to identify these mechanisms, but little is known presently on the reasons of specific regional vulnerability. Moreover, the neurons that are lost leave no information on the causes of their death. Microscopic observation of the brain does not only show neuronal loss ("negative" signs) but can also reveal "positive" alterations. Most of them are characterized by accumulation of proteins in the cell (so-called "inclusions"). For instance, Lewy bodies associated with IPD, consist in the accumulation of α-synuclein in the cell body of neurons. Tau protein fills the processes of so-called "tufted astrocytes" found in PSP or accumulates at the tip of these processes in the "astrocytic plaques," considered to be one of the characteristic lesions of CBD.

Just as are clinical "signs," these positive alterations (Lewy bodies, tufted astrocytes, astrocytic plaques, etc.) are "signs" in the sense that they are but an observable change caused by the disease. What are they the sign of? Some inclusions are seen in a large number of disorders or even in otherwise normal cases: amylaceous bodies belong to that category. Others are encountered but in a subset of disorders: they are described as "markers." Lewy bodies, for instance, are found in only a few circumstances *(15)*, most often IPD or dementia with Lewy bodies (DLB) but also Hallervorden–Spatz disease (NBIA-1 or neurodegeneration with brain iron accumulation type 1). The presence of the same marker in several diseases strongly suggests that the same metabolic dysfunction occurs in the various disorders where they are found. Obviously, two disorders looking clinically alike, e.g., IPD and parkinsonism owing to parkin mutations, may not share the same marker. In these two disorders the same cell populations are affected, explaining why they are clinically similar, but two different mechanisms lead to cell death. In IPD, α-synuclein accumulates in Lewy bodies because it is overproduced or not correctly consumed or destroyed. By contrast, the accumulation of α-synuclein does not take place in parkin mutation, perhaps because of a defect in ubiquitination, as it has been suggested *(16)* (Fig. 3). It is unfortunate that the same label (Parkinson's disease, ref. *17*) was applied to the two diseases with the logical (but in our view unjustified) conclusion that Lewy bodies, lacking in some cases of Parkinson disease (i.e., those with Parkin mutations), are just an insignificant byproduct. There is no reason to believe that all the morphologic markers play the same pathogenic role. Some may be toxic, others beneficial or innocent bystanders. Markers (or even neuronal loss) are lacking in some disorders (Fig. 4). Neuroleptics, for instance, cause spectacular extrapyramidal syndromes without causing any observable change.

Markers are useful in that they may give important information concerning physiopathology and, as such, contribute to the classification of neurodegenerative diseases. Molecular biology has shown in several cases that there is a direct relationship between the mutated gene and the protein accumulated in the inclusions. To take two striking examples, α-synuclein, which is mutated in some familial cases of IPD, is also present in the Lewy body, the marker of IPD. Tau accumulates in neurons and glia in hereditary fronto-temporal dementia with parkinsonism linked to chromosome 17 (FTDP-17); the mutations causing these disorders affect precisely the tau gene. There are many other examples, which suggest that one should "take the markers seriously" and consider them, at the least, as an indication of a pathogenic mechanism (either its cause or its consequence, ref. *18*), and at the most as indispensable evidence of a specific disease.

In the majority of cases, the lesions, which are observed in degenerative parkinsonism, consist in the accumulation of α-synuclein or of tau protein. α-Synuclein accumulates in the neuronal cell body (Lewy body) and in the neurites (Lewy neurites) of IPD. It may also accumulate in the glial inclusions of MSA. Although α-synuclein accumulates in both IPD and MSA, there is presently no evidence that these two disorders are otherwise linked in any way. Tau accumulates in neurons or glia of many neurodegenerative disorders: PSP, CBD, postencephalitic parkinsonism (PEP), amyotrophic lateral sclerosis parkinsonism–dementia complex of Guam (PDC), and tau mutations. In these diseases, the cellular type and the region of the cell where tau accumulates are important determinants of the inclusions.

SYNUCLEINOPATHY: IPD AND DLB—MULTIPLE SYSTEM ATROPHY

The Lewy Body

The inclusions that Friedrich H. Lewy observed in the brain of IPD patients are illustrated in the epoch-making monograph that he devoted to that disorder in 1923, titled "Die Lehre vom Tonus und der Bewegung" [The science of tonus and movement]. The variety of their shapes and of their topography, in those illustrations, demonstrates that F. Lewy had, in a certain sense, a remarkably modern view of the disorder: he had seen inclusions in the cell processes of the neurons (a lesion now described as "Lewy neurite") and in locations such as the nucleus basalis of Meynert, the hypothalamus, and the vegetative centers of the medulla. Historically, the term Lewy body, coined by Tretiakoff *(19)*, came to mean a spherical inclusion underlined by a clear halo located in the cell body of the neuron. This is indeed their manifestation in the substantia nigra where Tretiakoff observed them. The inclusion appears red with standard hematoxylin and eosin (H&E) stain since it exhibits a special affinity for eosin (eosinophilia). This type of Lewy bodies is mainly observed in the brainstem and is today considered the indispensable accompaniment of IPD *(15,20)*.

Lewy bodies were also identified in the cerebral cortex but almost 50 yr after their first description. The initial observation was due to Okazaki and his coworkers *(21)* who found them in two cases of dementia with quadriparesis in flexion. The peculiar aspect of cortical Lewy bodies explains why they were discovered much later than their brainstem counterparts. They are also eosinophilic, but lack the clear halo seen in the brainstem inclusions. Therefore, they may be mistaken for an abnormal, homogenized cytoplasm. The nucleus of the cell that contains the inclusion is often clear and may lack the large nucleolus typical of neurons: the cell may erroneously be identified as an astrocyte.

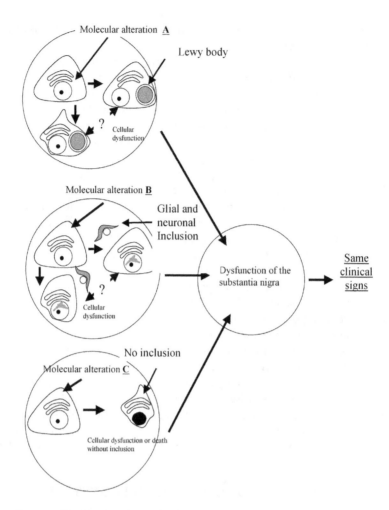

Fig. 3. Three diseases affecting the substantia nigra, with similar clinical consequences. Diagram showing, in the upper panel, the presence of Lewy bodies in the substantia nigra, causing idiopathic Parkinson's disease, in the middle panel, α-synuclein containing oligodendroglial and neuronal inclusions characteristic of striato-nigral degeneration (MSA), and in the lower panel, neuronal death associated with parkin mutations. The clinical signs may be quite similar although the pathogenic mechanisms, and possibly the markers, may be different.

The mechanism of formation of Lewy bodies and neurites is still unknown. With electron microscopy, they appear to be made of a dense, osmiophilic center in which vesicles and fibrils, 8–10 nm in diameter, can be identified *(22)*. At the periphery of the inclusion, the fibrils are radially oriented. The first histochemical studies showed that the inclusion was essentially made of proteins. Immunohistochemistry revealed the presence of many epitopes. Pollanen et al. *(23)* listed as many as 26 epitopes, among which neurofilaments were the most regularly found before ubiquitin and α-synuclein, the two constituents thought to be the most significant, were identified.

Anti-ubiquitin antibodies strongly label Lewy bodies and Lewy neurites *(24)*. Ubiquitination of proteins depends on the activity of specific ubiquitin ligases, which target proteins that have to be degraded. Several ubiquitin molecules make a polyubiquitin chain that serves as a signal to direct the protein to the proteasome, a large proteolytic complex located outside the lysosome. Epitopes of the proteasome are also found in the Lewy body *(25)*. Ubiquitin and proteasome components are present in the Lewy body, most likely because the inclusion is enriched in a protein that they are unable to degrade or one that is degraded at a slower pace than it is produced.

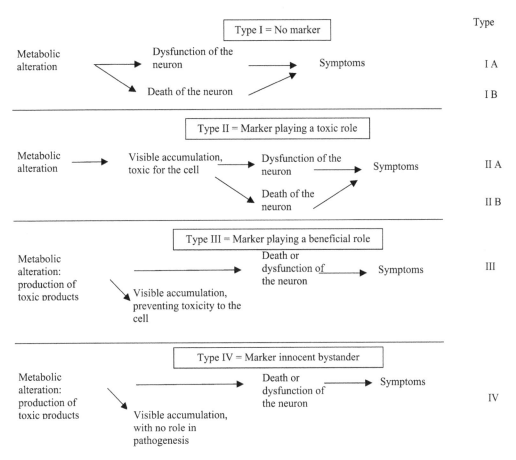

Fig. 4. Various potential effects of the cellular inclusions used as markers. Although the pathophysiology of most neurodegenerative diseases remains elusive, observational evidences suggest that at least four types of relationship may exist between the molecular process causing the neurodegenerative disorders and the cellular inclusions that may (or may not) be found in those disorders. An arbitrary number was given to each of them to facilitate their description. Data, supporting the view that each of these mechanisms is indeed encountered in pathology, are still circumstantial: neuroleptics lead to parkinsonism without neuronal death nor detectable lesion (type IA). Parkin mutation leads to neuronal death, most of the time without any identified markers (type IB). Many data indicate that the number of NFTs is correlated with the severity of the symptoms, for instance in Alzheimer's disease *(225–227)*, suggesting their direct toxic role (type II). Preventing the formation of nuclear inclusions in polyglutamine disease may, in some experimental conditions, aggravate neuronal toxicity *(228,229)*, an observation compatible with their beneficial effect (type III).

α-Synuclein was initially isolated from the torpedo fish electric organ that Marotaux et al. *(26)* screened for presynaptic proteins. A fragment of α-synuclein was found to be present in an extract of senile plaques and called NAC (non-amyloid component of the senile plaque) *(27)*. The precursor of this protein, called NACP, is identical to α-synuclein. A similar protein, called synelfin, has been identified in the bird *(28)*. Years after the identification of α-synuclein, the finding of mutations in the α-synuclein gene in IPD patients from four families living around the Mediterranean Sea came as a surprise *(29)*. The presence of α-synuclein in the Lewy body was demonstrated shortly after this initial observation *(30)*. The intensity of the labeling by anti-α-synuclein antibody and its sensitivity suggest that it is, indeed, a major component of the Lewy body. α-Synuclein immunohistochemistry facilitates the identification of the lesions and makes it clear that their distribution is more widespread than initially thought *(5)*.

There is indirect evidence that Lewy bodies could be responsible for neuronal death. They are, indeed, associated with neuronal loss in all the subcortical nuclei where they are found. The existence of a neuronal loss in the cerebral cortex is more difficult to ascertain *(31)*. It could be lacking *(32)*.

Distribution of Lewy Bodies and Lewy Neurites

Lewy body disease is the term proposed by Kosaka *(33–35)* to describe the disorders in which Lewy bodies are abundant, regardless of the clinical symptoms and signs. It is a neuropathological term that cannot be considered as the final diagnosis, which has to integrate, as we shall see, the clinical data. The distribution of the inclusions is not random. In the brainstem, they selectively involve the pigmented nuclei (substantia nigra, locus coeruleus, dorsal nucleus of the Xth nerve). They are abundant in subcortical nuclei such as the basal nucleus of Meynert, the amygdala, the hypothalamus, and the limbic nuclei of the thalamus *(36)*. In the cerebral cortex, they are predominantly found in the deep layers of the parahippocampal and the cingulate gyri, and in the insula *(32,37,38)*. They are also present in the peripheral nervous system, particularly in the stellate ganglia *(39)*, and in the cardiac *(40)* and myenteric *(41)* plexuses.

According to Kosaka *(34,35)*, Lewy bodies may be found in the brainstem ("brainstem type" of Lewy body disease), the brainstem and the limbic cortices (transitional type), and the brainstem, limbic cortices, and the isocortex (diffuse type); see Table 1. The borders between these three types of Lewy body diseases are not as sharp as may appear. It has become apparent *(42)*, particularly with α–synuclein immunohistochemistry, that Lewy bodies were nearly always present in the isocortex when they were found in the substantia nigra.

Association of Cortical Lewy Bodies With Alzheimer's Type Pathology

The frequent association of Alzheimer's lesions and Lewy bodies has been mentioned in IPD as well as in Alzheimer's disease.

Alzheimer's Lesions in IPD Cases

Alzheimer's lesions are often found in cases of IPD *(42–48)*. They have long been considered the principal cause of parkinsonism dementia, the intellectual deficit occurring at the late stages of IPD. The importance of Alzheimer's lesions may, however, have been exaggerated. Recent data, obtained with α-synuclein immunohistochemistry, tend to emphasize the responsibility of cortical Lewy pathology in the cognitive deficit *(49)*.

Lewy Bodies in Alzheimer's Disease

Lewy bodies have often been associated with senile plaques in large postmortem studies of cases with initial or predominant dementia *(50–53)*. They are particularly abundant in the amygdala, where the co-occurrence of a neurofibrillary tangle and of a Lewy body in the same neurone has been reported *(54)*. The low density of neurofibrillary tangles, when Lewy bodies are added to Alzheimer's-type pathology *(55)*, could be owing to a more rapid fatal outcome than in pure Alzheimer's disease. This would explain why Braak stage is usually lower at death in the cases with combined pathology *(56)*. The presence of Lewy bodies in cases suffering from a disorder that is, in many clinical and neuropathological aspects, comparable to Alzheimer's disease, explains terms such as "Lewy body variant of Alzheimer's disease" *(57)* or "senile dementia of Lewy body type" *(58)*, now replaced by the general appellation "dementia with Lewy bodies" *(59,60)*. A high prevalence of Lewy bodies is not only found in the sporadic form of Alzheimer's disease, but has also been mentioned in familial cases *(61,62)* or in trisomy 21 *(63)*.

Why are Alzheimers-type and Lewy-type pathology so frequently associated? Alzheimer's disease and IPD are frequent but not to the point of explaining the high prevalence of their common occurrence. The hypothesis, according to which IPD and Alzheimer's disease are extremes of a spectrum of neurodegeneration sharing the same pathogenic mechanism, has been put forward *(64)*. It

Table 1
The Three Types of Lewy Body Disease According to Kosaka

	Brainstem Type	Transitional Type	Diffuse Type
Brainstem	X	X	X
Basal nucleus of Meynert	X	X	X
Limbic Areas		X	X
Isocortex			X

According to Kosaka *(34,35)*, the topography of the Lewy bodies is organized in three different distributions. An "X" rectangle means presence of Lewy bodies. The brainstem type is commonly found in Parkinson's disease. The diffuse type is usually associated with DLB. In the transitional type, cognitive symptoms are common; they may be primary or complicate IPD. The borders between the three types may be difficult to draw. It has been shown that even in cases of apparently uncomplicated IPD, the presence of a few Lewy bodies in the isocortex is common *(42)*.

should, however, be stressed that there are differences in the genetic background of IPD and Alzheimer's disease cases. The prevalence of the ApoE4 allele, a known risk factor for Alzheimer's disease, is normal in IPD cases even with dementia *(65,66)*, but is increased in cases of dementia even with Lewy bodies *(67)*. Moreover, the mutations causing Alzheimer's disease are clearly different from those related to IPD, indicating that at least some causal factors are not shared by the two disorders: they cannot simply be considered as phenotypic variants of the same disease. At the cellular level, direct interaction between tau and α-synuclein proteins could enhance their fibrillization *(68)*.

Clinico-Pathological Correlations

The final diagnosis in cases with Lewy bodies is clinico-pathological since long-standing IPD and DLB may present with similar, or possibly identical, neuropathological phenotype. The most characteristic diagnostic combinations are the following (*see* Table 2):

1. The initial and main complaints concern the motor system. The disorder slowly progresses during decades. Lewy bodies and Lewy neurites are mainly found in the brainstem (brainstem type of Lewy body disease). The diagnosis of IPD should be made.
2. The initial and main complaints concern the motor system but in the late stages of the disease, visual hallucinations occur and a cognitive deficit was present. Lewy bodies are found not only in the brainstem and in the limbic cortices, but also in large numbers in the cerebral cortex, often associated with Alzheimer's lesions (diffuse type of Lewy body disease). The diagnosis of PD with dementia is then warranted.
3. Finally, the disease starts with a fluctuating cognitive deficit that remains as the main symptom and is associated with visual hallucinations. Numerous Lewy bodies are found not only in the brainstem and in the limbic cortices, but also in the isocortex. The diagnosis of dementia with Lewy bodies should be made.

Multiple System Atrophy

Striatonigral degeneration *(69,70)* was initially an autopsy finding since the symptoms are very similar to those of IPD, except that there is a resistance to treatment by L-dopa *(71)*. The gross examination shows a peculiar and often severe atrophy along with a green discoloration of the putamen that is distinctive of the disease. The substantia nigra is pale. As already mentioned by Adams et al. ("Dégénérescences nigro-striées et cérébello-nigro-striées"), the cerebellum is often atrophic *(69)*. This introduces a second group of disorders, which were identified at the beginning of the 20th century by Dejerine and Thomas under the descriptive term of olivopontocerebellar atrophy. The sporadic nature of this atrophy contrasted with familial cases previously described by Menzel. Here, the severity of the cerebellar syndrome is striking. Again, the progression of the disease is relentless, but it had been noticed since the initial descriptions that parkinsonism may develop secondarily (*see*

Table 2
Various Types of Lewy Body Disease Are Clinico-Pathological Diagnoses

Symptoms	Distribution of Lewy Bodies	Diagnosis
Parkinsonism	Brainstem type of Lewy body disease	Idiopathic Parkinson's disease
Initial parkinsonism. Late cognitive symptoms	Diffuse type of Lewy body disease +/– Alzheimer lesions	Idiopathic Parkinson disease with dementia
Initial and predominant cognitive symptoms.	Diffuse type of Lewy body disease +/– Alzheimer's lesions	Dementia with Lewy bodies
?	Brainstem type of Lewy body disease	Probable idiopathic Parkinson's disease, possibly incipiens
?	Diffuse type of Lewy body disease	Idiopathic Parkinson's disease with dementia *or* dementia with Lewy bodies

The diagnosis of the common diseases with Lewy bodies is clinico-pathological. It mainly relies on the chronological order in which the motor symptoms and the cognitive deficit appear (*see* first column) and on the distribution of the Lewy bodies, which can be classified, according to Kosaka, into three types (brainstem, transitional, diffuse)—see second column. When only the pathological information is available (? in the first column), the final diagnosis is ambiguous in case of diffuse type of Lewy body disease.

e.g., ref. *72*). Parkinsonism, when present, masks the cerebellar symptoms. Finally, orthostatic hypotension is frequently associated both with striatonigral degeneration and olivopontocerebellar atrophy. Autonomic failure may be the main symptom. Primary autonomic failure is also known under the eponym of Shy–Drager syndrome.

The frequent association of the three disorders (striatonigral degeneration, olivopontocerebellar atrophy, and primary autonomic failure) led Graham and Oppenheimer, in a case report, to suggest that they were in fact syndromes belonging to the same disease. They tentatively named it multiple system atrophy (MSA) *(73)*, the name that is still in use today *(71)* (*see* Fig. 5).

An unexpected validation of this concept came from neuropathology. In many of the cases that were recorded as suffering from MSA, peculiar inclusions were identified by Papp and Lantos *(74)*. They were initially demonstrated by Gallyas staining method but were perfectly visible with other silver impregnations *(75)*. They mainly involve the cell body of the oligodendrocytes but may also affect neurons or astrocytes (*see* Chapter 4, Neuropathology of Atypical Parkinsonian Disorders, for detailed description). The high frequency of oligodendroglial lesions helps to understand why the myelin appears so massively affected in MSA.

It is by chance that these inclusions were found to include α-synuclein epitopes that were identified by immunohistochemistry. The expression of α-synuclein in glia is poorly explained but can probably occur normally *(76)*. The attempt of reproducing the disease by introducing an α-synuclein transgene under the control of an oligodendroglial promoter has, so far, been unsuccessful *(77)*.

THE TAUOPATHIES

Tau Protein: 3R and 4R Tau

A large group of neurodegenerative diseases (including Alzheimer's disease, PSP, CBD, argyrophilic grain disease, Pick's disease, PDC, PEP) are characterized by the accumulation of tau protein. Tau is a phospho-protein that is normally involved in the regulation of tubulin assembly. Tau accumulation is always intracellular and gives rise to inclusions with a variety of shapes, depending on the disease in which they occur. This diversity in the morphology of the inclusions is not understood at the present time. It is obviously related to the cellular type in which the accumulation takes place

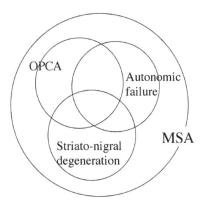

Fig. 5. Multiple system atrophy. This Venn diagram illustrates the way in which the three syndromes (olivopontocerebellar atrophy or OPCA, striato-nigral degeneration, and primary autonomic failure) may be diversely associated. The pure syndromes, as well as their various associations, all belong to multiple system atrophy or MSA. Areas are not proportional to prevalence in this diagram.

(astrocytes, oligodendrocytes, and neurons), but even within a given cell type, tau protein may aggregate in inclusions of different shapes. This suggests that tau protein interacts with different cofactors or occupy different subcellular compartments. This could be related to the isoforms of tau: six of them have been identified *(78)* that are generated by alternative splicing. These tau isoforms may include three or four of the repetitive motives that bind to the microtubules (respectively three or four repeats tau: 3R or 4R tau). In 3R tau the second repeat (encoded by exon 10) has been spliced out. Western blot analysis reveals three main patterns of migration of tau protein in neurodegenerative diseases explained by different ratios of tau isoforms *(79,80)*. The accumulation of tau involves:

- 3R and 4R tau: This is the case in Alzheimer's disease *(81,82)*, PEP *(83)*, and PDC).
- 4R tau: This occurs in PSP, CBD *(79,84)*, and argyrophilic grain disease *(85)*.
- 3R tau: As in Pick's disease *(86)*.

Several transgenic mice expressing tau transgenes under various promoters have been produced. Tau-positive inclusions in neurons and glia have been observed in some of these lines *(87)*. The clinical deficit is related to the site of expression of the tau transgene *(88)*.

We will now consider the diseases in which tau-enriched inclusions are observed either in neurons or in glia (so called "tauopathy"). The isoform(s) of tau that accumulate and the shape of the inclusions are characteristic of each one of these disorders. Four-R, 3R, and 3&4R tauopathies are the diseases in which, respectively, 4R tau, 3R tau, and 3&4R tau accumulate.

The 4R Tauopathies: PSP, CBD, and Argyrophilic Grain Disease—Their Borders and Overlaps

In PSP, CBD *(89)*, and argyrophilic grain disease *(85)*, it is predominantly the tau protein containing four repetitive motives that accumulates. Parkinsonism is prominent in both PSP and CBD, whereas dementia is the main symptom of argyrophilic grain disease. Although parkinsonism is lacking in this last disorder, we shall briefly deal with it, since it may be associated with the other two.

The initial description of PSP and CBD *(90–92)* suggested that their neuropathology was quite different: neurofibrillary tangles (NFTs) were seen in the brainstem of PSP and ballooned neurons in the cerebral cortex of CBD, two clearly different neuropathological lesions. The realization that tau pathology was prominent in both disorders made their borders less sharply defined. Moreover, PSP and CBD share a common genetic risk factor: several polymorphisms have indeed been identified in the tau gene *(93)* and may be grouped in two haplotypes, H1 and H2. The H1 haplotype, is frequent in the general population (frequency of that haplotype in the general population, around 77%) but this frequency reaches nearly 94% in PSP cases and 92% in CBD *(94,95)*. Despite this resemblance, PSP and CBD have characteristics of their own that we will now discuss.

Progressive Supranuclear Palsy

There were various reports of cases with hypertonia and gaze palsy of voluntary movements before the classical description of Steele et al. *(90)*. At the time of that paper, a major issue was to differentiate postencephalitic parkinsonism from PSP, since both disorders were initially defined by the presence of NFTs in the brainstem *(96)*. The distinction still remains difficult today, on either clinical *(97)* or pathological grounds *(98)*.

Soon after the identification of tau protein epitopes in the NFTs of Alzheimer's disease *(99,100)*, NFTs in PSP were also found to be reactive with tau antibody *(101)*. Tau immunohistochemistry, but also a particular silver method (Gallyas silver impregnation; *see* ref. *102*), expanded the span of the morphological alterations thought to be characteristic of PSP. It was discovered that fibrillar structures, especially in the basal ganglia, were intensely reactive with tau antibody. They were called "neuropil threads" *(103)* by analogy with morphologically similar lesions found in Alzheimer's disease. However, electron microscopy revealed that the accumulation of tau protein, in PSP, occurred in the myelin rather than in the axon itself *(104–106)*. Tau is initially present in the cytoplasm of the oligodendrocytes, and follows the cytoplasm while it wraps around the axon in the process of myelin formation *(106)*. In the cell body of the oligodendrocytes, tau precipitates in fibrillar structures, which seem to coil around the oligodendrocyte nucleus, hence the term "coiled body" proposed by Braak and Braak *(107)*. Coiled bodies were initially described in argyrophilic grains disease (another 4R tauopathy mainly responsible for cognitive deficits, as previously mentioned). Coiled bodies are actually present in a range of diseases: not only PSP, but also argyrophilic grains disease, Pick's disease and CBD.

Oligodendrocytes are not the only glial cells in which tau protein accumulates. Astrocytes are also altered. Although this astrocytic lesion happened to be identified much later than the NFTs, it now seems to be the best marker of PSP *(108)*. Tau accumulation in astrocytes was initially suspected on the shape of the cell bearing the inclusion: the nucleus was clear and the immunoreactivity filled the entire length of the cellular processes, which appeared to be equally distributed in all directions—hence the name "tuft(ed) astrocyte" that was applied to this lesion *(109,110)*. Double labeling showed a colocalization of tau and glial fibrillary acid protein (GFAP) *(108,111–113)*. Tufted astrocytes are particularly abundant in the putamen and caudate nucleus; they are also found in the red nucleus and in the superior colliculus *(114)*.

There are still some discussions concerning the ultrastructural aspect of PSP lesions. The first descriptions concluded that NFTs were made of straight filaments 15 nm in diameter, straight tubules *(115,116)* clearly different from the paired helical filaments (PHFs) as seen in Alzheimer's disease. Other reports mention twisted structures, 22 nm in diameter, reminiscent of PHFs and described as "twisted tubules" *(117,118)*. A more recent study *(119)* suggests that straight filaments are present in glia, either in oligodendrocytes (coiled bodies) where they are 15 nm thick and have a smooth appearance or in astrocytes (tufted astrocytes), where they have jagged contours and their diameter reaches 22 nm. The twisted filaments (22 nm wide) are most commonly seen in neurons (NFTs).

In the initial paper of Steele et al. *(90)*, the pathology was described as largely confined to subcortical structures. Increased sensitivity of the staining procedures and of immunohistochemistry allowed for the conclusion that the cerebral cortex was not spared and often contained NFTs *(109,120,121)*. Astrocytic tufts are also present in the cortex, particularly in the precentral and premotor areas *(108,114)*.

Tau accumulation takes place in selective regions of the brain and the balance between the three major alterations (tuft astrocytes, neuropil threads, and NFTs) is variable according to the regions *(110,122)* (see Chapter 4).

The diagnosis of PSP was previously clinico-pathological and although cases without gaze palsy had been reported *(123,124)*, the clinical syndrome appeared fairly homogeneous. The recent tendency of relying mainly on morphological markers to make the diagnosis deeply modified the clinical aspect of the disease and greatly expanded its scope (Table 3). Prominent frontal syndrome (already mentioned by Cambier et al. in ref. *125*) and cognitive decline *(126–128)* probably related to the severity of the cortical involvement *(129,130)*, progressive aphasia *(131)*, limb apraxia, focal dystonia, and arm levitation more common in CBD *(126,132–135)* have been reported in pathologically confirmed PSP cases. On the other hand, supranuclear gaze palsy, initially considered to be the clinical hallmark of the disease, may be absent in as many as half the cases *(123,124)*.

A focus of atypical parkinsonism resembling PSP has also been identified in Guadaloupe, French West Indies *(136)*. Three cases have been published up to now. In two cases, the diagnosis of PSP could be reliably made. One case had an unusual tauopathy characterized by pretangles, tangles, and a large number of threads, without tufted astrocytes nor glial plaques. Tau gene was found normal *(136)*. In the three cases, the Western blot showed 4R-tau accumulation. The high prevalence of atypical parkinsonism in Guadaloupe has been attributed to environmental factor. Herbal tea or fruits of tropical plants, traditionally used by African-Caribbeans, contain alkaloid toxins, which could play a pathogenic role *(137)*.

Corticobasal Degeneration

Apraxia is an inability of carrying on a purposive movement, not explained by a motor deficit, a sensory loss, or ataxia. In the absence of a space-occupying or vascular lesion, progressive apraxia of relentless course is a striking and uncommon clinical sign, which helped to identify the disorder now known as CBD *(91,92)*. In the first three cases that were published, the emphasis was put on two basic features of the disorder:

1. The neuronal loss had a peculiar topography for which the forbidding label of "corticodentatonigral degeneration" was proposed.
2. A special lesion of the neurons was observed in the involved areas: having lost their Nissl granules, their cell body appeared abnormally pale.

In the first days of neuropathology, when Nissl stain was the most commonly used technique in neuropathology, Nissl granules were the only structures that were stained in the neuronal cell body. A neuron without Nissl granules was said to be chromatolytic (chroma = color); chromatolysis is, for instance, the consequence of axon section. Rebeiz, Kolodny, and Richardson *(91,92)* coined the new term "achromatic" to define the neurons that were found in this new disorder and that might, indeed, be slightly different from those seen in chromatolysis *(92)*. "The appearance of these swollen nerve cells was reminiscent of the central chromatolysis that typifies the retrograde cell change (axonal reaction) and the neuronal change typical of pellagra but differed in that there was total disappearance of Nissl granules, rather than sparseness or peripheral displacement of them" *(92)*.

Strangely enough, CBD, as judged by published reports, remained exceptionally diagnosed for many years. It was felt at that time that the major difficulty was to distinguish achromatic neurons of CBD from the ballooned neurons (also called Pick's cells) found in Pick's disease. Although Pick's disease is essentially a frontal dementia, cases were reported with a predominant parietal syndrome characterized by a progressive apraxia *(138,139)*. The border with CBD appeared thus difficult to draw. This may still be the case today but for other reasons.

The diagnosis of CBD has experienced a renaissance when a new name was given to the disease to emphasize the peculiar distribution of the lesions: they indeed involve both the cortex and the basal ganglia—hence corticobasal degeneration *(140)*. Scrutiny of the lesions of the substantia nigra sug-

Table 3
Typical and Atypical Clinical Forms of Progressive Supranuclear Palsy and Corticobasal Degeneration

	Clinical Symptoms	Distinctive Neuropathological Features	Common Histopathological Features	Common Genetic Risk Factor	Common Biochemical Characteristic
PSP — Typical form	Gait disturbance Severe rigidity without tremor Poor Dopa responsiveness Gaze supranuclear palsy	Abundant NFTs (straight filaments) in brainstem & pallidum Astrocytic tufts in putamen, premotor, and prefrontal cortex.	NFTs in substantia nigra		
PSP — Atypical clinical forms	Prominent frontal syndrome Cognitive decline Limb apraxia Progressive apraxia	Generally linked with the severity of the involvement of specific areas. Astrocytic tuft used as a diagnostic marker.	Coiled bodies Tau-positive threads of glial origin (more in CBD than in PSP)	High prevalence of the H1 haplotype of tau protein	Accumulation of tau protein with four repetitive motives (4R-tau), i.e., with the sequence corresponding to exon 10
CBD — Typical form	Absence of supranuclear palsy Progressive apraxia	? Ballooned neurons principally in cortex. Astrocytic plaque in cortex and caudate.	Ballooned neurons in limbic system (especially in PSP if argyrophilic grain disease associated)		
CBD — Atypical clinical forms	Supranuclear gaze palsy Frontal syndrome Progressive aphasia	Generally linked with the severity of the involvement of specific areas. Astrocytic plaque used as a diagnostic marker.			

PSP and CBD were initially clinicopathological diagnoses (a typical clinical syndrome was associated with a characteristic neuropathology). Since pathological markers have been used to define them—astrocytic tuft for PSP and astrocytic plaque for DCB—their clinical phenotype has changed ("atypical clinical forms"). PSP and CBD have a common genetic risk factor (tau haplotype H1). In both diseases, it is mainly tau 4-R that accumulates.

gested that some type of inclusion could help identifying the disorder: they were basophilic, poorly argyrophilic with Bielschowsky stain, and filled the neuronal cell body *(140)*. But those "corticobasal inclusions" did not survive tau immunohistochemistry, which demonstrated that they were, in fact, true NFTs.

It may be surprising that it took more than 25 yr to realize that a severe cytoskeletal pathology occurred in CBD *(141–144)*. Such a long delay between the initial description of the disease and the elucidation of its typical lesions is probably related to the poor reactivity of CBD alterations to standard silver stain (Gallyas stain, which exquisitely labels them, is an exception) *(142)*. Immunohistochemistry now reveals a whole range of tau accumulations in neurons, glia, and processes. In neurons, it shows inclusions that resemble Pick's bodies, a resemblance that has suggested overlaps between the two disorders *(145,146)*. However, Pick's bodies and neuronal inclusions of CBD may be distinguished *(147)*: one important difference is the low reactivity of Pick's bodies to Gallyas stain in contrast to the neuronal inclusions of CBD. This contrast in staining properties could be due to a difference in the isoforms of the tau protein that accumulates: Pick's bodies are made of 3R-tau whereas neuronal inclusions of CBD contain 4R-tau *(148,149)*. The high density of tau-positive threads in the subcortical white matter and in the deep layers of cortex is quite distinctive of CBD *(150,151)*. As in PSP, these threads appear to be related to the presence of tau in myelin inner and outer loops *(104)*. Another lesion is now considered to be more specific of CBD: the "astrocytic plaque" (or "glial plaque") characterized by "an annulus of tau-positive structures surrounding a clear central core" *(144)*. This lesion has been interpreted as the accumulation of tau in the distal processes of the astrocyte *(144,152)*: this interpretation is based on double-labeling experiments using tau and CD44 antibodies. CD44 is a membrane protein found in leukocytes and activated astroglia. Colocalization is not found with GFAP *(144)*. Astrocytic plaques are particularly abundant in the prefrontal and premotor areas of the cerebral cortex and in the caudate nucleus *(114)*.

Tau-positive threads, coiled bodies, and tangles are shared lesions of CBD and PSP. Thus, although it was, initially, with Pick's disease that the border of CBD was considered difficult to draw, it was, later on, with PSP that the differences seemed to be most elusive. Komori et al. proposed using astrocytic plaques and tufted astrocytes as diagnostic hallmarks, respectively of CBD and PSP *(153,154)*, an opinion that was essentially endorsed by the diagnostic criteria of CBD *(155)*. When these neuropathologic markers are taken as diagnostic tools, the clinical presentation of both diseases appears to be more diverse than initially thought: there are indeed cases of supranuclear gaze palsy *(156)*, progressive aphasia *(131,147,157)*, or frontal dementia *(158,159)*, which exhibit the typical lesions of CBD, whereas some patients who meet the neuropathologic diagnostic criteria of PSP present, as we have seen, with progressive apraxia, reminiscent of CBD.

The use of astrocytic plaques and of tufted astrocytes as the diagnostic markers of CBD and PSP, respectively, modifies the spectrum of the clinical phenotype of both diseases and makes any prediction concerning the pathology, at least presently, particularly difficult. There are distinctive features at neuropathological examination (they are fully reviewed in ref. *160)*, but even at this stage doubts concerning the diagnosis may remain; cases have been described with neuropathological characteristics of both disorders *(161)*.

Argyrophilic Grain Disease and Neurofibrillary Degeneration of CA2

Argyrophilic grain disease is characterized by the presence of small, spindle-shaped structures loosely scattered in the neuropil of the hippocampus, entorhinal cortex, and amygdala. It was originally found in cases with dementia and was frequently associated with Alzheimer's disease-type pathology. Parkinsonism is not a feature of this disease but since the grains are the focal accumulation of 4R-tau *(85)* in dendritic spines, it is useful to mention here that association of argyrophilic grain disease and PSP seems particularly frequent *(162)*. Also common to 4R tauopathy is the neurofibrillary degeneration in CA2 sector of the hippocampus, an unusual alteration found in argyrophilic grain disease, PSP, and CBD *(163)*.

The 3 and 4R Tauopathies

We turn now to a set of disorders in which tau protein that makes up the inclusions is a various mix of 3R and 4R isoforms. Alzheimer's disease belongs to that category and because of its frequency is the first disorder to be considered in this chapter.

Alzheimer's Disease

Alzheimer's-type pathology is the only detectable lesion in a significant proportion of cases in which the diagnosis of IPD has been made premortem *(20,164,165)*. This observation raises the possibility that Alzheimer's disease, in the absence of dementia, causes the parkinsonian symptoms by a direct involvement of the nigrostriatal pathway *(165)*. It is not the place to review here the pathology of Alzheimer's disease: suffice it to say that extracellular deposition of Aβ peptide and intracellular accumulation of both 3R and 4R tau isoforms are the principal lesions. Tau accumulates in three compartments: the neuronal cell body (NFT), the dendrites (neuropil threads), and the axonal component of the corona of the senile plaques (their "neuritic" component). Aβ deposition, without a neuritic component, does not correlate with symptoms or only weakly, whereas tau pathology usually strongly does. The abundance of Aβ peptide deposits in the striatum has been known for a long time *(166)* but it is doubtful, in view of what has just been said, that they explain the clinical signs. It is more likely that the NFTs found in many large and in a few medium-size neurons of the same nucleus *(166)* play a role. There is also evidence that the NFTs present in the substantia nigra *(167)* are the main culprit; their abundance is indeed linked with the severity of the extrapyramidal signs *(168)*. The existence and the severity of the neuronal loss in this nucleus is discussed *(168–170)*.

The involvement of the substantia nigra could be more severe in the common type of DLB, in which Lewy bodies and NFTs combine their effects. Extrapyramidal symptoms belong to the cardinal signs, which should raise the possibility of DLB in cases of dementia. However, as already mentioned, it is difficult to differentiate on a clinical basis Alzheimer's disease with and without Lewy bodies *(171)* from DLB cases with and without Alzheimer's lesions *(37)*.

Dementia pugilistica, the dementia that develops in boxers, is characterized by a severe extrapyramidal syndrome. Its pathology resembles Alzheimer's disease pathology *(172)*. Quite intriguing is the finding of isolated neocortical NFTs in a young boxer who died early in his career *(173)*. This suggests that head trauma could, by itself, induce the formation of NFTs, preceding amyloid deposition *(174)* (*see* Chapter 4 for further developments).

The two disorders that are considered next, PEP and PDC, are rare. The epidemic at the origin of PEP ended a long time ago. PDC is confined to one small geographic area. Data from these disorders may help answer two questions: Are the differences in the ratio of tau isoforms between tauopathy explained by the cell types in which tau accumulates? Are tauopathies explained by a specific etiology? (1) To explain that different tau isoforms accumulate in various diseases, the hypothesis has been put forward that their relative abundance depends on the cellular type, neuronal or glial, in which the inclusions are found. PEP and PDC show that this is probably not the case: tau accumulates only in neurones in Alzheimer's disease, a 3&4R tauopathy. PEP and PDC are also 3&4R tauopathies but the inclusions are not limited to the neurones. (2) PEP also indicates that NFTs cannot be considered as indicating a specific etiology. It is indeed observed in disorders caused by mutations, head traumas (dementia pugilistica), or, as shown by PEP, an infectious disease of the brain. NFTs could be a "process specific" marker, the evidence of a stereotyped reaction of the neurone to injury.

Postencephalitic Parkinsonism

Parkinsonism, and other movement disorders, followed acute episodes of encephalitis lethargica, initially described by von Economo during an outbreak of the disease in 1916–1917 in Vienna. Cases were reported in 1918 in France, England, and North America. The disease presented with a variety of symptoms such as somnolence, ophthalmoplegia, hyperkinesias, and akinesia. Parkinsonism, described as the chronic form of the episode, could appear years after the acute episode *(175)*. Most salient clinical characteristics of PEP are onset below middle age, symptom duration lasting more than 10 yr, presence of oculogyric crisis, and obviously a history of encephalitis *(176)*. The disease has been linked to the "Spanish" influenza pandemic that occurred at approximately the same time. The influenza virus responsible for the Spanish flu has been isolated from an archival 1918 autopsy lung sample; its RNA was not detected in archival brain tissues from acute encephalitis lethargica. These data make the connection between Spanish flu and encephalitis lethargica doubtful *(177)*.

In the acute phase, the disease was characterized by a severe inflammation, with perivascular cuffing and neuronophagia, in the mesencephalon, particularly the substantia nigra, and in the diencephalon. Pathology is characterized by abundant neurofibrillary tangles present in a wide range of regions, the substantia nigra being usually massively involved and showing severe neuronal loss. Of more recent notice is the presence of glial fibrillary tangles or astrocytic tufts *(178)*, characterized by the presence of tau protein in astrocytes, not necessarily found in the regions most affected by tangle formation *(179)*.

In the absence of clinical history, the distinction between PSP and PEP may be particularly difficult. Subtle differences in the distribution of the lesions have been described *(180)*, but the ultrastructural aspect of the tangles (more often PHFs similar to Alzheimer's disease tangles than straight filaments common in PSP) as well as the biochemical signature of tau accumulation (both 3R and 4R tau *[83]* in PEP; 4R tau in PSP) are ways of differentiating both disorders, despite their morphologic resemblance.

Parkinsonism Dementia Complex of Guam

This disease appears so tightly related to a geographical area that the island of Guam, where it was initially described, is mentioned in its very name. However, a similar disorder is probably found in other foci of the world—the Kii peninsula, in Japan, being one (*see* refs. *181–183* for a review of the pathology).

The neuropathologist Harry Zimmerman, assigned by the U.S. Navy to Guam during World War II, was the first to notice there a high incidence of amyotrophic lateral sclerosis (ALS). ALS was said to affect 10% of the population and the number of deaths attributed to ALS was 100 times higher in Guam than in other countries *(184)*. It was secondarily noted that another degenerative disease, combining parkinsonism and dementia, was also highly prevalent. The neuropathology of this Guam "parkinsonism dementia complex" (PDC) was described by Hirano et al. *(184,185)*. Hirano et al. divided the cases into three groups: Parkinsonism and dementia; Parkinsonism, dementia, and involvement of the upper motor neuron; cases with symptoms of lower motor neuron disease. The opinion has recently been expressed that ALS in Guam is not different from ALS in other parts of the world *(181)*. The presence of Bunina bodies, the marker of classical ALS, in the Guam cases is one of the data in favor of this view *(186)*.

The neuropathology of PDC combines NFTs and neuronal loss. Most of the tangles are made of paired helical filaments, similar to those seen in Alzheimer's disease. They are tau- and, for some of them, ubiquitin-positive and have the same immunological profile as Alzheimer's tangles. According to one study *(187)*, they could occupy the cell body of the neuron for 2.5 yr before causing its death. They are then freed in the neuropil (ghost tangle). The distribution of the NFTs is widespread: isocortex and hippocampus, striatum and pallidum, hypothalamus, amygdala, substantia nigra, periaqueductal gray, pontine nuclei, dorsal nucleus of the vagus nerve, reticular formation, anterior and posterior horns of the spinal cord are among the affected structures. Neuronal loss explains the cerebral atrophy and is usually marked in the substantia nigra and locus coeruleus. The cerebellum is usually spared. Aβ pathology and tau-positive threads are *not* features of PDC. Glial pathology, shown by Gallyas stain and tau immunohistochemistry, has been observed more recently. It consists in "granular hazy inclusions" found in the cell body of the astrocytes and "crescent/coiled inclusions" in oligodendrocytes *(188)*. Hirano bodies, i.e., eosinophilic rodlike inclusions adjacent to neuronal cell bodies (and occasionally within them), in the Sommer sector of the hippocampus, were initially described in Guam patients but were also found later in other degenerative diseases.

Guam ALS/PDC has raised many still unanswered questions. Since the disease seemed to be confined to the Chamorro population, the native people of Guam, a hereditary disorder was initially suspected. However, several facts argue against an etiologic role of heredity. The incidence of Guam ALS has been dramatically decreasing in the last decades (although the incidence of PDC not so markedly), a change that heredity cannot explain. The risk of developing the disease is lower in Chamorros that have left Guam but with inertia (a latency of several decades). Finally, Filipinos and a few Caucasians have also developed the disease (*see* review in ref. *183*).

Many attempts made to identify the cause of Guam ALS/PDC have failed. The principal etiologies that have been considered are infectious (by a process similar to PEP after encephalitis lethargica) and toxic. The possibility that cycad, the seed of the false sago palm traditionally used in Chamorro food, contained toxic species, was put forward by P. Spencer *(189)*. However the amount of seed necessary to obtain a toxic effect in the monkey seems incompatible with the common use of cycad by Chamorros *(190)*. More recently, Perl et al. have shown a high concentration of aluminum and iron in the NFTs of Guam ALS/PDC and have suggested that these metals could play a role in the pathogenesis (*see* review in ref. *183*). Although the identification of the etiological factor should be easier for a rare disorder developing in a circumscribed environment than for common diseases that are geographically widespread, the etiology of Guam ALS/PDC remains elusive.

The Use of the Terms Pick's Disease and Pick's Complex

Although parkinsonism in Pick's disease (in the restricted sense) is a secondary symptom and raises little diagnostic difficulty, the extensive use of the term Pick's disease and the recently introduced Pick's complex (which may include conditions otherwise defined as CBD) requires some explanation.

The clinical symptoms of frontal involvement, which are seen at the onset in some cases of dementia, contrast strongly with the initial memory problems typical of Alzheimer's disease. In the old literature *(191–193)*, those cases were grouped under the heading of Pick's disease. The term was historically incorrect since Pick had initially described cases with focal cortical deficit owing to "circumscribed atrophy" (in the language of the time) *(194–196)*. Cases of frontal syndrome are not included in his main articles, which described cases of progressive aphasia *(197)* and of progressive apraxia *(196)*. Alzheimer performed the neuropathological examination of cases of circumscribed atrophy (probably of the frontal lobe but this is barely mentioned in his paper) and found a new inclusion *(198)* (English translation in ref. *199*), which was later known as Pick's body. It is a spherical accumulation of tau-positive and argyrophilic material, approximately the size of the nucleus, located in the cell body of the neurons. Pick's body is generally considered as almost exclusively made of 3R tau *(148,149,200)*, although some doubts have been recently expressed concerning the selectivity of the isoform *(201)*. Pick's bodies are particularly abundant in the dentate gyrus, where they are considered to be constant. They are generally associated with ballooned, chromatolytic neurons, called Pick's cells. Ramified astrocytes and small Pick's body-like inclusions, discovered more recently, are evidence that the disease does not spare the glia *(202)*. Pick's bodies are generally found in cases of dementia with a predominant frontal syndrome.

The meanings of Pick's disease have been shaped by the various historical contexts in which the term has been used (focal cortical syndrome or "circumscribed atrophy"; frontal syndrome owing to a degenerative disease with or without Pick's bodies; dementia, generally of the frontal-lobe type, with Pick's bodies). A Venn diagram may visualize the relationship between these different meanings, from the least to the most specific ones, and helps explain why Pick's disease has come to be such a confusing label (*see* Fig. 6). The recent attempt to introduce the term Pick's complex for a large set of disorders with various neuropathology *(203–209)* may, in our view, be discussed since it

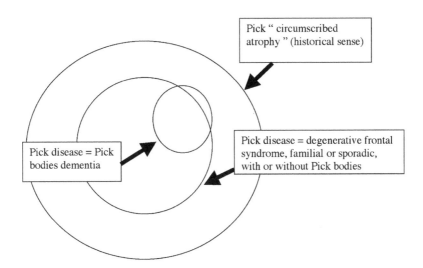

Fig. 6. The different meanings of Pick's disease. The different meanings of the term Pick's disease cover overlapping subsets of disorders. The concept of Pick's complex, more recently proposed *(205)*, would probably include most of the cases that were historically described under the heading of "Pick's circumscribed atrophy." From the point of view adopted in this chapter, it seems more adequate to restrict the use of the term to its most specific meaning of "Pick's bodies dementia." Pick's bodies are generally found in sporadic cases with a predominant frontal syndrome. Cases with progressive aphasia *(139,209,230)* or apraxia *(139)* have been described, explaining why the last circle ("Pick's bodies dementia") overlaps the set of "circumscribed atrophies" (focal cortical syndromes). The surface areas enclosed in the three circles are subjective evaluations of the prevalence of the various disorders: the figure does not rely on objective data.

lumps diseases that all the recent data tend to separate. We would rather recommend restricting the use of Pick's disease to the cases of dementia with Pick bodies *(210,211)*, as most neurologists and neuropathologists would *(212)*. In this use, Pick's disease is a rare sporadic disease.

The Familial Tauopathies: Frontotemporal Dementia With Parkinsonism

Besides the sporadic cases with Pick's bodies, a large number of patients present with a frontal syndrome of progressive course. A fair proportion of them are familial. Among them, several exhibit parkinsonian symptoms. A consensus meeting identified some of those families with linkage to chromosome 17 and grouped those cases under the heading of frontotemporal dementia with parkinsonism linked to chromosome 17 or FTDP-17 *(213)*. Shortly after, a mutation of the tau gene was found in some of these families *(214,215)*. Tau mutations are very diverse and so is the neuropathology. The isoforms of tau, which accumulate depend on the mutation. Both 3R and 4R tauopathy are met in this group of disorders. It is not the place here to review the complex picture of FTDP-17 neuropathology (analyzed in details in ref. *216*). It is useful however to emphasize here the phenotypic mimicry of some specific mutations. The neuropathology of the sporadic diseases that we have previously considered, more specifically PSP *(217)*, CBD *(218,219)*, and Pick's disease *(220,221)*, can, indeed, be mimicked by tau mutations. This observation suggests that the cellular type in which tau accumulation occurs, and its subcellular topography, are highly dependent on the tau molecule itself. The presence of ballooned neurons, NFTs, Pick's bodies, and glial inclusions may, indeed, be determined by one single change in the molecular structure of tau. This is not to say that all the diseases that were considered here have a genetic origin: PSP, CBD, and Pick's disease are, in the great majority of cases, sporadic. But the similarity of the phenotypes suggests that the pathogenic mechanism involves directly tau protein in the sporadic as well as in the hereditary tauopathies.

OTHERS CAUSES

This review did not consider drug-induced parkinsonism, probably its most common etiology and usually related to neuroleptics. Suffice it to say that up to now, no lesions have been identified in those cases. Toxic causes (MPTP induced or related to manganese poisoning) are dealt with in Chapter 4. Several hereditary disorders—among which are spinocerebellar ataxia (SCA), Huntington's disease (related to an expansion of the triplet cytosine adenine guanine coding for a long polyglutamine stretch in the mutated protein), Wilson's disease, neurodegeneration with brain iron accumulation (formerly Hallervorden–Spatz disease)—may cause extrapyramidal symptoms. They are considered in Chapter 4.

FUTURE DIRECTIONS

The nosology of neurodegeneration will ultimately rely on the understanding of mechanisms. Mechanism, in this context, means the intricate relationship between the cause of a disease and the beneficial or detrimental processes that the organism triggers in response. A number of neurodegenerative diseases will probably give their secret in the decades to come, with the help of molecular biology and of the animal models that are rapidly generated. What will then be the place of pathology? Will its role be reduced to that of classifying details? Will it still be used as an important way to unravel the complexity of the postgenomic processes? Time will tell. For the present time, the morphological markers are important indications that should help both the doctor to reach a specific and precise diagnosis and the scientist to focus his or her investigations.

REFERENCES

1. Martin JP. The basal ganglia and posture. London: Pitman Medical Publishing, 1967.
2. Fahn S. Description of Parkinson's disease as a clinical syndrome. Ann N Y Acad Sci 2003;991:1–14.
3. Lewy FH. Die Lehre vom Tonus und der Bewegung zugleich systematische Untersuchungen zur Klinik, Physiologie, Pathologie und Pathogenese der Paralysis Agitans. Berlin: Julius Springer, 1923.
4. Falck B, Hillarp NA, Thieme G, Torp A. Fluorescence of catecholamine and related compounds condensed with form-aldehyde. J Histochem Cytochem 1962;10:348–354.
5. Del Tredici K, Rub U, De Vos RA, Bohl JR, Braak H. Where does Parkinson disease pathology begin in the brain? J Neuropathol Exp Neurol 2002;61:413–426.
6. Jellinger KA. Post mortem studies in Parkinson's disease—is it possible to detect brain areas for specific symptoms? J Neural Transm Suppl 1999;56:1–29.
7. Jellinger KA, Mizuno Y.Parkinson's disease. In: Dickson D, eds. Neurodegeneration: The Molecular Pathology of Dementia and Movement Disorders. Basel: ISN Neuropath Press, 2003.
8. Hunter R, Smith J, Thomson T, Dayan AD. Hemiparkinsonism with infarction of the ipsilateral substantia nigra. Neuropathol Appl Neurobiol 1978;4:297–301.
9. Gherardi R, Roualdes B, Fleury J, Prost C, Poirier J, Degos JD. Parkinsonian syndrome and central nervous system lymphoma involving the substantia nigra. A case report. Acta Neuropathol (Berl) 1985;65:338–343.
10. Josephs KA, Ishizawa T, Tsuboi Y, Cookson N, Dickson DW. A clinicopathological study of vascular progressive supra-nuclear palsy: a multi-infarct disorder presenting as progressive supranuclear palsy. Arch Neurol 2002;59:1597–1601.
11. Wilson SAK. An experimental research into the anatomy and physiology of the corpus striatum. Brain 1914;36:437.
12. Russmann H, Vingerhoets F, Ghika J, Maeder P, Bogousslavsky J. Acute infarction limited to the lenticular nucleus: clinical, etiologic, and topographic features. Arch Neurol 2003;60:351–355.
13. Chang CM, Yu YL, Ng HK, Leung SY, Fong KY. Vascular pseudoparkinsonism. Acta Neurol Scand 1992;86:588–592.
14. Adhiyaman V, Meara J. Meningioma presenting as bilateral parkinsonism. Age Ageing 2003;32:456–458.
15. Gibb WRG, Lees AJ. The significance of the Lewy body in the diagnosis of idiopathic Parkinson's disease. Neuropathol Appl Neurobiol 1989;15:27–44.
16. Shimura H, Schlossmacher MG, Hattori N, et al. Ubiquitination of a new form of α–synuclein by parkin from human brain: implications for Parkinson's disease. Science 2001;293:263–269.
17. Calne D. Parkinson's disease is not one disease. Parkinsonism Relat Disord 2000;7:3–7.
18. Armstrong RA, Cairns NJ, Lantos PL. Are pathological lesions in neurodegenerative disorders the cause or the effect of the degeneration? Neuropathology 2002;22:133–146.

19. Tretiakoff C. Contribution à l'étude de l'anatomie pathologique du locus niger de Soemmering avec quelques déductions relatives à la pathogénie des troubles du tonus musculaire et de la maladie de Parkinson; Medical Thesis, Paris: Jouve et Cie, 1919:124p.

20. Hughes AJ, Daniel SE, Kilford L, Lees AJ. Accuracy of clinical diagnosis of idiopathic Parkinson's disease : a clinicopathological study of 100 cases. J Neurol Neurosurg Psychiatry 1992;55:181–184.

21. Okazaki H, Lipkin LE, Aronson SM. Diffuse intracytoplasmic inclusions (Lewy type) associated with progressive dementia and quadriparesis in flexion. J Neuropathol Exp Neurol 1961;20:237–244.

22. Duffy PE, Tennyson VM. Phase and electron microscopic observations of Lewy bodies and melanin granules in the substantia nigra and locus caeruleus in Parkinson's disease. J Neuropathol Exp Neurol 1965;24:398–414.

23. Pollanen MS, Dickson DW, Bergeron C. Pathology and biology of the Lewy body. J Neuropathol Exp Neurol 1993;52:183–191.

24. Lowe J, Blanchard A, Morrell K, et al. Ubiquitin is common factor in intermediate filament inclusion bodies of diverse type in man, including those of Parkinson's disease, Pick's disease, and Alzheimer's disease, as well as Rosenthal fibres in cerebellar astrocytomas, cytoplasmic bodies in muscle, and Mallory bodies in alcoholic liver disease. J Pathol 1988;155:9–15.

25. Ii K, Ito H, Tanaka K, Hirano A. Immunocytochemical co-localization of the proteasome in ubiquitinated structures in neurodegenerative diseases and the elderly. J Neuropathol Exp Neurol 1997;56:125–131.

26. Maroteaux L, Campanelli JT, Scheller RH. Synuclein: a neuron-specific protein localized to the nucleus and presynaptic nerve terminal. J Neurosci 1988;8:2804–2815.

27. Ueda K, Fukushima H, Masliah E, et al. Molecular cloning of cDNA encoding an unrecognized component of amyloid in Alzheimer disease. Proc Natl Acad Sci USA 1993;90:11282–11286.

28. George JM, Jin H, Woods WS, Clayton DF. Characterization of a novel protein regulated during the critical period for song learning in the zebra finch. Neuron 1995;15:361–372.

29. Polymeropoulos MH, Lavedan C, Leroy E, et al. Mutation in the α–synuclein gene identified in families with Parkinson's disease. Science 1997;276:2045–2047.

30. Spillantini MG, Crowther RA, Jakes R, Hasegawa M, Goedert M. A–synuclein in filamentous inclusions of Lewy bodies from Parkinson's disease and dementia with Lewy bodies. Proc Natl Acad Sci U S A 1998;95:6469–6473.

31. Uchikado H, Iseki E, Tsuchiya K, et al. Dementia with Lewy bodies showing advanced Lewy pathology but minimal Alzheimer pathology—Lewy pathology causes neuronal loss inducing progressive dementia. Clin Neuropathol 2002;21:269–277.

32. Gomez-Isla T, Growdon WB, McNamara M, et al. Clinicopathologic correlates in temporal cortex in dementia with Lewy bodies. Neurology 1999;53:2003–2009.

33. Kosaka K, Tsuchiya K, Yoshimura M. Lewy body disease with and without dementia: a clinicopathological study of 35 cases. Clin Neuropathol 1988;7:299–305.

34. Kosaka K, Yoshimura M, Ikeda K, Budka H. Diffuse type of Lewy body disease: progressive dementia with abundant cortical Lewy bodies and senile changes of varying degree—a new disease? Clin Neuropathol 1984;3:185–192.

35. Kosaka K. Diffuse Lewy body disease in Japan. J Neurol 1990;237:197–204.

36. Braak H, Braak E, Yilmazer D, Schultz C, Devos RAI, Jansen ENH. Nigral and extranigral pathology in Parkinson's disease. J Neural Transm 1995;Supp 46:15–31.

37. Gomez-Tortosa E, Newell K, Irizarry MC, Albert M, Growdon JH, Hyman BT. Clinical and quantitative pathologic correlates of dementia with Lewy bodies. Neurology 1999;53:1284–1291.

38. Marui W, Iseki E, Nakai T, et al. Progression and staging of Lewy pathology in brains from patients with dementia with Lewy bodies. J Neurol Sci 2002;195:153–159.

39. Rajput AH, Rozdilsky B. Dysautonomia in Parkinsonism: a clinicopathological study. J Neurol Neurosurg Psychiatry 1976;39:1092–1100.

40. Iwanaga K, Wakabayashi K, Yoshimoto M, et al. Lewy body-type degeneration in cardiac plexus in Parkinson's and incidental Lewy body diseases. Neurology 1999;52:1269–1271.

41. Wakabayashi K, Takahashi H, Takeda S, Ohama E, Ikuta F. Parkinson's disease: the presence of Lewy bodies in Auerbach's and Meissner's plexuses. Acta Neuropathol (Berl) 1988;76:217–221.

42. Hughes AJ, Daniel SE, Blankson S, Lees AJ. A clinicopathologic study of 100 cases of Parkinson's disease. Arch Neurol 1993;50:140–148.

43. Hakim AM, Mathieson G. Dementia in Parkinson disease: a neuropathologic study. Neurology 1979;29:1209.

44. Boller F, Mizutani R, Roessmann U, Gambetti P. Parkinson's disease, dementia and Alzheimer's disease: clinicopathological correlations. Ann Neurol 1980;1:329–355.

45. Gaspar P, Gray F. Dementia in idiopathic Parkinson disease. A neuropathological study of 32 cases. Acta Neuropathol (Berl) 1984;64:43–52.

46. Mattila PM, Roytta M, Torikka H, Dickson DW, Rinne JO. Cortical Lewy bodies and Alzheimer-type changes in patients with Parkinson's disease. Acta Neuropathol (Berl) 1998;95:576–582.

47. Jendroska K, Kashiwagi M, Sassoon J, Daniel SE. Amyloid beta-peptide and its relationship with dementia in Lewy body disease. J Neural Transm Suppl 1997;51:137–144.
48. Jellinger KA, Seppi K, Wenning GK, Poewe W. Impact of coexistent Alzheimer pathology on the natural history of Parkinson's disease. J Neural Transm 2002;109:329–339.
49. Apaydin H, Ahlskog JE, Parisi JE, Boeve BF, Dickson DW. Parkinson disease neuropathology: later-developing dementia and loss of the levodopa response. Arch Neurol 2002;59:102–112.
50. Gibb WR, Lees AJ. Prevalence of Lewy bodies in Alzheimer's disease. Ann Neurol 1989;26:691–693.
51. Bergeron C, Pollanen M. Lewy bodies in Alzheimer disease—one or two diseases? Alzheimer Dis Assoc Disord 1989;3:197–204.
52. Mirra SS. Neuropathological assessment of Alzheimer's disease: the experience of the Consortium to Establish a Registry for Alzheimer's Disease. Int Psychogeriatr 1997;9:263–268; discussion 269–272.
53. Heyman A, Fillenbaum GG, Gearing M, et al. Comparison of Lewy body variant of Alzheimer's disease with pure Alzheimer's disease: Consortium to Establish a Registry for Alzheimer's Disease, Part XIX. Neurology 1999;52:1839–1844.
54. Schmidt ML, Martin JA, Lee VM, Trojanowski JQ. Convergence of Lewy bodies and neurofibrillary tangles in amygdala neurons of Alzheimer's disease and Lewy body disorders. Acta Neuropathol 1996;91:475–481.
55. Hansen LA, Masliah E, Galasko D, Terry RD. Plaque-only Alzheimer disease is usually the Lewy body variant and vice versa. J Neuropathol Exp Neurol 1993;52:648–654.
56. Gearing M, Lynn M, Mirra SS. Neurofibrillary pathology in Alzheimer disease with Lewy bodies: two subgroups. Arch Neurol 1999;56:203–208.
57. Hansen L, Salmon D, Galasko D, et al. The Lewy body variant of Alzheimer's disease : a clinical and pathologic entity. Neurology 1990;40:1–8.
58. Perry RH, Irving D, Blessed G, Fairbairn A, Perry EK. Senile dementia of Lewy body type. A clinically and neuropathologically distinct form of Lewy body dementia in elderly. J Neurol Sci 1990;95:119–139.
59. McKeith IG, Galasko D, Kosaka K, et al. Consensus guidelines for the clinical and pathologic diagnosis of dementia with Lewy bodies (DLB) : report of the consortium on DLB international workshop. Neurology 1996;47:1113–1124.
60. McKeith IG, Perry EK, Perry RH. Report of the second dementia with Lewy body international workshop: diagnosis and treatment. Consortium on Dementia with Lewy Bodies. Neurology 1999;53:902–905.
61. Lantos PL, Ovenstone IM, Johnson J, Clelland CA, Roques P, Rossor MN. Lewy bodies in the brain of two members of a family with the 717 (Val to Ile) mutation of the amyloid precursor protein gene. Neurosci Lett 1994;172:77–79.
62. Lippa CF, Fujiwara H, Mann DMA, et al. Lewy bodies contain altered α–synuclein in brains of many familiar Alzheimer's disease patients with mutations in presenilin and amyloid precursor protein genes. Am J Pathol 1998;153:1365–1370.
63. Lippa CF, Schmidt ML, Lee VM, Trojanowski JQ. Antibodies to α–synuclein detect Lewy bodies in many Down's syndrome brains with Alzheimer's disease. Ann Neurol 1999;45:353–357.
64. Perl DP, Olanow CW, Calne D. Alzheimer's disease and Parkinson's disease: distinct entities or extremes of a spectrum of neurodegeneration? Ann Neurol 1998;44:S19–S31.
65. Egensperger R, Bancher C, Kosel S, Jellinger K, Mehraein P, Graeber MB. The apolipoprotein E epsilon 4 allele in Parkinson's disease with Alzheimer lesions. Biochem Biophys Res Commun 1996;224:484–486.
66. Inzelberg R, Chapman J, Treves TA, et al. Apolipoprotein E4 in Parkinson disease and dementia: new data and meta-analysis of published studies. Alzheimer Dis Assoc Disord 1998;12:45–48.
67. Gearing M, Schneider JA, Rebeck GW, Hyman BT, Mirra SS. Alzheimer's disease with and without coexisting Parkinson's disease changes: apolipoprotein E genotype and neuropathologic correlates. Neurology 1995;45:1985–1990.
68. Giasson BI, Forman MS, Higuchi M, et al. Initiation and synergistic fibrillization of tau and α–synuclein. Science 2003;300:636–640.
69. Adams RD, Bogaert van L, Vander Eecken H. Dégénérescences nigro-striées et cérébello-nigro-striées. Psychiatria et Neurologia 1961;142:219.
70. Adams RD, Bogaert van L, Vander Eecken H. Striato-nigral degeneration. J Neuropathol Exp Neurol 1965;23:584–608.
71. Gilman S, Low PA, Quinn N, et al. Consensus statement on the diagnosis of multiple system atrophy. J Neurol Sci 1999;163:94–98.
72. Konigsmark BW, Weiner LP. The olivopontocerebellar atrophies: a review. Medicine (Baltimore) 1970;49:227–241.
73. Graham JG, Oppenheimer DR. Orthostatic hypotension and nicotine sensitivity in a case of multiple system atrophy. J Neurol Neurosurg Psychiatry 1969;32:28–34.
74. Papp MI, Kahn JE, Lantos PL. Glial cytoplasmic inclusions in the CNS of patients with multiple system atrophy (striatonigral degeneration, olivopontocerebellar atrophy and Shy–Drager syndrome). J Neurol Sci 1989;94:79–100.
75. Costa C, Duyckaerts C, Cervera P, Hauw J-J. Les inclusions oligodendrogliales, un marqueur des atrophies multisystématisées. Rev Neurol (Paris) 1992;148:274–280.

76. Mori F, Tanji K, Yoshimoto M, Takahashi H, Wakabayashi K. Demonstration of α-synuclein immunoreactivity in neuronal and glial cytoplasm in normal human brain tissue using proteinase K and formic acid pretreatment. Exp Neurol 2002;176:98–104.

77. Kahle PJ, Neumann M, Ozmen L, et al. Hyperphosphorylation and insolubility of α-synuclein in transgenic mouse oligodendrocytes. EMBO Rep 2002;3:583–588.

78. Goedert M, Wischik CM, Crowther RA, Walker JE, Klug A. Cloning and sequencing of the cDNA encoding a core protein of the paired helical filament of Alzheimer disease: identification as the microtubule-associated protein tau. Proc Natl Acad Sci U S A 1988;85:4051–4055.

79. Buée L, Delacourte A. Comparative biochemistry of tau in progressive supranuclear palsy, corticobasal degeneration, FTDP-17 and Pick's disease. Brain Pathol 1999;9:681–693.

80. Delacourte A, Buee L. Tau pathology: a marker of neurodegenerative disorders. Curr Opin Neurol 2000;13:371–376.

81. Vermersch P, Frigard B, Delacourte A. Mapping of neurofibrillary degeneration in Alzheimer's disease—evaluation of heterogeneity using the quantification of abnormal tau proteins. Acta Neuropathol (Berl) 1992;85:48–54.

82. Delacourte A, Defossez A. Alzheimer's disease: Tau proteins, the promoting factors of microtubule assembly are major components of paired helical filaments. J Neurol Sci 1986;76:173–186.

83. Buee-Scherrer V, Buee L, Leveugle B, Perl DP, Vermersch P, Hof PR, Delacourte A. Pathological tau proteins in postencephalitic parkinsonism: comparison with Alzheimer's disease and other neurodegenerative disorders. Ann Neurol 1997;42:356–359.

84. Flament S, Delacourte A, Verny M, Hauw J-J, Javoy-Agid F. Abnormal tau proteins in progressive supranuclear palsy. Similarities and differences with the neurofibrillary degeneration of the Alzheimer type. Acta Neuropathol (Berl) 1991;591–596.

85. Togo T, Sahara N, Yen SH, et al. Argyrophilic grain disease is a sporadic 4-repeat tauopathy. J Neuropathol Exp Neurol 2002;61:547–556.

86. Buée-Scherrer V, Hof PR, Buée L, et al. Hyperphosphorylated tau proteins differentiate corticobasal degeneration and Pick's disease. Acta Neuropathol (Berl) 1996;91:351–359.

87. Lin WL, Lewis J, Yen SH, Hutton M, Dickson DW. Filamentous tau in oligodendrocytes and astrocytes of transgenic mice expressing the human tau isoform with the P301L mutation. Am J Pathol 2003;162:213–218.

88. Allen B, Ingram E, Takao M, et al. Abundant tau filaments and nonapoptotic neurodegeneration in transgenic mice expressing human P301S tau protein. J Neurosci 2002;22:9340–9351.

89. Sergeant N, Wattez A, Delacourte A. Neurofibrillary degeneration in progressive supranuclear palsy and corticobasal degeneration: tau pathologies with exclusively "exon 10" isoforms. J Neurochem 1999;72:1243–1249.

90. Steele JC, Richardson JC, Olszewski J. Progressive supranuclear palsy; a heterogeneous degeneration involving the brain stem, basal ganglia and cerebellum with vertical gaze and pseudobulbar palsy, nuclear dystonia and dementia. Arch Neurol 1964;10:333–359.

91. Rebeiz JJ, Kolodny EH, Richardson EP. Corticodentatonigral degeneration with neuronal achromasia: a progressive disorder of late adult life. Transact Am Neurol Assoc 1967;92:23–26.

92. Rebeiz JJ, Kolodny EH, Richardson EP. Corticodentatonigral degeneration with neuronal achromasia. Arch Neurol 1968;18:20–33.

93. Conrad C, Andreadis A, Trojanowski JQ, et al. Genetic evidence for the involvement of tau in progressive supranuclear palsy. Ann Neurol 1997;41:277–281.

94. Baker M, Litvan I, Houlden H, et al. Association of an extended haplotype in the tau gene with progressive supranuclear palsy. Hum Mol Genet 1999;8:711–715.

95. Houlden H, Baker M, Morris HR, et al. Corticobasal degeneration and progressive supranuclear palsy share a common tau haplotype. Neurology 2001;56:1702–1706.

96. Steele JC. Progressive supranuclear palsy. Historical notes. J Neural Transm Suppl 1994;42:3–14.

97. Wenning GK, Jellinger K, Litvan I. Supranuclear gaze palsy and eyelid apraxia in postencephalitic parkinsonism. J Neural Transm 1997;104:845–865.

98. Geddes JF, Hugues AJ, Lees AJ, Daniel SE. Pathological overlap in cases of Parkinsonism associated with neurofibrillary tangles. A study of recent cases of postencephalitic parkinsonism and comparison with progressive supranuclear and Guamanian parkinsonism-dementia complex. Brain 1993;116:1–22.

99. Brion JP, Passareiro H, Nunez J, Flament-Durand J. Mise en évidence immunologique de la protéine tau au niveau des lésions de dégénérescence neurofibrillaire de la maladie d'Alzheimer. Arch Biol (Brux) 1985;95:229–235.

100. Grundke-Iqbal I, Iqbal K, Tung YC, Quinlan M, Wiesniewski HM. Abnormal phosphorylation of the microtubule associated protein (tau) in Alzheimer cytoskeletal pathology. Proc Natl Acad Sci USA 1986;83:4913–4917.

101. Bancher C, Lassmann H, Budka H, et al. Neurofibrillary tangles in Alzheimer's disease and progressive supranuclear palsy; antigenic similarities and differences. Acta Neuropathol (Berl) 1987;74:39.

102. Gallyas F. Silver staining of Alzheimer's neurofibrillary changes by means of physical development. Acta Morphol Acad Sci Hung 1971;19:1–8.

103. Probst A, Langui D, Lautenschlager C, Ulrich J, Brion JP, Anderton BH. Progressive supranuclear palsy: extensive neuropil threads in addition to neurofibrillary tangles. Very similar antigenicity of subcortical neuronal pathology in progressive supranuclear palsy and Alzheimer's disease. Acta Neuropathol (Berl) 1988;77:61–68.

104. Ikeda K, Akiyama H, Haga C, Kondo H, Arima K, Oda T. Argyrophilic thread-like structure in corticobasal degeneration and supranuclear palsy. Neurosci Letters 1994;174:157–159.

105. Ikeda K, Akiyama H, Aral T, Nishimura T. Glial tau pathology in neurodegenerative diseases; their nature and comparison with neuronal tangles. Neurobiol Aging 1998;19:S85–S91.

106. Arima K, Nakamura M, Sunohara N, et al. Ultrastructural characterization of the tau-immunoreactive tubules in the oligodendroglial perikarya and their inner loop processes in progressive supranuclear palsy. Acta Neuropathol (Berl) 1997;93:558–566.

107. Braak H, Braak E. Cortical and subcortical argyrophilic grains characterize a disease associated with adult onset dementia. Neuropathol Appl Neurobiol 1989;15:13–26.

108. Matsusaka H, Ikeda K, Akiyama H, Arai T, Inoue M, Yagishita S. Astrocytic pathology in progressive supranuclear palsy: significance for neuropathological diagnosis. Acta Neuropathol (Berl) 1998;96:248–252.

109. Hauw J-J, Verny M, Delaère P, Cervera P, He Y, Duyckaerts C. Constant neurofibrillary changes in the neocortex in progressive supranuclear palsy. Basic differences with Alzheimer's disease and aging. Neurosci Lett 1990;119:182–186.

110. Hauw J-J, Agid Y. Progressive Supranuclear Palsy (PSP) or Steele–Richardson–Olszewski Disease. In: Dickson D, eds. Neurodegeneration: the molecular pathology of dementia and movement disorders. Basel: ISN Neuropath Press, 2003.

111. Abe H, Yagishita S, Amano N, Bise K. Ultrastructural and immunohistochemical study of "astrocytic tangles" (ACT) in patients with progressive supranuclear palsy. Clin Neuropathol 1992;5:278.

112. Yamada T, McGeer PL, McGeer EG. Appearance of paired nucleated, Tau positive glia in patients with progressive supranuclear palsy brain tissue. Neurosci Lett 1992;135:99–102.

113. Yamada T, Calne DB, Akiyama H, McGeer PL. Further observations on tau-postive glia in the brains with progressive supranuclear palsy. Acta Neuropathol (Berl) 1993;85:308–315.

114. Hattori M, Hashizume Y, Yoshida M, et al. Distribution of astrocytic plaques in the corticobasal degeneration brain and comparison with tuft-shaped astrocytes in the progressive supranuclear palsy brain. Acta Neuropathol 2003;106:143–149.

115. Tellez-Nagel I, Wisniewski HM. Ultrastructure of neurofibrillary tangles in Steele–Richardson–Olszewski syndrome. Arch Neurol 1973;29:324–327.

116. Bugiani O, Mancardi GL, Brusa A, Ederli A. The fine structure of subcortical neurofibrillary tangles in progressive supranuclear palsy. Acta Neuropathol (Berl) 1979;45:147–152.

117. Tomonaga M. Ultrastructure of neurofibrillary tangles in progressive supranuclear palsy. Acta Neuropathol (Berl) 1977;37:177–181.

118. Yagishita S, Itoh Y, Amano N, Nakano T, Saitoh A. Ultrastructure of neurofibrillary tangles in progressive supranuclear palsy. Acta Neuropathol (Berl) 1979;48:27–30.

119. Takahashi M, Weidenheim KM, Dickson DW, Ksiezak-Reding H. Morphological and biochemical correlations of abnormal tau filaments in progressive supranuclear palsy. J Neuropathol Exp Neurol 2002;61:33–45.

120. Verny M, Duyckaerts M, Delaère M, He Y, Hauw J-J. Cortical tangles in progressive supranuclear palsy. J Neural Transm 1994;(Suppl)42:179–188.

121. Verny M, Duyckaerts C, Agid Y, Hauw J-J. The significance of cortical pathology in progressive supranuclear palsy. Brain 1996;119:1123–1136.

122. Hauw J-J, Daniel SE, Dickson D, et al. Preliminary NINDS neuropathologic criteria for Steele–Richardson–Olszewski syndrome (progressive supranuclear palsy). Neurology 1994;44:2015–2019.

123. Dubas F, Gray F, Escourolle R. Maladie de Steele–Richardson–Olszewski sans ophtalmoplégie; six cas anatomo-cliniques. Rev Neurol (Paris) 1983;139:407–416.

124. Birdi S, Rajput AH, Fenton M, et al. Progressive supranuclear palsy diagnosis and confounding features: report on 16 autopsied cases. Mov Disord 2002;17:1255–64.

125. Cambier J, Masson M, Viader J, Limodin J, Strube A. Le syndrome frontal de la paralysie supranucléaire progressive. Rev Neurol (Paris) 1985;141:537–545.

126. Davis PH, Bergeron C, McLachlan DR. Atypical presentation of progressive supranuclear palsy. Ann Neurol 1985;17:337–343.

127. Litvan I. Cognitive disturbances in progressive supranuclear palsy. J Neural Transm 1994;42(Suppl):69–78.

128. Bergeron C, Davis A, Lang AE. Corticobasal ganglionic degeneration and progressive supranuclear palsy presenting with cognitive decline. Brain Pathol 1998;8:355–365.

129. Bigio EH, Brown DF, White CL, III. Progressive supranuclear palsy with dementia: cortical pathology. J Neuropathol Exp Neurol 1999;58:359–364.

130. Foster NL, Sima AAF, D'Amato C, et al. Cerebral cortical pathology in progressive supranuclear palsy is correlated with severity of dementia. Neurology 1996;46:A363.

131. Boeve B, Dickson D, Duffy J, Bartleson J, Trenerry M, Petersen R. Progressive nonfluent aphasia and subsequent aphasic dementia associated with atypical progressive supranuclear palsy pathology. Eur Neurol 2003;49:72–78.

132. Rafal RD, Friedman JH. Limb dystonia in progressive supranuclear palsy. Neurology 1987;37:1546–1549.

133. Bergeron C, Pollanen MS, Weyer L, Lang AE. Cortical degeneration in progressive supranuclear palsy. A comparison with cortico-basal ganglionic degeneration. J Neuropathol Exp Neurol 1997;56:726–735.

134. Cordato NJ, Halliday GM, McCann H, Davies L, Williamson P, Fulham M, Morris JG. Corticobasal syndrome with tau pathology. Mov Disord 2001;16:656–67.

135. Leiguarda RC, Pramstaller PP, Merello M, Starkstein S, Lees AJ, Marsden CD. Apraxia in Parkinson's disease, progressive supranuclear palsy, multiple system atrophy and neuroleptic-induced parkinsonism. Brain 1997;120:75–90.

136. Caparros-Lefebvre D, Sergeant N, Lees A, Camuzat A, Daniel S, Lannuzel A, Brice A, Tolosa E, Delacourte A, Duyckaerts C. Guadeloupean parkinsonism: a cluster of progressive supranuclear palsy-like tauopathy. Brain 2002;125:801–811.

137. Caparros-Lefebvre D, Elbaz A. Possible relation of atypical parkinsonism in the French West Indies with consumption of tropical plants: a case-control study. Caribbean Parkinsonism Study Group. Lancet 1999;354:281–286.

138. Cambier J, Masson M, Dairou R, Henin D. Etude anatomo-clinique d'une forme pariétale de maladie de Pick. Rev Neurol (Paris) 1981;137:33–38.

139. Tsuchiya K, Ikeda M, Hasegawa K, et al. Distribution of cerebral cortical lesions in Pick's disease with Pick bodies: a clinicopathological study of six autopsy cases showing unusual clinical presentations. Acta Neuropathol (Berl) 2001;102:553–571.

140. Gibb WRG, Luthert PJ, Marsden CD. Corticobasal degeneration. Brain 1989;112:1171–1192.

141. Horoupian DS, Chu PL. Unusual case of corticobasal degeneration with tau/Gallyas-positive neuronal and glial tangles. Acta Neuropathol (Berl) 1994;88:592–598.

142. Uchihara T, Mitani K, Mori H, Kondo H, Yamada M, Ikeda K. Abnormal cytoskeletal pathology peculiar to corticobasal degeneration is different from that of Alzheimer's disease or progressive supranuclear palsy. Acta Neuropathol (Berl) 1994;88:379–383.

143. Mori H, Nishimura N, Namba Y, Oda M. Corticobasal degeneration: a disease with widespread appearance of abnormal tau and neurofibrillary tangles, and its relation to progressive supranuclear palsy. Acta Neuropathol (Berl) 1994;88:113–121.

144. Feany MB, Dickson DW. Widespread cytoskeletal pathology characterizes corticobasal degeneration. Am J Pathol 1995;146:1388–1396.

145. Daniel SE, Geddes F, Revesz T. Clinicopathological overlap between cases of Pick's disease and corticobasal degeneration. Brain Pathology 1994;4:516.

146. Feany MB, Mattiace LA, Dickson DW. Neuropathologic overlap of progressive supranuclear palsy, Pick's disease and corticobasal degeneration. J Neuropathol Exp Neurol 1996;55:53–67.

147. Ikeda K, Akiyama H, Iritani S, et al. Corticobasal degeneration with primary progressive aphasia and accentuated cortical lesion in superior temporal gyrus: case report and review. Acta Neuropathol (Berl) 1996;92:534–539.

148. Arai T, Ikeda K, Akiyama H, et al. Different immunoreactivities of the microtubule-binding region of tau and its molecular basis in brains from patients with Alzheimer's disease, Pick's disease, progressive supranuclear palsy and corticobasal degeneration. Acta Neuropathol (Berl) 2003;105:489–498.

149. de Silva R, Lashley T, Gibb G, et al. Pathological inclusion bodies in tauopathies contain distinct complements of tau with three or four microtubule-binding repeat domains as demonstrated by new specific monoclonal antibodies. Neuropathol Appl Neurobiol 2003;29:288–302.

150. Komori T, Arai N, Oda M, et al. Morphologic difference of neuropil threads in Alzheimer's disease, corticobasal degeneration and progressive supranuclear palsy: a morphometric study. Neurosci Lett 1997;233:89–92.

151. Dickson DW. Neuropathologic differentiation of progressive supranuclear palsy and corticobasal degeneration. J Neurol 1999;246 Suppl 2:II6–II15:

152. Tolnay M, Probst A. Tau protein pathology in Alzheimer's disease and related disorders. Neuropathol Appl Neurobiol 1999;25:171–187.

153. Komori T, Shibata N, Kobayashi M. Plaque-like structures in the cerebral cortex of corticobasal degeneration: a histopathological marker? Neuropathology 1995;15:175–176.

154. Komori T, Arai N, Oda M, et al. Astrocytic plaques and tufts of abnormal fibers do not coexist in corticobasal degeneration and progressive supranuclear palsy. Acta Neuropathol (Berl) 1998;96:401–408.

155. Dickson DW, Bergeron C, Chin SS, et al. Office of rare diseases neuropathologic criteria for corticobasal degeneration. J Neuropathol Exp Neurol 2002;61:935–46.

156. Shiozawa M, Fukutani Y, Sasaki K, et al. Corticobasal degeneration: an autopsy case clinically diagnosed as progressive supranuclear palsy. Clin Neuropathol 2000;19:192–199.

157. Mimura M, Oda T, Tsuchiya K, et al. Corticobasal degeneration presenting with nonfluent primary progressive aphasia: a clinicopathological study. J Neurol Sci 2001;183:19–26.

158. Tsuchiya K, Ikeda K, Uchihara T, Oda T, Shimada H. Distribution of cerebral cortical lesions in corticobasal degeneration: a clinicopathological study of five autopsy cases in Japan. Acta Neuropathol (Berl) 1997;94:416–424.

159. Grimes DA, Lang AE, Bergeron CB. Dementia as the most common presentation of cortical-basal ganglionic degeneration. Neurology 1999;53:1969–1974.

160. Dickson D, Litvan I. Corticobasal degeneration. In: Dickson D, ed. Neurodegeneration: The Molecular Pathology of Dementia and Movement Disorders. Basel: ISN Neuropath Press, 2003.

161. Katsuse O, Iseki E, Arai T, et al. 4-repeat tauopathy sharing pathological and biochemical features of corticobasal degeneration and progressive supranuclear palsy. Acta Neuropathol 2003;11:11.

162. Togo T, Dickson DW. Ballooned neurons in progressive supranuclear palsy are usually due to concurrent argyrophilic grain disease. Acta Neuropathol (Berl) 2002;104:53–56.

163. Ishizawa T, Ko LW, Cookson N, Davias P, Espinoza M, Dickson DW. Selective neurofibrillary degeneration of the hippocampal CA2 sector is associated with four-repeat tauopathies. J Neuropathol Exp Neurol 2002;61:1040–1047.

164. Morris JC, Drazner M, Fulling K, Grant EA, Goldring J. Clinical and pathological aspects of parkinsonism in Alzheimer's disease. A role for extranigral factors? Arch Neurol 1989;46:651–657.

165. Daniel SD, Lees AJ. Neuropathological features of Alzheimer's disease in non-demented parkinsonian patients. J Neurol Neurosurg Psychiatry 1991;54:971–975.

166. Braak H, Braak E. Alzheimer's disease: striatal amyloid deposits and neurofibrillary changes. J Neuropathol Exp Neurol 1990;49:215–224.

167. Schneider JA, Bienias JL, Gilley DW, Kvarnberg DE, Mufson EJ, Bennett DA. Improved detection of substantia nigra pathology in Alzheimer's disease. J Histochem Cytochem 2002;50:99–106.

168. Liu Y, Stern Y, Chun MR, Jacobs DM, Yau P, Goldman JE. Pathological correlates of extrapyramidal signs in Alzheimer's disease. Ann Neurol 1997;41:368–374.

169. Kemppainen N, Roytta M, Collan Y, Ma SY, Hinkka S, Rinne JO. Unbiased morphological measurements show no neuronal loss in the substantia nigra in Alzheimer's disease. Acta Neuropathol (Berl) 2002;103:43–47.

170. Lyness SA, Zarow C, Chui HC. Neuron loss in key cholinergic and aminergic nuclei in Alzheimer disease: a meta-analysis. Neurobiol Aging 2003;24:1–23.

171. Stern Y, Jacobs D, Goldman J, et al. An investigation of clinical correlates of Lewy bodies in autopsy-proven Alzheimer disease. Arch Neurol 2001;58:460–465.

172. Corsellis JAN, Bruton CJ, Freeman-Browne D. The aftermath of boxing. Psychol Med 1973;3:270–303.

173. Geddes JF, Vowles GH, Robinson SFD, Sutcliffe JC. Neurofibrillary tangles, but not Alzheimer-type pathology, in a young boxer. Neuropathol Appl Neurobiol 1996;22:12–16.

174. Geddes JF, Vowles GH, Nicoll JA, Revesz T. Neuronal cytoskeletal changes are an early consequence of repetitive head injury. Acta Neuropathol (Berl) 1999;98:171–178.

175. Reid AH, McCall S, Henry JM, Taubenberger JK. Experimenting on the past: the enigma of von Economo's encephalitis lethargica. J Neuropathol Exp Neurol 2001;60:663–670.

176. Litvan II, Jankovic J, Goetz CG, et al. Accuracy of the clinical diagnosis of postencephalitic parkinsonism: a clinicopathologic study. Eur J Neurol 1998;5:451–457.

177. Taubenberger JK, Reid AH, Krafft AE, Bijwaard KE, Fanning TG. Initial genetic characterization of the 1918 "Spanish" influenza virus. Science 1997;275:1793–1796.

178. Ikeda K, Akiyama H, Kondo H, Ikeda K. Anti-tau-positive glial fibrillary tangles in the brain of postencephalitic parkinsonism of Economo type. Neurosci Lett 1993;162:176–178.

179. Haraguchi T, Ishizu H, Terada S, et al. An autopsy case of postencephalitic parkinsonism of von Economo type: some new observations concerning neurofibrillary tangles and astrocytic tangles. Neuropathology 2000;20:143–148.

180. Geddes JF, Hughes AJ, Lees AJ, Daniel SE. Pathological overlap in cases of parkinsonism associated with neurofibrillary tangles. A study of recent cases of postencephalitic parkinsonism and comparison with progressive supranuclear palsy and Guamanian parkinsonism-dementia complex. Brain 1993;116:281–302.

181. Oyanagi K. Parkinsonism-dementia complex of Guam. In: Dickson D, ed. Neurodegeneration: the Molecular Pathology of Dementia and Movement Disorders. Basel: ISN Neuropath Press, 2003.

182. Oyanagi K, Wada M. Neuropathology of parkinsonism-dementia complex and amyotrophic lateral sclerosis of Guam: an update. J Neurol 1999;246(Suppl 2):19–27.

183. Perl DP. Amyotrophic lateral sclerosis-parkinsonism-dementia complex of Guam. In: Markesbery WR, ed. Neuropathology of Dementing Disorders. London: Arnold, 1998.

184. Hirano A, Kurland LT, Krooth RS, Lessell S. Parkinsonism-dementia complex, an endemic disease on the island of Guam. I. Clinical features. Brain 1961;84:642–661.

185. Hirano A, Malamud N, Kurtland LT. Parkinsonism-dementia complex, an endemic disease of island of Guam. II.-Pathological features. Brain 1961;84:662–679.

186. Morris HR, Al-Sarraj S, Schwab C, et al. A clinical and pathological study of motor neurone disease on Guam. Brain 2001;124:2215–2222.

187. Schwab C, Schulzer M, Steele JC, McGeer PL. On the survival time of a tangled neuron in the hippocampal CA4 region in parkinsonism dementia complex of Guam. Neurobiol Aging 1999;20:57–63.

188. Oyanagi K, Makifuchi T, Ohtoh T, Chen KM, Gajdusek DC, Chase TN. Distinct pathological features of the gallyas- and tau-positive glia in the Parkinsonism-dementia complex and amyotrophic lateral sclerosis of Guam. J Neuropathol Exp Neurol 1997;56:308–316.

189. Spencer PS, Nunn PB, Hugon J, et al. Guam amyotrophic lateral sclerosis-parkinsonism-dementia linked to a plant excitant neurotoxin. Science 1987;237:517–522.

190. Duncan MW, Steele JC, Kopin IJ, Markey SP. 2-Amino-3-(methylamino)-propanoic acid (BMAA) in cycad flour: an unlikely cause of amyotrophic lateral sclerosis and parkinsonism-dementia of Guam. Neurology 1990;40:767–772.

191. Lüers T, Spatz H. Picksche Krankheit (Progressive umschriebene Grosshirnatrophie). In: Lubarsch O, Henke F, Rössle R, eds. Hanbuch der speziellen pathologischen Anatomie und Histologie. Berlin: Springer-Verlag, 1957.

192. Onari K, Spatz H. Anatomische Beiträge zur Lehre von der Pickschen umschriebenen Grosshirnrinde-Atrophie ("Picksche Krankheit"). Z ges Neurol 1926;101:470–511.

193. Escourolle R. La maladie de Pick. Etude critique d'ensemble et synthèse anatomo-clinique. Paris: R.Foulon, 1958.

194. Pick A. Beiträge zur Pathologie und pathologischen Anatomie des Zentralnervensystems. Berlin: S. Karger, 1898.

195. Pick A. Senile Hirnatrophie als Grundlage von Herderscheinungen. Wiener klinische Wschr 1901;14:16–17.

196. Pick A. Uber einen weiteren Symptomencomplex im Rahmen der Dementia senilis, bedingt durch umschriebene stärkere Hirnatrophie (gemischte Apraxie). Mschr Psychiat Neurol 1906;19:97–108.

197. Pick A. Ueber die Beziehungen der senilen Hirnatrophie zur Aphasie. Prager Med Wschr 1892;17:15–17.

198. Alzheimer A. Uber eigenartige Krankheitsfälle des späteren Alters. Zentralblatt Gesam Neurol Psychiat 1911;4:356–385.

199. Alzheimer A, Förstl H, Levy R. On certain peculiar diseases of old age. Hist Psychiatry 1991;2:71–101.

200. Arai T, Ikeda K, Akiyama H, et al. Distinct isoforms of tau aggregated in neurons and glial cells in brains of patients with Pick's disease, corticobasal degeneration and progressive supranuclear palsy. Acta Neuropathol (Berl) 2001;101:167–73.

201. Zhukareva V, Mann D, Pickering-Brown S, et al. Sporadic Pick's disease: a tauopathy characterized by a spectrum of pathological tau isoforms in gray and white matter. Ann Neurol 2002;51:730–739.

202. Komori T. Tau-positive glial inclusions in progressive supranuclear palsy, corticobasal degeneration and Pick's disease. Brain Pathol 1999;9:663–679.

203. Kertesz A, Hudson L, Mackenzie IRA, Munoz DG. The pathology and nosology of primary progressive aphasia. Neurology 1994;44:2065–2075.

204. Kertesz A, Munoz D. Clinical and pathological characteristics of primary progressive aphasia and frontal dementia. Neural Transm (Suppl) 1996;47:133–141.

205. Kertesz A. Pick complex and Pick's disease, the nosology of frontal lobe dementia, primary progressive aphasia, and corticobasal ganglionic degeneration. Eur J Neurol 1996;3:280–282.

206. Kertesz A, Munoz D. Clinical and pathological overlap between frontal dementia, progressive aphasia and corticobasal degeneration. The Pick complex. Neurology 1997;48:293.

207. Kertesz A. Frontotemporal dementia, Pick disease, and corticobasal degeneration. One entity or 3? Arch Neurol 1997;54:1427–1429.

208. Kertesz A, Munoz D. Pick's disease, frontotemporal dementia, and Pick complex: emerging concepts. Arch Neurol 1998;55:302–304.

209. Kertesz A, Munoz DG. Primary progressive aphasia and Pick complex. J Neurol Sci 2003;206:97–107.

210. Duyckaerts C, Dürr A, Uchihara T, Boller F, Hauw J-J. Pick complex: too simple? Eur J Neurol 1996; 3:283–286.

211. Duyckaerts C, Hauw JJ. Diagnostic controversies: another view. Adv Neurol 2000;82:233–240.

212. Kertesz A, Munoz DG, Hillis A. Preferred terminology. Ann Neurol 2003;54(Supp 5):S3–S6.

213. Foster NL, Wilhelmsen K, Sima AA, Jones MZ, D'Amato CJ, Gilman S. Frontotemporal dementia and parkinsonism linked to chromosome 17: a consensus conference. Ann Neurol 1997;41:706–715.

214. Hutton MJ, Lendon CL, Rizzu P, et al. Association of missense and 5'-splice-site mutations in tau with the inherited dementia FTDP-17. Nature 1998;393:702–705.

215. Spillantini MG, Murrell JR, Goedert M, Farlow MR, Klug A, Ghetti B. Mutation in the tau gene in familial multiple system tauopathy with presenile dementia. Proc Natl Acad Sci U S A 1998;95:7737–7741.

216. Ghetti B, Hutton ML, Wszolek ZK. Fronto-temporal dementia and parkinsonism linked to chromosome 17 associated with tau gene mutations (FTDP-17T). In:Dickson D, eds. Neurodegeneration: the molecular pathology of dementia and movement disorders. Basel: ISN Neuropath Press, 2003.

217. Morris HR, Osaki Y, Holton J, et al. Tau exon 10 +16 mutation FTDP-17 presenting clinically as sporadic young onset PSP. Neurology 2003;61:102–104.

218. Spillantini MG, Yoshida H, Rizzini C, et al. A novel tau mutation (N296N) in familial dementia with swollen achromatic neurons and corticobasal inclusion bodies. Ann Neurol 2000;48:939–943.

219. Bugiani O, Murrell JR, Giaccone G, et al. Frontotemporal dementia and corticobasal degeneration in a family with a P301S mutation in tau. J Neuropathol Exp Neurol 1999;58:667–677.

220. Neumann M, Schulz-Schaeffer W, Crowther RA, et al. Pick's disease associated with the novel Tau gene mutation K369I. Ann Neurol 2001;50:503–513.
221. Rosso SM, van Herpen E, Deelen W, et al. A novel tau mutation, S320F, causes a tauopathy with inclusions similar to those in Pick's disease. Ann Neurol 2002;51:373–376.
222. Bumke O, Foerster O. Allgemeine Neurologie I Anatomie. Berlin: Julius Springer, 1935.
223. Truex RC, Carpenter MB. Human Neuroanatomy. Baltimore: Williams & Wilkins, 1969.
224. Carpenter MB. Human neuroanatomy. Baltimore: Williams & Wilkins, 1976.
225. Arriagada PV, Growdon JH, Hedley-Whyte ET, Hyman BT. Neurofibrillary tangles but not senile plaques parallel duration and severity of Alzheimer's disease. Ann Neurol 1992;42:631–639.
226. Bierer LM, Hof PR, Purohit DP, et al. Neocortical neurofibrillary tangles correlate with dementia severity in Alzheimer's disease. Arch Neurol 1995;52:81–88.
227. Duyckaerts C, Bennecib M, Grignon Y, et al. Modeling the relation between neurofibrillary tangles and intellectual status. Neurobiol Aging 1997;18:267–273.
228. Saudou F, Finkbeiner S, Devys D, Greenberg ME. Huntingtin acts in the nucleus to induce apoptosis but death does not correlate with the formation of intranuclear inclusions. Cell 1998;95:55–66.
229. Sisodia SS. Nuclear inclusions in glutamine repeat disorders: are they pernicious, coincidental, or beneficial? Cell 1998;95:1–4.
230. Graff-Radford NR, Damasio AR, Hyman BT, et al. Progressive aphasia in a patient with Pick's disease: a neuropsychological, radiologic and anatomic study. Neurology 1990;40:620–626.

9

Genetics of Atypical Parkinsonism

Implications for Nosology

Thomas Gasser

INTRODUCTION

Parkinson's disease (PD) is traditionally defined as a clinico-pathologic entity, characterized by a core syndrome of akinesia, rigidity, tremor, and postural instability, and pathologically by a more or less selective degeneration of dopaminergic neurons of the substantia nigra, leading to a deficiency of dopamine in the striatal projection areas of these neurons. Characteristic eosinophilic inclusions, the Lewy bodies (LBs), are found in surviving dopaminergic neurons but also, although less abundantly, in other parts of the brain in most cases *(1)*.

Approximately 20–30% of patients with parkinsonism exhibit additional clinical features and a neuropathological picture clearly different from idiopathic PD. These disorders are collectively called "atypical parkinsonism." The most common clinico-pathological entities of this group are dementia with LBs (DLB), multiple system atrophy (MSA), progressive supranuclear palsy (PSP), corticobasal degeneration (CBD), and frontotemporal dementia with parkinsonism (FTDP). In addition, a number of other rare familial or sporadic diseases may present with parkinsonism and different atypical features.

The nosologic classification of these entities, however, is not always easy. Considerable overlap exists, both clinically and pathologically, between some of these syndromes, but also, for example, between DLB and Alzheimer's disease (AD), leading to the concept of the "neurodegenerative overlap syndromes" *(2)*. Although the majority of cases appears to be sporadic in all atypical parkinsonian syndromes, it was the recent progress in molecular genetics that has provided an "Archimedes point" in the search for a nosologic classification, by identifying the genetic cause of several rare, monogenic variants.

These findings have brought several key molecules into the focus of research, particularly α-synuclein and the microtubule-associated protein tau, providing the first rational basis for a very broad molecular classification of neurodegenerative diseases: in those disorders associated with α-synuclein accumulation (synucleinopathies: PD, DLB, MSA, and neurodegeneration with brain iron accumulation type 1, NBIA-1), and those characterized by an abnormal accumulation of the microtubule-associated protein tau (MAPT), the tauopathies such as frontotemporal dementia with parkinsonism linked to chromosome 17 (FTDP-17), PSP, and CBD *(3)*. The most common neurodegenerative disease, AD, has possible links to both groups of disorders, as will be seen below.

Although those findings have greatly advanced our understanding of the etiology of neurodegenerative diseases, the relationship between genes, mutations, and the associated molecular pathways (the "genotype") on the one hand, and the clinical and pathologic features observed in patients and families (the "phenotype") on the other hand, is increasingly recognized to be highly complex.

From: *Current Clinical Neurology: Atypical Parkinsonian Disorders*
Edited by: I. Litvan © Humana Press Inc., Totowa, NJ

This review will attempt to give an overview of the current knowledge on these issues, focussing not on PD, but on atypical parkinsonian syndromes. Genetic findings in individual diseases will be discussed, and the range of phenotypic presentations related to particular genetic causes will be reviewed.

SYNUCLEINOPATHIES: PARKINSONISM RELATED TO α-SYNUCLEIN AGGREGATION

α-Synuclein: Its Physiologic Function and Role in Disease

A major breakthrough in the molecular dissection of parkinsonism was the discovery of mutations in the gene for α-synuclein on the long arm of chromosome 4 as the cause for a dominantly inherited disorder that resembles idiopathic PD in many ways both clinically and pathologically *(4)*.

α-Synuclein is a relatively small, natively unfolded protein that is abundantly expressed in many parts of the brain and localized mostly to presynaptic nerve terminals. Many aspects of the normal function of α-synuclein are still unknown. The protein may functionally be involved in brain plasticity and has been shown to bind to brain vesicles *(5)* and other cell membranes *(6)*. However, knock-out mice for α-synuclein show only very subtle alterations in dopamine release under certain experimental conditions, but no other phenotype *(7)*.

The central role of α-synuclein in the neurodegenerative process became clear when it was discovered that fibrillar aggregates of this protein are not only found in those rare families with mutations of the α-synuclein gene, but also constitute the primary component of the LB, the well-known pathologic hallmark of idiopathic PD and in DLB. Furthermore, α-synuclein aggregates are also found in oligodendrocytes in patients with MSA in the form of so-called "glial cytoplasmic inclusions" (GCIs) *(8)* and, although less consistently, in NBIA-I *(9)*, the disorder formerly called Hallervorden–Spatz disease. All those disorders have therefore been collectively termed "synucleinopathies."

The currently favored hypothesis states that through a hydrophobic 12 amino acid domain in the center of the protein, α-synuclein has the tendency to form fibrillar structures *(10)*, which go on to form aggregates in a nucleation-dependent manner. It is assumed that the amino acid changes in the α-synuclein protein associated with pathogenic mutations may favor the β-pleated sheet conformation, which in turn may lead to an increased tendency to form aggregates. This has been demonstrated in vitro *(11–13)*. As most cases of synucleinopathies express wt-α-synuclein and not a mutated form, other factors must be assumed to also promote aggregate formation. In fact, this has been shown for oxidative stress *(14)*, which is thought to be particulary high in dopaminergic neurons, and also for dopamine itself *(15)*, possibly explaining the selectivity of the neurodegenerative process.

The precise relationship between the formation of aggregates and cell death is unknown. It is possible that a failure of proteasomal degradation of α-synuclein and other proteins may lead to an accumulation of toxic compounds, ultimately leading to cell death *(16)*. Formation of α-synuclein-containing aggregates would then be only a secondary effect *(17)*. However, other mechanisms of pathogenesis may also be important. Known α-synuclein mutations appear to alter the vesicle-binding properties of the protein *(5)*, and the functional homology of α-synuclein to the 14-3-3 protein, a ubiquitously expressed chaperone, may indicate a more profound role for this protein in cellular metabolism and suggests still other possible pathogenic mechanisms, which might also differ between the various synucleinopathies.

Parkinsonism Caused by Mutations Affecting the Gene for α-Synuclein (PARK1 and PARK4)

The first mutation of the α-synuclein gene was recognized in a large family with autosomal-dominantly inherited parkinsonism, the "Contursi-kindred." It consisted of a point mutation leading to the exchange of the amino acid alanine to threonine at position 53 of the protein. A second point mutation (Ala39Pro) was later discovered in a small German pedigree *(18)*. Patients suffer from L-dopa-responsive parkinsonism, and neuropathological studies in individuals with the Ala53Thr mutation showed the characteristic pattern of neuronal degeneration with α-synuclein-positive LBs in the substantia nigra. In the early descriptions it appeared that only the relatively early age at onset (with a mean 44 yr in the large "Contursi" kindred) distinguished this disease from typical sporadic PD *(19)*. As more families with this mutation are being studied, however, it became clear that it is associated with a broader range of phenotypes and that patients frequently also exhibit clinical features that clearly exceed what is usually found in typical PD, including prominent dementia, hypoventilation, and severe autonomic disturbances *(20)*. There are also differences in the pathologic picture that distinguish cases with α-synuclein mutations from typical PD. In the inherited cases, extensive pathology with α-synuclein-positive Lewy neurites are found in brainstem pigmented nuclei, but also in the hippocampus and the temporal neocortex *(20)*. Unexpectedly, neuritic and less frequent perikaryal inclusions of tau were also observed *(21)*. Interestingly, the presence of tau immunoreactivity has been suggested to distinguish between LBs of typical PD and those seen in DLB *(22)*.

Point mutations in the α-synuclein gene clearly appear to be a very rare cause of parkinsonism. Only three mutations have been recognized *(4,18,22a)*. The mutation that was found in the original Contursi family (Ala53Thr) has also been identified in several Greek kindreds *(4,23,24)*. Haplotype analyses support the hypothesis that this is owing to a founder effect *(24)*, pointing to a single mutational event.

Very recently, a different type of mutation affecting the α-synuclein gene was identified in another family with widespread synuclein pathology. One branch of this family, now called the "Iowa-kindred," was originally described by Spellman, and later in more detail by Muenter and colleagues *(25)*. A different branch of the family was identified by Waters and Miller *(26)*.

The clinical picture of affected family members is variable, ranging from relatively pure PD to parkinsonism with prominent dementia, autonomic disturbances, and hypoventilation *(25)*. Age at onset is rather uniformly in the fourth decade and progression is rapid with a disease duration of less than 10 yr. Pathologic examination showed nigral cell loss and LBs in pigmented brainstem nuclei, resembling typical PD, but also extensive neuritic changes and α-synuclein inclusions with vacuolization in neocortical areas, most prominent in the superior temporal gyrus *(27)*, remarkably similar to the findings in the Contursi kindred just described.

The gene locus had originally been mapped to the short arm of chromosome 4 (4p13, PARK4; *see* ref. 28), and thus thought to be distinct from the α-synuclein locus on chromosome 4q. It is now known that this chromosomal assignment was actually because of a typing error, and that the causative mutation is in fact a triplication of a 2 Mb region containing (in addition to 19 other genes) the entire α-synuclein gene on chromosome 4q26 *(28a)*. The triplication was associated with a twofold increase of α-synuclein expression in the brain, determined at both the RNA and the protein level. This important finding shows that not only a pathogenic alteration of the protein, but also a mere increase in its expression level, is sufficient to cause neurodegeneration and disease with profound Lewy pathology. The situation is therefore similar to AD, where point mutations in several genes (APP, presenilin 1 and 2) but also an increase of expression of the normal APP gene, as in trisomy 21 (Down syndrome) can cause AD pathology.

Taken together, these findings also show that mutations affecting the α-synuclein protein or its expression level can result, within single families, in a spectrum of phenotypes that can variably share many clinical and pathologic features with PD (L-dopa-responsive parkinsonism with LBs and neurodegeneration more or less restricted to brainstem nuclei) as well as with other synucleinopathies, which should more appropriately be classified as atypical parkinsonism, particularly DLB (dementia, Lewy pathology in limbic and cortical areas) and even MSA (orthostatic hypotension).

Dementia With Lewy Bodies

Although the recognition of α-synuclein mutations has extremely important implications for the understanding of the underlying disease process, it must be recognized that the vast majority of cases of the common "synucleinopathies," such as PD, DLB, and MSA, are sporadic and are not a result of a recognized α-synuclein gene mutation. It is therefore assumed that in these cases other genetic or non-genetic factors may lead to an abnormal processing of α-synuclein. As the tried and tested tools of molecular genetics, such as linkage analysis and positional cloning, are not easily applied to sporadic disorders, the identification of these factors may turn out to be a major challenge of future research. Nevertheless, recent findings have begun to shed some light also on these still enigmatic diseases.

DLB is a disorder characterized by dementia and parkinsonism with several additional characteristic features, such as formed visual hallucinations, fluctuating levels of alertness, as well as frequent falls and increased sensitivity to neuroleptic treatment *(29)*. Neuropathologically, α-synuclein-positive LBs, Lewy neurites, and neuronal degeneration are found in pigmented brainstem nuclei, but also, to a variable degree, in limbic and neocortical regions. In addition, a profound cholinergic deficit occurs owing to degeneration of brainstem and basal forebrain cholinergic projection neurons *(30)*.

The question whether PD and DLB are separate entities or rather different manifestations of a single disease process has been widely debated. There is in fact considerable evidence suggesting that PD and DLB are both parts of a continuum of LB diseases. With sensitive α-synuclein immunostaining, cortical LBs are found in the majority of patients with typical PD *(31)*. Furthermore, the findings in families with α-synuclein mutations described in the previous subheading indicate that the pathology associated with a single mutation can be restricted to the brainstem (clinically pure PD) or affect limbic and cortical areas as in DLB (clinically PD plus dementia).

However, the situation in sporadic cases is more complex. Density of cortical LBs is not always correlated with the degree of dementia *(32)*. Pure Lewy pathology is actually found only in a minority of patients with DLB, whereas Alzheimer's-type changes are found, in addition to Lewy pathology, in the majority of cases. This AD-like pathology differs to some degree from that found in "typical" AD. Senile plaques, composed of the Aβ-fragment of the amyloid precursor protein (APP) are found in similar density and distribution as in AD, but neurofibrillary tangles, consisting of hyperphosphorylated tau protein are less prominent and are often not sufficient to allow the diagnosis of AD according to accepted criteria.

It has therefore been a matter of considerable debate whether to consider DLB a "variant" of AD, a variant of PD, or a disease entity of its own. In any case, the overlapping clinical and neuropathologic spectrum suggests that common pathogenic mechanisms may be operating. The identification of common genetic risk factors could potentially clarify this complex relationship.

Familial DLB

Several large families with parkinsonism and dementia have been published in the literature, but as far as can be told from the family descriptions, only a few would fulfill the clinical criteria for the diagnosis of DLB, with dementia preceding or occurring within 1 yr of parkinsonism, and even fewer with neuropathologic confirmation. However, as shown earlier for the families with α-synuclein mutations, families who had originally been described as suffering from PD may actually resemble more closely DLB, both clinically and neuropathologically. It remains to be determined whether the less than a handful of other families, who have been described under the heading of "familial DLB" *(33,34)*, will prove to have α-synuclein mutations.

Families With Coexistence of AD and LB Pathology

The emergence of α-synuclein as the most sensitive histologic marker for Lewy pathology has revealed unexpected findings in AD: Lewy bodies are found in 20–40% of cases of AD, not in brainstem nucei, but rather in the amygdala *(35)*. Even more striking, in more than half of the patients developing early-onset familial AD because of a mutation in the APP gene (APP717), LBs are found in the brainstem and in the neocortex. LBs have also been found in patients with other APP mutations and with mutations in presenilin 1 *(3)*. The extent and distribution of Lewy pathology varies within families with the identical APP mutation, indicating that Alzheimer and Lewy pathology are closely related, but dependent on factors other than the primary APP mutation.

Other dominant families have been described with parkinsonism and a variable degree of dementia, who showed coexisting Lewy and Alzheimer pathology at postmortem examination *(36)*. In two of these families, the gene has been mapped to chromosome 2p13 *(37)*, but not yet identified. As affecteds from those families presented clinically with L-dopa-responsive parkinsonism *(38)* and developed dementia only later during the course of the disease *(36)*, these kindreds were classified as dominantly inherited PD (PARK3). Again, follow-up examination and postmortem analysis demonstrated that the phenotype associated with single mutations may be more variable than initially thought, and that clinical dementia and plaque-predominant AD and LB changes occur in affecteds and may share a common genetic susceptibility.

Taken together, family studies in dominant families with mutations in the genes for α-synuclein, APP, and in as yet unidentified genes indicate that three possible scenarios exist (Fig. 1):

- A continuum of restricted brainstem to widespread cortical Lewy pathology without significant AD changes in families with mutations in α-synuclein.
- The occurrence of limbic and cortical AD changes on top of a brainstem LB disorder as the consequence of single, as yet unidentified gene mutations (e.g., PARK3).
- The appearance of LBs, in addition to AD-type changes, in patients with a primary "AD-mutation" (APP717).

These findings indicate that the underlying mutation may be viewed as a port of entry to a disease process, which involves different molecular pathways that lead to overlapping pathologic changes with disease progression.

Genetic Risk Factors for DLB

As mentioned in the previous subheading, dominantly inherited monogenic cases of PD, AD, and DLB are very rare. Therefore, no single genetic cause can be identified in the majority of cases.

Nevertheless it is assumed that genetic risk factors are modulating the susceptibility to and the course of these disorders even in sporadic cases. If common genetic risk factors could be identified for AD, PD, and DLB, this would strengthen the argument for a common molecular disease process.

The ε4-allele of the apolipoprotein E gene (ApoE4) is the only confirmed risk factor for sporadic AD. ApoE4 has been shown to increase the risk for, and decrease the age of onset of AD *(39)*. This has been confirmed in a large number of studies. By contrast, the majority of studies does not find an association of PD with the ApoE4 allele *(40,41)*.

Studies on the influence of ApoE4 on DLB have produced conflicting results, which can in part be explained by differences in the study design and small sample sizes *(42–46)*. Koller *(44)* and Egensperger *(47)* did not find a difference between PD patients with or without dementia, as compared to controls, whereas in the study of Hardy et al. *(43)* ApoE4 allele frequencies in patients with DLB were intermediate between controls and AD. A higher proportion of ApoE4 alleles was also found in patients with PD and concomitant AD changes ("B and C" according to the CERAD [Consortium to Establish a Registry for Alzheimer's Disease] criteria) as compared to PD patients without such changes *(48)*. The association of neuritic plaques with ApoE4 was confirmed by Olechney *(49)*, whereas another study supported a role of the ApoE4 allele in the density of cortical LBs, but not AD changes *(50)*.

A single formal meta-analysis has been published *(51)* that confirmed a higher rate of ApoE4 alleles in DLB, but did not distinguish between "pure" DLB and DLB with AD-plaques (which would

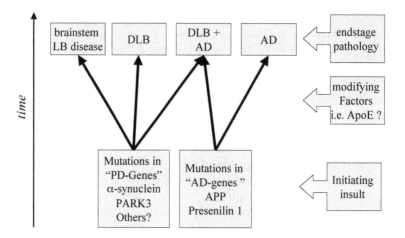

Fig. 1. Hypothetical scheme of the evolution of inherited PD, DLB, and AD. The underlying mutation and mostly modifying factors act together to determine distribution and type of pathology.

also be very difficult in a meta-analysis because of the heterogeneity of the populations examined and ambiguous descriptions in the original populations).

Overall the studies seem to indicate that ApoE4 is likely to be a risk factor for dementia in patients with parkinsonism, although not quite as clearly as in "pure" AD. It remains unresolved whether this is because of an increase of AD changes or to the cortical or limbic LB load.

Another risk factor for DLB may be an as yet unidentified gene in the pericentromeric region of chromosome 12. Linkage with this locus was identified in a genome-wide screen in a group of families with late-onset AD *(52)*. Further analysis of this region showed that much of the evidence was derived from a subset of families with affected individuals with the neuropathologic diagnosis of DLB *(53)*. Interestingly, linkage to this region was also found in a Japanese family with autosomal-dominant parkinsonism (PARK8; *see* ref. *54*), and this locus has been confirmed in other families with dominant parkinsonism *(54a)*. The clinical and neuropathologic spectrum in these families is variable, including brainstem and diffuse Lewy pathology, again indicating that mutations in a single gene can cause a range of phenotypes that may be determined more specifically by other genetic or nongenetic factors.

Multiple System Atrophy (MSA)

MSA is the second most common parkinsonian syndrome after idiopathic PD. In a majority of patients with MSA, parkinsonism predominates (MSA-P), whereas a smaller proportion have prominent cerebellar disturbances (MSA-C). Regardless of the predominant clinical picture, MSA has been classified among the synucleinopathies, since it was discovered that a key pathologic feature is the aggregation of α-synuclein in the form of flame-shaped cytoplasmic inclusions in oligondendrocytes and in neurons. It is still enigmatic why α-synuclein should accumulate in oligodendrocytes, as these cells usually express only very low levels of this protein.

By contrast to all other atypical parkinsonian syndromes, no clearly familial cases with MSA have been described in the literature. It is still conceivable that genetic factors may influence the susceptibility to the disease. Only a few association studies have been performed with polymorphisms in genes, which were considered candidate genes for MSA, including dopamine beta hydroxylase *(55)*, apolipoprotein E *(56)*, and debrisoquine hydroxylase *(57)*, without any consistent positive findings.

TAU-RELATED DISORDERS

Several neurodegenerative disorders appear to be related to the abnormal deposition of the microtubule-associated protein tau (MAPTau). A detailed discussion of this complex group of disorders is beyond the scope of this chapter. Excellent reviews on the clinical *(58)* and molecular *(59)* aspects of tauopathies have been published. The brief discussion here will be restricted to aspects directly related to their presentation as atypical parkinsonian syndromes.

Tau: Normal Function and Role in Disease

The normal function of tau is to bind to tubulin, to promote its polymerization, and to maintain the stability of microtubules. As also explained in other chapters of this book, the tau gene gives rise to six isoforms of the tau protein, generated by alternative splicing of exons 2, 3, and 10. Tau contains four imperfect repeat sequences in the carboxy terminal part of the protein, referred to as the microtubule binding domains. The fourth domain is encoded by exon 10. Therefore, alternative splicing of exon 10 determines whether the protein contains three or four copies of repeated sequence. Under normal conditions, three-repeat and four-repeat tau are present in roughly equal amounts in the brain.

Tau is found as fibrillar aggregates in AD (then called neurofibrillary tangles), but also in a number of other neurodegenerative disorders, such as PSP, CBD, the parkinsonism dementia complex of Guam, postencephalitic and posttraumatic parkinsonism, and others. The analysis of mutations of the tau gene and their functional consequences in inherited tauopathies has provided important information on the molecular mechanisms of tau-associated neurodegeneration.

Inherited Tauopathies With Mutations in the MAPTau Gene

The term "frontotemporal dementia with parkinsonism linked to chromosome 17," or FTDP-17, has been adopted for a familial disorder characterized by behavioral and cognitive disturbances, usually beginning between the ages of 40 and 50, progressing to dementia, and a variable degree of extrapyramidal, pyramidal, oculomotor, and lower motorneuron signs. Pathologically, atrophy of frontal and temporal lobes is most prominent, together with involvement of the substantia nigra, the amygdala, and the striatum *(60)*. Only about 10% of all cases of frontotemporal dementia are inherited in an autosomal-dominant manner, but of these, a substantial subset of 10–40% turned out to be genetically linked to a locus on the long arm of chromosome 17 (17q21-22) *(60,61)*. As the tau gene is located in this region, it had to be considered a primary candidate gene, and in fact, mutations in this gene have been identified *(62)* in many families with FTDP-17 *(63)*.

Mutations are clustered around the part of the gene encoding the microtubule binding domain and have been found in exons 9, 10, 12, and 13, or in adjacent intronic sequences. The variability of the clinical phenotype is accounted for, at least in part, by the fact that tau mutations appear to lead to pathology by different mechanisms.

Intronic mutations flanking exon 10, as well as some exonic exon 10 mutations affect the alternative splicing of this exon, and as a consequence alter the relative abundance of three-repeat and four-repeat tau, the two major classes of the protein present in the brain *(62)*. Other exon 10 and exon 9 mutations seem to impair the ability of tau to bind microtubules or to promote microtubule assembly, as shown by functional in vitro assays *(64)*. Whereas mutations affecting exon 10 splicing lead to the deposition of predominantly four-repeat tau, non-exon 10 coding mutations result in tau aggregates consisting of three-repeat and four-repeat tau *(65)*.

To some extent, the different functional consequences of the mutations result in a characteristic clinical picture. If mutations affect exon 10 splicing (and thus lead to the deposition of predominantly four-repeat tau) L-dopa unresponsive parkinsonism tends to be a a prominent clinical feature *(66–68)* (reviewed in ref. *58*). This is particularly striking in the family described by Wszolek et al. clinically and pathologically as pallido-ponto-nigral degeneration (PPND) *(69)*. Affected subjects present with rapidly progressive L-dopa-unresponsive parkinsonism with supranuclear gaze palsy, with dementia, frontal-lobe release signs, and perseverative vocalizations developing later. This family was found to harbor a mutation (N279K) increasing the activity of an exoning splice enhancer of exon 10, thus leading to increased production of four-repeat tau *(70,71)*.

However, behavioral disturbances may also be prominent in families with this class of mutations. In the first family linked to chromosome 17 (and in whom the disease had been named "disinhibition-dementia-parkinsonism-amyotrophy complex; *see* ref. *61*) personality changes begin at an average age of 45, accompanied by hypersexuality and hyperphagia. L-dopa-unresponsive parkinsonism is a consistent feature. This family bears an intronic mutation adjacent to exon 10.

In other families, a more typical picture of frontotemporal dementia with cognitive and behavioral disturbances predominates, followed by parkinsonism, and other neurological disturbances such as supranuclear gaze palsy, pyramidal tract dysfunction, and urinary incontinence to a variable degree during the later course of the disease. These phenotypes are more commonly associated with missense mutations in the constitutively spliced exons 9, 12, and 13 *(58)*. Other mutations have been associated with dementia with epilepsy *(72)*, progressive subcortical sclerosis *(73)*, or "familial multiple system tauopathy" *(74)*.

The same mutation may lead to different clinical manifestations in different families and also within single pedigrees. The most common mutation, P301L, has been found to be associated with a variety of clinical phenotypes, more or less closely resembling Pick's disease *(75)*, CBD *(76)*, or PSP. The considerable variability within single families *(77,78)* indicates that other factors in addition to tau mutations are influencing the clinical characteristics of the disease in a given patient.

Although a reduced penetrance of tau mutations has been reported *(62)*, heterozygous (dominant) mutations are almost exclusively found in individuals with a clearly positive dominant family history and are very rare in series of patients with sporadic dementing syndromes (< 0.2%) *(79)*. However, recent evidence raises the possibility of autosomal-recessive mutations causing an apparently sporadic PSP-like phenotype *(80)* (*see* below).

The relationship between the tau gene, FTDP-17, and PSP is particularly interesting. As will be discussed below, typical PSP is nearly always a sporadic disorder, but the prominent accumulation of four-repeat tau strongly suggests that the tau protein, and hence possibly also the tau gene, is intimately involved in the disease process. Given the high variability of the clinical picture in families with tau mutations and the predominance of extrapyramidal symptoms associated with some of them, it is not too surprising that, as noted above, some tau mutations lead to a phenotype more or less resembling typical PSP. One interesting mutation causing a PSP-like phenotype, the S305S-mutation, is located in exon 10 of the tau gene and forms part of a stem-loop structure at the 5' splice donor site *(81)*. Although the mutation does not give rise to an amino acid change in the tau protein, functional exon-trapping experiments show that it results in a significant 4.8-fold increase in the splicing of exon 10, resulting in the overproduction of tau containing four microtubule-binding repeats. Although the clinical phenotype in this family, as well as in other families with mutations that affect splicing of exon 10, share features of PSP, both clinically and neuropathologically, others have emphazised the differences that distinguish those families from typical PSP and have questioned whether the disorder should be called "familial PSP" *(82)*. Regardless of terminology, this finding emphasizes the close relationship between FTDP-17 and PSP.

Another interesting observation strengthening this link is that in rare cases, homozygous or compound heterozygous mutations of the tau gene can cause a PSP-like syndrome *(80,83)*, whereas heterozygous mutation carriers were either unaffected or showed only mild parkinsonism with late onset. Again, although this "recessive" form of FTDP-17 shared several features with PSP, both cases also differed from typical PSP by their early onset (40 yr or less) and by the presence of additional neurologic deficits, such as apraxia, cortical sensory deficits, or speech disturbances.

Other Diseases Associated With Tau Deposits

As in the synucleinopathies, the majority of cases of neurodegeneration with tau deposition is sporadic. Two disease entities are usually distinguished, but as will become apparent, are probably closely related: PSP and CBD.

Progressive Supranuclear Palsy (PSP)

PSP is a disease characterized by predominantly axial, L-dopa-unresponsive parkinsonism, early postural instability, supranuclear gaze palsy, and subcortical dementia *(84)*.

PSP is, with exception of the cases described above, a sporadic disorder. It is pathologically characterized by the deposition of abnormally phosphorylized tau protein as neurofibrillary tangles and neuropil threads, consisting predominantly of four-repeat tau. Tangles are also present in astrocytes ("tufted astrocytes") and oligodendroglia (coiled bodies). Based on this pathologic pattern and on the insights gained into the molecular mechansims from the inherited tauopathies described in the previous subheading, it seems likely that an abnormality of the splicing of the tau gene may be the underlying molecular defect.

Although no coding region or splice site mutations in the tau gene can be identified in typical PSP, there appears to be a genetic susceptibility to the disease that is related to the tau gene. Initially, Conrad and coworkers observed that one particular allele (which they called the "A0" allele) of a dinucleotide repeat marker within the tau gene is highly associated, in homozygous form, with PSP *(85)*. This allele was later found to be part of an extended haplotype (the H1-haplotype) of more than 100 kb, that is usually inherited *en bloc (86,87)*. It is unclear why no recombinations occur within this region in the human population.

As the H1-haplotype is common in the general population (~ 60% of chromosomes) it does *per se* not carry a high risk for the development of a tau-related disorder. It is possible, however, that a more recent mutation that has occurred on the background of this haplotype is responsible, or that the H1-haplotype is merely "permissive" for the development of typical PSP, although the ultimate cause remains unknown.

Corticobasal Degeneration

Much of what has been said for PSP also holds true for CBD. CBD is in most instances a sporadic syndrome that shares with PSP the relentless progression of L-dopa-unresponsive parkinsonism and predominantly subcortical cognitive disturbances, but differs in the additional presence of a usually marked asymmetry of signs, dystonia and irregular reflex myoclonus in the most affected limb, as well as cortical sensory loss and, in about 40% of cases, the characteristic "alien limb sign." In addition to the subcortical changes, asymmetric cortical atrophy is often observed. Neuropathology reveals characteristic tau accumulation in the form of neuropil threads throughout gray and white matter. Tau filaments in CBD include both paired helical filament (PHF)-like filaments and straight tubules *(59)*. As in PSP, the filaments are composed predominantly of four-repeat tau.

As was also described for PSP, in a few families with dominant tau mutations, the disease resembles CBD *(76)*. It is probably a matter of semantics whether the disease in these cases should be called "familial CBD" or "FTDP resembling CBD," as long as it is kept in mind that there are similarities and differences: sporadic CBD is not caused by detectable exonic or splice site mutations in the tau gene, but it shares the same tau-related genetic background with PSP, the homozygocity for the H1-haplotype, supporting the close relationship between these two disorders *(88,89)*.

TAUOPATHIES, SYNUCLEINOPATHIES, AND BEYOND

Although recent genetic and pathologic evidence lead to the distinction of two major groups of neurodegenerative disorders, the tauopathies and the synucleinopathies, based on the predominant pathology and on mutations of the respective genes in rare familial forms of these diseases, there is also evidence accumulating that the pathogenic mechanisms may in fact be related.

As detailed above, there appears to be considerable overlap both clinically and pathologically between PD, DLB, and AD. Various combinations of Lewy pathology and AD-type pathology are found even in monogenically inherited forms.

However, there is also neuropathologic and genetic evidence linking Lewy pathology to alterations of tau: LBs in DLB have been distinguished from LBs in PD by tau staining (22). Similarly, some LBs found in the brain of patients with the α-synuclein mutation A53T could be stained with antibodies to the tau protein (21).

An association of the H1 haplotype, which is present in homozygous form in the great majority of PSP-patients, with idiopathic PD has been reported (90) but not confirmed (91). However, in a total genome screen in a large number of sib pairs and small families with PD, the tau locus on chromosome 17 was identified as one of the five loci with suggestive lod scores (although not reaching statistical significance) (92).

Finally, in a recent report, Wszolek et al. describe a family with autosomal-dominant inheritance, initially presenting with pure L-dopa-responsive parkinsonism (93). Some affecteds progressed to show symptoms of atypical parkinsonism, including supranuclear gaze palsy. Interestingly, pathology in different members of this family varied, from typical brainstem LB disease to diffuse LB disease to a tauopathy resembling PSP (106). The gene locus in this family most likely maps to the PARK8 locus on chromosome 12. If in fact the disease in all affected subjects of this family is owing to a mutation in a single gene, this would bridge the gap between the two major categories of neurodegenerative disease recognized today, and strongly argue for a common pathogenic process.

OTHER GENETIC DISEASES OCCASIONALLY PRESENTING WITH ATYPICAL PARKINSONISM

Huntington's Disease

Huntington's disease (HD) is an autosomal-dominantly inherited disorder, usually characterized by a hyperkinetic movement disorder, personality changes, and dementia. It is caused by the pathologic expansion of a CAG-trinucleotide repeat sequence in the gene for Huntingtin on chromosome 4 (94). The fact that particularly cases of early onset frequently present with dystonia and parkinsonism, rather than with chorea, has long been recognized (95). In addition, the widespread use of molecular diagnosis for HD has shown that the phenotypic spectrum may even include late-onset levodopa-responsive parkinsonism (96) and atypical parkinsonian syndromes (97).

Spinocerebellar Ataxias

Like HD, the spinocerebellar ataxias (SCAs) are caused by expansions of CAG repeat sequences. The core syndrome is usually that of a progressive cerebellar ataxia with or without additional neurologic features. Particularly in SCA1, 2, and 3, extrapyramidal symptoms are relatively common, and have been described in 10–50% of patients (98). Patients with SCA3 have occasionally been found to present with parkinsonism (99). This has recently been confirmed in another family (100) and extended to a family with SCA2 (101). It is therefore not unlikely that other forms of SCA might also, occasionally, mimic parkinsonian syndromes. The reason for the variable expressivity of the genes with expanded CAG repeat expansion is still largely unknown.

Neurodegeneration With Brain Iron Accumulation Type 1 (NBIA-1)

NBIA-1 (formerly called Hallervorden–Spatz disease) is an autosomal-recessive disorder presenting during childhood or adolescence with a progressive syndrome of parkinsonism, dystonia, spasticity, epileptic seizures, and cognitive decline. The characteristic iron accumulations in the basal ganglia are visible on magnetic resonance imaging (MRI) as hypointensities with a central region of hyperintensity reflecting gliosis (eye of the tiger sign). The disease gene maps to chromosome 20, and has been identified to code for pantothenate kinase 2 (PANK2), an enzyme catalyzing an impor-

Table 1
Genes and Mutations Associated With Atypical Parkinsonian Syndromes

Name	Chromosomal Region	Gene Mutation	Range of Age of Disease Onset (Mean), in Years	Phenotype	Response to Levodopa	Pathology
Autosomal dominant						
PARK 1/4	4q21	α-synuclein three missense mutations one triplication	20–85 (46)	PD, some cases with dementia	Good	Lewy bodies in brainstem, Lewy neurite, and vacuolization in temporal cortex
PARK 3	2p13	Unknown	36–89 (58)	PD, some cases with dementia	Good	Lewy bodies and amyloid plaques
PARK 8	12p11.2- q13.11	Unknown	38–68 (51)	PD	Good	Variable: pure nigral degeneration, Lewy body, tau pathology
FTDP-17	17q21-22	tau/multiple mutations	25–76 (49)	FTD, PD, PSP, CBgD, ALS	Poor	Tau pathology
DYT12	19q13	Unknown	12–45 (23)	Rapid-onset dystonia-parkinsonism	Poor	Unknown
Autosomal recessive						
NBIA I	20p12.3	Pantothenate kinase/ multiple mutations	4–64	Parkinsonism, dystonia, spasticity, dementia	Poor	Iron accumulation, Lewy bodies
PARK 9	1p36	Unknown	11–16 (10's)	PD, dementia, gaze palsy	Good	Unknown
X-linked recessive						
DYT3	Xq13.1	Unknown	12–48 (35)	Dystonia-parkinsonism	Poor	No Lewy bodies

tant step in the acyl-CoA-metabolism *(102)*. As with many other diseases, the discovery of the gene led to the appreciation of a broader phenotype, including cases of adult-onset atypical parkinsonism. It seems that all cases show the typical MRI changes, leading to the correct diagnosis.

CONCLUSIONS: IMPACT OF GENETICS ON NOSOLOGY

The identification of several genes that lead to monogenic forms of the major neurodegenerative disorders has greatly advanced our understanding of the molecular mechanisms involved. However, the careful analysis of their clinical and pathologic features reveals that, although they share many features with the respective sporadic diseases, there are clearly also important differences. Therefore, those disorders should be viewed as natural models, recapitulating some, but certainly not all features of their molecular pathogenesis. Perhaps most remarkably, both the variability of the phenotypes associated with single gene mutations, as well as the similarities and overlap between disorders caused by alterations in different genes appear to indicate that we are dealing in fact not with strictly distinct pathways, but rather with a complex metabolic network, consisting of pathogenic mutations, genetic modifiers, and probably also environmental influences, which defines the course of the disease in a given patient.

FUTURE RESEARCH

In order to better understand the relationship between genetic alterations on one hand, and pathologic and clinical phenotypes on the other, further research will be needed: (1) To identify additional loci and genes in large informative pedigrees with monogenically inherited forms of parkinsonism. (2) To study the role of genes identified in monogenic forms also in large, well-characterized patient populations. (3) To identify the metabolic pathways involved in the disease process in monogenic forms, in order to identify new candidate genes for the sporadic disease.

REFERENCE

1. Gibb WR, Lees AJ. The significance of the Lewy body in the diagnosis of idiopathic Parkinson's disease. Neuropathol Appl Neurobiol 1989;15(1):27–44.
2. Perl DP, Olanow CW, Calne D. Alzheimer's disease and Parkinson's disease: distinct entities or extremes of a spectrum of neurodegeneration? Ann Neurol 1998;44(3 Suppl 1):S19–S31.
3. Hardy J, Duff K, Hardy KG, Perez-Tur J, Hutton M. Genetic dissection of Alzheimer's disease and related dementias: amyloid and its relationship to tau. Nat Neurosci 1998;1(5):355–358.
4. Polymeropoulos MH, Lavedan C, Leroy E, Ide SE, Dehejia A, Dutra A, et al. Mutation in the α-synuclein gene identified in families with Parkinson's disease. Science 1997;276:2045–2047.
5. Jensen PH, Nielsen MS, Jakes R, Dotti CG, Goedert M. Binding of alpha-synuclein to brain vesicles is abolished by familial Parkinson's disease mutation. J Biol Chem 1998;273(41):26292–26294.
6. McLean PJ, Kawamata H, Ribich S, Hyman BT. Membrane association and protein conformation of alpha-synuclein in intact neurons. Effect of Parkinson's disease–linked mutations. J Biol Chem 2000;275(12):8812–8816.
7. Abeliovich A, Schmitz Y, Farinas I, Choi-Lundberg D, Ho WH, Castillo PE et al. Mice lacking alpha-synuclein display functional deficits in the nigrostriatal dopamine system. Neuron 2000;25(1):239–252.
8. Spillantini MG, Crowther RA, Jakes R, Cairns NJ, Lantos PL, Goedert M. Filamentous alpha-synuclein inclusions link multiple system atrophy with Parkinson's disease and dementia with Lewy bodies. Neurosci Lett 1998;251(3):205–208.
9. Neumann M, Adler S, Schluter O, Kremmer E, Benecke R, Kretzschmar HA. Alpha-synuclein accumulation in a case of neurodegeneration with brain iron accumulation type 1 (NBIA-1, formerly Hallervorden–Spatz syndrome) with widespread cortical and brainstem-type Lewy bodies. Acta Neuropathol (Berl) 2000;100(5):568–574.
10. Giasson BI, Uryu K, Trojanowski JQ, Lee VM. Mutant and wild type human alpha-synucleins assemble into elongated filaments with distinct morphologies in vitro. J Biol Chem 1999;274(12):7619–7622.
11. Biere AL, Wood SJ, Wypych J, Steavenson S, Jiang Y, Anafi D, et al. Parkinson's disease-associated alpha-synuclein is more fibrillogenic than beta- and gamma-synuclein and cannot cross-seed its homologs. J Biol Chem 2000;275(44):34574–34579.
12. Conway KA, Lee SJ, Rochet JC, Ding TT, Williamson RE, Lansbury PTJ. Acceleration of oligomerization, not fibrillization, is a shared property of both alpha-synuclein mutations linked to early-onset Parkinson's disease: implications for pathogenesis and therapy. Proc Natl Acad Sci USA 2000;97(2):571–576.

13. Conway KA, Harper JD, Lansbury PT. Accelerated in vitro fibril formation by a mutant alpha-synuclein linked to early-onset Parkinson disease. Nat Med 1998;4(11):1318–1320.

14. Hashimoto M, Hsu LJ, Xia Y, Takeda A, Sisk A, Sundsmo M, et al. Oxidative stress induces amyloid-like aggregate formation of NACP/alpha-synuclein in vitro. Neuroreport 1999;10(4):717–721.

15. Conway KA, Rochet JC, Bieganski RM, Lansbury PT, Jr. Kinetic stabilization of the alpha-synuclein protofibril by a dopamine-alpha-synuclein adduct. Science 2001;294(5545):1346–1349.

16. McNaught KS, Olanow CW, Halliwell B, Isacson O, Jenner P. Failure of the ubiquitin-proteasome system in Parkinson's disease. Nat Rev Neurosci 2001;2(8):589–594.

17. McNaught KS, Jenner P. Proteasomal function is impaired in substantia nigra in Parkinson's disease. Neurosci Lett 2001;297(3):191–194.

18. Krüger R, Kuhn W, Müller T, Woitalla D, Graeber M, Kösel S, et al. Ala39Pro mutation in the gene encoding α-synuclein in Parkinson's disease. Nat Genet 1998;18:106–108.

19. Golbe LI, Di Iorio G, Sanges G, Lazzarini A, LaSala S, Bonavita V, et al. Clinical genetic analysis of Parkinson's disease in the Contursi kindred. Ann Neurol 1996;40:767–775.

20. Spira PJ, Sharpe DM, Halliday G, Cavanagh J, Nicholson GA. Clinical and pathological features of a Parkinsonian syndrome in a family with an Ala53Thr alpha-synuclein mutation. Ann Neurol 2001;49(3):313–319.

21. Duda JE, Giasson BI, Mabon ME, Miller DC, Golbe LI, Lee VM et al. Concurrence of alpha-synuclein and tau brain pathology in the Contursi kindred. Acta Neuropathol (Berl) 2002;104(1):7–11.

22. Galloway PG, Bergeron C, Perry G. The presence of tau distinguishes Lewy bodies of diffuse Lewy body disease from those of idiopathic Parkinson disease. Neurosci Lett 1989;100(1–3):6–10.

22a. Zarranz JJ, Alegre J, Gomez-Esteban JC, et al. The new mutation, E46K, of alpha-synuclein causes Parkinson and Lewy body dementia. Ann Neurol 2004;55(2):164–173.

23. Markopoulou K, Wszolek ZK, Pfeiffer RF. A Greek-American kindred with autosomal dominant, levodopa-responsive parkinsonism and anticipation. Ann Neurol 1995;38(3):373–378.

24. Papadimitriou A, Veletza V, Hadjigeorgiou GM, Patrikiou A, Hirano M, Anastasopoulos I. Mutated alpha-synuclein gene in two Greek kindreds with familial PD: incomplete penetrance? Neurology 1999;52(3):651–654.

25. Muenter MD, Forno LS, Hornykiewicz O, Kish SJ, Maraganore DM, Caselli RJ et al. Hereditary form of parkinsonism—dementia. Ann Neurol 1998;43(6):768–781.

26. Waters CH, Miller CA. Autosomal dominant Lewy body parkinsonism in a four-generation family. Ann Neurol 1994;35(1):59–64.

27. Gwinn-Hardy K, Mehta ND, Farrer M, Maraganore D, Muenter M, Yen SH, et al. Distinctive neuropathology revealed by alpha-synuclein antibodies in hereditary parkinsonism and dementia linked to chromosome 4p. Acta Neuropathol (Berl) 2000;99(6):663–672.

28. Farrer M, Gwinn-Hardy K, Muenter M, Wavrant DF, Crook R, Perez-Tur J, et al. A chromosome 4p haplotype segregating with Parkinson's disease and postural tremor. Hum Mol Genet 1999;8(1):81–85.

28a. Singleton AB, Farrer M, Johnson J, et al. Alpha-synuclein locus triplication causes Parkinson's disease. Science 2003;302(5456):841.

29. McKeith IG. Dementia with Lewy bodies. Br J Psychiatry 2002;180(2):144–147.

30. Dickson DW, Davies P, Mayeux R, Crystal H, Horoupian DS, Thompson A, et al. Diffuse Lewy body disease. Neuropathological and biochemical studies of six patients. Acta Neuropathol (Berl) 1987;75(1):8–15.

31. Hughes AJ, Daniel SE, Blankson S, Lees AJ. A clinicopathologic study of 100 cases of Parkinson's disease. Arch Neurol 1993;50(2):140–148.

32. Colosimo C, Hughes AJ, Kilford L, Lees AJ. Lewy body cortical involvement may not always predict dementia in Parkinson's disease. J Neurol Neurosurg Psychiatry 2003;74(7):852–856.

33. Tsuang DW, Dalan AM, Eugenio CJ, Poorkaj P, Limprasert P, La Spada AR, et al. Familial dementia with lewy bodies: a clinical and neuropathological study of 2 families. Arch Neurol 2002;59(10):1622–1630.

34. Wakabayashi K, Hayashi S, Ishikawa A, Hayashi T, Okuizumi K, Tanaka H, et al. Autosomal dominant diffuse Lewy body disease. Acta Neuropathol (Berl) 1998;96(2):207–210.

35. Arai Y, Yamazaki M, Mori O, Muramatsu H, Asano G, Katayama Y. Alpha-synuclein-positive structures in cases with sporadic Alzheimer's disease: morphology and its relationship to tau aggregation. Brain Res 2001;888(2):287–296.

36. Wszolek K, Gwinn-Hardy K, Wszolek K, Muenter D, Pfeiffer F, Rodnitzky L, et al. Neuropathology of two members of a German-American kindred (Family C) with late onset parkinsonism. Acta Neuropathol (Berl) 2002;103(4):344–350.

37. Gasser T, Müller-Myhsok B, Wszolek ZK, Oehlmann R, Calne DB, Bonifati V, et al. A susceptibility locus for Parkinson's disease maps to chromosome 2p13. Nat Genet 1998;18:262–265.

38. Wszolek ZK, Cordes M, Calne DB, Munter MD, Cordes I, Pfeifer RF. Hereditary Parkinson disease: report of 3 families with dominant autosomal inheritance. Nervenarzt 1993;64(5):331–335.

39. Corder EH, Saunders AM, Strittmatter WJ, Schmechel DE, Gaskell PC, Small GW, et al. Gene dose of apolipoprotein E type 4 allele and the risk of Alzheimer's disease in late onset families. Science 1993;261(5123):921–923.

40. Apolipoprotein E genotype in familial Parkinson's disease. The French Parkinson's Disease Genetics Study Group. J Neurol Neurosurg Psychiatry 1997;63(3):394–395.

41. Benjamin R, Leake A, Edwardson JA, McKeith IG, Ince PG, Perry RH, et al. Apolipoprotein E genes in Lewy body and Parkinson's disease [letter]. Lancet 1994;343(8912):1565–1565.

42. Arai H, Higuchi S, Muramatsu T, Iwatsubo T, Sasaki H, Trojanowski JQ. Apolipoprotein E gene in diffuse Lewy body disease with or without co-existing Alzheimer's disease [letter]. Lancet 1994;344(8932):1307–1307.

43. Hardy J, Crook R, Prihar G, Roberts G, Raghavan R, Perry R. Senile dementia of the Lewy body type has an apolipoprotein E epsilon 4 allele frequency intermediate between controls and Alzheimer's disease. Neurosci Lett 1994;182(1):1–2.

44. Koller WC, Glatt SL, Hubble JP, Paolo A, Troster AI, Handler MS, et al. Apolipoprotein E genotypes in Parkinson's disease with and without dementia. Ann Neurol 1995;37(2):242–245.

45. Lippa CF, Smith TW, Saunders AM, Crook R, Pulaski Salo D, Davies P, et al. Apolipoprotein E genotype and Lewy body disease. Neurology 1995;45(1):97–103.

46. St Clair D, Norrman J, Perry R, Yates C, Wilcock G, Brookes A. Apolipoprotein E epsilon 4 allele frequency in patients with Lewy body dementia, Alzheimer's disease and age-matched controls. Neurosci Lett 1994;176(1):45–46.

47. Egensperger R, Bancher C, Kosel S, Jellinger K, Mehraein P, Graeber MB. The apolipoprotein E epsilon 4 allele in Parkinson's disease with Alzheimer lesions. Biochem Biophys Res Commun 1996;224(2):484–486.

48. Mattila PM, Koskela T, Roytta M, Lehtimaki T, Pirttila TA, Ilveskoski E, et al. Apolipoprotein E epsilon4 allele frequency is increased in Parkinson's disease only with co-existing Alzheimer pathology. Acta Neuropathol (Berl) 1998;96(4):417–420.

49. Olichney JM, Hansen LA, Galasko D, Saitoh T, Hofstetter CR, Katzman R, et al. The apolipoprotein E epsilon 4 allele is associated with increased neuritic plaques and cerebral amyloid angiopathy in Alzheimer's disease and Lewy body variant. Neurology 1996;47(1):190–196.

50. Wakabayashi K, Kakita A, Hayashi S, Okuizumi K, Onodera O, Tanaka H, et al. Apolipoprotein E epsilon4 allele and progression of cortical Lewy body pathology in Parkinson's disease. Acta Neuropathol (Berl) 1998;95(5):450–454.

51. Bang OY, Kwak YT, Joo IS, Huh K. Important link between dementia subtype and apolipoprotein E: a meta-analysis. Yonsei Med J 2003;44(3):401–413.

52. Pericak-Vance MA, Bass MP, Yamaoka LH, Gaskell PC, Scott WK, Terwedow HA, et al. Complete genomic screen in late-onset familial Alzheimer disease. Evidence for a new locus on chromosome 12. JAMA 1997;278(15):1237–1241.

53. Scott WK, Grubber JM, Conneally PM, Small GW, Hulette CM, Rosenberg CK, et al. Fine mapping of the chromosome 12 late-onset Alzheimer disease locus: potential genetic and phenotypic heterogeneity. Am J Hum Genet 2000;66(3):922–932.

54. Funayama M, Hasegawa K, Kowa H, Saito M, Tsuji S, Obata F. A new locus for Parkinson's disease (PARK8) maps to chromosome 12p11.2-q13.1. Ann Neurol 2002;51(3):296–301.

54a. Zimprich A, Muller-Myhsok B, Farrer M, et al. The PARK8 locus in autosomal dominant Parkinsonism: confirmation of linkage and further delineation of the disease-containing interval. Am J Hum Genet 2004;74(1):11–19.

55. Cho S, Kim CH, Cubells JF, Zabetian CP, Hwang DY, Kim JW, et al. Variations in the dopamine beta-hydroxylase gene are not associated with the autonomic disorders, pure autonomic failure, or multiple system atrophy. Am J Med Genet 2003;120A(2):234–236.

56. Morris HR, Schrag A, Nath U, Burn D, Quinn NP, Daniel S et al. Effect of ApoE and tau on age of onset of progressive supranuclear palsy and multiple system atrophy. Neurosci Lett 2001;312(2):118–120.

57. Plante-Bordeneuve V, Bandmann O, Wenning G, Quinn NP, Daniel SE, Harding AE. CYP2D6-debrisoquine hydroxy-lase gene polymorphism in multiple system atrophy. Mov Disord 1995;10(3):277–278.

58. Reed LA, Wszolek ZK, Hutton M. Phenotypic correlations in FTDP-17. Neurobiol Aging 2001;22(1):89–107.

59. Lee VM, Goedert M, Trojanowski JQ. Neurodegenerative tauopathies. Annu Rev Neurosci 2001;24:1121–59.:1121–1159.

60. Foster NL, Wilhelmsen K, Sima AA, Jones MZ, D'Amato CJ, Gilman S. Frontotemporal dementia and parkinsonism linked to chromosome 17: a consensus conference. Conference Participants. Ann Neurol 1997;41(6):706–715.

61. Wilhelmsen KC, Lynch T, Pavlou E, Higgins M, Nygaard TG. Localization of disinhibition-dementia-parkinsonism-amyotrophy complex to 17q21-22. Am J Hum Genet 1994;55(6):1159–1165.

62. Hutton M, Lendon CL, Rizzu P, Baker M, Froelich S, Houlden H, et al. Association of missense and 5'-splice-site mutations in tau with the inherited dementia FTDP-17. Nature 1998;393(6686):702–705.

63. Hutton M. Missense and splice site mutations in tau associated with FTDP-17: multiple pathogenic mechanisms. Neurology 2001;56(11 Suppl 4):S21–S25.

64. Hong M, Zhukareva V, Vogelsberg-Ragaglia V, Wszolek Z, Reed L, Miller BI, et al. Mutation-specific functional impairments in distinct tau isoforms of hereditary FTDP-17. Science 1998;282(5395):1914–1917.

65. Spillantini MG, Bird TD, Ghetti B. Frontotemporal dementia and Parkinsonism linked to chromosome 17: a new group of tauopathies. Brain Pathol 1998;8(2):387–402.

66. Yasuda M, Takamatsu J, D'Souza I, Crowther RA, Kawamata T, Hasegawa M, et al. A novel mutation at position +12 in the intron following exon 10 of the tau gene in familial frontotemporal dementia (FTD-Kumamoto). Ann Neurol 2000;47(4):422–429.

67. Delisle MB, Murrell JR, Richardson R, Trofatter JA, Rascol O, Soulages X, et al. A mutation at codon 279 (N279K) in exon 10 of the Tau gene causes a tauopathy with dementia and supranuclear palsy. Acta Neuropathol (Berl) 1999;98(1):62–77.
68. Tsuboi Y, Uitti RJ, Delisle MB, Ferreira JJ, Brefel-Courbon C, Rascol O, et al. Clinical features and disease haplotypes of individuals with the N279K tau gene mutation: a comparison of the pallidopontonigral degeneration kindred and a French family. Arch Neurol 2002;59(6):943–950.
69. Wszolek ZK, Pfeiffer RF, Bhatt MH, Schelper RL, Cordes M, Snow BJ, et al. Rapidly progressive autosomal dominant parkinsonism and dementia with pallido-ponto-nigral degeneration. Ann Neurol 1992;32(3):312–320.
70. Clark LN, Poorkaj P, Wszolek Z, Geschwind DH, Nasreddine ZS, Miller B, et al. Pathogenic implications of mutations in the tau gene in pallido-ponto- nigral degeneration and related neurodegenerative disorders linked to chromosome 17. Proc Natl Acad Sci USA 1998;95(22):13103–13107.
71. Reed LA, Schmidt ML, Wszolek ZK, Balin BJ, Soontornniyomkij V, Lee VM, et al. The neuropathology of a chromosome 17-linked autosomal dominant parkinsonism and dementia ("pallido-ponto-nigral degeneration"). J Neuropathol Exp Neurol 1998;57(6):588–601.
72. Sperfeld AD, Collatz MB, Baier H, Palmbach M, Storch A, Schwarz J, et al. FTDP-17: an early-onset phenotype with parkinsonism and epileptic seizures caused by a novel mutation. Ann Neurol 1999;46(5):708–715.
73. Goedert M, Spillantini MG, Crowther RA, Chen SG, Parchi P, Tabaton M, et al. Tau gene mutation in familial progressive subcortical gliosis. Nat Med 1999;5(4):454–457.
74. Spillantini MG, Murrell JR, Goedert M, Farlow MR, Klug A, Ghetti B. Mutation in the tau gene in familial multiple system tauopathy with presenile dementia. Proc Natl Acad Sci U S A 1998;95(13):7737–7741.
75. Rizzini C, Goedert M, Hodges JR, Smith MJ, Jakes R, Hills R, et al. Tau gene mutation K257T causes a tauopathy similar to Pick's disease. J Neuropathol Exp Neurol 2000;59(11):990–1001.
76. Bugiani O, Murrell JR, Giaccone G, Hasegawa M, Ghigo G, Tabaton M, et al. Frontotemporal dementia and corticobasal degeneration in a family with a P301S mutation in tau. J Neuropathol Exp Neurol 1999;58(6):667–677.
77. Mirra SS, Murrell JR, Gearing M, Spillantini MG, Goedert M, Crowther RA, et al. Tau pathology in a family with dementia and a P301L mutation in tau. J Neuropathol Exp Neurol 1999;58(4):335–345.
78. Nasreddine ZS, Loginov M, Clark LN, Lamarche J, Miller BL, Lamontagne A, et al. From genotype to phenotype: a clinical pathological, and biochemical investigation of frontotemporal dementia and parkinsonism (FTDP-17) caused by the P301L tau mutation. Ann Neurol 1999;45(6):704–715.
79. Houlden H, Baker M, Adamson J, Grover A, Waring S, Dickson D, et al. Frequency of tau mutations in three series of non-Alzheimer's degenerative dementia. Ann Neurol 1999;46(2):243–248.
80. Pastor P, Pastor E, Carnero C, Vela R, Garcia T, Amer G, et al. Familial atypical progressive supranuclear palsy associated with homozygosity for the delN296 mutation in the tau gene. Ann Neurol 2001;49(2):263–267.
81. Stanford PM, Halliday GM, Brooks WS, Kwok JB, Storey CE, Creasey H, et al. Progressive supranuclear palsy pathology caused by a novel silent mutation in exon 10 of the tau gene: Expansion of the disease phenotype caused by tau gene mutations. Brain 2000;123(Pt 5):880–893.
82. Wszolek ZK, Tsuboi Y, Uitti RJ, Reed L, Hutton ML, Dickson DW. Progressive supranuclear palsy as a disease phenotype caused by the S305S tau gene mutation. Brain 2001;124(Pt 8):1666–1670.
83. Morris HR, Osaki Y, Holton J, Lees AJ, Wood NW, Revesz T, et al. Tau exon 10 +16 mutation FTDP-17 presenting clinically as sporadic young onset PSP. Neurology 2003;61(1):102–104.
84. Litvan I, Agid Y, Calne D, Campbell G, Dubois B, Duvoisin RC, et al. Clinical research criteria for the diagnosis of progressive supranuclear palsy (Steele–Richardson–Olszewski syndrome): report of the NINDS-SPSP international workshop. Neurology 1996;47(1):1–9.
85. Conrad C, Andreadis A, Trojanowski JQ, Dickson DW, Kang D, Chen X, et al. Genetic evidence for the involvement of tau in progressive supranuclear palsy. Ann Neurol 1997;41(2):277–281.
86. Baker M, Litvan I, Houlden H, Adamson J, Dickson D, Perez-Tur J, et al. Association of an extended haplotype in the tau gene with progressive supranuclear palsy. Hum Mol Genet 1999;8(4):711–715.
87. Pastor P, Ezquerra M, Tolosa E, Munoz E, Marti MJ, Valldeoriola F, et al. Further extension of the H1 haplotype associated with progressive supranuclear palsy. Mov Disord 2002;17(3):550–556.
88. Di Maria E, Tabaton M, Vigo T, Abbruzzese G, Bellone E, Donati C, et al. Corticobasal degeneration shares a common genetic background with progressive supranuclear palsy. Ann Neurol 2000;47(3):374–377.
89. Houlden H, Baker M, Morris HR, MacDonald N, Pickering-Brown S, Adamson J, et al. Corticobasal degeneration and progressive supranuclear palsy share a common tau haplotype. Neurology 2001;56(12):1702–1706.
90. Pastor P, Ezquerra M, Munoz E, Marti MJ, Blesa R, Tolosa E, et al. Significant association between the tau gene A0/A0 genotype and Parkinson's disease. Ann Neurol 2000;47(2):242–245.
91. de Silva R, Hardy J, Crook J, Khan N, Graham E, Morris C, et al. The tau locus is not significantly associated with pathologically confirmed sporadic Parkinson's disease. Neurosci Lett 2002;330(2):201.

92. Scott WK, Nance MA, Watts RL, Hubble JP, Koller WC, Lyons K, et al. Complete genomic screen in Parkinson disease: evidence for multiple genes. JAMA 2001;286(18):2239–2244.

93. Wszolek ZK, Pfeiffer B, Fulgham JR, Parisi JE, Thompson BM, Uitti RJ, et al. Western Nebraska family (family D) with autosomal dominant parkinsonism. Neurology 1995;45(3 Pt 1):502–505.

94. Huntington's Disease Collaborative Research Group. A novel gene containing a trinucleotide repeat that is expanded and unstable on Huntington's disease chromosomes. Cell 1993;72(6):971–983.

95. van Dijk JG, van der Velde EA, Roos RA, Bruyn GW. Juvenile Huntington disease. Hum Genet 1986;73(3):235–239.

96. Racette BA, Perlmutter JS. Levodopa responsive parkinsonism in an adult with Huntington's disease. J Neurol Neurosurg Psychiatry 1998;65(4):577–579.

97. Reuter I, Hu MT, Andrews TC, Brooks DJ, Clough C, Chaudhuri KR. Late onset levodopa responsive Huntington's disease with minimal chorea masquerading as Parkinson plus syndrome. J Neurol Neurosurg Psychiatry 2000;68(2):238–241.

98. Schols L, Amoiridis G, Buttner T, Przuntek H, Epplen JT, Riess O. Autosomal dominant cerebellar ataxia: phenotypic differences in genetically defined subtypes? Ann Neurol 1997;42(6):924–932.

99. Tuite PJ, Rogaeva EA, St George Hyslop PH, Lang AE. Dopa-responsive parkinsonism phenotype of Machado–Joseph disease: confirmation of 14q CAG expansion. Ann Neurol 1995;38(4):684–687.

100. Gwinn-Hardy K, Singleton A, O'Suilleabhain P, Boss M, Nicholl D, Adam A, et al. Spinocerebellar ataxia type 3 phenotypically resembling Parkinson disease in a black family. Arch Neurol 2001;58(2):296–299.

101. Gwinn-Hardy K, Chen JY, Liu HC, Liu TY, Boss M, Seltzer W, et al. Spinocerebellar ataxia type 2 with parkinsonism in ethnic Chinese. Neurology 2000;55(6):800–805.

102. Zhou B, Westaway SK, Levinson B, Johnson MA, Gitschier J, Hayflick SJ. A novel pantothenate kinase gene (PANK2) is defective in Hallervorden–Spatz syndrome. Nat Genet 2001;28(4):345–349.

103. Wszolek ZK, Pfeiffer RF, Tsuboi Y, et al. Autosomal dominant Parkinsonism associated with variable synuclein and tau pathology. Neurology 2004, in press.

10

Medical History and Physical Examination in Parkinsonian Syndromes

How to Examine a Parkinsonian Syndrome

Marie Vidailhet, Frédéric Bourdain, and Jean-Marc Trocello

The current chapter was prepared to help clinicians examine patients with parkinsonian syndromes and to detect clinical signs and clues that should alert to the appropriate diagnosis. For the main clinical diagnosis criteria of various parkinsonian syndromes (Parkinson's disease [PD], multiple system atrophy [MSA], progressive supranuclear palsy [PSP], corticobasal degeneration [CBD], and dementia with Lewy bodies [DLB],), the semiology will be detailed. The validity and reliability of these criteria will not be touched upon, as they were extensively reviewed recently in a reference paper by Litvan and colleagues *(1)*.

We will consider (a) medical history and clinical description of the cardinal signs and helpful clues and (b) how they relate to the established diagnostic criteria of various parkinsonian syndromes.

PARKINSONISM

Major signs are resting tremor, rigidity, akinesia, and postural instability *(2)*. Advanced PD rarely presents a diagnostic problem, but careful medical history and clinical examination is necessary at an early stage of a parkinsonian syndrome and in very old patients, especially because of other superimposed neurological or non-neurological disturbances (vascular lesions, musculoskeletal disease, vision and auditory problems).

Interview of Patient and Spouse or Family

- Lack of spontaneous gestures and smiling commented on by the family.
- Slowing of activities of daily living with increase in the length of time needed to get up and to get dressed, difficulties using the involved hand (buttons, toothbrush, lack of dexterity), slowness of gait, dragging of the involved leg, stooped posture; and insidious, and progressive and mistaken by the patient as related to "normal aging."
- Difficulties in sports (altered tennis and golf swing, lack of coordination while swimming).
- Micrographia and slowness of handwriting (the size of the handwriting progressively decreases after a few words or sentences in patients with PD; there is a fast micrographia with small letters from the beginning in PSP patients).
- Uncomfortable sensation of fatigue, tightness, stiffness of the limbs.

From: *Current Clinical Neurology: Atypical Parkinsonian Disorders*
Edited by: I. Litvan © Humana Press Inc., Totowa, NJ

- Mild depression and withdrawal.
- Resting tremor when sitting in an armchair or while walking.
- Miscellaneous: profuse sweating or dry skin; sleep disturbances; daytime sleepiness; pain, numbness, or tingling in the limbs; shoulder arthralgia; radiculopathy.

In all cases, the examiner has to obtain a complete drug history as drug-induced parkinsonism and PD can present with the same clinical signs.

Clinical Examination

Tremor

The 4–5 Hz tremor is most apparent when the arm is fully relaxed (supported and at rest, in an armchair). It is increased by mental calculation and stress and best seen during walking. It is reduced by action and intention (tricks used by the patients to hide the tremor). The classical description is the "pill-rolling" rhythmic alternating opposition of the thumb and forefinger. Some patients have postural tremor in particular conditions (holding a phone) with a different frequency (6 Hz).

Bradykinesia

This is the most disabling feature in PD as it involves the whole range of motor activity with a decrease in amplitude and rhythm of movement. Automatic movements disappear. Bradykinesia is well explored in the motor items of UPDRS III, the Unified Parkinson Disease Rating Scale (finger tapping, alternating pronation/supination movements, foot tapping, etc.), with rapid decline in amplitude and frequency.

Rigidity

Abnormal tone is observed when the patient is relaxed and the limb passively flexed and extended. Passive circling movements are better to test rigidity, as the patient cannot voluntarily "help" the passive movement (whereas active movement is sometimes superimposed to the passive movement during simple flexion–extension movements).

The Froment sign is classically described as an increase in tone of the limb during contralateral active movements. The actual sign, described by Jules Froment, was an increase of tone in the examined limb as the patient bent to reach a glass of water on the table (both postural adaptation and voluntary movement of the contralateral limb).

The cogwheel phenomenon is not pathognomonic of PD or parkinsonism and reflects the underlying tremor (can be observed in severe and disabling postural tremor) *(2,3)*.

Impairment of Postural-Reflexes

This is observed when the patient moves spontaneously (rising from a chair, pivoting when turning, etc.). The patient will take extra steps in pivoting and may have a careful gait. Postural challenge consists of a thrust to the shoulders (the examiner stays behind the patient to prevent a fall and the patient is instructed to resist the thrust). According to the UPDRS III score, one can observe a retropulsion (more than one step backward), but the patient recovers unaided (score 1); absence of postural response, the patient would fall if not caught by the examiner (score 2); the patient is very unstable, tends to lose balance spontaneously (score 3); the patient is unable to stand without assistance (score 4). This pull test is not standardized and each neurologist has his or her own technique. As a consequence, the examiner may adapt (consciously or not) the intensity of the thrust to the expected reaction of the patient! (*see* video segment 1.)

Only scores 0 (normal) and 1 are observed in PD until a later stage. In contrast, early postural instability is observed in MSA (with walking difficulties) and particularly in PSP (cardinal sign). Spontaneous falls (without warning or obstacle, occasional then frequent) occur in PSP *(4)* with loss of anticipatory postural reflexes, reactive postural responses, or rescue and protective reactions (the patient does not use his arms to keep balance and does not throw out his arms to break the fall and protect the head from injuries).

Gait Disorders

At an early stage of parkinsonism, slowing and shuffling of gait with dragging of the affected limb is common. A flexed posture of the arms (unilateral then bilateral) with a loss of arm swing is observed.

In contrast, in "vascular" parkinsonism or normal-pressure hydrocephalus, the arm swing is preserved or even exaggerated (to keep the balance) and the arms are not flexed. In that case, "parkinsonism" predominates in the lower limbs (thus the name of "lower body parkinsonism"). The "marche à petits pas" described by Déjerine is suitable for the description of these patients. The gait is characterized by short quick steps, initially without dragging or shuffling the feet on the ground (in contrast to PD), with start and turn hesitation (take several steps on turning), slight wide base (but can be narrow), and moderate disequilibrium (described by Nutt and colleagues as "frontal gait disorder") *(5)*. Visual clues (contrasted lines on the ground) do not help these patients (in contrast to PD). The diagnosis of vascular origin (differential diagnosis from degenerative parkinsonism) is made by the company it keeps: pyramidal signs, dysarthria and pseudo-bulbar signs, urinary disturbances, cognitive signs, and stepwise progression with past medical history of acute motor deficits. In time, patients may develop a magnetic gait (the feet are glued to the ground) and astasia-abasia (they do not know how to walk anymore). Overall, the gait is different from those of patients with late PD or even PSP or MSA.

Gait disorders in PSP have been described as "subcortical disequilibrium." This gait pattern is characterized by a severe postural instability, loss of postural reflexes (cf. supra), and inappropriate response to disequilibrium (e.g., when rising from a chair, the patient will extend the trunk and neck and fall backward). The gait is also impaired by the disequilibrium, and is characterized by a wide base. Some patients do not hesitate to walk briskly, and are careless of the risk of falls (as if they did not realize they were in danger of falling).

Freezing and gait ignition failure are defined by a marked difficulty with initiating gait and difficulties maintaining locomotion in front of various obstacles (door, modification of the pattern of the floor, turning). They are observed at a late stage in PD or at earlier stages in MSA patients. They may be associated with various gait disturbances. Pure gait ignition failure is a different disorder, still poorly defined and, to date, with few clinical-pathological correlations (mostly associated with PSP).

In summary, a parkinsonian syndrome is easily explored, and may take only a few minutes. Spontaneous movements (or the lack of them) are observed when the patient and spouse are providing the medical history. Clumsiness and slowness are detected when patients are searching for documents or glasses in their bag, and when they take off or put on their jacket and shirt (buttons). Writing a few sentences will demonstrate the micrographia; walking in the examination room or corridor will help to detect a resting tremor, loss of arm swing, flexed posture, general slowness, and difficulties of gait and turning. The pull test will explore postural instability. In the end, the UPDRS III motor score will give a quantification of the severity of the parkinsonian syndrome.

FRONTAL SYNDROME

Clinical Examination: Utilization and Imitation Behaviors (Video Segment 2)

The classic signs of frontal syndrome are usually well known. Distractibility and attentional disturbances are easy to detect when several people are present in addition to the patient and the examiner. Therefore, it is very important that all of them remain completely neutral and indifferent toward the patient, and do not react during the clinical examination.

As described by Lhermitte "the test begins with the solicitation of manual grasping behavior." The examiner places his or her hands on the patient's palms and stimulates them with slow and rapid rubbing movements. A bilateral grasping reflex is obtained, even if the patient is instructed not to take the hands of the examiner. Moreover, the patient holds the hands so tightly that the examiner can lift the patient from the chair.

Then, while the hands of the patient are free, the examiner displays various objects in the field of vision of the patient. The patient may grasp the object and collect as many objects as he or she can hold (collectionism). Moreover, he or she usually starts to use them in a proper manner (utilization behavior) *(6)*. When the patients are asked why they took them and used them, the answer is "because I thought I had to take them and use them." Normal subjects do not react this way.

Moreover, even when the examiner tells the patient "whatever I do, do not imitate me," the patient will still do it, all the same. The patient may copy funny behaviors, with or without actual objects (imitation behavior) *(7)*. When asked why they imitated the examiner, they answer, "Because I thought I had to imitate." Again, a normal subject never imitates the examiner (except to make fun of him!).

These tests are very sensitive, easy to do at the bedside and take only a few minutes.

EYE MOVEMENTS

Bedside Examination (Video Segments 3 and 4)

The patient may complain of problems with visual acuity as they cannot read properly anymore. Several pairs of glasses have been changed unsuccessfully. The upward- and downward-gaze impairment are rarely detected by the patient. In contrast, the family will observe "a reptilian" gaze, with a staring and terrified look.

The bedside examination will mainly explore the visually guided saccades in four directions (up, down, left, and right). The targets should be at a certain distance (arm length). The best way to have the right distance and to prevent movements of the head is to hold the chin of the patient at arm length. The targets should be clearly visible (colorful balls or pens). The midline target should be neutral (e.g., the switch of the light) and the lateral should be 25° from the midline target. Voluntary saccades are made after verbal instruction: "look at the switch," "look at the red pencil." Note the time taken to initiate the saccade, its speed, and its amplitude (the target is reached with the initial saccade or correction with additional small saccades are needed). In normal subjects, the displacement of the eyes cannot be detected by the examiner (who sees the initial and the final positions of the eyes). Any perception of the displacement (like in oil) is abnormal. People usually focus on vertical gaze (because of the diagnostic criteria of PSP). However, horizontal saccades are impaired at a early stage of the disease and bedside examination can also detect this abnormality.

In summary, as Drs. Leigh and Riley stated, "it is saccadic speed that counts and the key finding is slowing of the saccade" *(8)*. This can be observed before reduced amplitude is detected.

Testing visual pursuit is not very useful as pursuit is frequently altered (including by drugs). Moreover, testing pursuit is testing the velocity of the target, more than those of the eyes.

Vestibular ocular reflexes (VORs) are normal in PSP patients, by definition (supranuclear palsy).

In summary, eye movement examination is very helpful for the diagnosis of PSP *(9)*, and does not help as much for PD or MSA. Useful clues are:

- Slowing of vertical or horizontal saccades.
- Decreased amplitude of saccades (vertical and/or horizontal). Several small and slow saccades are needed to reach the target (steplike displacement of the eyes).
- Square-wave jerks can be observed in the neutral (central position), and better seen through the use of an ophtalmoscope (small movements take the eye away from the fixation point).
- Patients often blink before they move their eyes when they have mild supranuclear gaze palsy, or they use their VOR (vestibular ocular reflex) to help movement of the eyes at more severe stages.
- In all cases, the VORs are normal.

Although pathologically proven cases of PSP without "abnormal eye movements" have been described, eye movements were usually not quite "normal." Indeed, these patients did not have a downward oculomotor palsy, but Birdy and colleagues *(10)* observed that they had a slowed downward-command saccades, square-wave jerks, slow horizontal saccades, and blepharospasm. This should be considered probable PSP, even if the best specificity for PSP (NINDS-SPSP) criteria are postural instability leading to falls within the first year of onset coupled with a vertical supranuclear gaze paresis *(1,4)*.

DYSAUTONOMIA

Dysautonomia is characterized by urogenital and/or orthostatic dysfunction. Orthostatic hypotension is defined by an orthostatic fall in blood pressure by 20 mmHg systolic or 10 mmHg diastolic, but a 30-mmHg systolic or 15-mmHg diastolic is required for the consensus diagnosis criteria by Gilman *(11)*. Although this is considered to be a frequent and early sign in the disease *(12,13)*, it is rarely symptomatic (syncope or faintness), and autonomic nervous system testing may not distinguish MSA from PD *(14)*.

Urinary disturbances often appear early in the course of the disease, or are a presenting symptom (impotence common in men). Urinary incontinence (70% of MSA) or retention (30%) may be detected by medical history, leading to more refined explorations. MSA, PSP, as well as PD patients complain of urgency, frequent voiding, or dysuria. Some describe difficulties voiding but are not aware of chronic urinary retention. Incontinence is never observed in patients with PD and rarely in late stages in PSP. In all cases, additional laboratory tests such as urodynamic tests and sphincter electromyogram (EMG) may make the association between urinary symptoms and urinary tract denervation *(13)*. Patients with PD have less severe urinary dysfunction, by contrast with these common findings in MSA. However, sphincter EMG does not distinguish MSA from PSP.

In summary, the detection of autonomic and urinary features by medical history and, if necessary, laboratory tests, may be a good clue at early stages of the parkinsonian syndrome, but the diagnosis should take into account other clinical clues to reach the diagnostic criteria for PD, MSA, or PSP.

HALLUCINATIONS

Most of the time, the patient does not spontaneously report hallucinations and only a small portion of them are detected by the spouse (emerged part of the "iceberg"). Patients should be specifically questioned on the presence of minor, visual, and auditory hallucinations. As reported by Fénelon and colleagues, *(15)* the most frequent type are visual hallucinations. The patient has a vivid sensation of the presence of somebody either somewhere in the room or, less often, behind him or her. The presence is often a relative (alive or deceased) who is often perceived as benevolent like a "guardian angel." However, the patient is ready to accept that the "presence" is not real.

Formed visual hallucinations are more complex with vivid scenes "like a film," sometimes close to real (members of family), sometimes full of fantasy (ninja turtles, dancing Russians, medieval stories), but soundless. In some cases, the hallucinations may be frightening (house burning, wild animals). Auditory hallucinations are rare and tactile hallucinations often involve animals. As they are more frequent in the evening they may be associated with vivid dreams and sleep disorders *(15)*.

In all cases, the main risk factor for hallucinations is cognitive impairment. Therefore, it is important to detect them as they are among features used for the diagnostic criteria of dementia with Lewy bodies (DLB) in addition to cognitive impairment, attentional and visuospatial deficits, fluctuating cognition, and parkinsonism *(16)*.

MOVEMENT DISORDERS

Dystonia

Dystonia associated with parkinsonian syndromes is often manifested by dystonic postures (video segments 5 and 6) more than abnormal movements and they are rarely modified by a "geste

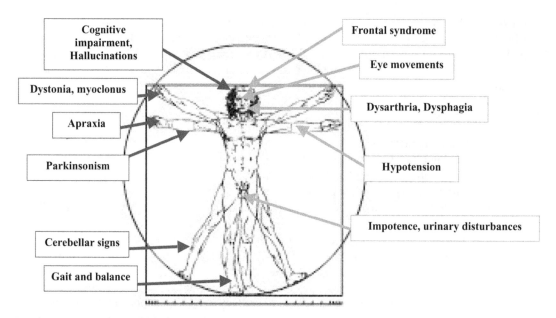

Fig. 1. Clinical examination at a glance from head to feet.

antagoniste." They include limb dystonia (from writer's cramp to a dystonic posture of the arm or foot), blepharospasm (and/or eyelid apraxia), orofacial dystonia, stridor, axial dystonia, and cervical dystonia. Axial dystonia is sometimes difficult to differentiate from rigidity, especially in the neck. In cervical dystonia, torticollis, retrocollis, or laterocollis are easy to define but antecollis can range from severe bent neck (considered to be a good clue for MSA) to abnormal neck flexion; in such cases, cervical dystonia can be found in up to 25% of MSA patients *(17)* and in most PSP patients *(18)*.

As a rule of thumb, dystonia predominantly affects cranio-cervical musculature in MSA and PSP, although limb dystonia may be observed in PSP (leading to misdiagnosis of CBD). In fact, in CBD, the best predictors for the diagnosis are limb dystonia, ideomotor apraxia, myoclonus, asymmetric akinetic-rigid syndrome with late-onset gait or balance disturbances *(19)*.

Levodopa-induced dyskinesias are observed in PD but are not infrequent in MSA. In MSA the presence of painful, dystonic, postural as well as orofacial and cervical dyskinesias are good clues for its diagnosis.

Myoclonus

Myoclonus is sometimes difficult to differentiate from irregular tremor by clinical examination. Stimulus-sensitive myoclonus is elicited by either pinprick or light touch of the skin. It can be observed in MSA and in CBD patients. In PD patients, myoclonus is rare and may be related to levodopa (levodopa-induced myoclonus). Electrophysiologic testing helps to differentiate the stimulus-sensitive myoclonus in CBD with a pattern characteristic of cortical myoclonus *(20)* (video segments 5 and 6).

CONCLUSION: EXAMINATION AT A GLANCE

Very simple tests will help to get the most out of the clinical examination and medical history. This is particularly true for the bedside neuropsychological examination and eye movement exploration, which appear complicated but are not (video segments 3 and 4). Moreover, a refined and precise evaluation will increase the accuracy of the diagnostic criteria in clinico-pathological studies. For example, the precision of the information in the "clinical vignettes" is of great importance. This may allow clinicians to rename probable criteria into clinically definite or clinically probable. This high specificity of criteria is important for research studies, especially genetics or therapeutic studies.

As a rule of thumb, we suggest examining the patient "from head to feet" (*see* Fig. 1) in order to check all the diagnostic features included in the criteria for PD, MSA (video segment 7), PSP (video segments 1–4), CBD (video segments 5 and 6), and DLB.

VIDEO LEGENDS

Video 1: Corticobasal degeneration with myoclonus. Right upper limb dystonia with shoulder abduction, and elbow + wrist + fingers flexion, associated with myoclonic jerks (at rest and triggered by posture and action). Polygraphic EMG recordings show brief and synchronous bursts on the upper arm muscles.

Video 2: Corticobasal degeneration with apraxia. Tremor, akinesia, myoclonic jerks and left hand dystonia. Symbolic motor sequences are not properly performed: cross sign is performed from right to left shoulder, thumbing one's nose is replaced by a kiss, showing that someone is a fool is done uncompletely and cross sign is not possible with left hand.

Video 3: Multiple system atrophy (MSA-P). At an early stage, DOPA-resistant akineto-rigid syndrome is associated with inability to walk without aid and postural instability.

Video 4: Progressive supranuclear palsy (Steele-Richardson-Olszewski syndrome). Vertical voluntary saccades are slow and with limitation of the amplitude of the saccades. Horizontal voluntary saccades are reduced and several ocular movements (several small saccades) are needed to move the eyes from side to side. Oculocephalic reflexes (VOR) are normal, demonstrating the supranuclear location of the dysfunction. Postural instability is observed.

Video 5: Abnormal eye movements in progressive supranuclear palsy. Vertical and horizontal voluntary saccades are reduced. Several saccades are needed to reach the target. Perseverations are observed, the patient looks at a previous target when asked to look to another direction. Frontalis muscle contractions are associated with upward saccades. Oculocephalic reflexes are normal (but difficult to perform because of distractibility and cervical stiffness), demonstrating the supranuclear location of the dysfunction.

Video 6: Frontal behavior in Progressive supranuclear palsy. As described by Lhermitte, frontal behavioral signs include grasping reflex (even when discouraged), utilization behavior and collection of the examiner's personal stuff without order, imitation behavior with imitation of all the gestural activities of the examiner, including nonsense as eating a metallic object.

Video 7: Postural instability in Progressive supranuclear palsy. Spontaneous postural instability. A gentle pulling test would make the patient fall, without any attempt or ability to recover his balance (loss of postural reflexes).

REFERENCES

1. Litvan I, Bhatia KP, Burn DJ, et al. SIC task force appraisal of clinical diagnostic criteria for parkinsonian disorders. Mov Disord 2003;18:467–486.
2. Gelb DJ, Oliver E, Gilman S. Diagnostic criteria for Parkinson disease. Arch Neurol 1999;56:33–39.
3. Rao G, Fisch L, Srinivasan S, et al. Does this patient have Parkinson disease? JAMA 2003;289:347–353.
4. Litvan I, Campbell G, Mangone CA, et al. Which clinical features differentiate progressive supranuclear palsy (Steele–Richardson–Olszewski syndrome) from related disorders? A clinicopathological study. Brain 1997;120:65–74.
5. Nutt JG, Marsden CD, Thompson PD. H walking and higher-level gait disorders particularly in the elderly. Neurology 1993;43:268–279.
6. Lhermitte F. Utilization behaviour and its relation to lesions of the frontal lobe. Brain 1983;106:237–255.
7. Lhermitte F, Pillon B, Serdaru M. Human autonomy and the frontal lobes. Part I: imitation and utilization behavior: a neuropsychological study of 75 patients. Ann Neurol 1986;19:326–334.
8. Leigh RJ, Riley DE. Eye movements in parkinsonism. It's saccadic speed that counts. Neurology 2000; 54:1018–1019.
9. Rivaud-Pechoux S, Vidailhet M, Gallouedec G, Litvan I, Gaymard B, Pierrot-deseilligny C. Longitudinal oculomotor study in corticobasal degeneration and progressive supranuclear palsy. Neurology 2000;54:1029–1032.

10. Birdi S, Rajput AH, Fenton M, et al. Progressive supranuclear palsy diagnosis and confounding features: report on 16 autopsied cases. Mov Disord 2002;17:1255–1264.
11. Gilman S, Low PA, Quinn N. Consensus statement on the diagnosis of multiple system atrophy. J Neurol Sci 1999;163:94–98.
12. Chaudhuri KR. Autonomic dysfunction in movement disorders. Curr Opin Neurol. 2001;14:505–511.
13. Wenning GK, Scherfler C, Granata R, et al. Time course of symptomatic orthostatic hypotension and urinary incontinence in patients with postmortem confirmed parkinsonian syndromes: a clinicopathological study. J Neurol Neurosurg Psychiatry 1999;67:620–623.
14. Riley DE, Chelimsky TC. Autonomic nervous system testing may not distinguish multiple system atrophy from Parkinson's disease J Neurol Neurosurg Psychiatry 2003;74:56–60.
15. Fenelon G, Mahieux F, Huon R, Ziegler M. Hallucinations in Parkinson's disease: prevalence, phenomenology and risk factors. Brain 2000;123:733–745.
16. McKeith IG, Galasko D, Kosaka K, et al. Consensus guidelines for the clinical and pathologic diagnosis of dementia with Lewy bodies (DLB): report of the consortium on DLB international workshop. Neurology 1996;47:1113–1124.
17. Boesch SM, Wenning GK, Ransmayr G, Poewe W. Dystonia in multiple system atrophy. J Neurol Neurosurg Psychiatry 2002;72:300–303.
18. Barclay CL, Lang AE. Dystonia in progressive supranuclear palsy. J Neurol Neurosurg Psychiatry 1997;62:352–356.
19. Litvan I, Grimes DA, Lang AE et al. Clinical features differentiating patients with postmortem confirmed progressive supranuclear palsy and corticobasal degeneration. J Neurol 1999;246(Suppl 2):II1–II5.
20. Monza D, Ciano C, Scaioli V, et al. Neurophysiological features in relation to clinical signs in clinically diagnosed corticobasal degeneration. Neurol Sci 2003;24:16–23.

11

Role of Neuropsychiatric Assessment in Diagnosis and Research

Dag Aarsland, Uwe Ehrt, and Clive Ballard

INTRODUCTION

Although the basal ganglia have traditionally been considered as primarily involved in the regulation of motor functioning, their role in the integration of emotions with cognitive and motor behavior is increasingly recognized. Psychiatric symptoms, including disturbance of affect (anxiety and depression), perception (hallucinations), thought (delusions), as well as behavioral and personality changes (apathy and disinhibition) are commonly observed in most basal ganglia diseases. They produce increased suffering and distress both for the patients themselves as well as for the caregivers, and are associated with increased need for care. Thus, psychiatric symptoms should not be viewed as a secondary or additional feature of the movement disorders, but rather, representing important and inherent aspects of these disorders. Although this is true for Parkinson's disease (PD), it is even more so for several of the atypical parkinsonian disorders, where psychiatric symptoms may represent key features of the clinical syndrome. For instance, in dementia with Lewy bodies, visual hallucinations are among the three cardinal features (1), and in focal lesions of the caudate, neuropsychiatric symptoms occur more commonly than motor disorders (2). Knowledge of the wide variety of psychiatric symptoms and having the diagnostic skills to identify and optimize treatment of these symptoms are thus of major importance in the management of patients with movement disorders. In addition to providing important diagnostic information, they help elucidate the relationship between key brain circuits and psychiatric symptoms.

The studies of patients with various parkinsonian disorders differ markedly with regard to diagnostic criteria used, the number and selection of patients with a high risk for random error and selection bias, the level of cognitive functioning within each diagnostic group and between the groups compared, and the use of instruments to measure neuropsychiatric symptoms. Thus, firm conclusions regarding comparisons of the frequency, severity, and profile of psychiatric symptoms in different parkinsonian disorders are premature.

This chapter will define the most common psychiatric symptoms in parkinsonian disorders and how they can be reliably measured, explore the relationship between basal ganglia structure and functioning with neuropsychiatric symptoms, and review studies of the frequency and characteristics, clinical implications as well as the so far limited data pertaining to treatment.

From: *Current Clinical Neurology: Atypical Parkinsonian Disorders*
Edited by: I. Litvan © Humana Press Inc., Totowa, NJ

DEFINITION AND IDENTIFICATION OF KEY NEUROPSYCHIATRIC SYMPTOMS

The definition of psychotic symptoms (i.e., delusions, delusional misidentification, and hallucinations) requires particular consideration as these symptoms are very frequent in some parkinsonian disorders, particularly in patients with dementia. In addition, as they are phenomenologically different from psychotic symptoms occurring in patients with functional psychoses and cannot be reliably observed or inferred from behavior, a specific method is required to identify these symptoms in patients with cognitive impairments. According to Burns, delusions are defined as false, unshakable ideas or beliefs that are held with extraordinary conviction and subjective certainty *(3)*. To minimize overlap with confabulation and delirium, they should be reiterated on at least two occasions more than 1 wk apart. Hallucinations are described as percepts in the absence of a stimulus, reported directly by either the patient or indirectly via an informant, and may occur in any modality. Typically, visual hallucinations are the most common type of hallucinations encountered in patients with parkinsonian disorders. Delusional misidentification, including the Capgras syndrome (the belief that a person, object, or environment has been replaced by a double or replica), delusional misidentification of visual images (whereby figures on television or in photographs are thought to exist in the real environment), delusional misidentification of mirror images (one's reflection is perceived as the image of a separate person), and the phantom boarder delusion (believing that strangers are living in or visiting the house) are also commonly encountered in parkinsonian patients.

The diagnosis of depression in parkinsonian disorders may be difficult, and both over- and underdiagnosis may occur. The motor symptoms may mask the affective features, leading to underdiagnosis, whereas the psychomotor slowing, apathy and masked facies may be erroneously interpreted as depression. Although most reports indicate that the symptoms of depression are broadly similar in people with or without a parkinsonian disorder, patients with PD may have more commonly dysphoria and pessisimism, but less commonly guilt, self-blame, and suicidal behavior than subjects without a parkinsonian disorder. Symptoms such as fatigue, apathy, sleep, and appetite disturbance may occur independently of mood as an intrinsic part of the neurodegenerative process. The nonsomatic symptoms of depression appear to be the most important for distinguishing between depressed and nondepressed patients with parkinsonism *(4)*. Dementia may further complicate the diagnosis of depression in these patients because patients are unable to verbalize their subjective experience. Despite this, there is evidence that depression can be reliably and validly diagnosed even in patients with a parkinsonian disorder using standardized depression-rating scales (see below).

Apathy consists of lack of motivation with diminished goal-directed behavior, reduced goal-directed cognition, and decreased emotional engagement. Apathy may accompany depression, but it is often an independent syndrome without the sadness, despair, and intense suffering typically experienced by depressed patients *(5)*. Apathy is commonly accompanied by evidence of executive dysfunction.

Anxiety is characterized by excessive and unjustified apprehension, feelings of foreboding, and thoughts of impending doom. Patients are tense and irritable, and frequently exhibit autonomic disturbances including sweating, palpitations, gastrointestinal distress, and shortness of breath. Both low-grade, free-floating anxiety and acute and intense panic attacks may occur.

Although less frequently reported, a number of other neuropsychiatric symptoms need to be mentioned. Agitation, such as aggression, restlessness, and shouting, can usually be observed, and thus the identification of these symptoms is less problematic. However, key symptoms of agitation are often secondary to other psychiatric syndromes. For example, anxiety may lead to restlessness, shouting, or trailing carers, or aggression may be secondary to delusional beliefs. Disinhibition is characterized by inappropriate social and interpersonal interactions. Elation/euphoria refers to an elevated mood with excessive happiness and overconfidence, and obsessional and compulsory symptoms, with recurrent thoughts, vocalizations, or rituals, may also occur in basal ganglia disorders.

MEASURING PSYCHIATRIC SYMPTOMS

The measurement of psychiatric disturbances in patients with neurological disorders presents unique challenges. Because of the commonly co-occurring cognitive deficits, patients may not remember or report their symptoms. Furthermore, since these symptoms may fluctuate, the patients may not exhibit the symptoms at the time of the examination. It may thus be useful to infer symptoms from behavior or ascertain symptoms from an informant interview referring to a specific time period, in addition to the direct observation and interview of the patient.

A number of different instruments have been used to measure neuropsychiatric symptoms in patients with parkinsonian disorders. These can be divided into clinical interviews that focus upon a broad range of symptoms or more focused scales. Examples of the first group include the Present Behavioural Examination (PBE) *(6)*, Neuropsychiatric Inventory (NPI) *(7)*, and Brief Psychiatric Rating Scale (BPRS) *(8)*. The PBE is a lengthy interview with a detailed assessment of behavior in patients with dementia, and requires a trained observer. The NPI is a highly structured, caregiver-based interview, which can be completed in a relatively short time depending on the amount of disturbances (see below). The BPRS was constructed essentially for schizophrenic states, and requires a trained rater. Examples of scales that assess specific syndromes in more detail are the Hamilton Depression Rating Scale (HAM-D) *(9)*; and self-rating scales completed by the patients themselves (i.e., Beck Depression Inventory [BDI]) *(10)* and Geriatric Depression Scale *(11)*. Acceptable psychometric properties of the PBE, BPRS, and NPI have been demonstrated in patients without parkinsonian disorders only, although interrater reliability of the NPI has been reported to be high in PD patients *(12)*. The depression scales HAM-D, Montgomery & Åsberg Depression Rating Scale (MADRS) *(13)*, BDI *(14)*, and Hospital Anxiety and Depression Scale (HAD) *(15)* have been validated in patients with PD. However, the cutoff scores may differ from nonparkinsonian subjects, and whereas lower cutoff scores are useful for screening purposes, higher scores are needed to make these scales good diagnostic instruments in these populations *(13,14)*. Although qualitative differences of depression prevalence and phenomenology may exist between different parkinsonian disorders *(16)*, it is reasonable to assume that the psychometric properties achieved in PD patients may apply for patients with atypical parkinsonian disorders as well.

The most widely used scale for the measurement of a broad range of psychiatric and behavioral symptoms among recently published studies in patients with neurological disorders is the NPI (*see* video). This is a highly structured, caregiver-based interview that rates frequency and severity of 10 psychiatric disturbances commonly observed in patients with different dementing conditions: delusions, hallucinations, agitation/aggression, dysphoria, anxiety, euphoria, disinhibition, apathy, irritability, and aberrant motor activity. The use of screening questions makes it easy to use in clinical practice, and the highly structured design suggests that the tool can be reliably used by individuals with low levels of training when provided with appropriate instruction regarding how to use the instrument. Since the NPI is scored on the basis of information provided by a caregiver, it avoids the problem inherent in observer-based strategies. On the other hand, it is subject to bias if the caregiver lacks or distorts information, and a caregiver with daily contact with the patient may not always be available.

THE NEUROPSYCHIATRY OF THE BASAL GANGLIA

The basal ganglia are involved in two major brain systems associated with the regulation of emotions, mood, and behavior: (a) the "limbic" structures with widely distributed brainstem, striatal, and paralimbic sites, with rich reciprocal connections to the basal ganglia, in particular between the amygdalae and caudate *(17)*; and (b) five frontosubcortical circuits, linking frontal lobe regions to subcortical structures, including the basal ganglia, and back to frontal lobe areas *(18)*. These circuits receive input from brainstem nuclei, including dopaminergic input from substantia nigra and pars compacta. In addition to motor and eye movement control, the frontosubcortical circuits subserve key behaviors including executive functioning, motivated behavior, and integration of emotional information into contextually appropriate behavior. Thus, the basal ganglia are interpositioned as an interface between internal personal drives (mood and motivation) and behavioral responses to external stimuli.

On the other hand, imaging studies have revealed that the basal ganglia are involved in "functional" psychiatric disorders. Magnetic resonance imaging (MRI) studies report reductions in caudate and putamen volume in unipolar and bipolar depression in addition to the prefrontal cortex, and positron emission tomography (PET) studies reveal hypermetabolism of globus pallidus in patients with unipolar and bipolar depression *(19)*. Similarly, in obsessive compulsive disorder *(20)*; changes in caudate activity have been reported. Thus, it is not surprising that diseases of the basal ganglia are associated with a wide range of neuropsychiatric disturbances. Furthermore, since the three frontosubcortical circuits mediating cognitive and emotional control transverse different regions of the basal ganglia, it is likely that the differential involvement of the basal ganglia in different diseases results in different patterns of neuropsychiatric symptoms.

Since parkinsonian disorders usually involve several subcortical structures, particularly at more advanced disease stages, focal lesions may provide a better opportunity to unravel the relationship between different basal ganglia regions and neuropsychiatric symptoms. In a literature review, Bhatia and Marsden reported the motor and behavioral changes in 240 patients with lesions affecting the basal ganglia *(2)*. Although publication bias and wide variations in the assessment of neuropsychiatric symptoms employed limit the generalizability of the findings, some interesting results emerged. First, "behavioral disturbances" were reported in 46% of the cases. Second, such disturbances occurred nearly exclusively in patients with lesions involving the caudate nucleus, whereas lesions confined to the putamen or globus pallidus, or the combination of these, rarely were associated with neuropsychiatric changes. Finally, in lesions involving the caudate nucleus, apathy (28%), disinhibition (11%), and depression (29%) were the most common neuropsychiatric symptoms. Notably, neuropsychiatric symptoms were more common than motor disturbances after such lesions *(2)*. Thus, lesions involving the caudate nucleus or other aspects of the three frontosubcortical circuits mediating behavior are associated with neuropsychiatric symptoms. Apathy, disinhibition, depression, and obsessive-compulsive symptoms are common behavioral correlates of such disturbances. Further empirical support for the involvement of basal ganglia in cognition and emotion was reported in a study of 143 patients with bilateral basal ganglia mineralization, which was associated with an increased risk for affective and paranoid disorders *(21)*.

Cummings proposed an integrating hypothesis linking observations from molecular biologic, neuropathologic, and neurochemical studies in neurodegenerative disorders to neuropsychiatric manifestations of these disorders. According to this model, proteinopathies, such as tauopathies and alpha-synucleinopathies, are associated with a distinct anatomic pattern of degeneration. Cell death in specific brain nuclei responsible for transmitter synthesis leads to deficits in a variety of transmitter systems. Specifically, α-synuclein disturbances, such as PD, dementia with Lewy bodies (DLB), and multiple system atrophy (MSA), mainly involve substantia nigra, brainstem, and limbic system neurons, whereas frontal and basal ganglionic neurons are predominantly affected in tau metabolism disturbances, such as progressive supranuclear palsy (PSP) and corticobasal degeneration (CBD), resulting in frontal and subcortical abnormalities *(22)*. These differential regional and transmitter involvements may result in differential patterns of motor, cognitive, and neuropsychiatric changes.

EPIDEMIOLOGY AND IMPLICATIONS OF NEUROPSYCHIATRIC FEATURES IN PARKINSONIAN DISORDERS

There are few epidemiological studies of neuropsychiatric symptoms in parkinsonian disorders. In one study of a relatively large, representative community-based sample of patients with PD, 61% had a positive score on at least one NPI item, and 45% had a positive score on at least two items. Patients in nursing homes, with more advanced parkinsonism, and with dementia had more frequent and severe neuropsychiatric symptoms *(12)*. Studies of patients with atypical parkinsonian disorders have typically involved small convenience samples from highly specialized movement disorder clinics, and thus may not necessarily be representative of the general population. The exception is DLB, and two studies, both including 98 patients with DLB, showed a high prevalence of neuropsychiatric symptoms *(23,24)*. In one study, 98% had at least one positive symptom as measured by the NPI *(24)* demonstrating the importance of neuropsychiatric symptoms in this common disorder, which affects 5% of the elderly aged 75 or more *(25)*. Unlike other dementias, neuropsychiatric symptoms in DLB are not associated with declining cognition *(23)*, nor with age or gender *(26)*. In PSP, 88% of patients had at least one positive NPI item *(27)* and 87% of CBD patients *(28)*, again underlining the importance of neuropsychiatric symptoms in patients with parkinsonian disorders. In PSP and CBD, there is little correlation between neuropsychiatric symptoms and motor and cognition scores, indicating that in these disorders, the frontosubcortical circuits mediating behavior and motor symptoms degenerate independently.

What are the clinical implications of neuropsychiatric symptoms in patients with parkinsonian disorders? Again, most research has been performed on patients with PD, and it seems reasonable to extrapolate the findings from these studies to patients with atypical parkinsonian disorders. First, several studies have consistently demonstrated that neuropsychiatric symptoms have strong negative influences on the quality of life, including physical, social, and psychological well-being of patients with PD, even after controlling for motor, functional, and cognitive disturbances. For instance, depression has consistently, and irrespective of instruments used to assess depression, been found to be among the most important independent predictors of impaired quality of life in PD patients *(29–31)*, and a longitudinal study reported that depression and insomnia were the most important factors associated with poor quality of life *(32)*. Although there is overlap between the symptoms of depression and quality of life, these findings highlight the need to diagnose and treat depression in patients with parkinsonian disorders.

Second, caring for a patient with a parkinsonian disorder is associated with considerable emotional, social, and physical distress *(33–35)*. Neuropsychiatric symptoms of PD patients, such as depression, cognitive impairment, delusions, and hallucinations, have been found to be significant and independent contributors to the perceived burden in spouses of these patients *(33)*. Third, a substantial proportion of patients with parkinsonian disorders are admitted to nursing homes *(36)*. In addition to motor symptoms and functional impairment, neuropsychiatric symptoms such as cognitive impairment and psychosis have been found to be independent predictors of nursing home admission in parkinsonsian patients *(37,38)*. Both higher need for care and increased caregiver burden may contribute to the relationship between nursing home admission and neuropsychiatric symptoms. Fourth, neuropsychiatric symptoms may increase the economic costs in patients with parkinsonism. In a recent study of patients with Alzheimer's disease (AD), health-related costs were substantially higher in patients with higher scores on the NPI compared to those with low levels *(39)*, and a similar relationship may exist in patients with parkinsonian disorders as well. Finally, there is some evidence that neuropsychiatric symptoms are associated with a more severe disease course. PD patients with depression have been related to a more rapid cognitive decline *(40)*, although other studies have not found a relationship between neuropsychiatric symptoms and cognitive decline *(41)* or mortality *(42)*. In summary, the importance of neuropsychiatric symptoms for the quality of life and prognosis of patients with parkinsonian disorders, perceived stress of their spouses as well as the need for health care resources is well established, highlighting the need for proper diagnosis and management of these aspects of the parkinsonian disorder.

THE ROLE OF NEUROPSYCHIATRIC ASSESSMENT IN DIAGNOSIS OF PARKINSONIAN DISORDERS

Methodological Considerations

Given the assumption that the neuropsychiatric profile of a neurological disorder reflects the underlying neuropathology, the neuropsychiatric assessment may also provide important information pertaining to the diagnosis. The differential neuropsychiatric profile may be most pronounced at early stages because of the disappearance during later stages of the relatively distinct anatomical involvement observed initially.

During the last decade an increasing number of studies describing the neuropsychiatric characteristics of patients with neurodegenerative disorders have been published. Among the group of movement disorders, however, the majority of studies have focused on patients with PD, and only few studies with a low number of participants have explored the pattern of neuropsychiatric symptoms in atypical parkinsonian disorders, and thus the knowledge of the neuropsychiatric characteristics of these disorders is still limited. In addition, there are several other methodological caveats to consider when comparing different studies of the neuropsychiatric profile of patients with parkinsonism. First, patients can be selected from different sources. Clinical and demographic characteristics of patients attending a specialized movement disorder clinic may differ from patients referred to a neuropsychiatric unit or residing in the community with regard to age, education, duration of disease, cognitive functioning, and social and economic status. Such differences may influence the frequency of neuropsychiatric symptoms. Second, the clinical diagnostic accuracy of movement disorders is not optimal as *(43–46)* clinico-pathologic studies have shown significant false-positive and false-negative rates for diagnosing parkinsonian disorders *(47)*. Studies using patients with autopsy confirmed diagnoses are rare, and the clinical diagnostic criteria employed may vary. Third, the assessment of neuropsychiatric symptoms varies. Some studies are retrospective chart reviews using unstructured clinical notes, whereas others have prospectively assessed patients using standardized instruments with established reliability and validity. In addition, different instruments may yield different results. For instance, highly different frequencies of depression may occur depending on whether a diagnosis of major depression according to the *DSM (Diagnostic and Statistical manual of Mental Disorders)* system IV is used, or whether rating scales such as NPI, HAM-D, or BDI, with different possible cutoff scores are used *(13,14)*. In addition, the time frame is of importance since the prevalence may differ depending on whether a point-prevalence, a 1-wk, 1-mo, or even lifetime diagnosis of depression is recorded. Finally, the neuropsychiatric profile may vary with disease duration. For example, psychosis is more common in later stages rather than in earlier stages of PD *(42,48,49)*, and thus comparative studies should control for disease duration or disease stage.

With these caveats in mind, some information with potential diagnostic value can nevertheless be drawn from the literature of neuropsychiatric symptoms in parkinsonian disorders. The interpretation of existing studies benefits from the fact that several studies have used the NPI to assess neuropsychiatric symptoms, and thus it is possible to compare the NPI profile of the different parkinsonian disorders.

NEUROPSYCHIATRIC SYMPTOMS IN PARKINSON'S DISEASE

The cardinal pathological feature of PD is Lewy body degeneration of the substantia nigra, causing loss of dopaminergic innervation of the striatum. In addition, other pigmented brainstem and cholinergic nuclei are involved, and Lewy bodies are found in the neocortex of most patients. The cardinal clinical features are resting tremor, bradykinesia, and rigidity.

Neuropsychiatric symptoms are common, and their prevalence, phenomenology, and clinical implications have been extensively studied during the last decade. The majority of PD patients develop dementia with cortical and subcortical features when disease duration exceeds 10 yr *(41)*. Depression is the most common psychiatric symptom in PD *(12,50)*, and may occur in up to 40% of patients *(51)*. Different studies report wide variations in prevalence rates, however, and population-based studies suggest that major depression according to the DSM system is uncommon, occurring in less than 10% of cases *(52,53)*.

The etiology of depression in PD is not yet determined. Although psychosocial factors, i.e., social support, psychological reaction to the disease, and coping strategies, certainly play a role *(54)*, biological factors are also thought to contribute. Serotonergic, dopaminergic, and noradrenergic deficits, cortical and subcortical neurodegeneration, and genetic factors may contribute to depression in PD *(55)*. Stefurak and Mayberg proposed a model for depression in PD based on clinical, imaging, treatment, and behavioral challenge studies, which involves cortical-limbic and frontostriatal pathways. According to this model, a dorsal-cortical compartment (prefrontal, premotor, and parietal cortices and dorsal and posterior cingulate) is postulated to mediate the cognitive aspects of depression (including apathy, attentional, and executive dysfunction), whereas a ventral-limbic compartment (ventral cingulate, hippocampus, and hypothalamus) mediates circadian, somatic, and vegetative aspects of depression (sleep, appetite, libidinal, and endocrine disturbances). Finally, the rostral cingulate, with reciprocal connections to both compartments, is suggested to serve a regulatory role, including a major role in determining the response to treatment *(19)*. Key neurotransmitters involved in these structures include dopamine and serotonin.

Is depression more prevalent in PD compared to other conditions with comparable functional impairment? If not, there is little reason to assume a disease-specific association between PD and depression. Studies of this question have usually included small samples subject to selection and participation biases. Nilsson et al. used the Danish registers of somatic and psychiatric in-patients to address this question. Data from more than 200,000 persons were analyzed, and more than 12,000 subjects with PD were identified. A significant increased risk for hospitalization owing to depression in patients with PD compared to subjects with osteoarthritis or diabetes mellitus was found, and the authors suggest that the increased risk was not a mere psychological reaction to the disease, but rather because of disease-specific brain changes in PD patients *(56)*.

Visual hallucinations are also common in PD, and typically involve people of normal size and configuration who do not communicate with the patient. A substantial proportion of patients report vague feelings of a presence *(57)*. The patients may or may not be aware of the abnormality of the experience, and the visions usually do not cause emotional disturbance. However, more severe psychotic symptoms with delusions and behavioral disturbances may occur as well, particularly in patients with dementia *(48)*. Although these symptoms have previously been considered secondary to dopaminergic treatment, there is evidence suggesting that other factors may be even more important. First, psychotic symptoms were described in PD before levodopa was introduced and in untreated patients. Second, most studies find that psychotic symptoms are not related to the dose, duration of treatment, or number of dopaminergic agents *(57)*. Third, hallucinations do not relate to levodopa plasma level or to sudden changes in plasma level *(58)*. Fourth, although dopaminergic agents may induce psychotic symptoms in non-PD patients, PSP patients treated with dopaminergic agents do not develop hallucinations *(49)*. Similarly, the phenomenology of well-formed images of people, usually not threatening to the patients and sometimes with insight retained, as well as the content of delusions, is very similar to the symptoms in DLB, which usually occur without dopaminergic treatment *(59)*. Thus, dopaminergic agents may provide a neurochemical milieu with a high risk for psychosis in PD, but are not necessary or sufficient to cause psychosis. The association between duration and severity of disease, dementia, depression, sleep disturbance, visual disturbances, and psychotic symptoms suggests a multifactorial etiology, including brain changes associated with the disease itself. Neurochemical changes potentially contributing to hallucinations in PD include limbic dopaminergic hypersensitivity and cholinergic and serotonergic changes. Sensory deprivation may also contribute, and patients with PD may process retinal images abnormally. In fact, there is evidence that visual hallucinations in PD and DLB arise as a result of abnormal activation of higher order. This would fit well with the finding that visual hallucinations are associated with Lewy bodies in the temporal lobe *(60)*.

The NPI profile of a community-based sample of 139 patients with PD was characterized by relatively high levels of depression (38%), hallucinations (27%), and anxiety (20%), whereas euphoria and disinhibition were uncommon *(12)* (Table 1). A positive score on at least one NPI item was

Table 1
Frequency of Neuropsychiatric Symptoms in Parkinsonian Disorders Using the NPI

	PD (ref. *12*)	PSP (ref. *49*)	CBD (ref. *28*)	DLB (ref. *71*)
N	139	61	15	93
Age	74.4 (7.9)	67.1 (6.5)	67.9 (SEM 2)	73.9 (6.4)
M/F	61/78	38/23	8/7	55/36
MMSE score	25.2 (5.9)	27.0 (4.2)	26.1 (SEM 1.2)	17.9 (4.6)
Delusion	16	3	7	62
Hallucinations	27	2	0	77
Agitation	17	21	20	58
Depression	38	25	73	72
Anxiety	20	18	13	67
Euphoria	1	0	0	17
Disinhibition	7	56	13	23
Irritability	10	20	20	55
Apathy	19	84	40	46
Aberrant motor behavior	11	9	7	52
Total with NPI symptom	61	88	87	98
Mean total NPI score	7.1 (12.0)	12.4 (9.4)	9.0 (SEM 3.2)	22.8 (15.4)

The numbers represent percentage with symptom present or mean (SD) values. NPI, Neuropsychiatric Inventory; PD, Parkinson's disease; PSP, progressive supranuclear palsy; CBD, corticobasal degeneration; DLB, dementia with Lewy bodies; MMSE, Mini Mental State Examination.

reported for 61%, and 45% had more than one symptom. Neither age, duration of disease, nor levodopa dosage correlated with NPI subscores. Hallucination, delusion, and agitation scores correlated with more advanced disease stage and cognitive impairment, and apathy with cognitive impairment. Compared with AD, PD patients with a similar level of dementia had significantly higher hallucination scores and a nonsignificant trend toward higher depression scores than AD patients, whereas AD patients had higher scores on most other items *(61)*. The NPI profile of this PD population has also been used for direct comparisons with DLB and PSP patients.

PSYCHIATRIC ASPECTS OF DEMENTIA WITH LEWY BODIES

DLB is characterized clinically by dementia, visual hallucinations, and fluctuating consciousness in addition to parkinsonism. Neuropathological characteristics include alpha-synucleinopathy, such as Lewy bodies and Lewy neurites in the brainstem, particularly the substantia nigra, subcortical structures, limbic cortex, and neocortex. Some amyloid deposition is also found in most patients. Neurochemically marked cholinergic deficits are reported in addition to a moderate nigro-striatal dopaminergic, and monoaminergic deficits have also been reported. It is estimated that at least 80% of DLB patients experience some form of neuropsychiatric symptoms *(23)*, such as visual hallucinations, auditory hallucinations, delusions, delusional misidentification, and depression. These visual hallucinations are consistently reported to be more frequent in DLB than in AD, also in samples diagnosed at autopsy, and constitute one of the key diagnostic features of the disorder. Although rates vary from 25% to 83%, most prospective studies indicate a frequency of more than 50%. Delusions, including delusional misidentifications, are also common in DLB patients (frequency 13–75%). The rate reported for depression has varied from 14% to 50% in patients with DLB depending upon the study definition, with a frequency of major depression that is probably greater than 30%.

Sleep disturbances, such as insomnia and increased daytime sleepiness, are more common in DLB than AD *(62)*, and are also pronounced in PD *(63)*. REM sleep behavior disorder (RBD) is characterized by loss of normal skeletal muscle atonia during REM sleep with prominent motor activity and dreaming. RBD is particularly common in DLB *(64)*. When associated with dementia or parkinsonism, RBD usually predicts an underlying synucleinopathy, and it has been proposed that RBD should be included in the clinical diagnostic criteria for DLB *(64)*. In PD, an association between RBD and visual hallucinations has been reported *(65)*. Interestingly, during clonazepam treatment, which may improve RBD, the frequency of visual hallucinations decreased, suggesting a causal link between RBD and halucinations *(65)*.

Autopsy studies have identified greater cholinergic deficits in the cortex of hallucinating patients when compared to nonhallucinating patients *(66,67)*. A provisional report of a prospective clinicopathological study *(68)* indicates an association between visual hallucinations and less severe neurofibrillary tangle pathology, the reverse association to that seen in AD, highlighting an important difference in the biological substrates of key neuropsychiatric symptoms in the two conditions. Recent neuropathological studies have also indicated a significantly higher number of Lewy bodies in the temporal cortex of DLB patients with visual hallucinations compared to those without *(60)*. Neuroimaging studies using SPECT (single photon emission computed tomography) report reduced blood flow to the primary visual areas in the occipital cortex as the main association of visual hallucinations *(69)*. Delusions have been less studied, but were associated with increased muscarinic M1 receptor binding *(70)*. One preliminary study has examined the neurochemical associations of depression, indicating that DLB patients with major depression had a relative preservation of 5HT reuptake sites, compared to those without *(68)*. The associations of other neuropsychiatric features await evaluation.

In a direct comparison with PD and dementia, DLB and PD patients showed very similar profiles of neuropsychiatric symptoms, although the frequency of most symptoms was higher in DLB than in PD patients *(59)*. The majority of DLB patients were diagnosed by autopsy, but the methods of assessing neuropsychiatric symptoms differed slightly in the two groups. In 93 DLB patients recruited to an international multicenter study of rivastigmine *(24)*, neuropsychiatric symptoms were assessed using the NPI. On most items, a positive score was reported in more than 50% of the patients, except euphoria, disinhibition, and apathy. The highest frequency was found for hallucinations, depression, and anxiety (*see* Table 1) (Janet Grace & Ian McKeith, personal communication) *(71)*, a pattern similar to that reported in PD. There was a trend toward higher NPI scores in patients with more cognitive impairment as measured with the Mini Mental State Examination (MMSE), and this was significant for the four-item NPI (the sum of hallucination, delusion, depression, and apathy items) *(24)*. In summary, psychiatric symptoms, in particular visual hallucinations, are extremely common in DLB, and help distinguish these patients from patients with AD and other disorders *(46)*, although DLB may be diagnosed also in the absence of visual hallucinations *(72)*. The profile of neuropsychiatric symptoms, as well as the cognitive profile *(73)* in DLB patients are similar to the symptoms observed in PD patients.

NEUROPSYCHIATRIC SYMPTOMS IN PROGRESSIVE SUPRANUCLEAR PALSY

Few studies have explored the neuropsychiatric symptoms of patients with PSP, a disorder characterized neuropathologically by abundant neurofibrillary tangles in several subcortical nuclei (striatum, pallidum, subthalamic nucleus), in addition to the substantia nigra *(74)*. Prefrontal and parahippocampal cortices may also be involved. Locus ceruleus and raphe nuclei are relatively preserved, and noradrenaline and serotonin concentrations are usually not affected *(28)*. Clinical symptoms include supranuclear vertical gaze palsy, akineto-rigid predominant parkinsonism, early postural instability, and subcortical dementia. Some studies of the clinical features in patients with PSP have included neuropsychiatric aspects, although most studies have employed only unstructured assessments based on retrospective review of clinical records. In one study of 52 patients, at the time of diagnosis

45% had memory impairment, 15% were depressed, 23% had personality changes, and 17% emotional lability *(75)*. In another study, caregivers of 437 of the 1184 members of the Society for Progressive Supranuclear Palsy (SPSP) *(76)* completed a structured questionnaire assessing common symptoms and signs, including cognitive and emotional/personality problems. Personality and emotional problems were uncommon 2 yr prior to the diagnosis. At the time of diagnosis, however, changes in personality appeared in 46% and depression in 44%. Other personality problems, such as losing control over emotions, lack of emotions, and excessive anger, were reported in less than 30% of patients at the time of diagnosis. A UK sample of 187 patients was diagnosed according to the National Institute of Neurological Disorders and Stroke (NINDS)–SPSP criteria for probable or possible PSP. Sixty-two patients were drawn from a prevalence study and examined by the investigators, 49 of these with a structured clinical examination. At onset, 15% had neuropsychiatric features, including memory impairment (7%), personality change (4%), and depression/anxiety/apathy (3%). Apathy was noted in 50% of the patients during the disease course *(77)*. Seven patients had responded to an antidepressive drug. In a group of 24 patients with an autopsy-confirmed diagnosis of PSP, frontal lobe symptomatology, including executive dysfunction and personality changes such as apathy and depression, was the presenting symptom in 8%, 55% had such symptoms at the first visit, and 58% at the last visit *(78)*.

A clinical series of 25 PSP patients were assessed for depression using the BDI. The majority of patients (55%) had scores above the cutoff for probable depression: mild (score 11–17, $n = 7$), moderate (18–23; $n = 3$) or severe depression (24 or above, $n = 3$) *(79)*. Depression scores did not correlate with neuropsychological performance. The proportion of subjects with a BDI score of 18 or more in PSP (24%) is identical to the findings in a large PD population *(52)*. A cutoff score of 16/17 has received empirical support for diagnosing clinically relevant depression in PD *(14)*.

Few studies have focused specifically on neuropsychiatric aspects using standardized assessment procedures. The NPI profile was reported in 61 patients with PSP *(49)*, 13 of whom were diagnosed as definite PSP according to the NINDS–PSP *(43)* (i.e., autopsy confirmed); the remaining met the criteria for probable ($n = 36$) or possible ($n = 12$) NINDS–SPSP criteria, which have high diagnostic specificity. The most common NPI items were apathy (positive score in 84%) and disinhibition (56%), whereas hallucinations and delusions were very rare (Table 1). Compared to age- and gender-matched PD patients, the severity of apathy and disinhibition was higher in PSP than PD patients, whereas hallucinations, delusions, and agitation scores were higher in PD than PSP patients. Interestingly, 44% of the PSP patients were taking at least one anti-parkinsonian agent, usually levodopa, at similar doses as the PD group. Thus, hallucinations and delusions do not seem to occur in PSP even when taking dopaminergic agents. The same group of PSP patients was compared with Huntington's disease and Gilles de la Tourette syndrome, both typical hyperkinetic movement disorders. Patients with PSP, a hypoactive movement disorder, had lower scores on NPI items assessing "hyperactive" behaviors (i.e., agitation, irritability, euphoria, and anxiety), but higher scores on apathy, a "hypoactive" behavior *(27,80)*. Thus, in summary, the neuropsychiatric profile of PSP is characterized by early subcortical dementia and frequent occurrence of apathy and disinhibition, whereas hallucinations, delusions, and agitation are rare, irrespective of whether the patients are treated with anti-parkinsonian agents.

NEUROPSYCHIATRIC SYMPTOMS IN CORTICOBASAL DEGENERATION

CBD is characterized pathologically by neurodegeneration of frontal and parietal cortices, substantia nigra, and several basal ganglia nuclei including subthalamic nucleus, striatum, and pallidum. Other brainstem nuclei, including locus ceruleus, raphe nucleus, and midbrain tegmentum, are also involved, with marked reductions of noradrenaline and serotonin in addition to the nigrostriatal dopamine deficiency *(81)*. Tau protein-positive inclusions and achromatic neurons are found. Several studies have characterized the motor and cognitive features of CBD, but the patient's neuropsychiatric symptoms have rarely been described.

The clinical studies have usually been retrospective chart reviews of clinically or neuropathologically diagnosed patients with CBD conducted at movement disorders clinics, focusing more on the motor than the neuropsychiatric features. Rinne et al. performed a retrospective chart review of 36 cases with a clinical or a pathological diagnosis of CBD *(82)*. Initially, seven (19%) patients showed slight generalized cognitive impairment, and one had prominent personality and behavioral changes with impulsiveness and excessive eating and drinking. Subsequently, nine (25%) patients had evidence of generalized higher mental function involvement. Further characterization of neuropsychiatric symptoms was not provided. In a study of neuropsychological functioning in 21 patients with CBD and 21 with AD, significantly more severe depression as measured by the Geriatric Depression Scale, a self-rating instrument, was reported in CBD (mean [SD] score 14.8 [8.6]) compared to AD (6.8 [6.2]). Both groups had a cognitive performance in the mildly demented range. Eight (38%) CBD patients exceeded the cutoff for "probable depression" (a score of 15 or greater), compared to only one (5%) of the AD patients *(83)*. In the CBD group, depression severity was correlated with duration of symptoms and verbal fluency and attention, but not with memory, language, and intellectual test scores.

In 14 patients with a neuropathological diagnosis of CBD selected from the research and neuropathological files of seven medical centers, the presenting symptom was dementia in 21%, frontal behavior (i.e., apathy, disinhibition, and irritability) in 21% and depression in 7%. Subsequently, dementia and depression had developed in 30–40%, and at the last visit, 58% showed frontal behaviors *(84)*. Dementia as a presenting symptom in CBD was also reported in another postmortem study *(85)*. A high prevalence of frontal behaviors was also reported in one of the few prospective studies reported. Kertesz et al. followed 35 patients with a clinical diagnosis of CBD and included a structured evaluation of language, cognition, and personality changes (Frontal Behavioral Inventory or FBI; *see* ref. *86*), which was specifically designed to assess the spectrum of apathy and disinhibition in frontotemporal dementias *(87)*. They found two groups of patients according to the initial presentation: 15 (43%) patients presented with the extrapyramidal or apractic symptoms, but later developed behavioral or language symptoms, and 20 cases (57%) presented with behavioral or language symptoms followed by movement disorder. During the disease course, 20 (57%) patients developed frontotemporal dementia. In the largest clinical series to date, a retrospective chart review was performed in 147 clinically diagnosed CBD patients from eight major movement disorder clinics *(88)*. Except for dementia, reported in 25%, neuropsychiatric symptoms were not described in detail. However, it was reported that antidepressants, used by 11%, "were not effective in treating depression." Of 92% who received dopaminergic drugs, hallucinations had occurred in five (3.7%) patients. Six patients had been exposed to neuroleptics, with "clinical improvement" in four, but the reasons for using neuroleptic drugs were not reported. One detailed case report documented the presence of depression and obsessive-compulsive symptoms in a patient with pathological confirmed CBD *(89)*.

In the only prospective and detailed study of neuropsychiatric symptoms in CBD to date, Litvan et al. administered the NPI to 15 CBD and 34 PSP patients *(28)*. The duration of disease of the CBD patients was relatively short, less than 2 yr, and the mean MMSE score was relatively high, 26.0. Patients with CBD exhibited depression (73%), apathy (40%), irritability (20%), and agitation (20%), but rarely delusions and hallucinations, and, surprisingly, disinhibition (13%) (Table 1). The depression and irritability of patients with CBD were significantly more frequent and severe than those of patients with PSP and normal controls, whereas PSP patients exhibited significantly more apathy. A pattern of high depression and irritability and low apathy scores correctly identified 88% of the CBD patients. In CBD patients, irritability was associated with disinhibition and apathy. Neuropsychiatric symptoms were not associated with motor or cognitive/executive functions, leading the authors to conclude that the various frontosubcortical pathways in CBD are not affected in parallel, at the relatively early stages of the disease. Thus, in conclusion, the neuropsychiatric profile in the early stages of CBD is characterized by depression and apathy, combined with a mild cognitive impairment. Later in the disease course, frontal-type behaviors predominate, with more severe apathy and disinhibition combined with a more severe dementia. In addition to the basal ganglia pathology, the involvement of prefrontal cortex and noradrenergic and serotonergic nuclei may contribute to this neuropsychiatric pattern. However, more detailed neuropsychiatric studies of patients at different stages of CBD are needed.

NEUROPSYCHIATRIC SYMPTOMS IN MULTIPLE SYSTEM ATROPHY

MSA is clinically characterized by the variable combination of autonomic failure, parkinsonism, cerebellar ataxia, and pyramidal signs, and includes the previously called striatonigral degeneration (parkinsonian features predominate), sporadic olivopontocerebellar atrophy (OPCA) (cerebellar features predominate), and the Shy–Drager syndrome (autonomic dysfunction predominates). Histologically, all subtypes of MSA show glial cytoplasmic inclusions in oligodendrocytes of the cerebral white matter, which contain alpha-synuclein. Therefore MSA ranks among the synucleinopathies, but the reason explaining the different cellular topography of α-synuclein (neuronal in PD, glial in MSA) is still unknown *(90)*.

The majority of data describing neuropsychiatric disturbances in MSA are case reports. Although these reports demonstrate that neuropsychiatric symptoms occur in MSA, few systematical studies have been published. In one of the largest retrospective chart reviews of pathologically proven MSA, clinical data of 203 patients were reported. Unfortunately, neuropsychiatric assessment was restricted to "bedside impressions" of cognition. Mild intellectual impairment was noted in 22%, moderate impairment in 2%, and only one patient had severe dementia *(91)*.

Several reports have described depressive symptoms in MSA *(16,92–95)*. In a study of 15 patients clinically diagnosed with Shy–Drager syndrome using the BDI, 86% scored in the depressed range (i.e., BDI score 10–15), and 29% scored in the moderately depressed range (BDI score 16–19). The mean BDI score was 14.4. This score is comparable to that reported in a community-based sample of patients with PD, who had a mean BDI score of 12.8, compared to 7.9 in patients with non-neurological chronic disease (diabetes mellitus) and 5.9 in healthy elderly controls *(52)*. Severity of depression did not correlate with disability or ability to perform activities of daily living (ADL) *(95)*. In another study using the BDI, 3 of 15 (20%) patients had a score over 15, and MSA patients had similar severity of depression as PD patients *(94)*. The importance of depression in MSA is underlined by reports showing that MSA patients may initially present with an affective disturbance *(92,96)*. Fetoni et al. compared 12 MSA with 12 PD patients matched for age and motor disability at baseline before and after levodopa therapy using the HAM-D and the BPRS. Only 1 of the 12 MSA patients had a HAM-D score of 18 (indicating a moderate-severe depression). At baseline patients with PD were more depressed and anxious than patients with MSA who, by contrast, showed apathy. After levodopa, depression and anxiety of patients with PD improved significantly, whereas the apathy in patients with MSA did not change *(16)*.

Psychotic symptoms have been described in MSA *(97–100)*, also as part of affective disturbances *(101)*. Of special interest for diagnostic thinking is the observation that paranoid-hallucinatory psychosis with organic character can be initial manifestation of MSA *(97,99)*. The patients described by Ehrt et al. also exhibited visual hallucinations, a symptom typically seen in other synucleinopathies such as DLB and PD. However, in a relatively large clinico-pathologic comparative study, "neuropsychiatric toxicity" was reported to be less common in MSA ($n = 38$) than PD patients *(102)*. However, this term included confusion or hallucinations or the combination of both, the proportion of dementia was higher in PD than MSA, the number and dosage of dopaminergic drugs in the two groups were not comparable, and the assessments were retrospective and unstructured. Thus, it is not yet proven that visual hallucinations are less common in MSA than PD.

Several studies have reported sleep disorders in MSA *(64,103–107)*. Wright et al. describe a polysomnographically confirmed RBD associated with Shy–Drager syndrome *(108)*. Motor dyscontrol in REM sleep has been described in 90% of patients with MSA *(104)*. Among 93 patients with RBD, 14 patients had MSA, 25 PD, and only 1 had PSP *(109)*. And similarly, in a recent study of 15 patients with RBD, the neuropathological diagnosis was DLB in 12 and MSA in 3 cases *(64)*. In a comparison of unselected patients with MSA (*n* = 57) with 62 age- and sex-matched PD patients, 70% of patients with MSA complained of sleep disorders compared with 51% of patients with PD, and RBD was present in 48% of the MSA patients *(106)*. Decreased nigrostriatal dopaminergic projections may contribute to RBD in MSA *(107)*.

In summary, MSA patients frequently suffer from depression and sleep disorders, including RBD, and visual hallucinations, also seem to be quite common. Thus, the neuropsychiatric pattern resembles that of DLB and PD, suggesting clinical similarities in disorders with α-synuclein pathology *(110)*. In fact, one patient with a clinical diagnosis of MSA turned out at autopsy to have diffuse Lewy body disease *(111)*, supporting the interrelationship of these disorders.

Summary

Although few studies have explored the neuropsychiatric symptoms of parkinsonian disorders other than PD and DLB, some preliminary hypotheses regarding the potential diagnostic value of the neuropsychiatric assessment can be postulated. The α-synucleinopathies DLB and PD, as well as MSA, are characterized by the frequent occurrence of hallucinations and delusions, which may be related to Lewy bodies in the temporal lobe or cholinergic deficits. In addition, depression and anxiety are common, and are possibly related to the additional involvement of monoaminergic brainstem nuclei. Finally, RBD seem to be a marker for these disorders. In contrast, tauopathies such as PSP and CBD are characterized by very high frequency of apathy, possibly related to the marked hypostimulation of orbital and medial frontosubcortical circuits owing to involvement of several basal ganglia nuclei, and disinhibition, possibly secondary to frontal lobe involvement. A high frequency of depression has been reported in CBD, which may be caused in part by involvement of brainstem monoaminergic nuclei. However, depression in parkinsonian disorders probably has a multifactorial etiology, including a wide range of neurological and neurochemical changes in combination, and interaction, with psychosocial factors. Future research should further explore the symptom pattern using standardized diagnostic instruments and the underlying brain pathology of neuropsychiatric features in patients with PSP, CBD, and MSA (*see* Future Research Issues).

MANAGEMENT OF NEUROPSYCHIATRIC SYMPTOMS

Pharmacological Treatment of PD

In light of the high prevalence and clinical importance of neuropsychiatric symptoms in patients with parkinsonian disorders, relatively few adequately designed clinical trials have been reported. In a recent evidence-based review of management of PD, including psychosocial treatments, produced by The Movement Disorder Society *(112)*, the only neuropsychiatric treatment that was concluded to be "efficacious" was the atypical antipsychotic agent clozapine for hallucinations/psychosis. In addition, the tricyclic antidepressant nortriptyline was considered to be "likely efficacious." Too few or methodologically inadequate studies precluded positive conclusions for other treatments.

To our knowledge, only nine randomized, placebo-controlled studies of neuropsychiatric symptoms in parkinsonian disorders have been reported: four trials with cholinergic agents in DLB (rivastigmine) *(113)*, PD (donepezil) *(114)*, and PSP (donepezil and RS-86, a cholinergic agonist) *(115,116)*, two trials with clozapine in PD *(117,118)*, and three trials with antidepressants in PD *(119–121)*. The studies have usually included few subjects, with a total number of 356 patients in the nine studies. Further details are provided in Table 2. In addition to the two studies showing efficacy of clozapine in PD with psychosis, rivastigmine improved neuropsychiatric symptoms in DLB *(113)*,

Table 2
Placebo-Controlled Studies of Neuropsychiatric Symptoms in Patients With Parkinsonian Disorders

Author	Disorder	Drug	Dose, mg/d	N	Duration, Weeks	Design	Main outcome Measures	Result
The Parkinson study group (118)	PD psychosis	clozapine	Mean 25	60	4	Parallel	BPRS	Positive
The French Clozapine Parkinson Study Group (117)	PD psychosis	clozapine	Mean 36	60	4	Parallel	PANSS, CGIC	Positive
Andersen 1980 (119)	PD depression	nortriptyline	Max 150	22	8 + 8	Cross-over	Andersen scale (119)	Positive
Wermuth 1998 (120)	PD depression	citalopram	65+: max 10 <65: max 20	37	6	Parallel	HDRS	Negative
Leentjens 2003 (121)	PD depression	sertraline	Max 100	12	10	Parallel	MADRS	Negative
Aarsland 2002 (114)	PD dementia	donepezil	10	14	10 + 10	Cross-over	CGIC, MMSE	Positive
McKeith 2000 (113)	DLB	rivastigmine	Mean 9,4	120	20	Parallel	CGIC, NPI	Positive
Litvan 2001 (116)	PSP	donepezil	10	21	6 + 4 + 6	Cross-over	NPI, AES*, HDRS, MMSE	Negative
Foster 1989 (115)	PSP + dementia	RS-86	4	10	4 + 1 + 4	Cross-over	Neuropsycholog Battery, MMSE POMS**	Negative

*Apathy Evaluation Scale (135).
**Profile of Mood States (136).
NPI, Neuropsychiatric Inventory; PD, Parkinson's disease; PSP, Progressive supranuclear palsy, DLB, Dementia with Lewy bodies; MMSE, Mini-Mental State Examination; BPRS, Brief Psychiatric Rating Scale; PANSS, Positive and Negative Syndrome Scale; CGIC, Clinical Global Impression of Change; HDRS, Hamilton Depression Scale; MADRS, Montgomery & Åsberg Depression Rating Scale.

donepezil improved cognition in PD *(114)* but not in PSP *(115,116)*, whereas nortriptyline *(119)* but neither citalopram *(120)* nor sertraline *(121)* were more effective than placebo for depression in PD. Two randomized studies suggest that in PD with psychosis, clozapine is better tolerated than olanzapine *(122)* and risperidone *(123)*. In addition, a range of case reports and case series reporting the use of cholinesterase inhibitors, antidepressants, and atypical antipsychotics have been published. The vast majority of these studies have included patients with PD or DLB. Although positive results have been reported, these should be interpreted with caution because of the open, uncontrolled design. The literature of treatment studies of the atypical parkinsonian disorders is reviewed below. (*See* recent excellent reviews for the treatment of neuropsychiatric symptoms in PD in refs. *55, 112,* and *124.*) Importantly, in patients with parkinsonism and neuropsychiatric symptoms, general measures, including counseling, education, and supportive measures, should be considered. Attention to general medical conditions that could contribute to neuropsychiatric symptoms, such as hypoxemia, infection, or electrolyte disturbances, and the taking of nonessential drugs are important in the management of patients with parkinsonian disorders and neuropsychiatric disorders. Anticholinergic agents can induce delirium and psychosis and should be discontinued. Curtailing doses of dopaminergic agents should also be considered in patients with psychotic or delirious symptoms.

PHARMACOLOGICAL TREATMENT OF DLB

Several open-label studies suggest that atypical antipsychotic agents can improve psychotic symptoms in DLB *(125,126)*. However, DLB sufferers seem to be particularly vulnerable to a specific type of adverse reaction to neuroleptic agents. Patients develop severe parkinsonism, impairment of consciousness, autonomic instability, and frequently experience falls and a marked drop in their level of cognitive performance and functioning *(127,128)*. Furthermore, even in DLB patients who do not experience severe neuroleptic sensitivity, there is some evidence that neuronal loss in the caudate and putamen may be exacerbated by neuroleptic treatment *(129)*. Given the major concerns regarding severe neuroleptic sensitivity reactions, neuroleptic agents cannot be considered to be the first-choice management approach for neuropsychiatric symptoms, but may possibly still have a role in severe and intractable cases with psychosis.

A number of case reports and case series indicate that cholinesterase inhibitors may improve not only the cognitive impairment, but also the psychiatric symptoms in approx 170% of DLB cases with good tolerability (with no exacerbation of parkinsonism in most reports). The first double-blind, placebo-controlled trial of cholinesterase inhibitor therapy for the treatment of DLB confirms these encouraging results *(113)*. The total NPI score improved in 61% of patients on rivastigmine compared with 28% in the placebo group. Hallucinations and delusions, apathy, anxiety, and motor overactivity were the symptoms that improved most markedly. Rivastigmine was well tolerated with no increase in adverse events requiring withdrawal in comparison with the placebo group. Furthermore, there was no deterioration in parkinsonism in the treatment group. Given the potential hazards of neuroleptic treatment, most specialists would now recommend cholinesterase inhibitor therapy as a first-line treatment for neuropsychiatric symptoms in DLB patients. The evidence is still however preliminary, and further double-blind, placebo-controlled trials are probably needed before confident, evidence-based practice guidelines could be developed.

A variety of other psychotropic drugs are used in the short-term clinical management of DLB. Anxiety and insomnia are common symptoms that may respond well to benzodiazepine sedatives and antidepressant, and anticonvulsants may be useful in controlling behavioral and psychotic symptoms. Most of these observations are based upon clinical experience and anecdote, rather than evidence; and given the poor tolerability of DLB patients to psychotropic drugs, it is probably best to avoid all pharmacological interventions with psychotropic agents other than cholinesterase inhibitors, unless the clinical situation makes it imperative. Given the potential adverse response to neuroleptics, studies evaluating the potential value of nonpharmacological treatment approaches are also needed. Another key issue for future trials is the management of depression in these patients (*see* Future Research Issues), since no pharmacological or nonpharmacological studies have been published so far.

TREATMENT OF PSP, CBD, AND MSA

Few trials of neuropsychiatric symptoms have been reported in PSP. In a recent placebo-controlled trial, the cholinesterase inhibitor donepezil did not improve neuropsychiatric symptoms. A slight improvement in memory was noted, but because of worsening of motor symptoms, a worsening of ADL was found in patients receiving donepezil *(116)*. Similarly, a small placebo-controlled trial with RS-86, a cholinergic agonist, did not improve cognition or mood in PSP patients with dementia *(115)*. In a clinical survey, it was reported that some PSP patients responded to antidepressive drugs *(77)*. In a chart review, 7 of 12 autopsy-diagnosed PSP patients responded to a dopaminergic drugs, and 1 of 3 to a tricyclic antidepressant. None of the patients responded markedly, however. The serotonergic agent trazodone, but not the neuroleptic drug thiotixine or carbamazepine, improved agitation in patients with PSP *(130)*. Another case report suggested that electroconvulsive therapy (ECT) could improve depression without affecting motor symptoms in PSP *(131)*. Similar findings have been reported in PD patients *(132)*. Very few reports of the treatment of neuropsychiatric symptoms exist for patients with CBD and MSA. In a large clinical survey of CBD patients, antidepressive therapy was reported not to improve depression, whereas four of six patients exposed to neuroleptics showed clinical improvement *(88)*. Further details of the treatments were not provided, however. In a patient with MSA, clozapine was reported to improve psychotic depression without aggravating neurological abnormalities *(98)*. ECT was reported to be a safe and effective treatment for major depression in some patients with MSA *(101,133)*, with long-term benefit in some *(134)*.

In summary, although some placebo-controlled drug trials of neuropsychiatric symptoms in parkinsonian disorders have been reported, there is limited evidence available to guide pharmacological treatment for patients with atypical parkinsonian disorders.

FUTURE RESEARCH ISSUES

1. Descriptive studies of the neuropsychiatric features in PSP, MSA, and CBD using standardized psychiatric rating scales.
2. Study the diagnostic properties of the neuropsychiatric profile in parkinsonian disorders.
3. Exploring the neurochemical underpinnings of neuropsychiatric symptoms in patients with parkinsonian disorders.
4. In DLB, placebo-controlled trials of antidepressive and antipsychotic agents, and further trials of cholinesterase inhibitors need to be conducted.
5. In PSP, MSA, and CBD, pilot studies of the potential benefit of psychotropic agents are needed.
6. Systematic studies of non-pharmacological strategies should be conducted for patients with parkinsonian disorders.

ACKNOWLEDGMENT

We want to thank Jeffrey L. Cummings for the permission to use the Neuropsychiatric Inventory video.

REFERENCES

1. McKeith IG, Galasko D, Kosaka K, et al. Consensus guidelines for the clinical and pathologic diagnosis of dementia with Lewy bodies (DLB): report of the consortium on DLB international workshop. Neurology 1996;47:1113–1124.
2. Bhatia KP, Marsden CD. The behavioural and motor consequences of focal lesions of the basal ganglia in man. Brain 1994;117(Pt 4):859–876.
3. Burns A, Jacoby R, Levy R. Psychiatric phenomena in Alzheimer's disease. I: Disorders of thought content. Br J Psychiatry 1990;157:72–76, 92–94.

4. Leentjens AF, Marinus J, Van Hilten JJ, Lousberg R, Verhey FR. The contribution of somatic symptoms to the diagnosis of depressive disorder in Parkinson's disease: a discriminant analytic approach. J Neuropsychiatry Clin Neurosci 2003;15:74–77.

5. Levy ML, Cummings JL, Fairbanks LA, et al. Apathy is not depression. J Neuropsychiatry Clin Neurosci 1998;10:314–319.

6. Hope T, Fairburn CG. The Present Behavioural Examination (PBE): the development of an interview to measure current behavioural abnormalities. Psychol Med 1992;22:223–230.

7. Cummings JL, Mega M, Gray K, Rosenberg-Thompson S, Carusi DA, Gornbein J. The Neuropsychiatric Inventory: comprehensive assessment of psychopathology in dementia. Neurology 1994;44:2308–2314.

8. Andersen J, Larsen JK, Schultz V, et al. The Brief Psychiatric Rating Scale. Dimension of schizophrenia—reliability and construct validity. Psychopathology 1989;22:168–176.

9. Hamilton M. A rating scale for depression. J Neurol Neurosurg Psychiatry 1960;23:56–62.

10. Beck AT, Ward CH, Mendelson M, Mock J, Erbaugh J. An inventory for measuring depression. Arch Gen Psychiatry 1961;4:561–571.

11. Yesavage JA, Brink TL, Rose TL, et al. Development and validation of a geriatric depression screening scale: a preliminary report. J Psychiatr Res 1982;17:37–49.

12. Aarsland D, Larsen JP, Lim NG, et al. Range of neuropsychiatric disturbances in patients with Parkinson's disease. J Neurol Neurosurg Psychiatry 1999;67:492–496.

13. Leentjens AF, Verhey FR, Lousberg R, Spitsbergen H, Wilmink FW. The validity of the Hamilton and Montgomery-Asberg depression rating scales as screening and diagnostic tools for depression in Parkinson's disease. Int J Geriatr Psychiatry 2000;15:644–649.

14. Leentjens AF, Verhey FR, Luijckx GJ, Troost J. The validity of the Beck Depression Inventory as a screening and diagnostic instrument for depression in patients with Parkinson's disease. Mov Disord 2000;15:1221–1224.

15. Marinus J, Leentjens AF, Visser M, Stiggelbout AM, Van Hilten JJ. Evaluation of the hospital anxiety and depression scale in patients with Parkinson's disease. Clin Neuropharmacol 2002;25:318–324.

16. Fetoni V, Soliveri P, Monza D, Testa D, Girotti F. Affective symptoms in multiple system atrophy and Parkinson's disease: response to levodopa therapy. J Neurol Neurosurg Psychiatry 1999;66:541–544.

17. Mega MS, Cummings JL, Salloway S, Malloy P. The limbic system: an anatomic, phylogenetic, and clinical perspective. J Neuropsychiatry Clin Neurosci 1997;9:315–330.

18. Cummings JL. Frontal-subcortical circuits and human behavior. Arch Neurol 1993;50:873–880.

19. Stefurak TL, Mayberg HS. Critical-limbic-striatal dysfunction in depression. In: Chouinard S, ed. Mental and Behavioral Dysfunction in Movement Disorders. Totowa, NJ: Humana, 2003:321–338.

20. Lucey JV, Costa DC, Busatto G, et al. Caudate regional cerebral blood flow in obsessive-compulsive disorder, panic disorder and healthy controls on single photon emission computerised tomography. Psychiatry Res 1997;74:25–33.

21. Forstl H, Krumm B, Eden S, Kohlmeyer K. What is the psychiatric significance of bilateral basal ganglia mineralization? Biol Psychiatry 1991;29:827–833.

22. Cummings JL. Toward a molecular neuropsychiatry of neurodegenerative diseases. Ann Neurol 2003;54:147–154.

23. Ballard C, Holmes C, McKeith I, et al. Psychiatric morbidity in dementia with Lewy bodies: a prospective clinical and neuropathological comparative study with Alzheimer's disease. Am J Psychiatry 1999;156:1039–1045.

24. Del Ser T, McKeith I, Anand R, Cicin-Sain A, Ferrara R, Spiegel R. Dementia with lewy bodies: findings from an international multicentre study. Int J Geriatr Psychiatry 2000;15:1034–1045.

25. Rahkonen T, Eloniemi-Sulkava U, Rissanen S, Vatanen A, Viramo P, Sulkava R. Dementia with Lewy bodies according to the consensus criteria in a general population aged 75 years or older. J Neurol Neurosurg Psychiatry 2003;74:720–724.

26. Del Ser T, Hachinski V, Merskey H, Munoz DG. Clinical and pathologic features of two groups of patients with dementia with Lewy bodies: effect of coexisting Alzheimer-type lesion load. Alzheimer Dis Assoc Disord 2001;15:31–44.

27. Litvan I, Paulsen JS, Mega MS, Cummings JL. Neuropsychiatric assessment of patients with hyperkinetic and hypokinetic movement disorders. Arch Neurol 1998;55:1313–1319.

28. Litvan I, Cummings JL, Mega M. Neuropsychiatric features of corticobasal degeneration. J Neurol Neurosurg Psychiatry 1998;65:717–721.

29. Schrag A, Jahanshahi M, Quinn N. What contributes to quality of life in patients with Parkinson's disease? J Neurol Neurosurg Psychiatry 2000;69:308–312.

30. Karlsen KH, Larsen JP, Tandberg E, Maland JG. Quality of life measurements in patients with Parkinson's disease: A community-based study. Eur J Neurol 1998;5:443–450.

31. Kuopio AM, Marttila RJ, Helenius H, Toivonen M, Rinne UK. The quality of life in Parkinson's disease. Mov Disord 2000;15:216–223.

32. Karlsen KH, Tandberg E, Arsland D, Larsen JP. Health related quality of life in Parkinson's disease: a prospective longitudinal study. J Neurol Neurosurg Psychiatry 2000;69:584–589.

33. Aarsland D, Larsen JP, Karlsen K, Lim NG, Tandberg E. Mental symptoms in Parkinson's disease are important contributors to caregiver distress. Int J Geriatr Psychiatry 1999;14:866–874.

34. Caap-Ahlgren M, Dehlin O. Factors of importance to the caregiver burden experienced by family caregivers of Parkinson's disease patients. Aging Clin Exp Res 2002;14:371–377.

35. Uttl B, Santacruz P, Litvan I, Grafman J. Caregiving in progressive supranuclear palsy. Neurology 1998;51:1303–1309.

36. Larsen JP. Parkinson's disease as community health problem: study in Norwegian nursing homes. The Norwegian Study Group of Parkinson's Disease in the Elderly. BMJ 1991;303:741–743.

37. Aarsland D, Larsen JP, Tandberg E, Laake K. Predictors of nursing home placement in Parkinson's disease: a population-based, prospective study. J Am Geriatr Soc 2000;48:938–942.

38. Goetz CG, Stebbins GT. Mortality and hallucinations in nursing home patients with advanced Parkinson's disease. Neurology 1995;45:669–671.

39. Murman DL, Chen Q, Powell MC, Kuo SB, Bradley CJ, Colenda CC. The incremental direct costs associated with behavioral symptoms in AD. Neurology 2002;59:1721–1729.

40. Starkstein SE, Mayberg HS, Leiguarda R, Preziosi TJ, Robinson RG. A prospective longitudinal study of depression, cognitive decline, and physical impairments in patients with Parkinson's disease. J Neurol Neurosurg Psychiatry 1992;55:377–382.

41. Aarsland D, Andersen K, Larsen JP, Lolk A, Kragh-Sorensen P. Prevalence and characteristics of dementia in Parkinson disease: an 8-year prospective study. Arch Neurol 2003;60:387–392.

42. Factor SA, Feustel PJ, Friedman JH, et al. Longitudinal outcome of Parkinson's disease patients with psychosis. Neurology 2003;60:1756–1761.

43. Litvan I, Agid Y, Calne D, et al. Clinical research criteria for the diagnosis of progressive supranuclear palsy (Steele–Richardson–Olszewski syndrome): report of the NINDS–SPSP international workshop. Neurology 1996;47:1–9.

44. Litvan I, Agid Y, Goetz C, et al. Accuracy of the clinical diagnosis of corticobasal degeneration: a clinicopathologic study. Neurology 1997;48:119–125.

45. Litvan I, Goetz CG, Jankovic J, et al. What is the accuracy of the clinical diagnosis of multiple system atrophy? A clinicopathologic study. Arch Neurol 1997;54:937–944.

46. Litvan I, MacIntyre A, Goetz CG, et al. Accuracy of the clinical diagnoses of Lewy body disease, Parkinson disease, and dementia with Lewy bodies: a clinicopathologic study. Arch Neurol 1998;55:969–978.

47. Litvan I, Bhatia KP, Burn DJ, et al. SIC Task Force appraisal of clinical diagnostic criteria for parkinsonian disorders. Mov Disord 2003;18:467–486.

48. Aarsland D, Larsen JP, Cummins JL, Laake K. Prevalence and clinical correlates of psychotic symptoms in Parkinson disease: a community-based study. Arch Neurol 1999;56:595–601.

49. Aarsland D, Litvan I, Larsen JP. Neuropsychiatric symptoms of patients with progressive supranuclear palsy and Parkinson's disease. J Neuropsychiatry Clin Neurosci 2001;13:42–49.

50. Aarsland D, Andersen K, Larsen JP, Lolk A, Nielsen H, Kragh-Sorensen P. Risk of dementia in Parkinson's disease: a community-based, prospective study. Neurology 2001;56:730–736.

51. Cummings JL. Depression and Parkinson's disease: a review. Am J Psychiatry 1992;149:443–454.

52. Tandberg E, Larsen JP, Aarsland D, Cummings JL. The occurrence of depression in Parkinson's disease. A community-based study. Arch Neurol 1996;53:175–179.

53. Hantz P, Caradoc-Davies G, Caradoc-Davies T, Weatherall M, Dixon G. Depression in Parkinson's disease. Am J Psychiatry 1994;151:1010–1014.

54. Brown R, Jahanshahi M. Depression in Parkinson's disease: a psychosocial viewpoint. Adv Neurol 1995;65:61–84.

55. Burn DJ. Beyond the iron mask: towards better recognition and treatment of depression associated with Parkinson's disease. Mov Disord 2002;17:445–454.

56. Nilsson FM, Kessing LV, Sorensen TM, Andersen PK, Bolwig TG. Major depressive disorder in Parkinson's disease: a register-based study. Acta Psychiatr Scand 2002;106:202–211.

57. Fenelon G, Mahieux F, Huon R, Ziegler M. Hallucinations in Parkinson's disease: prevalence, phenomenology and risk factors. Brain 2000;123(Pt 4):733–745.

58. Goetz CG, Leurgans S, Pappert EJ, Raman R, Stemer AB. Prospective longitudinal assessment of hallucinations in Parkinson's disease. Neurology 2001;57:2078–2082.

59. Aarsland D, Ballard C, Larsen JP, McKeith I. A comparative study of psychiatric symptoms in dementia with Lewy bodies and Parkinson's disease with and without dementia. Int J Geriatr Psychiatry 2001;16:528–536.

60. Harding AJ, Broe GA, Halliday GM. Visual hallucinations in Lewy body disease relate to Lewy bodies in the temporal lobe. Brain 2002;125:391–403.

61. Aarsland D, Cummings JL, Larsen JP. Neuropsychiatric differences between Parkinson's disease with dementia and Alzheimer's disease. Int J Geriatr Psychiatry 2001;16:184–191.

62. Grace JB, Walker MP, McKeith IG. A comparison of sleep profiles in patients with dementia with lewy bodies and Alzheimer's disease. Int J Geriatr Psychiatry 2000;15:1028–1033.

63. Larsen JP. Sleep disorders in Parkinson's disease. Adv Neurol 2003;91:329–334.

64. Boeve BF, Silber MH, Parisi JE, et al. Synucleinopathy pathology and REM sleep behavior disorder plus dementia or parkinsonism. Neurology 2003;61:40–45.

65. Nomura T, Inoue Y, Mitani H, Kawahara R, Miyake M, Nakashima K. Visual hallucinations as REM sleep behavior disorders in patients with Parkinson's disease. Mov Disord 2003;18:812–817.
66. Perry EK, Marshall E, Kerwin J, et al. Evidence of a monoaminergic-cholinergic imbalance related to visual hallucinations in Lewy body dementia. J Neurochem 1990;55:1454–1456.
67. Perry EK, Marshall E, Perry RH, et al. Cholinergic and dopaminergic activities in senile dementia of Lewy body type. Alzheimer Dis Assoc Disord 1990;4:87–95.
68. Ballard C, Johnson M, Piggott M, et al. A positive association between 5HT re-uptake binding sites and depression in dementia with Lewy bodies. J Affect Disord 2002;69:219–223.
69. Colloby SJ, Fenwick JD, Williams ED, et al. A comparison of (99m)Tc-HMPAO SPET changes in dementia with Lewy bodies and Alzheimer's disease using statistical parametric mapping. Eur J Nucl Med Mol Imaging 2002;29:615–622.
70. Ballard C, Piggott M, Johnson M, et al. Delusions associated with elevated muscarinic binding in dementia with Lewy bodies. Ann Neurol 2000;48:868–876.
71. Grace J, McKeith I. Personal Communication, 2003.
72. McKeith IG, Ballard CG, Perry RH, et al. Prospective validation of consensus criteria for the diagnosis of dementia with Lewy bodies. Neurology 2000;54:1050–1058.
73. Aarsland D, Litvan I, Salmon D, Galasko D, Wentzel-Larsen T, Larsen JP. Cognitive impairment in PD and dementia with Lewy bodies. Comparison with Progressive supranuclear palsy and AD. J Neurology Neurosurg Psychiatry 2003;74:1215–1220.
74. Litvan I. Progressive supranuclear palsy revisited. Acta Neurol Scand 1998; 98:73–84.
75. Maher ER, Lees AJ. The clinical features and natural history of the Steele-Richardson-Olszewski syndrome (progressive supranuclear palsy). Neurology 1986;36:1005–1008.
76. Santacruz P, Uttl B, Litvan I, Grafman J. Progressive supranuclear palsy: a survey of the disease course. Neurology 1998;50:1637–1647.
77. Nath U, Ben-Shlomo Y, Thomson RG, Lees AJ, Burn DJ. Clinical features and natural history of progressive supranuclear palsy: a clinical cohort study. Neurology 2003;60:910–916.
78. Litvan I, Mangone CA, McKee A, et al. Natural history of progressive supranuclear palsy (Steele–Richardson–Olszewski syndrome) and clinical predictors of survival: a clinicopathological study. J Neurol Neurosurg Psychiatry 1996;60:615–620.
79. Esmonde T, Giles E, Gibson M, Hodges JR. Neuropsychological performance, disease severity, and depression in progressive supranuclear palsy. J Neurol 1996;243:638–643.
80. Kulisevsky J, Litvan I, Berthier ML, Pascual-Sedano B, Paulsen JS, Cummings JL. Neuropsychiatric assessment of Gilles de la Tourette patients: comparative study with other hyperkinetic and hypokinetic movement disorders. Mov Disord 2001;16:1098–1104.
81. Gibb WR, Luthert PJ, Marsden CD. Corticobasal degeneration. Brain 1989;112(Pt 5):1171–1192.
82. Rinne JO, Lee MS, Thompson PD, Marsden CD. Corticobasal degeneration. A clinical study of 36 cases. Brain 1994;117(Pt 5):1183–1196.
83. Massman PJ, Kreiter KT, Jankovic J, Doody RS. Neuropsychological functioning in cortical-basal ganglionic degeneration: differentiation from Alzheimer's disease. Neurology 1996;46:720–726.
84. Wenning GK, Litvan I, Jankovic J, et al. Natural history and survival of 14 patients with corticobasal degeneration confirmed at postmortem examination. J Neurol Neurosurg Psychiatry 1998;64:184–189.
85. Grimes DA, Lang AE, Bergeron CB. Dementia as the most common presentation of cortical-basal ganglionic degeneration. Neurology 1999;53:1969–1974.
86. Kertesz A, Davidson W, Fox H. Frontal behavioral inventory: diagnostic criteria for frontal lobe dementia. Can J Neurol Sci 1997;24:29–36.
87. Kertesz A, Martinez-Lage P, Davidson W, Munoz DG. The corticobasal degeneration syndrome overlaps progressive aphasia and frontotemporal dementia. Neurology 2000;55:1368–1375.
88. Kompoliti K, Goetz CG, Boeve BF, et al. Clinical presentation and pharmacological therapy in corticobasal degeneration. Arch Neurol 1998;55:957–961.
89. Rey GJ, Tomer R, Levin BE, Sanchez-Ramos J, Bowen B, Bruce JH. Psychiatric symptoms, atypical dementia, and left visual field inattention in corticobasal ganglionic degeneration. Mov Disord 1995;10:106–110.
90. Duyckaerts C, Verny M, Hauw JJ. [Recent neuropathology of parkinsonian syndromes]. Rev Neurol (Paris) 2003;159:11–18.
91. Wenning GK, Tison F, Ben Shlomo Y, Daniel SE, Quinn NP. Multiple system atrophy: a review of 203 pathologically proven cases. Mov Disord 1997;12:133–147.
92. Kwentus JA, Auth TL, Foy JL. Shy–Drager syndrome presenting as depression: case report. J Clin Psychiatry 1984;45:137–139.
93. Rizzoli AA. Psychiatric disturbances in the Shy–Drager syndrome. Br J Psychiatry 1986;148:484.
94. Pilo L, Ring H, Quinn N, Trimble M. Depression in multiple system atrophy and in idiopathic Parkinson's disease: a pilot comparative study. Biol Psychiatry 1996;39:803–807.

95. Gill CE, Khurana RK, Hibler RJ. Occurrence of depressive symptoms in Shy–Drager syndrome. Clin Auton Res 1999;9:1–4.
96. Goto K, Ueki A, Shimode H, Shinjo H, Miwa C, Morita Y. Depression in multiple system atrophy: a case report. Psychiatry Clin Neurosci 2000;54:507–511.
97. Ehrt U, Brieger P, Broich K, Marneros A. [Psychotic symptoms as initial manifestation of a multiple system atrophy]. Fortschr Neurol Psychiatr 1999;67:104–107.
98. Parsa MA, Simon M, Dubrow C, Ramirez LF, Meltzer HY. Psychiatric manifestations of olivo-ponto-cerebellar atrophy and treatment with clozapine. Int J Psychiatry Med 1993;23:149–156.
99. Ziegler B, Tonjes W, Trabert W, Kolles H. [Cerebral multisystem atrophy in a patient with depressive hallucinatory syndrome. A case report]. Nervenarzt 1992;63:510–514.
100. Fukutani Y, Takeuchi N, Kobayashi K, et al. Striatonigral degeneration combined with olivopontocerebellar atrophy with subcortical dementia and hallucinatory state. Dementia 1995;6:235–240.
101. Hooten WM, Melin G, Richardson JW. Response of the Parkinsonian symptoms of multiple system atrophy to ECT. Am J Psychiatry 1998;155:1628.
102. Wenning GK, Ben-Shlomo Y, Hughes A, Daniel SE, Lees A, Quinn NP. What clinical features are most useful to distinguish definite multiple system atrophy from Parkinson's disease? J Neurol Neurosurg Psychiatry 2000;68:434–440.
103. Coccagna G, Martinelli P, Zucconi M, Cirignotta F, Ambrosetto G. Sleep-related respiratory and haemodynamic changes in Shy–Drager syndrome: a case report. J Neurol 1985;232:310–313.
104. Plazzi G, Corsini R, Provini F, et al. REM sleep behavior disorders in multiple system atrophy. Neurology 1997;48:1094–1097.
105. Boeve BF, Silber MH, Ferman TJ, Lucas JA, Parisi JE. Association of REM sleep behavior disorder and neurodegenerative disease may reflect an underlying synucleinopathy. Mov Disord 2001;16:622–630.
106. Ghorayeb I, Yekhlef F, Chrysostome V, Balestre E, Bioulac B, Tison F. Sleep disorders and their determinants in multiple system atrophy. J Neurol Neurosurg Psychiatry 2002;72:798–800.
107. Gilman S, Koeppe RA, Chervin RD, et al. REM sleep behavior disorder is related to striatal monoaminergic deficit in MSA. Neurology 2003;61:29–34.
108. Wright BA, Rosen JR, Buysse DJ, Reynolds CF, Zubenko GS. Shy–Drager syndrome presenting as a REM behavioral disorder. J Geriatr Psychiatry Neurol 1990;3:110–113.
109. Olson EJ, Boeve BF, Silber MH. Rapid eye movement sleep behaviour disorder: demographic, clinical and laboratory findings in 93 cases. Brain 2000;123(Pt 2):331–339.
110. Cummings JL. The Neuropsychiatry of Alzheimer's Disease and Related Dementias. London: Martin Dunitz, Taylor & Francis Group, 2003.
111. Pakiam AS, Bergeron C, Lang AE. Diffuse Lewy body disease presenting as multiple system atrophy. Can J Neurol Sci 1999;26:127–131.
112. Lang AE, Lees A. Management of Parkinson's disease: an evidence-based review. Movement Disorders 2002;17:1–166.
113. McKeith I, Del Ser T, Spano P, et al. Efficacy of rivastigmine in dementia with Lewy bodies: a randomised, double-blind, placebo-controlled international study. Lancet 2000;356:2031–2036.
114. Aarsland D, Laake K, Larsen JP, Janvin C. Donepezil for cognitive impairment in Parkinson's disease: a randomised controlled study. J Neurol Neurosurg Psychiatry 2002;72:708–712.
115. Foster NL, Aldrich MS, Bluemlein L, White RF, Berent S. Failure of cholinergic agonist RS-86 to improve cognition and movement in PSP despite effects on sleep. Neurology 1989;39:257–261.
116. Litvan I, Phipps M, Pharr VL, Hallett M, Grafman J, Salazar A. Randomized placebo-controlled trial of donepezil in patients with progressive supranuclear palsy. Neurology 2001;57:467–473.
117. Aarsland D, Karlsen K. Neuropsychiatric aspects of Parkinson's disease. Curr Psychiatry Rep 1999;1:61–68.
118. Low-dose clozapine for the treatment of drug-induced psychosis in Parkinson's disease. The Parkinson Study Group. N Engl J Med 1999;340(10):757–763.
119. Andersen J, Aabro E, Gulmann N, Hjelmsted A, Pedersen HE. Anti-depressive treatment in Parkinson's disease. A controlled trial of the effect of nortriptyline in patients with Parkinson's disease treated with L-DOPA. Acta Neurol Scand 1980;62:210–219.
120. Wermuth L, Sørensen P, Timm B. Depression in idiopathic Parkinson's disease treated with citalopram. A placebo-controlled trial. Nord J Psychiatry 1998;52:163–169.
121. Leentjens AF, Vreeling FW, Luijckx GJ, Verhey FR. SSRIs in the treatment of depression in Parkinson's disease. Int J Geriatr Psychiatry 2003;18:552–554.
122. Goetz CG, Blasucci LM, Leurgans S, Pappert EJ. Olanzapine and clozapine: comparative effects on motor function in hallucinating PD patients. Neurology 2000;55:789–794.
123. Ellis T, Cudkowicz ME, Sexton PM, Growdon JH. Clozapine and risperidone treatment of psychosis in Parkinson's disease. J Neuropsychiatry Clin Neurosci 2000;12:364–369.
124. Friedman JH, Factor SA. Atypical antipsychotics in the treatment of drug-induced psychosis in Parkinson's disease. Mov Disord 2000;15:201–211.

125. Walker Z, Grace J, Overshot R, et al. Olanzapine in dementia with Lewy bodies: a clinical study. Int J Geriatr Psychiatry 1999;14:459–466.
126. Fernandez HH, Trieschmann ME, Burke MA, Friedman JH. Quetiapine for psychosis in Parkinson's disease versus dementia with Lewy bodies. J Clin Psychiatry 2002;63:513–515.
127. McKeith I, Fairbairn A, Perry R, Thompson P, Perry E. Neuroleptic sensitivity in patients with senile dementia of Lewy body type. BMJ 1992;305:673–678.
128. Ballard C, Grace J, McKeith I, Holmes C. Neuroleptic sensitivity in dementia with Lewy bodies and Alzheimer's disease. Lancet 1998;351:1032–1033.
129. Court JA, Piggott MA, Lloyd S, et al. Nicotine binding in human striatum: elevation in schizophrenia and reductions in dementia with Lewy bodies, Parkinson's disease and Alzheimer's disease and in relation to neuroleptic medication. Neuroscience 2000;98:79–87.
130. Schneider LS, Gleason RP, Chui HC. Progressive supranuclear palsy with agitation: response to trazodone but not to thiothixine or carbamazepine. J Geriatr Psychiatry Neurol 1989;2:109–112.
131. Netzel PJ, Sutor B. Electroconvulsive therapy-responsive depression in a patient with progressive supranuclear palsy. J Ect 2001;17:68–70.
132. Moellentine C, Rummans T, Ahlskog JE, et al. Effectiveness of ECT in patients with parkinsonism. J Neuropsychiatry Clin Neurosci 1998;10:187–193.
133. Ruxin RJ, Ruedrich S. ECT in combined multiple system atrophy and major depression. Convuls Ther 1994;10:298–300.
134. Roane DM, Rogers JD, Helew L, Zarate J. Electroconvulsive therapy for elderly patients with multiple system atrophy: a case series. Am J Geriatr Psychiatry 2000;8:171–174.
135. Marin RS, Biedrzycki RC, Firinciogullari S. Reliability and validity of the Apathy Evaluation Scale. Psychiatry Res 1991;38:143–162.
136. McNair D, Lorr M, Droppleman L. Profile of Mood States. San Diego: Eucational and Industrial Testing Service, 1971.

12

Added Value of the Neuropsychological Evaluation for Diagnosis and Research of Atypical Parkinsonian Disorders

Bruno Dubois and Bernard Pillon

INTRODUCTION

Diseases with movement disorders may be difficult to diagnose, both at the onset when motor symptoms are mild and not sufficiently specific (e.g., difficulty in manipulating objects), or at the end stage when distinctive motor signs are diluted into a severe and polymorphous clinical picture (e.g., gait disorder with postural instability and cognitive decline in aged patients). Erroneous diagnoses are frequent *(1,2)*, even in the most common idiopathic Parkinson's disease (PD) *(3)*. Some of these errors may be avoided if the cognitive dysfunctions that often accompany these diseases are included in the diagnostic criteria.

Subtle but specific cognitive deficits can frequently be detected in patients with a variety of diseases accompanied by movement disorders. We used to say "except for essential tremor" but some cognitive changes have recently been reported even in this case *(4)*. This is explained by the fact that the neuronal pathways connecting the basal ganglia to the cortex project not only to regions involved in the control of movements (motor, premotor, supplementary motor areas) but also to cortical areas contributing to cognitive functions (prefrontal cortex) and to emotional-processing behavior (cingulum and orbitofrontal cortex). In each of these diseases, the loss of different specific populations of neurons in the basal ganglia produces not only a characteristic motor syndrome, but also a recognizable pattern of neuropsychological deficits. Why not include these cognitive and behavioral changes in diagnosis decision trees? Indeed, the use of appropriate neuropsychological tests or questionnaires to detect these deficits can contribute to the diagnosis of such diseases (Table 1).

In this review, we will (1) present the different types of deficits that can be usually encountered following lesions of the basal ganglia; (2) characterize the neuropsychological pattern of the main movement disorders: idiopathic PD, multiple system atrophy (MSA), progressive supranuclear palsy (PSP), corticobasal degeneration (CBD), and dementia with Lewy bodies (DLB); and (3) show that the contribution of neuropsychological deficits to diagnosis varies from one parkinsonian disorder to another.

From: *Current Clinical Neurology: Atypical Parkinsonian Disorders*
Edited by: I. Litvan © Humana Press Inc., Totowa, NJ

Table 1
Proposed Neuropsychological Battery to Evaluate Cognitive and Behavioral Deficits in Parkinsonian Disorders

Domain of Investigation	Proposed Tool
Global cognitive efficiency	Mattis Dementia Rating Scale *(5)*
Global executive syndrome	Frontal Assessment Battery *(6)*
Set elaboration and monitoring	Wisconsin Card Sorting Test *(7)*
Set maintenance	Lexical fluency *(8)*
Set shifting	Trail Making Test *(9)*
Inhibition of interferences	Stroop Test *(10)*
Motor programming	Graphic and motor series *(11)*
Resistance to environmental dependency	Imitation, prehension, utilization *(12)*
Strategic components of memory	California Verbal Learning Test *(13)*
Opposition between free and cued recall	Grober and Buschke Test *(14)*
Linguistic functions	Boston Diagnostic Aphasia Examination *(15)*
Gestures	Apraxia examination *(16)*
Emotional behavior	Neuropsychiatric Inventory *(17)*

WHAT ARE THE COGNITIVE AND BEHAVIORAL CHANGES CURRENTLY ENCOUNTERED IN PARKINSONIAN DISORDERS?

The neuropsychological picture of patients may vary from subtle behavioral abnormalities to florid dementia with delusions and hallucinations. The nature and severity of cognitive disorders, the type of impaired memory processes, the presence or absence of instrumental deficits, the precocity of the dysexecutive syndrome, and the frequency of behavioral disorders depend on the underlying neuronal lesions.

Dementia

According to *DSM-IV (Diagnostic and Statistical Manual of Mental Disorders*, 4th ed.) criteria *(18)*, dementia is defined by the development of multiple cognitive deficits, severe enough to interfere with social activity or personal relationships and representing a decline from a previously higher level of functioning. The term *dementia* needs to be used with caution in diseases in which motor impairment, mood, and behavioral disorders may be part of the clinical picture. In these patients the loss of intellectual capacities can, however, be evaluated by psychometric criteria, using global scales, such as the Mattis Dementia Rating Scale *(5)*, which is more appropriate than the Mini Mental State Exam for predominantly subcortical degenerative diseases, given the inclusion of tests evaluating attention and executive functions. Such tools provide cutoff scores that permit a psychometric distinction between demented and nondemented patients. Dementia is usually not observed in PD with early onset *(19)* or in the early stages of PD *(20)* or MSA *(21,22)*. Dementia may occur in patients with late-onset PD *(23)*, PSP *(24,25)*, or CBD *(26)*. It is a major feature of DLB, although there may be fluctuations of intellectual functioning from one day to another *(27)*.

Memory

Learning disorders in neurodegenerative diseases may be assessed by tools, such as the California Verbal Learning Test *(13)* or the Grober and Buschke Test *(14)* that make it possible to analyze specific memory processes and distinguish between storage and retrieval difficulties. The key for understanding the relationship between memory disorders and degenerative diseases implicates the functional "mediotemporal vs frontal dissociation." Encoding deficits, loss of information after a delay, low effect of cuing on recall, high number of extralist intrusions, and false positives in recognition characterize diseases associated with lesion of hippocampal and perihippocampal areas such as Alzheimer's disease (AD) *(28)*. By contrast, predominant retrieval deficits, manifested by the opposition between impaired free recall and correct cued recall and recognition, are present in diseases associated with dysfunction of striatofrontal neuronal circuits such as PSP or PD with dementia (PDD) *(29)*. Milder deficient activation of the frontal component of memory processes occurs in PD *(30,31)*, MSA *(22)*, and CBD *(32,33)*. Little has been published on learning disorders in DLB, but a study with autopsy-confirmed cases show that they are less severe than in AD *(34)*. Clinical evidence suggests that although cued recall is less efficient in DLB than in PD or PSP, it is better preserved than in AD. A similar contrast between a true loss of information in AD and retrieval deficits in PDD also applies to retrograde amnesia.

Instrumental Activities

Instrumental dysfunction, suggestive of temporoparietal lesions, include aphasia, apraxia, and visuospatial deficits. Aphasia and apraxia may be investigated by clinical batteries, such as the Boston Diagnostic Aphasia Examination *(15)* or the Heilman and Gonzalez Rothi battery for apraxia *(16)*. Visuospatial deficits are less clearly defined and do not allow the differential diagnosis of the different diseases, since various cognitive abilities, such as visuospatial perception, drawing, or constructive aptitude, and conceptual thinking may affect performance *(35)*. Impairment of instrumental activities is specific to neurodegenerative diseases with a cortical involvement. Aphasia may be observed in DLB *(27)*, whereas apraxia is more characteristic of CBD *(32,36)*. In contrast, instrumental functions are mildly disturbed in PSP *(37)* and PDD *(38)* and are preserved in PD *(39)* and MSA *(22)*.

Executive Functions

Executive functions, namely the mental processes involved in behavioral planning, particularly when the environment requires adaptation to a new situation, are under the control of striatofrontal circuits. These functions may be investigated at the patient's bedside *(6)* (*see* video) or by a neuropsychological evaluation assessing the main processes mediated by striatofrontal loops such as set elaboration, set maintenance, and set shifting, inhibition of interferences, motor programming, and environmental autonomy (Table 1). These functions are impaired at an early stage of all parkinsonian disorders, but are much less severe in PD and MSA than in the other parkinsonian syndromes *(25,40)*.

Behavioral Disorders

Delusions and hallucinations, as diagnosed in accordance with the *DSM–IV* criteria *(18)*, are common at early stages of DLB *(27)*. They occur in PD, particularly in demented patients or as a result of treatment with anticholinergic or dopaminergic drugs, but are not characteristic of MSA, PSP, or CBD *(41)*. Apathy and disinhibition may also be observed in parkinsonian disorders *(42)*. Apathy has been defined as a lack of motivation and responsiveness to both positive and negative events in the absence of emotional distress or negative thoughts. It can be distinguished from depression using new scales, such as the Neuropsychiatric Inventory *(17)*. Apathy is particularly frequent in PSP *(43)* and DLB *(44)*, whereas irritability predominates in CBD *(45)* and depression in PD *(44)* (*see* Chapter 11).

WHICH NEUROPSYCHOLOGICAL PATTERN CHARACTERIZES EACH OF THE MAIN PARKINSONIAN DISORDERS?

Well-characterized neuropsychological profiles can be drawn from the clustering of the cognitive and behavioral characteristics found in each parkinsonian disorder (Table 2). The absence of marked cognitive or behavioral changes makes more probable the diagnosis of PD or MSA, whereas a severe dysexecutive syndrome suggestive of a striatofrontal dysfunction reinforces the diagnosis of PSP and specific deficits related to a cortical involvement contribute to the diagnosis of CBD or DLB.

Table 2
Neuropsychological Pattern of Each Disease

	PD	MSA	PSP	PDD	CBD	DLB
Dementia						
Mattis DRS (144)	>130	>130	<130	<130	<130	<130
Fluctuations	-	-	-	+	-	+
Dysexecutive syndrome						
FAB (18)	16	14	11	11	11	11
Envt Dependency	±	±	++	+	±	+
Memory deficits						
Free recall (48)	25	22	16	12	19	10
Total recall (48)	46	46	44	42	42	34
Instrumental deficits						
Language	-	-	±	±	+	+
Gesture	-	-	±	±	++	±
Psychosis	-	-	-	+	-	++

Mean indicative values adapted from refs. *6, 22, 29, 32, 52.*

-, absent; ±, mild or discussed; +, moderate or present in a proportion of patients; ++, severe and present in a majority of patients.

Parkinson's Disease

Cognitive changes in the majority of patients with PD are subtle and mainly restricted to attentional and retrieval deficits. It is only by using appropriate neuropsychological tests that these cognitive changes can be detected. They mainly concern (a) the visuospatial domain, observed in visuospatial paradigms that require self-elaboration of the response or forward-planning capacity; (b) memory, that is, working memory and long-term memory, especially in tasks that involve self-organization of the to-be-remembered material, temporal ordering and conditional associative learning, and procedural learning; and (c) executive functions, namely concept formation and problem solving, set-maintenance and set-shifting (for a review, *see* ref. *46*).

Mood and behavioral changes are also described in PD. Depression is encountered in about 30% of patients and has been the focus of a large number of studies *(47)*. It is important to diagnose it because depression induces attention and memory disorders and, if sufficiently severe, impairs cognitive functions especially those of the executive system in relation to a significant decrease in frontal metabolism evidenced on positron emission tomography (PET) scan studies. More recently, attention has been drawn to apathy and its relation to basal ganglia disorders. Apathy is not infrequent in PD and has repercussions on cognitive functions, affect, and behavior *(48,49)*.

Unlike depression, anxiety symptoms almost always begin after the onset of the motor symptoms and are related to medication-induced on–off fluctuations and wearing-off condition in most of the cases. Drug-induced psychiatric disorders are frequently found in PD and mainly consist of hallucinations and delusions. These disorders are, however, much more frequent in PDD or DLB *(44)*.

To conclude, the clinical diagnosis of PD relies on the evidence of a parkinsonian syndrome responsive to levodopa in the absence of severe intellectual or memory dysfunction. This is the rule, at least, in the young-onset form of the disease. In the late-onset one, however, a subcorticofrontal dementia may occur after several years of evolution, which may result from the compounding effect of disease-related neuronal lesions and age-related neuronal changes *(50)*. PDD is characterized by a marked dysexecutive syndrome, accompanied by a severe amnesic syndrome with a persistent response to cuing, in the absence of true aphasia, apraxia, or agnosia, and may be difficult to diagnose. *DSM–IV* criteria of dementia *(18)* are well suited to AD, but less appropriate for PD because the severe motor deficits may themselves affect patient's autonomy. Moreover, an overestimation of the severity of cognitive impairment may result from nonspecific factors (akinesia, hypophonia, depression, anxiety, marked cognitive slowing with delay in responses, uncontrolled dyskinesias) that interfere with the evaluation of cognitive functions.

Multiple System Atrophy

Cognitive changes are mild in the parkinsonian variant of MSA (MSA-P, previously called striatonigral degeneration), at least in the early stage of the disease, before patients reach a severe akinetic state with dysarthria, which may affect the cognitive evaluation. The few studies of cognition in MSA, including the MSA-P variant, display few differences from the neuropsychological pattern of PD: some more severe deficits in the Stroop test *(51)* or in verbal fluency *(52)*. In our experience, neuropsychological testing does not help to distinguish between the two disorders. In contrast, when faced to an axial parkinsonian syndrome poorly responsive to levodopa, the absence of a severe subcorticofrontal syndrome strongly favors the diagnosis of MSA-P and decreases the probability for PSP *(22,53)*.

Psychiatric disorders have been poorly studied in MSA-P. Depression, anxiety, and emotional lability have been described, but not psychosis *(54)*.

Progressive Supranuclear Palsy

Cognitive and behavioral changes are consistent even in the early stages of the disease. Cognitive slowing and inertia occur in the first year in 52% of cases. As the disease progresses, these changes progressively worsen. From 24 patients who underwent two or more neuropsychological evaluations over time, 38% showed a global impairment at their first examination, and 70% 15 mo later. The changes may become severe enough to warrant the diagnosis of dementia, but the deficits still conform to the pattern of subcorticofrontal dementia. The dysexecutive syndrome of PSP is much more severe than that observed in any other subcortical disorders, and the memory deficit is dramatically improved in conditions that facilitate retrieval processing such as cueing and recognition.

Cognitive slowing appears evident in patients with PSP, who answer questions and solve even the simplest problems with delay. It is a genuine slowing of central-processing time unrelated to motor or affective disorders, as demonstrated experimentally using reaction time tasks *(55)* and event-related brain potentials *(56)*.

Cognitive slowing may contribute to decreased lexical fluency that is more severely impaired in patients with PSP than in patients with PD or AD, although naming is more affected in the latter *(25)*. The deficit is observed in different types of fluency, including semantic fluency, where patients have to list animal names or objects that can be found in a supermarket, phonemic fluency, where patients are required to produce words beginning with a given letter, and design fluency, where patients must produce abstract designs *(57)*.

A tendency to perseverate may also account for some of the deficits, particularly in tasks involving concept formation and shifting ability. In the Wisconsin Card Sorting Test, PSP patients complete a smaller number of categories than patients with PD or MSA-P. This lack of flexibility affects both categorical and motor sequencing, as shown by the poor performance of patients with PSP in the Trail Making Test and in the motor series of Luria. Patients with PSP also experience difficulty in conceptualization and problem-solving ability, which may account for their poor performance in similarities, interpretation of proverbs, comprehension of abstract concepts, arithmetic and lineage problems, tower tasks, and picture arrangement.

This severe dysexecutive syndrome contributes to the memory deficits and instrumental disorders observed in PSP. Short-term memory was found to be impaired using the Brown–Peterson paradigm, a working memory task in which the patients were more sensitive than controls to interference. Long-term memory is also disturbed in PSP, as shown by immediate and delayed recall of the subtests of the Wechsler Memory Scale, the Rey Auditory Verbal Learning Test, and the California Verbal Learning Test. However, when encoding is controlled by using semantic category cues and when recall is performed with the same cues, as in the Grober and Buschke procedure, recall performance of the patients dramatically improves, confirming that there is no genuine amnesia in the disease *(29)*.

Various speech disorders have been described in PSP. A severe reduction of spontaneous speech resembling dynamic aphasia is usually observed *(58)*, but abnormal loquacity has also been reported. Word-finding difficulty may occur, but it is generally less severe than in AD patients. Semantic or syntactic comprehension disorders are absent or mild. Dynamic apraxia may be found *(32)*. Bilateral apraxic errors for transitive and intransitive movements have been reported, but they are much less severe than in CBD *(59)*. Visual and auditory perception may be disturbed, but there is no evidence of object agnosia or alexia. Therefore, instrumental disorders of patients with PSP, when present, are rather considered to be a consequence of impaired executive and perceptual-motor functions or attentional disorders.

Besides cognitive impairment, patients with PSP exhibit behavioral disorders. They show severe difficulty in self-guided behavior and are abnormally dependent on stimuli from the environment. They involuntarily grasp all the objects presented in front of them; they imitate the examiner's gestures passively and use objects in the absence of any explicit verbal orders *(25)*. Such uncontrolled behaviors are never observed in normal control subjects in the absence of explicit demands and are considered to result from a lack of the inhibitory control normally exerted by the frontal lobes *(12)*. PSP patients also have difficulty in inhibiting an automatic motor program once it is initiated. This can easily be evaluated with the "signe de l'applaudissement" ["clapping sign"] *(60)*: when asked to clap their hands three times consecutively, as quickly as possible, these patients have a tendency to clap more (four or five times), sometimes initiating an automatic program of clapping that they are unable to stop, as if they had difficulty in programming voluntary acts that compete with overlearned motor skills. This sign seems to be specific to striatal dysfunction occurring in PSP *(61)*. Changes in mood, emotion, and personality have also been described: most frequently bluntness of affective expression and lack of concern about personal behavior or the behavior of others, but sometimes obsessive disorders or disinhibition with bulimia, inappropriate sexual behavior, or aggressiveness. These changes are difficult to investigate, given the lack of insight and the transient nature of the emotions expressed. The testimony of caregivers is therefore required. Administering the Neuropsychiatric Inventory (NPI) to patients' informants showed that patients with PSP exhibited apathy almost as a rule, since it was observed in 91% of the cases *(43)*. Apathy was more frequent in PSP than in any other parkinsonian syndrome.

Corticobasal Degeneration

The cognitive profile of this disease is distinct from that of PSP, because of the presence of signs suggestive of cortical involvement. Many patients present only limb clumsiness and gesture disorders at the first examination, without any—or with few—cognitive or behavioral symptoms *(26)*. In contrast, the disease may begin by other signs of cortical involvement, particularly nonfluent progressive aphasia *(62)*. Finally, a severe frontal cognitive and behavioral syndrome may initiate the disease in some patients *(63)*.

CBD is typically defined by unilateral rigidity of one arm with apraxic features, accounting for the proposition of the new term "progressive asymmetric rigidity and apraxia syndrome" *(64)*. Gesture disorders are so characteristic of the disease that the diagnosis can be suspected on the simple analysis of the motor disturbances. They consist, at first, of the patient experiencing difficulty or showing perplexity in the performance of delicate and fine movements of the fingers of one hand. At this stage, patients complain of clumsiness and loss of manual dexterity, reminiscent of "limb apraxia," variously described as "kinesthetic" in patients with lesions of the parietal cortex, or "kinetic" in patients with lesions of the premotor cortex. Systematic evaluation shows disorders of dynamic motor execution (impaired bimanual coordination, temporal organization, control, and inhibition) *(32)*. Asymmetric praxis disorders (difficulty in posture imitation, symbolic gesture execution, and object utilization) are also regularly observed, even at this stage. Ideomotor apraxia is frequent, especially in patients who have initial symptoms in the right limb, in agreement with the hypothesis of a predominant storage of "movement formulae" in the left hemisphere *(65)*. In addition, central deficits in action knowledge and mechanical problem solving have been linked to parietal lobe pathology *(66)*. "Alien limb phenomenon," in which a limb behaves in an uncooperative or foreign way, has been attributed to lesions affecting the supplementary motor area. Its occurrence, in the absence of a known callosal lesion, would be highly suggestive of the diagnosis of CBD.

Other signs of cortical involvement have been observed in CBD. Linguistic disturbances are found, consisting of word-finding difficulties, decreased lexical fluency, transcortical motor aphasia, or progressive phonetic disintegration *(67)*. These deficits resembling primary progressive nonfluent aphasia can even be an initial symptom of CBD. Neglect and visuospatial deficits have also been reported. Constructive apraxia is observed in patients with predominant right-hemisphere lesions, in relation with the well-known influence of this hemisphere on visuospatial function.

Other cognitive changes resemble the subcorticofrontal dysfunction of PSP: a dysexecutive syndrome and a learning deficit that can be alleviated by semantic cuing *(32)*. The environmental dependency syndrome, thought to be related to a release of the inhibition normally exerted by the frontal lobes on the activity of the parietal lobes *(12)*, is less frequent, however, in CBD than in PSP, probably because of the parietal lobe dysfunction in this disease. Early subcorticofrontal syndrome in CBD would predict a shorter survival.

In most of the clinical studies performed on CBD patients, the level of intellectual deterioration was mild or moderate until an advanced stage of the disease. In some cases, however, patients with a severe dysexecutive syndrome associated with memory disorders and impaired instrumental activities may reach the threshold of dementia in which both cortical and subcorticofrontal components play a role. Thus, dementia is not infrequent in CBD and may even be observed from the onset in unusual clinical presentation. In 10 out of 13 cases with pathologically proven CBD, dementia was noticed within 3 yr of onset of symptoms *(68)*.

Besides frontal lobe–type behavioral alterations, patients with CBD may present neuropsychiatric disorders. In a series of CBD patients, the NPI showed that depression, apathy, irritability, and agitation were the symptoms most commonly exhibited *(45)*. The depression and irritability of patients with CBD were more frequent and severe than those of patients with PSP, whereas patients with PSP exhibited more apathy.

Dementia With Lewy Bodies

The diagnosis of DLB can be suspected clinically on the basis of the early occurrence of a cognitive decline resembling a chronic confusional state with fluctuating cognitive signs and visual and/or auditive hallucinations in a patient with mild parkinsonism *(69)*. The rapidly progressive dementia is accompanied by aphasia, dyspraxia, or spatial disorientation, suggestive of temporoparietal dysfunction. The neuropsychological profile differs from that of patients with AD: cognitive deficits are more acute, attentional fluctuations more intense, and psychotic features appear earlier. Moreover, patients with DLB present a more severe dysexecutive impairment but less severe memory deficits than patients with AD *(34)*. The neuropsychological pattern of DLB can also be distinguished from the subcortical dementia of PD on the basis of the early occurrence of cognitive deficits and psychotic features, and the presence of linguistic and visuospatial disorders *(44,70)*. It is, however, controversial whether DLB constitutes a disorder different from or overlapping with PDD. By convention, DLB is only considered when the cognitive changes appear before, with or within 1 yr after the occurrence of parkinsonism and cannot be proposed when they appear several years later *(69)*. At a

Table 3
Diagnostic Contribution of Motor and Cognitive Deficits

	Motor Syndrome		Cognitive Changes		
	L-dopa React	Axial Synd	Severity	Occurrence	Cortical Signs
MDP	+	-	±	early	-
MSA	±	+	±	early	-
PDD	+	+	+	late	-
PSP	-	+	+	early	-
DLB	±	+	+	early	+
CBD	-	-	±	late	+

-, absent; ±, mild or discussed; +, moderate or present in a proportion of patients; ++, severe and present in a majority of patients.

first glance, the clinical and cognitive profiles of both diseases are rather different with cortical signs only in DLB. The profile of attentional impairments and fluctuating attention *(71)* and the cognitive pattern at the Mattis Dementia Rating Scale *(72)* would be, however, rather similar in PDD and DLB, and postmortem examination revealed cortical Lewy bodies in both diseases, suggesting that their differential diagnosis may be more difficult than previously thought *(73)*.

CONCLUSION

Appropriate tests may help to differentiate among diseases associated with parkinsonism (Table 3). Schematically, three categories can be distinguished. The first group is defined by mild cognitive deficits. It includes PD and MSA, which have a similar subcorticofrontal pattern of impairment. In the second group (PSP), striatofrontal dysfunction is so severe that it leads to dramatic planning, monitoring, and recall deficits, evolving toward dementia. The third group of diseases (CBD and DLB) is characterized by signs of cortical involvement with asymmetric instrumental disorders in CBD (praxic and linguistic deficits) and more severe dementia with hallucinations in DLB. The inclusion of PDD in the second or the third category is an object of debate and further studies are required.

The neuropsychological profiles described herein are valid when applied to a group of patients with a particular disease. To assess individuals is more difficult. The distribution of the subcortical lesions and the severity of the resulting denervation can vary. The association of cortical lesions with those of the basal ganglia can produce composite pictures. Age at onset and disease duration can alter the neuropsychological picture at different points in time. Nevertheless, appropriate neuropsychological testing is a useful technique for investigating the neuronal pathways affected in these diseases, and can contribute, not only to the diagnosis, but also to our understanding of the underlying pathology. A better clinical knowledge of these diseases will allow the progressive selection and elaboration of shorter and more discriminant tools. Longitudinal studies with pathological confirmation are necessary to attain this aim *(see* below).

RESEARCH TO BE DONE TO AMELIORATE THE NEUROPSYCHOLOGICAL EVALUATION OF ATYPICAL PARKINSONIAN DISORDERS

Three directions:

- Elaboration of diagnostic criteria for subcorticofrontal dementia.
- Validation of new neuropsychological tools more sensitive to the specific aspects of each disease.
- Longitudinal evaluation of each disease with the same tools to better evaluate their sensitivity and specificity and postmortem anatomo-pathological correlation when possible.

REFERENCES

1. Litvan I, Agid Y, Calne D, et al. Clinical research criteria for the diagnosis of progressive supranuclear palsy (Steele–Richardson–Olszewski syndrome): Report of the NINDS-SPSP International Workshop. Neurology 1996;47:1–9.
2. Litvan I, Agid Y, Goetz C, et al. Accuracy of clinical diagnosis of corticobasal degeneration. Neurology 1997;48:119–125.
3. Hughes AJ, Daniel SE, Kilford L, Lees AJ. The accuracy of clinical diagnosis of idiopathic Parkinson's disease: a clinicopathological study. J Neurol Neurosurg Psychiatry 1992;55:181–184.
4. Troster AI, Woods SP, Fields JA, et al. Neuropsychological deficits in essential tremor: an expression of cerebello-thalamo-cortical pathophysiology? Eur J Neurol 2002;9:143–151.
5. Mattis S. Dementia Rating Scale. Odessa, FL: Psychological Assessment Resources Inc., 1988.
6. Dubois B, Slachevsky A, Litvan I, Pillon B. The FAB: a Frontal Assessment Battery at bedside. Neurology 2000;55:1621–1626.
7. Nelson HE. A modified Card Sorting Test sensitive to frontal lobe defect. Cortex 1976;12:313–324.
8. Benton AL. Differential behavioral effects in frontal lobe disease. Neuropsychologia 1968;6:53–60.
9. Reitan RM. Validity of the Trail Making Test as an indication of organic brain damage. Percept Mot Skills 1958;8:271–276.
10. Golden CJ. Stroop Color and Word Test. Chicago: Stoelting Company, 1978.
11. Luria AR. Higher Cortical Functions in Man. New York, NY: Basic Books, 1966.
12. Lhermitte F, Pillon B, Serdaru M. Human autonomy and the frontal lobes, I: imitation and utilization behaviors: a neuropsychological study of 75 patients. Ann Neurol 1986;19:326–334.
13. Delis DC, Kramer JH, Kaplan E, Ober BA. California Verbal Learning Test: Research Edition. New York: Psychological Corporation, 1987.
14. Grober E, Buschke H. Genuine memory deficits in dementia. Dev Neuropsychol 1987;3:13–36.
15. Goodglass H, Kaplan E. The Assessment of Aphasia and Related Disorders. Philadelphia: Lea & Febiger, 1976.
16. Heilman KM, Gonzalez Rothi LJ. Apraxia. In: Heilman KM, Valenstein E, eds. Clinical Neuropsychology, 2nd ed. Oxford: Oxford University Press, 1985:131–150.
17. Cummings JL, Mega M, Gray K, Rosenberg-Thompson S, Carusi DA, Gornbein J. The Neuropsychiatric Inventory: comprehensive assessment of psychopathology in dementia. Neurology 1994;44:2308–2314.
18. American Psychiatric Association. Diagnostic and Statistical Manual of Mental Disorders, 4th ed. Washington, DC: American Psychiatric Association, 1994.
19. Quinn N, Critchley P, Marsden CD. Young onset Parkinson's disease. Mov Disord 1987; 2:73–91.
20. Cooper JA, Sagar HJ, Jordan N, Harvey NS, Sullivan EV. Cognitive impairment in early untreated Parkinson's disease and its relationship to motor disability. Brain 1991;114:2095–2122.
21. Robbins TW, James M, Lange KW, Owen AM, Quinn NA, Marsden CD. Cognitive performance in Multiple System Atrophy. Brain 1992;115:271–291.
22. Pillon B, Gouider-Khouja N, Deweer B, et al. Neuropsychological pattern of striatonigral degeneration: comparison with Parkinson's disease and progressive supranuclear palsy. J Neurol Neurosurg Psychiatry 1995;58:174–179.
23. Zetusky WJ, Jankovic J, Pirozzolo FJ. The heterogeneity of Parkinson's disease: clinical and prognostic implications. Neurology 1985;35:522–526.
24. Maher ER, Lees AJ. The clinical features and natural history of the Steele–Richardson–Olszewski syndrome (progressive supranuclear palsy). Neurology 1986;36:1005–1008.
25. Pillon B, Dubois B, Ploska A, Agid Y. Severity and specificity of cognitive impairment in Alzheimer's, Huntington's, and Parkinson's diseases and progressive supranuclear palsy. Neurology 1991;41:634–643.
26. Wenning GK, Litvan I, Jankovic J, et al. Natural history and survival of 14 patients with corticobasal degeneration confirmed at postmortem examination. J Neurol Neurosurg Psychiatry 1998;64:184–189.
27. Byrne EJ, Lennox G, Lowe J, Godwin-Austen RB. Diffuse Lewy body disease: clinical features in 15 cases. J Neurol Neurosurg Psychiatry 1989;52:709–717.
28. Tounsi H, Deweer B, Ergis AM, et al. Sensitivity to semantic cuing: An index of episodic memory dysfunction in early Alzheimer's disease. Alzheimer disease and associated disorders 1999;13:38–46.
29. Pillon B, Deweer B, Michon A, Malpand C, Agid Y, Dubois B. Are explicit memory disorders of progressive supranuclear palsy related to damage to striatofrontal circuits? Comparison with Alzheimer's, Parkinson's, and Huntington's diseases. Neurology 1994;44:1254–1270.
30. Taylor AE, Saint-Cyr JA, Lang AE. Memory and learning in early Parkinson's disease: evidence for a "frontal lobe syndrome." Brain Cogn 1990;13:211–232.
31. Buytenhuijs EJ, Berger JC, van Spaendonck KP, Horstink MW, Borm GF, Cools AR. Memory and learning strategies in patients with Parkinson's disease. Neuropsychologia 1994;32:335–342.
32. Pillon B, Blin J, Vidailhet M, et al. The neuropsychological pattern of corticobasal degeneration. Comparison with progressive supranuclear palsy and Alzheimer's disease. Neurology 1995; 45:1477–1483.
33. Massman PJ, Kreiter KT, Jankovic J, Doody RS. Neuropsychological functioning in cortical-basal ganglionic degeneration: differenciation from Alzheimer's disease. Neurology 1996;46:720–726.

34. Connor DJ, Salmon DP, Sandy TJ, Galasko D, Hansen LA, Thal L. Cognitive profiles of autopsy-confirmed Lewy body variant vs pure Alzheimer's disease. Arch Neurol 1998; 55:994–1000.
35. Brown RG, Marsden CD. "Subcortical dementia": the neuropsychological evidence. Neurosci 1988;25:363–387.
36. Leiguarda R, Merello M, Nouzeilles MI, Balej J, Rivero A, Nagues M. Limb-kinetic apraxia in corticobasal degeneration: clinical and kinematic features. Mov Disord 2003;18:49–59.
37. Maher ER, Smith EM, Lees AJ. Cognitive deficits in the Steele–Richardson–Olszewski syndrome (progressive supranuclear palsy). J Neurol Neurosurg Psychiatry 1985;48:1234–1239.
38. Ross GW, Mahler ME, Cummings JL. The dementia syndromes of Parkinson's disease: cortical and subcortical features. In: Huber SJ, Cummings JL, eds. Parkinson's Disease: Neurobehavioral Aspects. Oxford: Oxford University Press,1992:132–148.
39. Taylor AE, Saint-Cyr JA, Lang AE. Frontal lobe dysfunction in Parkinson's disease. Brain 1986;109:845–883.
40. Owen AM, Robbins TW. Comparative neuropsychology of Parkinsonian syndromes. In: Wolters EC, Scheltens P, eds. Mental Dysfunction in Parkinson's Disease. Proceedings of the European Congress on Mental Dysfunction in Parkinson's Disease held in Amsterdam on 20–23 October 1993. Amsterdam: Vrije Universiteit, 1993:221–241.
41. Cummings JL. Psychosis in basal ganglia disorders. In: E Wolters E, Scheltens P, eds. Mental Dysfunction in Parkinson's Disease. Proceedings of the European Congress on Mental Dysfunction in Parkinson's Disease held in Amsterdam on 20–23 October 1993. Amsterdam: Vrije Universiteit, 1993:257–268.
42. Litvan I, Paulsen JS, Mega MS, Cummings JL. Neuropsychiatric assessment of patients with hyperkinetic and hypokinetic movement disorders. Arch Neurol 1998;55:1313–1319
43. Litvan I, Mega MS, Cummings JL, Fairbanks L. Neuropsychiatric aspects of progressive supranuclear palsy. Neurology 1996;47:1184–1189.
44. Aarsland D, Ballard G, Larsen JP, McKeith I. A comparative study of psychiatric symptoms in dementia with diffuse Lewy body disease and Parkinson's disease with and without dementia. Int J Geriatr Psychiatry 2001;16:528–536.
45. Cummings JL, Litvan I. Neuropsychiatric aspects of corticobasal degeneration. In: Litvan I, Goetz CG, Lang AE, eds. Corticobasal Degeneration. Advances in Neurology, vol. 82. Philadelphia: Lippincott, Williams & Wilkins, 2000:147–152.
46. Pillon B, Boller F, Levy R, Dubois B. Cognitive deficits and dementia in Parkinson's disease. In: Boller F, Grafman J (eds.). Handbook of Neuropsychology, vol 6. Aging and Dementia. Amsterdam: Elsevier, 2001:311–371.
47. Slaughter JR, Slaughter KA, Nichols D, Holmes SE, Martens MP. Prevalence, clinical manifestations, etiology, and treatment of depression in Parkinson's disease. J Neuropsychiatry Clin Neurosci 2001;13:187–196.
48. Pluck GC, Brown RG. Apathy in Parkinson's disease. J Neurol Neurosurg Psychiatry 2002;73:636–642.
49. Czernecki V, Pillon B, Houeto JL, Pachon JB, Levy R, Dubois B. Motivation, reward, and Parkinson's disease: influence of dopatherapy. Neuropsychologia 2002;40:2257–2267.
50. Katzen HL, Levin BE, Llabre ML. Age of disease onset influences cognition in Parkinson's disease. J Int Neuropsychol Soc 1998;4:285–290.
51. Meco G, Gasparini M, Doricchi F. Attentional functions in multiple system atrophy and Parkinson's disease. J Neurol Neurosurg Psychiatry 1996;60:393–398.
52. Soliveri P, Monza D, Paridi D, et al. Neuropsychological follow-up in patients with Parkinson's disease, striatonigral degeneration-type multisystem atrophy, and progressive supranuclear palsy. J Neurol Neurosurg Psychiatry 2000;69:313–318.
53. Brown RG, Pillon B, Uttner I, and Members of the Neuropsychology Working Group and NNIPPS Consortium, France, Germany, UK. Cognitive function in patients with progressive supranuclear palsy and multiple system atrophy. The Movement Disorder Society, 7th International Congress of Parkinson's disease and Movement Disorders, November 2002. Book of Abstracts, 2002, P706.
54. Ghika J. Mood and behavior in disorders of the basal ganglia. In: Bogousslavsky J, Cummings JL, eds. Behavior and Mood Disorders in Focal Brain Lesions. Cambridge: Cambridge University Press, 2000:122–200.
55. Dubois B, Pillon B, Legault F, Ajid Y, Lhermitte F. Slowing of cognitive processing in progressive supranuclear palsy. A comparison with Parkinson's disease. Arch Neurol 1988;45:1194–1199.
56. Johnson R. Event-related brain potentials. In: Litvan I, Agid Y, eds. Progressive Supranuclear Palsy. Oxford: Oxford University Press, 1992:122–154.
57. Grafman J, Litvan I, Stark M. Neuropsychological features of progressive supranuclear palsy. Brain Cogn 1995;28:311–320.
58. Esmonde T, Giles E, Xuereb J, Hodges J. Progressive supranuclear palsy presenting with dynamic aphasia. J Neurol Neurosurg Psychiatry 1996;60:403–410.
59. Pharr V, Uttl B, Stark M, Litvan I, Fantie B, Grafman J. Comparison of apraxia in corticobasal degeneration and progressive supranuclear palsy. Neurology 2001;56:957–963.
60. Dubois B, Défontaines B, Deweer B, Malapani C, Pillon B. Cognitive and behavioral changes in patients with focal lesions of the basal ganglia. In: Weiner WJ, Lang AE, eds. Behavioral Neurology of Movement Disorders. Advances in Neurology, vol. 65. New York: Raven, 1995: 29–41.

61. Slachevsky A, Pillon B, Beato R, et al. The "Signe de l'Applaudissement" in PSP. American Academy of Neurology 54th Annual Meeting, Denver, April 13–20, 2002. Neurology 2002;58(Suppl 3):P06.139.

62. Kertez A, Martinez-Lage P, Davidson W, Munoz DJ. The corticobasal degeneration syndrome overlaps progressive aphasia and frontotemporal dementia. Neurology 2000;55:1368–1375.

63. Bergeron C, Davis A, Lang AE. Corticobasal ganglionic degeneration and progressive supranuclear palsy presenting with cognitive decline. Brain Pathology 1998;8:355–365.

64. Lang AE, Maragonore D, Marsden CD, et al. Movement Disorder Society Symposium on cortico-basal ganglionic degeneration (CBGD) and its relationship to other asymmetrical cortical degeneration syndromes. Mov Disord 1996;11:346–357.

65. Leiguarda R, Lees AJ, Merello M, Starkstein S, Marsden CD. The nature of apraxia in corticobasal degeneration. J Neurol Neurosurg Psychiatry 1994;57:455–459.

66. Spatt J, Bak T, Bozeat S, Patterson K, Hodges JR. Apraxia, mechanical problem solving and semantic knowledge: contributions to object usage in corticobasal degeneration. J Neurol 2002;249:601–608.

67. Frattali CM, Grafman J, Patronas N, Makhlouf MS, Litvan I. Language disturbances in corticobasal degeneration. Neurology 2000;54:990–992.

68. Grimes DA, Lang AE, Bergeron C. Dementia is the most common presentation of corticobasal ganglionic degeneration. Neurology 1999;53:1969–1974.

69. Barber R, Panikkar A, McKeith IG. Dementia with Lewy bodies: diagnosis and management. Int J Geriatr Psychiatry 2001;16(Suppl 1):12–18.

70. Gnanalingham K, Byrne E, Thornton A, Samabrook MA, Bannister P. Motor and cognitive function in Lewy body dementia: comparison with Alzheimer's and Parkinson's disease. J Neurol Neurosurg Psychiatry 1997;62:243–252.

71. Ballard CG, Aarsland D, McKeith I, et al. Fluctuations in attention: PD dementia vs DLB with parkinsonism. Neurology 2002;59:1714–1720.

72. Aarsland D, Litvan I, Salmon D, Galasko D, Wentzel-larsen T, Larsen JP. Performance on the dementia rating scale in Parkinson's disease with dementia and dementia with Lewy bodies: comparison with progressive supranuclear palsy and Alzheimer's disease. J Neurol Neurosurg Psychiatry 2003;74:1215–1220.

73. Apaydin H, Ahlskog JE, Parisi JE, Boeve BF, Dickson DW. Parkinson disease neuropathology: later-developing dementia and loss of the levodopa response. Arch Neurol 2002;59:102–112.

13

Role of Praxis in Diagnosis and Assessment

Ramón Leiguarda

INTRODUCTION

Apraxia is a term used to denote a wide spectrum of higher-order motor disorders that result from acquired brain disease affecting the performance of skilled and/or learned movements with or without preservation of the ability to perform the same movement outside the clinical setting in the appropriate situation or environment. The disturbance of purposive movements cannot be termed apraxia, however, if the patient suffers from any elementary motor or sensory deficit (i.e., paresis, dystonia, ataxia) that could fully explain the abnormal motor behavior or if it results from a language comprehension disorder or from dementia *(1,2)*. Nevertheless, praxic errors are at present much better defined clinically and kinematically and may be distinguished from other nonpractic motor behaviors *(3,4)*. Praxic disturbances may affect specific parts of the body (i.e., limb apraxia, facial apraxia) and may involve both sides of the body (i.e., ideational [IA] and ideomotor apraxias [IMA]), preferentially one side (i.e., limb-kinetic apraxia [LKA]), or alternatively, interlimb coordination, as in the case of gait apraxia.

Apraxias are poorly recognized but common disorders that can result from a wide variety of focal or diffuse brain damage. There are two main reasons why apraxia may go unrecognised. First, many patients with apraxia, particularly IMA, show a voluntary-automatic dissociation, which means that the patient does not complain about the deficit because the execution of the movement in the natural context is relatively well preserved, and the deficit appears mainly in the clinical setting when the patient is required to represent explicitly the content of the action outside the situational props. Secondly, although in apraxic and aphasic patients specific functions are selectively affected, language and praxic disturbances frequently coexist and the former may interfere with the proper evaluation of the latter *(5)*.

Limb apraxia is a hallmark clinical feature and one of the presenting clinical manifestations of corticobasal degeneration (CBD); it is seen in about 80% of patients *(6–12)*. Roughly 25 and 65% of patients with Parkinson's disease (PD) and progressive supranuclear palsy (PSP), respectively, may exhibit limb apraxia *(13)*. It also seems to be a relatively frequent motor-behavioral deficit in Huntington's disease (HD) *(14)*, but very rare indeed or an absent clinical feature in multiple system atrophy (MSA) *(13,15)*. Moreover, not only the incidence of apraxia differs among different diseases but also and more important, there are specific features that characterize the praxic deficits observed in some of these diseases. Therefore, the adequate assessment of apraxia is essential because it may lead to the proper clinical diagnosis of the disease. In the present chapter, I will first describe the assessment of apraxia and the classical types of praxic disorders, as well as their putative physiopathological mechanisms, to thereafter present the characteristic features of the praxic deficit observed in patients with atypical parkinsonisms, in particular CBD and PSP.

From: *Current Clinical Neurology: Atypical Parkinsonian Disorders*
Edited by: I. Litvan © Humana Press Inc., Totowa, NJ

Table 1
Assessment of Limb Praxis

Intransitive movements	nonrepresentational (e.g., touch your nose, wriggle your fingers). representational (e.g., wave goodbye, hitch-hike)
Transitive movements	(e.g., use a hammer, use a screwdriver) under verbal, visual, and tactile modalities
Imitation of meaningful and meaningless movements, postures, and sequences.	
Tool[a] selection tasks	to select the appropriate tool to complete a task, such as a hammer for a partially driven nail
Alternative tool selection tasks	to select an alternative tool such as pliers to complete a task as pounding a nail, when the appropriate tool (i.e., hammer) is not available
Mechanical problem-solving task	(e.g., select the appropriate one of three novel tools for lifting a wooden cylinder out of a socket).
Multiple step tasks	(e.g., prepare a letter for mailing)
Gesture recognition and discrimination tasks	to assess the capacity to comprehend gestures, verbally (to name gestures performed by the examiner), as well as nonverbally (to match a gesture performed by the examiner with cards depicting the tool/object[b] corresponding to the pantomime); and to assess the ability to discriminate a well- from a wrongly performed gesture.

[a]Tool: implement with which an action is performed (e.g., hammer, screwdriver).
[b]Object: the recipient of the action (e.g., nail, screw).
From refs. *2*, *3*, and *39*.

ASSESSMENT OF LIMB PRAXIS

A systematic evaluation of praxis is critical in order: (a) to identify the presence of apraxia; (b) to classify correctly the nature of praxis deficit according to the errors committed by the patient and through the modality by which the errors are elicited; and (c) to gain an insight into the underlying mechanism of the patient's abnormal motor behavior (Table 1).

Patients' performance should be assessed in both forelimbs if an elementary motor-sensory deficit does not preclude testing the limb contralateral to the damaged hemisphere. Intransitive and transitive movements should be evaluated. The sample of intransitive gestures tested has to include movements performed toward or on the body (salute, crazy) vs away from the body (okay sign, wave goodbye), repetitive (beckon, go away) or nonrepetitive (sign of victory), since the dimensions of spatial location relative to the body and repetitiveness contribute to the overall complexity of the task and may be differentially influenced by the disorder. Likewise, several types of transitive movements have to be evaluated since it is not an uncommon finding that apraxic patients perform some but not all movements in a particularly abnormal fashion and/or that individual differences appear in some but not all components of a given movement. Therefore, the dissimilar complexity and features of transitive movements should also be considered in order to analyze and interpret praxic errors accurately. For instance, (a) movements may or may not be repetitive in nature (e.g., hammering vs using a bottle opener to remove the cap); (b) an action may be composed of sequential movements (e.g., to reach for a glass and take it to the lips in drinking); (c) a movement may primarily reflect proximal limb control (transport) such as transporting the wrist when carving a turkey, proximal and distal limb control such as reaching and grasping a glass of water, or primarily distal control as when the patient is asked to manipulate a pair of scissors; and (d) movements may be performed in the peripersonal space (e.g., carving a turkey), in body-centered space (e.g., tooth brushing), or require the integration of both, such as the drinking action *(4)*.

Transitive movements should be assessed under different modalities, including verbal, visual (seeing the tool or the object upon which the tool works), and tactile (using actual tools and/or objects) as well as on imitation, since impairment can be seen under some performance conditions but not others. Nevertheless, the most sensitive test for apraxia is asking patients to pantomime to verbal commands because this test provides the least cues and is almost entirely dependent on stored movement representations. In addition to the specific praxis assessment tasks listed in Table 1, it is important to evaluate other cognitive functions, since they may contribute to understand the neural mechanisms of some praxic deficits. Thus, the evaluation of conceptual tool and object knowledge, such as correct naming, descriptions, or correct associative semantic judgement, may help to discern the specific nature of an object/tool use deficit. Knowledge about body image, body structural description, and the effects of changing viewing angles when matching gestures as well as tests of body rotation are necessary to establish the involvement of the processes coding the dynamic position of the body parts of self and others, that is, the body schema, which may also facilitate the comprehension of the praxic defect *(16)*.

Analysis of a patient's performance is based on both accuracy and error patterns (Table 2). One problem with many investigations of apraxia is that the analysis of gestural performance may be insensitive to subtle apraxic deficits, which may have led to an uncorrected estimation about the frequency and degree of apraxia. Therefore, detailed error analysis is crucial to unveil and to properly classify an apraxic disorder. The patient with IA has difficulty mainly is sequencing actions (e.g., making coffee) and exhibits content errors or semantic parapraxias (e.g., mimicking a hammer use when requested to use a knife). Ideomotor apraxia patients show primarily temporal and spatial errors, which are more evident when they perform transitive than intransitive movements. Errors in LKA represent slowness, coarseness, and fragmentation of finger and hand movements *(4,17)*.

Three-dimensional analysis of different types of movements has provided a better and more accurate method to capture objectively the nature of the praxis errors observed in clinical examination. Patients with IMA, due to focal left-hemisphere lesions *(18,19)*, different asymmetric cortical degenerative syndromes *(20,21)*, CBD, PSP, and PD *(21,22)*, have shown several kinematic abnormalities of dissimilar severity, such as slow and hesitant build-up of hand velocity, irregular and non-sinusoidal velocity profiles, abnormal amplitudes, alterations in the plane of motion and in the direction and shapes of wrist trajectories, decoupling of hand speed and trajectory curvature, and loss of interjoint coordination. All these studies have evaluated gestures, such as carving a turkey or slicing a loaf of bread, which mainly explore the transport or reaching phase of the movement. However, the majority of transitive gestures included in most apraxia batteries include prehension (reaching and grasping) movements that reflect proximal (transport) as well as distal limb control (grasping). The kinematic analysis of aiming movements in apraxic patients has demonstrated spatial deficits, in particular when visual feedback is unavailable *(23)*, whereas the analysis of prehension movements in CBD has shown disruption of both the transport and grasp phases of the movements as well as transport-grasping uncoupling *(21,24)*. Furthermore, the study of manipulating finger movements in patients with CBD and LKA has disclosed several abnormalities, which more fully unveil the nature of the deficit. The workspace is highly irregular and of variable amplitude, there is breakdown of the temporal profiles of the scanning movements, and overall, a severe interfinger uncoordination is found *(25)*. Thus, exploration into the kinematics of reaching, grasping, and manipulating may provide useful information regarding the specific neural subsystems involved in patients with different types of limb praxic disorders.

Most of the errors exhibited by IMA cases are equally seen in left- or right-hemisphere-damaged patients when they pantomime nonrepresentative and representative/intransitive gestures, but are observed predominantly in left-hemisphere-damaged patients when they pantomime transitive movements, because it is this action type that is performed outside the natural context *(25)*. The left hemisphere would not only be dominant for the "abstract" performance (i.e., pantomiming to verbal command) of transitive movements but also for learning and reproducing novel movements such as meaningless actions and sequences *(27)*, as well as for action selection *(28)* and motor attention *(29)*.

Table 2
Types of Praxis Errors

I. Temporal

S = sequencing: some pantomimes require multiple positionings that are performed in a characteristic sequence. Sequencing errors involve any perturbation of this sequence including addition, deletion, or transposition of movement elements as long as the overall movement structure remains recognizable.

T = timing: this error reflects any alterations from the typical timing or speed of a pantomime and may include abnormally increased, decreased, or irregular rate of production or searching or groping behavior.

O = occurrence: pantomimes may involve either single (i.e., unlocking a door with a key) or repetitive (i.e., screwing in a screw with a screwdriver) movement cycles. This error type reflects any multiplication of single cycles or reduction of a repetitive cycle to a single event.

II. Spatial

A = amplitude: any amplification, reduction, or irregularity of the characteristic amplitude of a target pantomime.

IC = internal configuration: when pantomiming, the fingers and hand must be in specific spatial relation to one another to reflect recognition and respect for the imagined tool. This error type reflects any abnormality of the required finger/hand posture and its relationship to the target tool. For example, when asked to pretend to brush teeth, the subject's hand may close tightly into a fist with no space allowed for the imagined toothbrush handle.

BPO = body-part-as-object: the subject uses his or her finger, hand, or arm as the imagined tool of the pantomime. For example, when asked to smoke a cigarette, the subject might puff on his or her index finger.

ECO = external configuration orientation: when pantomiming, the fingers/hand/arm and the imagined tool must be in a specific relationship to the "object" receiving the action. Errors of this type involve difficulties orienting to the "object" or in placing the "object" in space. For example, the subject might pantomime brushing teeth by holding his hand next to his mouth without reflecting the distance necessary to accommodate an imagined toothbrush. Another example would be when asked to hammer a nail, the subject might hammer in differing locations in space reflecting difficulty in placing the imagined nail in a stable orientation or in a proper plane of motion (abnormal planar orientation of the movement).

M = movement: when acting on an object with a tool, a movement characteristic of the action and necessary to accomplish the goal is required. Any disturbance of the characteristic movement reflects a movement error. For example, a subject, when asked to pantomime using a screwdriver, may orient the imagined screwdriver correctly to the imagined screw but instead of stabilizing the shoulder and wrist and twisting at the elbow, the subject stabilizes the elbow and twists at the wrist or shoulder.

III. Content

P = perseverative: the subject produces a response that includes all or part of a previously produced pantomime.

R= related: the pantomime is an accurately produced pantomime associated in content with the target. For example, the subject might pantomime playing a trombone for a target of a bugle.

N = nonrelated: the pantomime is an accurately produced pantomime not associated in content with the target. For example, the subject might pantomime playing a trombone for a target of shaving.

H = the patient performs the action without benefit of a real or imagined tool. For example, when asked to cut a piece of paper with scissors, he or she pretends to rip the paper.

IV. Other

C = concretization. The patient performs a transitive pantomime not on an imagined object but instead on a real object not normally used in the task. For example, when asked to pantomime sawing wood, the patient pantomimes sawing on his or her leg.

NR = no response.

UR= unrecognizable response: the response shares no temporal or spatial features of the target.

From ref. *3*.

TYPES OF LIMB APRAXIA

Ideational Apraxia

Liepmann defined IA as impairment in tasks requiring a sequence of several acts with tools and objects *(17)*. However, other authors use the term to denote a failure to use single tools appropriately *(2)*. To overcome this confusion, Ochipa et al. have suggested restricting the term IA to a failure to conceive a series of acts leading to an action goal, and introduced the term conceptual apraxia (CA) to denote loss of diverse types of tool-action knowledge *(30)*. However, patients with IA not only fail on tests of multiple-object use but also when using single objects *(31)*; thus, a strict difference between IA and CA is not always feasible. Therefore, according to Freund *(5)* and following Liepmann *(17)*, IA could be defined as a deficit in the conception of the movement so that the patient does not know what to do *(5,17)*. Patients with IA or CA exhibit primarily content errors, in the performance of transitive movements (Table 2) or semantic parapraxias (e.g., use a comb as a toothbrush). They may also lose the ability to associate tools with the object that receives their action; thus, when a partially driven nail is shown, the patient may select a pair of scissors rather than a hammer from an array of tools to perform the action. Not only are patients unable to select the appropriate tool to complete an action, but they may also fail to describe a function of a tool or point to a tool when the function is described by the examiner, even when the patient names the tool properly when shown to him or her and may have difficulties in matching objects for shared purposes as well as being unable to solve novel mechanical problems *(30,32)*. However, selection and application of novel tools seem to rely on the direct influence of structure on function, which in turn would depend upon a parietal lobe-based system of nonsemantic sensorimotor representation that may be triggered by object affordance rather than conceptual knowledge *(33)*. These patients may also be impaired in the sequencing of tool/object use *(2,17)*. Patients with IA or CA are disabled in everyday life, because they use tools/objects improperly, misselect tools/objects for an intended activity, perform a complex sequential activity (e.g., make express coffee) in a mistaken order, or entirely fail to complete the task *(3)*.

Ideational apraxia was traditionally allocated to the left parieto-occipital and parieto-temporal regions *(2,17)*, although frontal and frontotemporal lesions may also cause CA *(32)*. Nevertheless, semantic or conceptual errors are particularly observed in patients with temporal lobe pathology (e.g., semantic dementia); these patients are impaired in the use of objects for which they have lost conceptual knowledge *(34)*.

Ideomotor Apraxia

IMA has been defined as "a disturbance in programming the timing, sequencing and spatial organisation of gestural movements" *(3)*. Patients with IMA exhibit mainly temporal and spatial errors. Movements are incorrectly produced but the goal of the action can usually be recognized, though on occasion performance is so severely deranged that the examiner cannot recognize the movement. Transitive movements are more affected than intransitive ones on pantomiming to command. Patients usually improve on imitation when performance is compared to responses to verbal command and acting with tools/objects is usually carried out better than pantomiming their use, but even so, movements are not normal *(2,3)*.

IMA is commonly associated with damage to the parietal association areas, less frequently with lesions of the premotor (PM) cortex and supplementary motor area (SMA), and usually with disruption of the intrahemispheric white matter bundles interconnecting them, as well as with basal ganglion and thalamic damage *(4)*. Although small lesions of the basal ganglia may cause IMA, most patients sustained larger lesions to the basal ganglia and/or thalamus together with the internal capsule and periventricular and peristriatal white matter, interrupting association fibers, in particular those of the superior longitudinal fasciculus and frontostriatal connections *(35)*. Most studies examining possible clinico-anatomical correlation for IMA have found a strong association of apraxia with large cortico-subcortical lesions in the suprasylvian, perirolandic region of the left-dominant hemisphere, but no specific lesion site correlating with apraxia *(4,36)*. However, a recent study using quantitative structural image analysis to determine the location and greatest lesion overlap in patients with left-hemisphere stroke and IMA—as determined by assessing spatiotemporal errors on imitating meaningful and meaningless gestures—found that damage to the left middle frontal gyrus (BA 46, 9, 8, and 6) and left superior and inferior parietal cortex surrounding the intraparietal sulcus (BA 7, 39, and 40) more commonly produce IMA than damage to other areas *(37)*. Some patients with apraxia commit errors only, or predominantly, when the movement is evoked by one but not all modalities (modality-specific or dissociation apraxias) *(3)*. The most frequent dissociation found in apraxic patients is related with movement and posture imitation; unlike those with the classic form of ideomotor apraxia, these patients are more impaired when imitating than when pantomiming to command, or could not imitate but performed flawlessly under other modalities. Deficits may be restricted solely to the imitation of meaningless gestures with preserved imitation to meaningful gestures *(38,39)*.

IMA may coexist with LKA; nevertheless, both types of apraxia can be clinically distinguished on the basis of the following aspects. First, though usually asymmetric IMA is invariably bilateral, whereas LKA is always contralateral to the affected hemisphere. Second, all movements in LKA, whether symbolic or nonsymbolic, intransitive or transitive, are affected irrespective of the modality (i.e., verbal, visual, tactile) through which they are evoked, whereas in IMA intransitive are less compromised than transitive movements and these are unequally involved depending on the modality under which they are tested. Third, finger and hand movements and posture errors typical of LKA are readily distinguished from temporospatial errors (i.e., external configuration, movement trajectory, body part as object) exhibited by patients with IMA, which predominantly involve the arm and hand rather than the fingers, although internal configuration type of errors may be common to both disorders; however, such errors in IMA are usually characterized by abnormal postures and movements of the whole hand but fail to reflect the severe distortion of individual finger movements and postures so typical of LKA *(25)*.

There are several possible physiopathological mechanisms underlying the ideomotor type of praxic deficits that depend on lesion location and are disclosed by the specific gesture evaluated and the modality through which they are evoked. The most common subgroup of patients with IMA are those who usually commit spatial and temporal errors when performing transitive as well as intransitive symbolic or communicative movements under all modalities of elicitation (i.e., verbal command, imitation, seeing and handling the object), although performance usually improves on imitation and with object use. These patients also exhibit errors when imitating meaningless postures and novel motor sequences. We originally suggested that the crucial underlying neural mechanism in this group of IMA patients was a disruption of the parallel parieto-frontal circuits and their subcortical connection *(4)*, subserving the computations required to translate an action goal into movements by integrating sensory input with central representation of actions based on prior experience *(37)*. Damage to circuits devoted to sensorimotor transformation for grasping, reaching, and posture, for transformation of body part location into information required to control body part movements, as well as for coding extrapersonal space, would produce incorrect finger and hand posture and abnormal orientation of the tool/object, inappropriate arm configuration, and faulty movement orientation (with respect to both the body and the target of the movement in extrapersonal space) as well as movement trajectory abnormalities. These patients usually complain of disability on everyday activities.

In another subgroup of patients, the ideomotor type of praxic deficits may be a result of disruption of action selection processes *(28)*; they exhibit spatial and temporal errors predominantly when pantomiming to verbal command with the left hand, i.e., outside the appropriate context; they markedly improve on imitation and performance is usually normal when handling the object. These patients do not complain of difficulties in everyday activities; there is an automatic-voluntary dissociation.

There are also patients who are particularly impaired when using familiar objects and on tasks requiring selection and use of novel tools, but with preserved semantic knowledge of object functions

(33,40,41). Most patients with difficulties in mechanical problem solving (novel tool selection), which unveil the incapacity to infer functions from structure, also fail on pantomime of object use and commit errors on actual use of familiar tools, so they are disabled in everyday life. Errors are mainly of the spatiotemporal type, usually characterized by marked abnormal hand postures, but without semantic parapraxias *(33,40)*. Defective tool selection is particularly seen in patients with parietal damage *(41)*. Thus, this type of apraxic deficit can be ascribed to the disruption of a parietal lobe base system specialized for visuomotor interaction with the environment, which may be triggered by visual and perhaps tactile object affordance *(33,40)*.

Neuroimaging and neuropsychological data support the existence of at least two partly independent routes for imitation of meaningful and meaningless actions *(42,43)*. Briefly, (a) imitation of a meaningful movement/posture activates the dorsal pathway extending to the premotor cortex from MT/V5 (BA 18/19) and always involving the inferior parietal lobule (IPL), with the participation of the temporal cortex; whereas (b) imitation of a meaningless movement/posture also involves the dorsal pathway, with predominant activation of the left IPL (area 40), with hand gestures, and right intraparietal sulcus (IPS) and medial visual association areas (BA 18/19) for finger gestures; the lateral occipito-temporal junction is activated by both hand and finger postures *(42,43)*. Thus, imitation of a meaningful movement/posture uses the temporal cortex for gestural meaning, whereas the imitation of a meaningless ones seems to be more body part specific; the gesture's visual appearance is translated into categories of body part relationships mainly in the left IPL when hand postures are to be imitated, and the addition of the right occipito-parietal cortex for precise perceptual analysis and spatial attention for finger gesture imitation *(43,44)*.

Finally, patients with IMA may exhibit several types of errors such as omissions, deletions, additions, transpositions, and perseverations when performing sequential limb movements *(1–4)*. Abnormalities in movement sequencing have been reported more commonly in patients with left parietal lobe lesions, but also with left frontal and basal ganglion involvement. Several clinical studies have shown that impairment in sequencing is particularly apparent for the left-hemisphere-damaged patients when the tasks place demands on memory; or when the temporal aspects of sequencing are considered, when patients have to select movements in a sequence, or when the process of motor attention is involved *(4)*.

Which are the putative roles of basal ganglia in praxis? All the motor areas of the cerebral cortex, as well as of the prefrontal cortex, send projections as part of parallel segregated circuits to diverse regions of the basal ganglia *(46)*. The parietal areas reciprocally interconnected with such areas of the motor cortex making up the parietofrontal circuits also send extensive projections to the basal ganglia *(47)*. Thus, it seems likely that the basal ganglia are an integral part of a series of specialized circuits for sensorimotor transformation. As regards reaching, Burnod et al. have recently suggested that the basal ganglia could provide the cortex with gating signals capable of triggering the sequence of movements at the appropriate time and in the appropriate order, when several outputs are possible for a given task and when the decision has to be made between concurrent tasks *(48)*. In addition to their putative roles in sensorimotor transformation for reaching and grasping, the basal ganglia may participate in praxis in other ways, whether in the selection of the kinematics and direction of arm movements, by encoding peripersonal space for limb movements, by contributing to diverse mechanisms of response selection, including inhibition of competing input from cortex, or by acting as an integral part of brain systems involved in the representation of action sequences *(36)*.

Limb-Kinetic Apraxia

This type of apraxia was originally described by Kleist, who called it "innervatory apraxia" to stress the loss of hand and finger dexterity owing to inability to connect and to isolate individual innervation and attributed it to damage to the PM cortex *(47,48)*. The deficit is mainly confined to finger and hand movements contralateral to the lesion, regardless of its hemispheric side, with preservation of power and sensation. Manipulatory finger movements are predominantly affected, but in most cases all movements, whether complex or routine, independently of the evoking modality, are coarse and mutilated. The virtuosity given to movements by practice is lost and they become clumsy, awkward, and "amorphous." Fruitless attempts usually precede wrong movements, which in turn are often contaminated by extraneous movements. Imitation of finger postures is also abnormal and some patients use the less affected or normal hand to reproduce the requested posture. The deficit clearly interferes with daily activities *(25,47,49,50)*.

LKA has been scantily reported with focal lesions. There are basically two potential explanations: first, most PM lesions also involve the precentral cortex, so that the contralateral paresis or paralysis precludes expression of the praxic deficit; and second, bilateral activation of the PM cortex is often observed with unilateral movements. Thus, a unilateral lesion would not be enough for the deficit to become clearly manifested, since bilateral involvement would be most likely necessary. As a matter of fact, all recently pathologically confirmed cases of LKA had undergone a degenerative process such as CBD and Pick's disease, involving frontal and parietal cortices, or predominantly, the PM cortex *(4)*.

DISTRIBUTION OF THE APRAXIAS IN OTHER BODY PARTS

Face apraxia refers to a disturbance of upper and lower face movements not explained by elementary motor or sensory deficits. Patients exhibit spatial and temporal errors of similar quality to those observed in the limbs when performing representational and nonrepresentational movements such as sticking out the tongue, blowing out a match, smiling, blowing a kiss, showing the teeth, blinking the left or right eye, looking down, or sucking on a straw. Although lower face or buccofacial apraxia often coexists with Broca's aphasia, and thus is more frequently observed with left-hemisphere lesions, in particular involving the frontal and central operculum, insula, centrum semiovale, and basal ganglia *(51)*, it can also be seen with lesions confined to left posterior cortical regions as well as with right-hemisphere damage *(52)*.

Apraxia of eyelid opening has been defined as a nonparalytic inability to open the eyes at will, in the absence of visible contraction of the orbicularis oculi muscle owing to involuntary palpebral levator inhibition *(53)*. Many patients show a forceful contraction of the frontalis muscle and/or a backward thrusting of the head on attempting eyelid opening and use different types of maneuvers to help open the eyes including opening the mouth, massaging the lids, and manual elevation of the lids. However, apraxia of eyelid opening can hardly be considered a "true" apraxia but rather a subclinical form of blepharospasm because (a) most patients exhibit abnormal persistence of orbicularis oculi activity detected at electromyography; (b) it is commonly associated with overt blepharospasm; and (c) it is particularly observed in patients with basal ganglion disorders *(54)*.

Truncal or whole body apraxia is a disorder of axial movements neither attributable to elementary motor (e.g., extrapyramidal) or sensory deficit nor to dementia. Patients have difficulties dancing or turning around and may be unable to adapt the body to the furniture; patients have difficulty sitting down in a chair, showing hesitation, sitting in a wrong position (e.g., on the edge of the chair) and in incorrect directions (e.g., facing the back of the chair). When lying in bed, their body is not aligned parallel to the major axis of the bed and they place the pillow in an unusual position. Patients may have minimal or no difficulty in standing or getting up, in contrast to features of some basal ganglion disorders such as parkinsonism. Truncal apraxia is seen with bilateral hemispheric damage involving the parietal or parieto-temporal cortex or affecting parieto-frontal connections *(55,56)*.

THE NATURE OF APRAXIA IN ATYPICAL PARKINSONISMS

Corticobasal Degeneration

Limb apraxia is a prominent clinical feature and the most widely studied cognitive deficit in CBD. It is almost invariably asymmetric and more frequent in patients whose initial symptoms were in the right limb (left-hemisphere dominance) than in the left limb (right-hemisphere dominance), in agreement with the fact that most right-handers develop IMA as well as IA predominantly with left-hemisphere lesions *(10,21)*. In CBD, IMA is the most common type of limb praxic deficit. Patients exhibit temporal and spatial errors more frequently when performing transitive than intransitive movements. Spatial errors such as incorrect positioning of the hand to grasp the tool (internal configuration errors), difficulty in orienting the hand with respect to the body and the tool with respect to the object receiving the tool's action in extrapersonal space (external configuration errors), abnormal movement trajectories, and timing errors were those more frequently found whereas body-part-as-object and sequencing errors were not so common (videotapes 1 and 2). All these patients have difficulties when imitating meaningful and meaningless postures and movements and some exhibited even more errors when imitating than pantomiming gestures to command. Thus, there is no consistent pattern when comparing performance on gestures to command with imitation and the use of the real object/tool, since some patients may have more difficulties when imitating than pantomiming gestures and occasional patients perform worse when handling the objects than pantomiming to command or the reverse, show a dramatic improvement when holding the tool/object *(10,21,57–63)*.

CBD patients may not only exhibit spatiotemporal errors when handling objects but in addition may often show impairment in the selection and usage of novel tools in the mechanical problem-solving task *(63)*; on occasion, they may also commit content errors and perform wrongly the sequential arm movement test, displaying errors such as omissions, misuse, mislocations, and intrusions, as well as pantomime recognition deficits *(10)*. Therefore, a consistent production or executive deficit may frequently combine with mechanical problem-solving impairment and less commonly with semantic knowledge breakdown as well *(63)*. However, disruption of conceptual knowledge and IA (content errors or semantic parapraxias) are uncommon in CBD patients; this type of praxic deficit is particularly observed in patients with cognitive impairment including aphasia and dementia *(10,64)*, or in the presence of primitive reflexes *(10)*. The combination of several types of limb praxic deficits relevant for object use clearly explains why CBD patients are far more disabled in everyday life than any patients with other atypical parkinsonian diseases.

The limb-kinetic type of apraxia has also been frequently reported in CBD *(21,25,49,50,65)*. Patients show slow, awkward, and mutilated finger and hand movements; on occasion, movements are amorphous and contaminated by extraneous movements. Difficulties are particularly evident with motor skills requiring fractionated or sequential fingers movements. Imitation of finger postures is abnormal and some patients use the other hand to move the abnormal one to reproduce the requested posture. At times, the fingers and hand remain in an abnormal posture while the patient performs other tasks with the contralateral hand. Perseveration of postures and movements is commonly observed. Patients are aware of the poor performance but are unable to correct their errors *(21)* (video 3). Kinematic studies in these patients showed severe disruption of manipulative movements with marked interfinger uncoordination *(25)*.

The prevalence of facial (buccofacial) apraxia in CBD is unclear. Pillon et al. *(58)* found orofacial apraxia in their patients though milder than limb apraxia. We only demonstrated orofacial apraxia in 4 out of 16 patients *(21)* but other authors failed to mention it in their studies *(57,59)*. However, in a recent study by Ozsancak et al., orofacial apraxia, as evaluated by means of simple and sequential gestures, was found in 9 of 10 patients with a clinical diagnosis of CBD *(66)*. Lastly, truncal apraxia has also been recorded in CBD patients *(56)*.

The brunt of the pathology in CBD is located in the superior frontal gyrus, which is more often affected than the middle and inferior gyri, the pre- and postcentral regions, the anterior corpus callosum, the caudate, putamen, globus pallidus, thalamus, and substantia nigra, with atypical asymmetric distribution *(67)*. Functional brain-imaging studies have disclosed decreased metabolism in the frontoparietal region, particularly in the superior prefrontal cortex, lateral and mesial premotor areas, in the sensorimotor and parietal association cortices, as well as in the caudate, lenticular, and thalamic regions with striking interhemispheric asymmetries, the hemisphere contralateral to the more affected limb proving more severely involved *(68)*.

The particular distribution of the pathological process in patients with CBD clearly explains the disruption of the cortical and subcortical components of the multiple, parallel, sensorimotor transformation circuits, and hence the severe IMA observed in these patients. An action selection deficit owing to involvement of parietal and premotor cortices and basal ganglia on the left hemisphere may further aggravate the praxic disorder. Moreover, frequent breakdown in mechanical problem solving as a result of parietal lobe pathology and the occasionally observed impairment in object-specific conceptual knowledge, probably related to temporofrontal pathology, explain the IA disorder and the rarely observed gesture recognition deficit *(10)*. The limb-kinetic type of praxic deficit is mainly related to damage to the circuits subserving grasping and manipulation; in addition, it may be further aggravated by derangement of independent finger movements and by dysfunction of somatosensory control of manipulation *(25)*. Involvement of inhibitory areas in the inferior and superior frontal gyri and damage to subcortical structures may reduce facilitation of inhibitory interneurones, causing defective cortical inhibition, which in turn may also interfere with the selection and control of finger muscle activity. We found reduced cortical inhibition, as reflected by a short silent period, in CBD patients with LKA *(25)*. Finally, an associated sensory defect because of parietal damage may interfere with the kinaesthetic and tactile information necessary for somatosensory control of manipulation; however, as a defect in somaesthesis may not be present and parietal involvement may be absent in patients with CBD, LKA may basically result from bilateral dysfunction of nonprimary cortical motor areas *(25)*.

APRAXIA IN OTHER ATYPICAL PARKINSONIAN DISORDERS

Although frequent *(13,62)*, limb apraxia is not a clinical feature included in the diagnostic criteria of PSP *(69,70)*. Bilateral IMA mainly for transitive movements, slightly asymmetric, and almost always more pronounced in the nondominant limb is the most consistent finding. IMA for intransitive movements is usually less frequent and severe. The praxic deficit is particularly evident when patients pantomime under verbal command, improve on imitation and more with the use of the tool/object *(13,58,62)*. Spatial (i.e., internal and external configuration, trajectory) are more prominent than temporal errors (i.e., hesitation, delay); perseveration and sequencing errors are uncommon; content errors are not found *(13)* (video 4). PSP patients rarely develop abnormal motor behavior compatible with LKA *(13,58)*. Ideomotor apraxia seems to correlate significantly with cognitive deficits as measured with Mini Mental State Examination (MMSE). Recognition of pantomimes is normal, but on occasion patients may fail on the multiple-step task *(13)*. Facial (orofacial) apraxia may be found, though it may be difficult to interpret the exact nature of the abnormal performance given the unique facial appearance usually present in PSP patients *(13)*. In turn, apraxia of eyelid opening is common and may be very disabling *(70)*.

The ideomotor type of praxic deficit is qualitatively similar in PSP and PD patients, though more frequent and usually more severe in the former *(13)*, as also demonstrated by the use of three-dimensional motor analysis *(22)*.

Limb apraxia is not observed *(13)*, or exceptionally found with MSA *(15)* and has not been systematically studied in patients with demential Lewy bodies (DLB). However, we have found IMA with predominantly imitative deficits in three patients with mild to moderate DLB as clinically diagnosed by McKeith et al. criteria *(72)* (*see also* Abeleyra et al., in preparation) (videotape 5).

Limb apraxic deficits in PSP seem to correlate with low MMSE, whereas in PD they appear to correlate with neuropsychological tests reflecting frontal lobe dysfunction and visuospatial cognitive deficits *(13)*. Since focal lesions restricted to the basal ganglia only rarely cause apraxia and patients with MSA, which is characterized by severe basal ganglion and slight cortical involvement, fail to exhibit praxic deficits, we suggested that apraxia in PSP and PD reflect combined corticostriatal dysfunction *(13)*. Cortical degeneration is now recognized to be common in PSP and identified mainly in the cingulate, superior, and medial frontal gyri *(72,74)*. However, in PSP patients with limb apraxia cortical pathology may predominate in motor cortices or coexist with Alzheimer's disease pathology *(74)*.

Table 3

Comparison of Different Types of Praxic Disorders Among CBD, PSP, MSA, and DLB

Praxic Disorder	CBD	PSP	MSA	DLB
Limb Apraxia				
Ideomotor				
Transitive gestures				
Pantomiming to verbal commands	+++	++	+/–	++
Object use	++	–	–	+
Imitation	++	+	–	+/++
Intransitive gestures	++	+/–	–	+
Asymmetry	+++	+	+	+
Voluntary / automatic dissociation	++	–	–	–
Mechanical problem solving	+++	–	–	Unknown
Ideational				
Conceptual errors	+	–	–	–
Sequencing	+	+/–	–	–
Limb-kinetic	+++	+	–	–
Pantomime recognition / discrimination	+	–	–	Unknown
Facial apraxia	++	+	–	–
Apraxia eyelid opening	+/–	++	–	–
Truncal apraxia	++	Unknown	Unknown	Unknown

+++, severe; ++, moderate; +, mild; –, absent.

In PD patients, impairment of neuropsychological tests reflecting frontal lobe function correlated with reduced fluorodopa uptake in caudate nucleus *(75)*, and proton magnetic resonance spectroscopy (MRS) may detect temporoparietal cortical dysfunction in nondemented patients with PD *(76)*. Therefore, it seems plausible that the subgroups of PD patients developing limb apraxia and more severe kinematic abnormalities in the spatial precision of movements and interjoint coordination *(22)* are those with greater caudate nucleus and frontal lobe involvement with or without temporoparietal cortical dysfunction *(36)*. Thus, basal ganglion pathology *per se* would not cause overt apraxia. However, when combined with dysfunction of the cortical components of the neural circuits devoted to sensorimotor transformation, sequencing, and action selection, various types of praxic deficits would become clinically manifested *(36)*.

CONCLUSION

The main clinical features of the diverse types of praxic disorders observed in CBD, PSP, MSA, and DLB are summarized in Table 3. IMA and LKA are both particularly severe in CBD. Compared with PSP and DLB, IMA is more asymmetric and intransitive movements are invariably affected. CBD patients are more severely disabled with object use, although some may exhibit deficits mainly in gesture imitation. Unlike PSP and probably DLB, there is no voluntary automatic dissociation in CBD. Ideational praxic deficit and pantomime recognition defects may be seen in CBD but neither in PSP nor in MSA. Facial apraxia is more severe in CBD than in PSP and truncal apraxia has not yet been properly described in the latter. Apraxia of eyelid opening is a salient feature in PSP. Further studies are required to characterize the nature of apraxia in DLB.

However, the design of clinical studies regarding specific apraxic deficits in patients with atypical parkinsonism first requires improving our knowledge of the neural components that subserve the multiple processes involved in limb praxis and their precise distribution over the large cortical and subcortical network of neural structures, made up by many interrelated systems pertaining to dissimilar levels of action representation. In turn, this will require the separate study of the functional neuroanatomical correlates of each of the different manifestations of limb apraxia (i.e., pantomiming to verbal command, imitation of meaningful and meaningless movements, tool/object use in real life, everyday actions, and action recognition, among others). Thus, a more refined cognitive neuroanatomical model of limb praxis will guide an accurate assessment and diagnosis of apraxia subtypes and allow developing rehabilitation programs to target specific apraxic deficits.

SOME AREAS FOR FUTURE RESEARCH IN LIMB PRAXIS

1. Clinical and kinematical studies correlating disruption of specific spatiomotor or sensorimotor processes with lesion location in patients with restricted focal cortical and subcortical damage.
2. Functional neuroimaging studies exploring distinct praxis processes in normal subjects and in patients with specific apraxic deficits and acute lesions, as well as following recovery.
3. To study the clinical implications of several cognitive processes, such as motor attention and action selection, in patients with diverse subtypes of apraxic disorders.
4. To study through motor imagery the "premovement" neural processes involved in limb praxis.

VIDEO LEGENDS

*Sequence 1
Patient with CBD and severe bilateral IMA.

1. When pantomiming to use a screwdriver, the patient exhibits diverse types of errors: irregular production rate, variable amplitude, abnormal arm posture, and abnormal hand orientation. Instead of twisting at the elbow, the patient moves the wrist and/or fingers. Performance improves with object use but remains abnormal.
2. When requested to pantomime drinking a glass of water, he places the hand in an abnormal posture, and there is no place for the glass between the hand and the mouth.

*Sequence 2
Patient with CBD and bilateral IMA.

Note the abnormal posture of the hand, the incorrect orientation, and variable amplitude of the movement when pantomiming to use a hammer.

*Sequence 3
Patient with CBD and unilateral LKA.

Note the difficulty for coordinating finger movements when requested to oppose the thumb against the other fingers, to throw pebbles, and to make the sign of victory. Movements are slow, coarse, and fragmented and on occasion amorphous. Finger selection is wrong and fingers fail to act in concert. He uses his normal hand to achieve the requested posture.

*Sequence 4
Patient with PSP and IMA.

When pantomiming to use a screwdriver, the patient shows hesitation, uses the wrong joints (wrist instead of elbow), and perseveres in the wrong movement.

*Sequence 5
Patient with Lewy Body dementia, IMA, and severe imitation deficits.
Note the abnormal hand configuration and position when requested to imitate meaningless hand posture.

REFERENCES

1. Roy EA, Square PA. Common considerations in the study of limb, verbal, and oral apraxia. In Roy EA, ed. Neuropsychological Studies of Apraxia and Related Disorders. Amsterdam: North-Holland, 1985:111–161.
2. De Renzi E. Apraxia. In Boller F, Grafman J, eds. Handbook of Neuropsychology. Amsterdam: Elsevier Science , 1989:245–263.
3. Rothi LJ, Heilman KM, eds. Apraxia: The Neuropsychology of Action. East Sussex: Psychology Press, 1997.

4. Leiguarda R, Marsden CD. Limb apraxias: higher-order disorders of sensorimotor integration [Review]. Brain 2000;123:860–879.
5. Freund HJ. The apraxias. In: Asbury Ak, McKhann GM, McDonald WJ, eds. Diseases of the Nervous System. Clinical Neurobiology, 2nd ed. Philadelphia: Saunders, 1992:751–767.
6. Rebeiz JJ, Kolodny EH, Richardson EP. Corticodentatonigral degeneration with neuronal achromasia. Arch Neurol 1968;18:20–33.
7. Riley DE, Lang AE, Lewis A, et al. Corticobasal ganglionic degeneration. Neurology 1990;40:1203–1212.
8. Gibb WR, Luthert PJ, Marsden CD. Corticobasal degeneration. Brain 1989;112:1171–1192.
9. Rinne J, Lee M, Thompson P, Marsden CD. Corticobasal degeneration: A clinical study of 36 cases. Brain 1994;117:1183–1196.
10. Leiguarda R, Lees AJ, Merello M, Starkstein S, Marsden CD. The nature of apraxia in corticobasal degeneration. J Neurol Neurosurg Psychiatry 1994;57:455–459.
11. Kampoliti K, Goetz CG, Boeve BF, et al. Clinical presentation and pharmacological therapy in corticobasal degeneration. Arch Neurol 1998;55:957–961.
12. Litvan I, Agid Y, Goetz C, et al. Accuracy of the clinical diagnosis of corticobasal degeneration: a clinicopathologic study. Neurology 1997;48:119–125.
13. Leiguarda R, Pramstaller P, Merello M, Starkstein S, Lees AJ, Marsden CD. Apraxia in Parkinson's disease, progressive supranuclear palsy, multiple system atrophy, and neuroleptic induced parkinsonism. Brain 1997;120:75–90.
14. Hamilton JM, Haaland KY, Adair JC, Brandt J. Ideomotor limb apraxia in Huntington's disease: implications for corticostriatal involvement. Neuropsychologia 2003;41:614–621.
15. Monza D, Soliveri P, Radice D, et al. Cognitive dysfunction and impaired organization of complex mobility in degenerative parkinsonian syndromes. Arch Neurol 1998;55:372–378.
16. Buxbaum LJ, Giovannetti, Libon D. The role of the dynamic body schema in praxis: evidence from primary progressive apraxia. Brain Cog 2000;44:166–191.
17. Liepmann H. Apraxia. Ergeb Gesamten Medizin 1920;1:516–543.
18. Clark MA, Merians AS, Kothari A, et al. Spatial planning deficits in limb apraxia. Brain 1994;117:1093–1106.
19. Poizner H, Clark MA, Merians AS, Macauley B, Gonzalez Rothi LJ, Heilman KM. Joint coordination deficits in limb apraxia. Brain 1995;118:227–242.
20. Leiguarda R, Starkstein S. Apraxia in the syndromes of Pick Complex. In Kertesz A, Muñoz DG, eds. Pick's Disease and Pick Complex. New York: Wiley-Liss, 1998:129–143.
21. Leiguarda R, Merello M, Balej J. Apraxia in corticobasal degeneration. In: Litvan I, Goetz CG, Lang A, eds. Corticobasal Degeneration and Related Disorders. Advances in Neurology, vol. 82. Philadelphia: Lippincott Williams &Wilkins, 2000:103–121.
22. Leiguarda R, Merello M, Balej J, Starkstein S, Nogués M, Marsden C. D. Disruption of spatial organization and interjoint coordination in Parkinson's disease, progressive supranuclear palsy and multiple system atrophy. Mov Disord 2000;15:627–640.
23. Haaland KY, Harrington DL, Knight RT. Spatial deficits in ideomotor limb apraxia. A kinematic analysis of aiming movements. Brain 1999;122:1169–1182.
24. Caselli RJ, Stelmach GE, Caviness JV, et al. A kinematic study of progressive apraxia with and without dementia. Mov Disord 1999;14:276–287.
25. Leiguarda R, Merello M, Nouzeilles MI, Balej J, Rivero A, Nogués M. Limb-kinetic apraxia in corticobasal degeneration: clinical and kinematic features. Mov Disord 2003;18(1):49–59.
26. Haaland KY, Flaherty D. The different types of limb apraxia errors made by patients with left vs. right hemisphere damage. Brain Cog 1984;3:370–384.
27. Rapcsak SZ, Ochipa C, Beeson PM, Rubens A. Apraxia and the right hemisphere. Brain Cog 1993;23:181–202.
28. Rushworth MFS, Nixon PD, Wade DT, Renowden S, Passingham RE. The left hemisphere and the selection of learned actions. Neuropsychologia 1998;36:11–24.
29. Rushworth MFS, Krams M, Passingham RE. The attentional role of the left parietal cortex: the distinct lateralization and localization of motor attention in the human brain. J Cogn Neurosci 2001;13(5):698–710.
30. Ochipa C, Rothi LJG, Heilman KM. Conceptual apraxia in Alzheimer's disease. Brain 1992;115:1061–1071.
31. De Renzi E, Lucchelli F. Ideational apraxia. Brain 1988;113:1173–1188.
32. Heilman KM, Maher LH, Greenwald L, Rothi LJ. Conceptual apraxia from lateralized lesions. Neurology 1997;49:457–464.
33. Hodges JR, Spatt J, Patterson K. "What" and "how": Evidence for the dissociation of object knowledge and mechanical problem-solving skills in the human brain. Proc Natl Acad Sci USA 1999;96:9444–9448.
34. Hodges J, Bozeat S, Lambon Ralph M, Patterson K, Spatt J. The role of conceptual knowledge in object use evidence from semantic dementia. Brain 2000;123:1913–1925.
35. Pramstaller PP, Marsden CD. The basal ganglia and apraxia [Review]. Brain 1996;119:319–340.
36. Leiguarda R. Limb-apraxia: cortical or subcortical. Neuroimage 2001;14:S137–S141.

37. Haaland KY, Harington DL, Knight RT. Neural representations of skilled movement. Brain 2000;123:2306–2313.
38. Ochipa C, Rothi LJ, Heilman KM. Conduction apraxia. J Neurol Neurosurg Psychiatry 1994;57:1241–1244.
39. Goldenberg G, Hagmann S. The meaning of meaningless gestures: a study of visuo-imitative apraxia. Neuropsychologia 1997;35:333–341.
40. Spatt J, Bak T, Bozeat S, Patterson K, Hodges JR. Apraxia, mechanical problem solving and semantic knowledge. Contribution to object usage in corticobasal degeneration. J Neurol 2002;249:601–608.
41. Goldenberg G, Hagmann S. Tool use and mechanical problem solving in apraxia. Neuropsychologia 1998;36:581–589.
42. Grèzes J, Costes N, Decety J. The effects of learning and intention on the neural network involved in the perception of meaningless actions. Brain 1999;122:1875–1887.
43. Hermsdörfer J, Goldenberg G, Wachsmuth C, et al. Cortical correlates of gesture processing: clues to the cerebral mechanisms underlying apraxia during the imitation of meaningless gestures. Neuroimage 2001;14:149–161.
44. Goldenberg G, Straus S. Hemisphere asymmetries for imitation of novel gestures. Neurology 2002;59:893–897.
45. Alexander GE, DeLong MR, Strick PL. Parallel organization of functionally segregated circuits linking basal ganglia and cortex. Ann Rev Neurosci 1986;9:357–381.
46. Yeterian EH, Pandya DN. Striatal connections of the parietal association cortices in rhesus monkeys. J Comp Neurol 1993;332:175–197.
47. Kleist K. Kortikate (innervatorische) Apraxie. J Psychiat Neurol 1907;25:46–112.
48. Kleist K. Gehirnpathologische und lokalisatorische Ergebnisse: das Stirnhirn im engeren Sinne und seine Störungen. Zeitschrift ges Neurologie und Psychiatrie 1931;131:442–448.
49. Denes G, Mantovan MC, Gallana A, Cappelletti JV. Limb-kinetic apraxia. Mov Disord 1998;13:468–476.
50. Blasi V, Labruna L, Soricelli A, Carlomagno S. Limb-kinetic apraxia: a neuropsychological description. Neurocase 1999;5:201–211.
51. Raade AS, Rothi LJG, Helman KM. The relationship between buccofacial and limb apraxia. Brain Cog 1991;16:130–146.
52. Bizzozero I, Costato D, Della Sala S, Papagno C, Spinnler H, Venneri A. Upper and lower face apraxia: role of the right hemisphere. Brain 2000;123:2213–2230.
53. Boghen D. Apraxia of lid opening: a review. Neurology 1997; 48:1491–1494.
54. Tozlovanu V, Forget R, Iancu A. Boghen D. Prolonged orbicularis oculi activity. A major factor in apraxia of lid opening. Neurology 2001;57:1013–1018.
55. Kase CS, Troncoso JF, Court JE, Tapia JF, Mohr JP. Global spatial disorientation: clinico-pathologic correlations. J Neurol Sci 1977;34:267–278.
56. Okuda B, Tanaka H, Kawabata K, Tachibana H, Sugita M. Truncal and limb apraxia in corticobasal degeneration. Mov Disord 2001;16:760–762.
57. Jacobs DH, Adair JC, Macauley BL, Gold M, Gonzalez Rothi LJ, Heilman KM. Apraxia in corticobasal degeneration. Brain Cogn 1999;40:336–354.
58. Pillon B, Blin J, Vadailhet M, et al. The neuropsychological pattern of corticobasal degeneration: comparison with supranuclear palsy and Alzheimer's disease: Neurology 1995;45:1477–1483.
59. Blondel A, Eustache F, Schaeffer S, Maire R, Lechvalier B, Sayette V. Etudie clinique et cognitive de l'apraxie dans l'atrophie cortico-basale. Rev Neurol (Paris) 1997;153:737–747.
60. Peigneux P, Van Der Linden M, Andres-Benito P, Sadzot B, Franck G, Salmon E. Exploration neuropsychologique et par imagerie fonctionnalle cérébrale d'une apraxia visuo-imitative. Rev Neurol (Paris) 2000;156(5):459–472.
61. Graham NL, Zenan A, Young AW, Patterson K, Hodges JR. Dyspraxia in a patient with corticobasal degeneration: the role of visual and tactile inputs to action. J Neurol Neurosurg Psychiatry 1999;67:334–344.
62. Pharr V, Utte B, Stark M, Litvan I, Fantie B, Grafman J. Comparision of apraxia in corticobasal degeneration and progressive supranuclear palsy. Neurology 2001;56:957–963.
63. Spatt J, Bak T, Bozeat S, Patterson K, Hodges JR. Apraxia, mechanical problem solving and semantic knowledge. Contributions to object usage in corticobasal degeneration. J Neurol 2002;249:601–608.
64. Kertesz A, Martínez-Lange P, Davidson W, Muñoz DG. The corticobasal degeneration syndrome overlaps progressive aphasia and frontotemporal dementia. Neurology 2000;14:1368–1375.
65. Okuda B, Tachibana H, Kawabata K, Takeda M, Sugita M. Slowly progressive limb-kinetic apraxia with a decrease in unilateral cerebral blood flow. Acta Neurol Scand 1992;86:76–81.
66. Ozsancak C, Auzou P, Hannequin D. Dysarthria and orofacial apraxia in corticobasal degeneration. Mov Disord 2000;15:905–910.
67. Dickson DW, Liu WK, Reding HK, Yen SH. Neuropathologic and molecular considerations, in corticobasal degeneration and related disorders. In: Litvan I, Goetz CG, Lang AE, eds. Advances in Neurology, vol. 82. Philadelphia: Lippincott Williams & Wilkins, 2000:9–28.
68. Brooks DJ. Functional imaging studies in corticobasal degeneration, in corticobasal degeneration and related disorders. In: Litvan I, Goetz CG, Lang AE, eds. Advances in Neurology, vol. 82. Philadepphia: Lippincott Williams & Wilkins, 2000:209–216.

69. Litvan I, Agid I, Calue D, et al. Clinical research criteria for the diagnosis of progressive supranuclear palsy (Steele–Richardson–Olszewski syndrome): report of the NINDS–SPSP international workshop. Neurology 1996;47:1–9.
70. Nath U, Ben-Shlomo Y, Thomson RG, Lees AJ, Buru DJ. Clinical features and natural history of progressive supranuclear palsy. Neurology 2003;60:910–916.
71. McKeith IG, Galasco D, Kosaba K. Consensus guidelines for the clinical and pathological diagnosis of dementia with lewy bodies (DLB): report of the consortium on DLB international work shop. Neurology 1996;47:113–124.
72. Daniel SE, de Bruin V, Lees AJ. The clinical and pathological spectrum of Steele–Richardson–Olszewski syndrome (progressive supranuclear palsy): a reappraises [Review]. Brain 1995;118:759–770.
73. Abeleyra C, Marello, M, Manes F, Leiguarda R. Defective imitation of limbgestures in Lewy body dementia, in preparation.
74. Bergeron C, Pollamen MS, Weyer L, Lang AE. Cortical degeneration in progressive supranuclear palsy. A comparison with cortical-basal ganglionic degeneration. J Neuropathol Exp Neurol 1997;56:726–734.
75. Rinne J, Portin R, Routtinen H, et al. Cognitive impairment and the brain dopaminergic system in Parkinson disease. Arch Neurol 2000;57:470–475.
76. Hu MTM, Taylor-Robinson SD, Ray Chaudhuri K, et. al. Evidence for cortical dysfunction in clinically non-demented patients with Parkinson's disease: a proton MR spectroscopy study. J Neurol Neurosurg Psychiatry 1999;67:20–26.

14

Role of Visuospatial Cognition Assessment in the Diagnosis and Research of Atypical Parkinsonian Disorders

Paolo Nichelli and Anna Magherini

INTRODUCTION

Visuospatial abilities play a pivotal role in our daily living. Indeed, our survival depends, to a great extent, on our ability to navigate sensory space. This means our ability to use spatial maps dependent on visual, tactile, and auditory information to form and guide motor programs. Visuospatial abilities are complex brain operations requiring integration of occipital, parietal, and frontal lobe function, as well as the contribution of subcortical structures. Consequently, it is not surprising that visuospatial skills are often impaired in diseases with movement disorders—an impairment that depends both on the type and on the stage of the disease in question.

Investigating visuospatial skills is helpful not only for differentiating among various diseases with movement disorders, but also for analyzing the source of patients' everyday life impairment, as this can, in turn, generate useful pointers for the development of remedial strategies.

Also, in the detailed analysis of visuospatial performance in patients with movement disorders, particular care must be taken to separate motor from cognitive components. In the devising of neuropsychological tools that can help us to gain a new insight into cortical and subcortical contributions to these activities, this represents a constant challenge.

The aim of this chapter is to review the contribution of visuospatial assessment in the differential diagnosis of movement disorders. After presenting a classification of visuospatial skills, we will discuss the evidence of visuospatial dysfunction in Parkinson's disease (PD) and in the various atypical parkinsonian disorders. We will then advance our own proposal for visuospatial assessment in this group of patients.

CLASSIFICATION OF VISUOSPATIAL DISORDERS

Visuospatial activities have been classified according to different criteria. O'Keefe and Nadel (1) divided them on the basis of the sensorimotor responses of persons moving in their own environment, classifying them as "position (or egocentric) responses" when subjects use their body as a reference, as "cued responses" when movements are guided by external cues, and as "place responses" when movements are guided by relationships between external references. Grüsser (2) classified the space around the subject as consisting of three functionally different "subspaces": the *body surface*, the *grasping space*, and the *distal space*. It seems that different brain regions are responsible for directing attention to different regions of space. For example, experimental studies on monkeys have local-

From: *Current Clinical Neurology: Atypical Parkinsonian Disorders*
Edited by: I. Litvan © Humana Press Inc., Totowa, NJ

ized the representation of personal space to parietal area 7a and postarcuate frontal area 6. Peripersonal space seems to be encoded by parietal areas 7a and 7b and frontal areas 6 and 8. Extrapersonal space is represented in frontal area 8, parietal area 7a, and the superior colliculus *(3)*.

For the purpose of this review we present a classification of visuospatial abilities that divides them into spatial perception, visuomotor coordination, visuospatial attention, perception of size, spatial memory, and visuospatial imagery. Although any classification of this sort is somewhat arbitrary, we believe it is useful to list the different domains to be examined during neuropsychological testing. Furthermore, the various parkinsonian disorders can affect some of these skills while leaving others intact.

Spatial Perception

Spatial perception is the ability to analyze the spatial relationships both between the stimulus and the observer and between different stimuli. Visual, tactile, and auditory information can contribute to spatial perception. However, visual-perceptual skills predominate disproportionately over the other perceptual skills. According to current theories *(4,5)* visual information is processed by two distinct pathways: the occipito-temporal (ventral) pathway, which conveys information about shape and patterns, and the occipito-parietal (dorsal) pathway, which is involved in spatial analysis. Three fundamental aspects of spatial perception are stimulus localization, perception of line orientation, and depth perception. All can be impaired after brain damage.

Stimulus Localization

Different methods have been proposed to examine stimulus localization. Warrington and Rabin *(6)* presented two cards, either simultaneously or in succession, and asked subjects to evaluate whether the position of a point was the same or different on the two cards. Hannay et al. *(7)* projected onto a screen one or two dots for 300 ms, then, after a 2-s delay, they presented a display showing 25 numbers in different positions: the subject's task was to read aloud the numbers corresponding to the correct dot positions. The performances of right-posterior brain-damaged patients are typically impaired.

Perception of Line Orientation

The most widely used instrument in the assessment of this component of visuospatial perception is the Benton's Judgement of Line Orientation Test *(8)*. This test requires subjects to identify the orientation of a pair of lines on an 11-line multiple-choice display. A number of studies have used this test to assess visuospatial abilities in PD patients, and given varying results. Boller et al. *(9)* demonstrated that PD patients with a normal IQ are impaired in line orientation judgement. Similar results were obtained by Goldenberg et al. *(10)*. However, Richards, Cote, and Stern *(11)* did not find differences between 14 patients with idiopathic PD and 12 normal controls matched for age and education. Similarly Levin and colleagues *(12,13)* did not identify line orientation abnormalities in their mildly and moderately affected PD patients. In a large sample (76 patients and an equal number of matched normal controls), Montse et al. *(14)* demonstrated that, in line orientation judgment, PD patients make proportionally more complex intraquadrant and horizontal line errors, but fewer simple intraquadrant errors than controls. Girotti et al. *(15)* reported that when PD patients were divided into those with and those without dementia, the line orientation test was one of the few tasks that distinguished the nondemented PD patients from controls, whereas many tasks differentiated the demented PD patients from controls. In conclusion, the line orientation test is often abnormal in PD patients but may be normal in patients in whom the disease is less advanced.

Depth Perception

The perception of depth is based on both monocular and binocular sources *(16,17)*. Monocular cues include apparent size of familiar objects, texture and brightness gradient, linear perspective, occluding contours, shading, and monocular parallax (i.e., the ability to analyze disparate retinal images successively produced by the same object on the retina). Stereopsis is the ability to discriminate depth on the basis of binocular information. Stereoacuity is commonly tested using the quantitative Titmus stereotest, which requires the subject, who is wearing appropriately polarized lenses, to detect circles that appear on a closer plane with respect to the background. Global stereopsis is tested using Julez's random dot stereograms, geometric forms that can—if viewed stereoscopically—be seen from below or above the background plane.

Both the striate and the peristriate and parietal visual areas play a pivotal role in depth perception based on binocular cues *(18–20)*. To the best of our knowledge, no systematic study of depth perception in patients with parkinsonian disorders has to date been conducted.

Visuomotor Coordination

The impaired ability to reach for visually presented stimuli, not related to motor, somatosensory, visual-acuity, or visual-field deficits, is named *optic (visuomotor) ataxia*. To detect subtle visuomotor ataxia, the subject is asked to reach for an object that requires a precision grip (i.e., true opposition of thumb and index finger). In a clinical setting, the examiner will hold the object (a coin or a paper clip) by its edge while the patient attempts to grasp it between the index finger and thumb. In the most severe cases, the disorder is apparent even when the patient is fixating when reaching for the object. More frequently, the impairment is only apparent when the target is located at the periphery of the visual field, or when the patient is not allowed to look at his reaching arm *(21)*.

Reaching for an object is a movement that can be divided into two components: the proximal component (the reaching or transportation phase) and the distal component (the grasping or manipulation phase). This dichotomy has received particular attention because it reveals the difference between two pathways of visuospatial perception respectively devoted to determining the target coordinates in a body-centered space (the occipito-parietal pathway) and to computing shape, size, and weight of the target object (the occipito-temporal pathway) *(4)*.

Examining in detail the different components of reaching for an object requires frame-by-frame analysis of a video recording of the movement. Studies of visuomotor coordination in PD patients show no deficit in the "transportation" and in the "manipulation" components of the reaching-to-grasp movement *(22)*. On the contrary, PD patients demonstrate some dysfunction when they are required to respond appropriately to modification of object size and location *(23,24)*. Rearick et al. *(25)* demonstrated that global features observed in five-digit grasping are preserved in PD patients. However, more subtle aspects of the coordination between digits, as revealed by frequency domain analysis, are not preserved, possibly owing to action tremor.

Visuospatial Attention

When we move in the environment, we are confronted with a vast array of sensory information that the nervous system cannot deal with on an equal basis. Thus, the brain must select which information to process. Visuospatial attention refers to the processes engaged by the nervous system in the selection of relevant information from the mass of information presented by the visual environment.

The neglect syndrome has been characterized as a failure to report, respond to, or orient attention to novel or meaningful stimuli presented to the side opposite to a brain lesion, when this failure cannot be attributed to either sensory or motor defects *(26)*. In severe neglect, patients may behave as though one-half of the world had suddenly ceased to exist. They may fail to eat the food on the left side of their plate, or omit to shave, groom, and dress the left side of the body. In other patients, the symptoms are much subtler and might not be detected by observation of their spontaneous behavior. In the latter cases, special maneuvers may be needed in order to disclose the presence of neglect.

Cancellation tasks are often used for diagnosis of the syndrome. Albert *(27)* developed the simplest form of these tasks, a test in which subjects are required to cancel each item in an array of 40 scattered lines. In the Bells Test *(28)*, rather than scattered lines, 315 small, silhouetted objects are distributed in a pseudorandom manner on the page, with 35 bells scattered among them. Despite their apparently random positions, the bells are actually arranged in seven columns with five bells to a column. The subjects' task is to circle the bells as quickly as possible. Similarly, Mesulam *(29)*, with the purpose of enhancing the method's sensitivity to inattention to the right as well as to the left side, devised verbal and nonverbal cancellation tasks consisting of four sheets, two (nonverbal) with various shapes, and two (verbal) with randomized letters.

A different technique for investigating unilateral inattention is to ask the patient to bisect a line. In the traditional version, patients are asked to mark the midpoint of a horizontal line drawn on a sheet of paper. Normal subjects tend to bisect the line 1–2 mm left of its true center *(30,31)*. Patients with left hemineglect tend to place their mark rightward of the center. To interpret this finding, both space representation and premotor impairment have been invoked. Assuming perceptual factors are responsible, bisection toward the right would be a result of underestimation of the length of the left part of the line, whereas the influence of premotor factors would result in reduced action toward the left (directional hypokinesia) or in reduced amplitude movement toward the left (directional hypometria). Different modifications of the line bisection paradigm have been devised to disentangle the representational and premotor component of bisecting a line. In the landmark test *(32)*, the subject's task is to point to the shorter side of a correctly prebisected line: when patients choose the left side as the shorter their neglect can be attributed to a representational deficit. In the line extension test *(33)*, patients are requested to extend a horizontal line leftward to double its original length. If premotor factors dominate, they should cause a relative left underextension (compared to the right) because of left hypokinesia-hypometria.

Animal studies have shown a central role of the dopaminergic system in the regulation of directional attention. Some authors believe that these circuits are purely premotor *(34)*, whereas others maintain that dopaminergic circuits also mediate perceptual aspects *(35,36)*. In humans, some case reports have shown significant improvement of patients with chronic neglect syndrome after therapy with dopaminergic drugs *(37,38)*. Asymmetric degeneration of the dopaminergic nigrostriatal pathways is the major mechanism underlying the motor symptoms of PD.

A number of early studies have found that patients with left hemi-PD tend to neglect the left side of space *(13,39–41)*. However, the rightward bias of left hemi-PD is at most mild and some authors *(42,44)* were not able to demonstrate visual neglect in their patients. In a more recent study Lee et al. *(43)* examined PD patients with two line bisection tasks. One was a conventional paper- and pencil-test. In the other, subjects were required to bisect a line presented on a computer screen by adjusting the position of a cursor operated by two pushbuttons, one in each hand. No significant differences were found on the paper-and-pencil test. On the contrary, predominantly left-sided PD patients showed significant rightward bias in their setting of the cursor. The same bias was found when subjects repeated the task with the pushbuttons switched between the hands, so that the cursor was moved to the left by the right hand and vice versa, thus suggesting a perceptual rather than a premotor bias.

Adopting a different approach, Ebersbach et al. *(44)* demonstrated that patients with predominantly right-sided PD, as well as normal controls, were more likely to start visual exploration on the left side of texture arrays requiring attentive oculomotor scanning. On the contrary, PD patients with predominantly left-sided disease showed a rightward directional bias for initial exploration, a behavior similar to that demonstrated by patients affected by visuospatial neglect following cortical lesions of the right parietal lobe.

Work by Posner and colleagues *(45)* has provided a theoretical framework within which the different processes involved in orienting attention might be interpreted. They distinguish between two distinct modes of spatial orienting. "Overt" orienting involves turning the eyes toward a particular location of interest, whereas "covert" orienting requires attention to be shifted to this location while the eyes remain fixated elsewhere. Several studies have examined overt orienting in PD patients, and there is a general consensus that internal control of eye movements through voluntary saccades (remembered, delayed, and predictive saccades and antisaccades) is deficient in PD patients *(46–49)*. At the same time there appears to be no deficit in PD patients for purely reflexive (or visually guided) saccades *(46,47,50,51)*. Thus, studies in PD patients suggest deficits in voluntary (internal) control, but no deficit in reflexive (external) control of overt orienting of attention. To evaluate covert orienting, subjects, all the time maintaining central fixation, are asked to press a key as soon as a peripheral stimulus appears. At the beginning of each trial subjects are given a visual cue, meant to draw their attention to the side where the stimulus is to appear. In most trials the target is presented where it was cued to appear (valid trials), but in some it appears on the opposite side (invalid trials). As it might be expected, normal subjects are significantly faster on valid than invalid trials. Patients with parietal lesions, even if nearly as good as normal controls on valid trials, are severely impaired on invalid trials, which require them to respond to a stimulus contralateral to the lesion. This impairment indicates defective attentional disengagement from a cued location. A number of researchers have reported conflicting results regarding the performance of PD patients in covert orienting tasks, with some studies reporting small covert orienting effects in PD patients *(52,53)*, and others finding no difference *(54–56)*. It turns out that, as for overt attention, it is important to distinguish between voluntary and reflexive control of spatial attention. Voluntary covert attention is assessed by using symbolic cues (e.g., arrows) presented at a central location. The purpose of these cues is to make the subject shift his or her attention to the intended location. Reflexive covert attention is evaluated by presenting a brief cue stimulus in the visual periphery that automatically draws attention to the location of the cue. A couple of studies *(57,58)* compared voluntary and reflexive covert control of spatial attention in PD patients. Both reported relatively normal cuing effects with voluntary (i.e., internally controlled) cues at short (250 ms) and intermediate (500 ms) intervals between cue and target. However, in PD patients facilitatory effects were eliminated with longer (800–1000 ms) intervals, thus demonstrating defective voluntary control of covert attention. On the contrary, PD patients appear to be significantly faster than control subjects on covert reflexive orienting *(59)*. Progressive supranuclear palsy (PSP) and corticobasal degeneration patients (CBD) can show specific impairments in visual-orienting tasks that will be discussed later in this chapter.

Perception of Size

In human perception theories, it is commonly assumed that size is processed independently of shape. Experimental animal studies in monkeys *(60,61)* have confirmed that object size is processed in the brain independently of other stimulus characteristics. An important consequence of this distinction between form and size concerns our general ability to identify objects of different size as identically shaped. The disorder of size perception of which patients are aware is termed *dysmetropsia* (also called dysmegalopsia or metamorphopsia). Objects can appear either shrunk (micropsia) or enlarged (macropsia), compared to their actual size *(62)*. Size perception can be also distorted in visuospatial neglect *(63)*, but in this case patients are unaware of the symptom.

It has recently been demonstrated *(64)* that predominantly left PD patients, probably because of right-hemisphere impairment, perceive a rectangle presented in the left and upper visual space as smaller compared to rectangles presented in different regions of space. The same authors *(65)* have raised the possibility that perceptual errors might have a causal role in determining PD patients' difficulties in negotiating doorways, narrow corridors, and other confined spaces. They asked PD patients to judge whether or not they would fit through a life-size schematic doorway shown on a large screen. Predominantly left PD patients obtained an increased ratio between the door width for which 50% of the judgments were positive and the width of the participant's body at the shoulders. This finding was interpreted as suggesting that the visual representation of the doorway (or of its relationship to perceived body size) is compressed in left PD. However, the clinical implications of this finding are not yet clear, since the authors could not demonstrate a causal role of these perceptual distortions in freezing episodes experienced by PD patients.

Spatial Memory

Within *spatial memory* it is possible to identify *short-* and *long-term* components.

Short-Term Spatial Memory

According to a widely accepted theoretical model *(66)* short-term memory is viewed as a "working memory," where information can be temporarily stored and accessed for use in a wide range of cognitive tasks. Working memory, on the other hand, is made up of an attentional system of limited capacity (the so-called "central executive") and of at least two "slave" subsystems: the "articulatory loop" and the "visuospatial sketchpad," respectively dealing with phonological and visuospatial items. In this scheme, the visuospatial sketchpad would appear to keep visuospatial information "on line" for subsequent processing by the "central executive." This hierarchical organization could allow the concurrent performance of phonological and visual tasks as long as they remain within the capacity limits of the two "slave" systems, whereas the "central executive" would be called upon should the information to be processed exceed these limits. A series of neuroimaging studies *(67)* has determined that spatial working memory is mediated by a network of predominantly right-hemisphere regions that include posterior parietal (BA 40 and BA 7), anterior occipital (BA 19), and inferior prefrontal (BA 47) sites. It has been hypothesized that the premotor area and the superior parietal area might mediate spatial rehearsal, whereas the inferior posterior parietal area and the anterior occipital area might mediate storage of spatial information *(67,68)*.

A simple way to test the visuospatial short-term memory is to measure its span with the Corsi Block Tapping Test *(69)*. The test consists of nine blocks arranged on a board. The examiner taps the blocks in sequences of increasing length, and after each one the subject is requested to copy the sequence just tapped out. The longest sequence correctly tapped out by the subject constitutes his or her visuospatial memory span. An important limitation regarding use of this task in a clinical setting with parkinsonian patients is the fact that it requires a motor response: the spatial span might be underestimated owing to the presence of bradykinesia. Nonetheless, studies that have used Corsi's test *(70)* failed to find any difference between PD patients and normal controls. On the contrary, Bradley, Welch, and Dick *(71)* found that PD patients are slower that normal controls when performing complex visuospatial memory, but not verbal memory, tasks. Postle et al. *(72)* also found a selective impairment of spatial (but not object) delayed response in PD, indicating a selective disruption of spatial working memory. A selective impairment of spatial working memory was also demonstrated in PD patients by Owen et al. *(73)* using a computerized battery of tests designed to assess spatial, verbal, and visual working memory. In the spatial working memory task, subjects were required to search systematically through a number of boxes to find "tokens" while avoiding those boxes in which tokens had previously been found. In the visual and verbal conditions, the subjects were required to search in exactly the same manner, but through a number of abstract designs or surnames, respectively, avoiding designs or names in which a token had previously been found. Medicated PD patients with severe clinical symptoms were impaired on all three tests of working memory. In contrast, medicated patients with mild clinical symptoms were impaired on the test of spatial working memory, but not on the verbal or visual working memory tasks. Nonmedicated patients with mild clinical symptoms were unimpaired on all three tasks. Further investigations by the same group *(73–76)* focused on the cognitive heterogeneity in PD. Taken together, the results demonstrate that impairment of spatial working memory can occur in the early stages of the disease in a subgroup of PD patients with frontostriatal circuitry involvement.

Using the dual-task paradigm to measure the ability to cope with concurrent task demands, a number of investigators *(77–80)* have hypothesized that the "central executive" is impaired in PD patients. Le Bras et al. *(81)*, using a specifically designed testing procedure, concluded that PD patients are impaired in all steps of executive information processing involved in spatial working memory (stimulus encoding, storage, and response programming). More recently, Lewis et al. *(76)* have found that PD patients performing badly on the Tower of London Test (a standard visuospatial task of executive functioning) were specifically impaired in manipulating information within verbal working memory.

Recent functional magnetic resonance imaging studies *(82)* have implicated the rostral caudate nucleus in the transformation of spatial information in memory to guide the action. Dorsal premotor cortex *(82)* and premotor cortex (Brodmann's areas 46 and 9) are also involved *(83–85)* in performing spatial memory tasks. PD patients are known to suffer loss of dopaminergic input to the rostral caudate. Extensive two-way connections link the striatum, the premotor, and the dorsolateral prefrontal cortices. It is therefore conceivable that the functional impairment of these brain regions is the basis of spatial working memory impairment in PD patients.

Long-Term Spatial Memory

Memory for location is commonly tested by presenting a sheet showing a number of figures, representing objects, and then asking patients, after various time intervals, to relocate them on another sheet in exactly the same position *(86)*. Using a similar procedure Pillon et al. *(87)* demonstrated that, compared to controls, PD patients show significantly impaired spatial location of pictures, a result that contrasts with their relatively preserved verbal memory and only mildly impaired perceptual visuospatial and executive functions. Subsequently, the same group *(88,89)* carried out a number of experiments specifically aimed at determining the nature of the deficit and its relationship with the dopaminergic depletion that characterizes the disease. Results suggested that the memory deficit for spatial location observed in PD patients is a consequence of a disturbance of strategic processing and of decreased attentional resources, which may be a result of dopaminergic depletion and related striatofrontal dysfunction.

Postle et al. *(72)* examined the performances of PD patients and normal controls on a visual delayed-response test with a spatial condition and a (nonspatial) object condition, equating the perceptual difficulty of the tests for each participant. The stimuli were irregular polygons presented at different locations on a computer screen. Results revealed a disruption of spatial memory unconfounded by sensory processing difficulties. The authors hypothesized that the selectivity of this deficit might reflect the circumscribed nature of pathophysiological change affecting the caudate nucleus in early PD.

Maze learning can also be used to evaluate long-term spatial learning. Wallesch et al. *(90)*, to analyze spatial learning and cognitive processes described as impaired in PD, used a computerized maze task that allowed only partial vision of the maze. Results demonstrated that PD patients require more trials than controls to solve the maze problems. Differences between the performances of patients and controls were interpreted as owing to a response bias in the PD patients that resulted in a tendency to repeat the previous action and in impaired multistep plan generation.

Spatial Imagery

The ability to create and manipulate images plays a central role in many daily activities: from navigation to memory and to creative problem solving. According to Kosslyn *(91)* imagery abilities fall into at least four categories: image generation, image inspection, image maintenance, and image transformation. Several neuroimaging studies *(92–94)* have provided strong evidence that visuospatial imagery activates the same brain areas that are involved in visuospatial processing. In line with this finding Levin et al., on the basis of the double dissociating performance of two patients, demonstrated that the distinction between the "what" and "where" cortical visual systems extends to mental imagery tasks. An open question is whether or not image generation, besides being associated with activation of the same representations that are involved in visuospatial processing, also involves the activation of circuits specifically devoted to mental image generating *per se*. In investigating visuospatial impairments of patients with movement disorders, imagery tasks have the advantage that they do not involve overt motor components liable to interfere with the recording of subjects' responses.

Image generation was investigated by Jacobs et al. *(95)*. These authors demonstrated that PD patients are impaired on a task of emotional facial imagery but not on an object imagery control task. They are also impaired on tasks of perceiving and making emotional faces. Performance on both the perceptual and motor tasks of facial expression correlated significantly with performance on the emotional facial imagery task.

Image transformation was investigated in Brown and Marsden's study *(96)*. They employed a mental rotation task that required subjects to align mentally an arrow with one arm of a Maltese cross and to decide whether a dot was on the left or the right of the arrow. PD patients, although slower than controls, did not perform differentially worse in the conditions that required a greater amount of reorientation (e.g., when the arrow was pointing down), thus demonstrating lack of a generalized visuospatial deficit in PD. However, in a subsequent study, Lee et al. *(97)*, using both two- and three-dimensional visual rotation tasks, demonstrated that PD patients make more errors on mental rotations involving larger rotations in depth (or three-dimensional rotations). Furthermore, when three-dimensional rotation is involved, they showed a pattern of reaction time suggesting a specific impairment with larger rotations, thus indicating that PD patients may indeed have some problems in extrapersonal space image transformation.

Disorders of Topographical Orientation

An individual's successful navigation of the environment depends on his or her ability to establish an integrated viewpoint from which objects are represented spatially in relation to her or himself and to each other. To achieve this, visual inputs have to be processed and the results of visuospatial processing associated with information already stored in long-term memory *(2)*. Disorders at any of these levels may affect route finding. Bowen et al. *(98)* demonstrated that a standardized "route walking test" yields deficiencies in PD patients, especially those with left-sided or bilateral symptoms. However, natural environments usually provide a subject with a much richer supply of external cues, which have been shown to facilitate performance *(99)*. Indeed, there is one report in the literature that may account for the thesis that mild-to-moderate PD patients' object-in-location memory does not show spatial deficits when tested in a natural setting *(100)*. Yet, Montgomery et al. *(101)* compared the ability of mild and moderate PD patients and controls to remain oriented to the starting position after being transported passively in a wheelchair. They examined subjects under the condition of either visual or vestibular processing. The moderate PD group demonstrated the poorest performance in both sensory conditions. The visual condition discriminated between the mild PD group and the controls, but both groups gave similar performances in the vestibular condition. Poor performance in the visual condition correlated significantly with poor performance on judgment of line orientation in the mild PD group. The authors concluded that spatial updating, or maintaining a sense of orientation while being moved in the environment, is impaired in PD. More recently, Leplow et al. *(102)* corroborated the view that PD patients show spatial memory deficits also in real-life settings. They devised a "search through" locomotor task incorporating the basic features of two paradigms (the radial maze and the water maze) widely used to assess spatial behavior in animal research *(103,104)*. The participants had to find and remember 5 out of 20 hidden locations within a completely controlled environment. The performances of PD patients were found to worsen if the starting position was moved by 90° and the proximal cues were deleted simultaneously. The results were interpreted as indicating patients' inability to generate rules that can be used flexibly in changing environments.

VISUOSPATIAL DISORDERS IN PARKINSON DISEASE

Visuospatial abnormalities have often been reported in PD patients. Early in 1964, Proctor et al. *(105)* demonstrated that PD patients have difficulty in determining when a rod is vertical if they are in a darkened room. Later, this abnormality was confirmed both in patients seated in a chair that is tilted either to the right or to the left *(13)*, and in patients who are upright *(106)*. Subsequently, as we have already documented, a number of authors reported that PD is associated with disproportionate impairments in visuospatial abilities. However, for a long time, consensus on the specificity and significance of experimental data was lacking. Part of the debate stemmed from methodological inadequacies of early studies that did not account for factors such as motor speed, dexterity, and presence or absence of pharmacological treatment. On this basis, it was suggested *(107)* that impaired visuospatial ability in PD patients may be owing to "generic" increase in reaction time or other aspects of attentional disorders.

More refined neuropsychological studies both in *de novo* PD patients *(88)* and using tasks either requiring no motor response or minimizing the dexterity, speed, and coordination, provided insight into the existence of visuospatial disturbances free of such confounding motor factors. In addition, statistical techniques were used to explore relationships between motor and visuospatial deficits and helped to determine whether or not spatial deficits are of the same magnitude as, or in excess of, those attributable to motor abnormalities.

Since degeneration of dopaminergic neurons constitutes the main biochemical abnormality found in PD, dopamine depletion has been considered to account for most of the symptoms, including behavioral abnormalities and cognitive deficits *(89)*. If striatal dopamine deficiency plays a role in PD patients' cognitive deficit, specialized hemispheric functions contralateral to the motor symptoms should be altered in patients with hemiparkinsonism, providing a unique opportunity to study the effect of asymmetrical subcortical degeneration on cognitive functions *(108)*. Yet, the results of these studies have been controversial. A number of studies were not able to demonstrate a specific pattern of difference between patients with predominantly left and right symptoms *(9,109–111)*. However, a number of more recent studies *(43,44)* did find a specific directional bias related to the side of the predominant symptoms. On the other hand, Pillon et al. *(112)* demonstrated that cognitive impairment is poorly correlated with symptoms responding well to levodopa treatment (e.g., akinesia and rigidity) and is strongly related to axial symptoms (such as gait disorders and dysarthria), which respond little if at all to levodopa treatment. This finding was interpreted as suggesting that cognitive impairment in PD patients is, to a great extent, a result of dysfunction of non-dopaminergic neuronal systems. A further suggestion that the visuospatial deficits of PD patients do not always depend on the same mechanisms subserving motor impairments derives from the observation that patients treated with bilateral deep brain stimulation of the subthalamic nucleus, despite obtaining clinical motor benefits, show a significant decline in their ability to encode visuospatial material *(113)*. According to this study, the decline was more consistently observed in patients over the age of 69 yr and it led to a mental state that the authors describe as similar to that observed in progressive supranuclear palsy (PSP) patients.

In conclusion, it is still possible that striatal dopamine deficiency, even if it is not the major determinant of visuospatial deficits, could play a role in determining attentional bias underlying the subtle neglect phenomena that are encountered in predominant left-sided PD patients.

PROGRESSIVE SUPRANUCLEAR PALSY

The most striking feature of PSP patients is the fixity of gaze that, resulting from supranuclear ophthalmoplegia, gives the disease its name. However, far from being a purely oculomotor problem, PSP patients' ocular movement difficulties are accompanied by a severe deficit in orienting attention. Rafal *(114)* has outlined very well the difficulties that PSP patients encounter in everyday life and how these difficulties interact with other components of the disease (gait disorder, dysphagia, and nuchal dystonia). When conversing with others, reaching for objects, eating, or dressing, PSP patients typically tend not to look at what they are doing. This failure to orient spontaneously the lower visual field contributes to gait disequilibrium (the source of falls) and to the ingestion of boluses that are too large to swallow (the source of *ab ingestis*). Loss of spontaneous social orienting is also a striking feature of PSP and it is kind of unique to this disease. Relatives tend to note this as an early sign and often attribute it to a change of mood or to carelessness.

A further characteristic trait of visuomotor impairment in some PSP patients is, conversely, difficulty in inhibiting orienting responses in situations in which orienting is disadvantageous. One need only think of patients who, as they walk, tend to orient toward the door or a wall mirror or TV set they have just passed, as if they were magnetically attracted to and fixed upon that object in the environment. This visual behavior, also called "visual grasping" by Ghika et al. *(115)*, is associated with repeated backward head movements while walking and is, consequently, a further cause of backward falls *(114)*.

As early as 1981, Kimura et al. *(116)* demonstrated that PSP patients are impaired in visual search and scanning tasks. Subsequently, Fisk et al. *(117)* performed systematic observations in an attempt to relate the performances of PSP patients on visual search and scanning tasks to the pattern of their oculomotor deficits. In one of these tasks, subjects were required to scan lines composed of a variable number of dots and dashes and to report either the number of dashes or the number of dots. Scanning in each of the four directions was measured: left to right, right to left, top to bottom, and bottom to top. PSP patients were less accurate than controls only when scanning along the vertical plane. This confirmed that bradykinesia and psychomotor retardation could not account for impaired performance and that some specific defect of visual search and scanning along the vertical plane had to be assumed.

Impaired performance on a visual search task, as well as on the Benton's Judgement of Line Orientation Test *(8)*, was also demonstrated by Soliveri and coworkers, in comparison with both normal controls *(118)* and PD patients *(119)*. The same authors could not demonstrate any difference on these tasks between PSP and CBD patients *(119)*.

In a detailed study of 25 patients, Esmonde et al. *(120)* confirmed a severe visuo-perceptual deficit in PSP. They found marked differences between patients and controls in two subtests of the Visual Object and Space Perception Battery *(121)*, (the Fragmented Letter and Cube analysis tests) which were explicitly chosen to minimize the effect of oculomotor scanning on performance.

Subsequently, in a series of experiments, Rafal, Posner, and colleagues *(45,122,123)* demonstrated that PSP patients are not only slow in scanning and searching when allowed to move their eyes, but also in covertly shifting their visual attention, especially in the vertical plane. However, unlike PD patients, who demonstrate defective voluntary control of covert attention, PSP patients are especially impaired in reflexive orienting.

The authors came to this conclusion after comparing attentional movements from both endogenous and exogenous cues. In both cases the subjects' task was to press a button upon detecting a target. In these tasks, targets are preceded by cues that may orient the attention to the target location (valid cue) or to another location (invalid cue), or may have only an alerting value and provide no spatial information (neutral cue). For testing voluntary control of attention, the (endogenous) cue is typically an arrow in the center of the display, instructing the subject where to expect the forthcoming target. Reflexive orienting is tested by an exogenous cue, e.g., lighting up of the box where the target might appear. In this case, unlike the case of the central cue paradigm, the cue has no predictive value and the target is equally likely to appear in an uncued as in the cued location. Results demonstrated that PSP patients show no "validity effect" on reflexive orienting of attention along the vertical plane: i.e., they are no faster in responding to a target when it is preceded by a valid exogenous cue. A similar trend for smaller orienting effects in the vertical plane is also seen in endogenous orienting but it is not as dramatic as in reflexive orienting. In other words PSP patients have problems in "shifting" attention, especially in the vertical plane and especially in response to exogenous signals.

Kertzman et al. *(124)* also provided evidence consistent with the conclusion that PSP has little or no effect on endogenous orienting of attention. In their experiment the cue was lighting up of a peripheral box that predicted the location of the forthcoming target. Vertical and horizontal attention movements were tested in separate blocks, thus giving the subjects maximum opportunity to use the cue to shift attention. Under these conditions the PSP patients did not show a smaller effect of cue validity in the vertical plane. This demonstrated that PSP patients' attentional deficit can be contrasted with that of inferior parietal lobe patients. These latter patients are typically impaired in the presence of endogenous cues, in the horizontal plane, and in the invalid cue condition, i.e., when they have to "disengage" attention that was cued by a central signal to the side opposite the target.

Rafal et al. *(114)* demonstrated quite convincingly that PSP attentional deficit is likely to be a result of the degenerative damage to the superior colliculus and the adjacent tectal nuclei. This part of the midbrain constitutes the phylogenetically older retinotectal pathway, which retains important functions for regulating visual attention and visually guided behavior. The frontal eye fields are also important in controlling saccadic eye movements *(125)*, show dramatic hypometabolism in PSP patients *(126)*, and might also be responsible for visual attention deficits. Nonetheless, patients with lesions restricted to the dorsolateral prefrontal cortex (including the frontal eye fields) perform normally in covert orienting of attention *(127)*, even if they show increased latencies for endogenous saccades to targets contralateral to the lesion *(128)*. Furthermore, converging evidence from normal subjects *(129)* and from hemianopic patients *(130)* demonstrates that the midbrain retinotectal pathway is important in reflexive orienting to exogenous signals and corroborate the view that it is decisive in determining the visuomotor and attentional deficit typically found in PSP patients.

CORTICOBASAL DEGENERATION

Corticobasal degeneration (CBD) is clinically characterized by the combination of motor with cognitive disorders. Neuropathologically, it features circumscribed parietal or frontoparietal atrophy, associated with basophilic and tau-postive inclusions in the neurons of the substantia nigra and basal ganglia.

Reflecting this definite pattern of neuronal damage, neuropsychological deficits of CBD patients most commonly include deficits of executive functions and of retrieval processes (in relation to the damage of the prefrontal cortex and the striatum) and apraxia (owing to the involvement of the parietal cortex). Leiguarda et al. *(131)* described the nature of apraxia in CBD. To minimize the confounding effects of the primary motor disorder, they examined the least affected limb. They found that ideomotor apraxia is the most frequent type of apraxia in CBD patients and they hypothesized that it was because of the dysfunction of the supplementary motor area (SMA). They also examined a subgroup of CBD patients with severe (ideomotor and ideational) apraxia, correlating this with global cognitive impairment, and attributed it to additional parietal or diffuse cortical damage. Several authors have hypothesized that SMA dysfunction underlies limb apraxia in CBD *(132,133)*, but a similar role has also been attributed to the lateral premotor cortex *(133,134)* and to the parietal regions *(135,136)*.

Indeed, the left supplementary motor cortex has been repeatedly implicated in the genesis of apraxia *(137–140)*. However, the role of the left posterior parietal lobe in determining ideomotor *(141,142)* and ideational *(143)* apraxia is well documented. Furthermore, the assumption that ideational apraxia is an extreme form of ideomotor apraxia (a result of brain damage superimposed on that causing the latter form of apraxia) is disproved by the lack of correlation between the two deficits *(144)*.

A couple of studies have tried to determine the origin of apraxia in CBD patients. Blondel et al. *(132)* tried to characterize the different processes underlying apraxic disorders in these patients according to a theoretical framework postulating a two-step system controlling limb gestures: the conceptual system and the production system. The results, extremely similar in the three patients they studied, showed a sparing of the conceptual system and an impairment of the production system with a dramatic deficit in the control of the temporal and spatial aspects of the gestures. The authors interpreted these results as suggesting a dysfunction of the SMA. Similarly, Jacobs et al. *(133)* reported the results of testing three nondemented CBD subjects on tasks requiring the production of meaningful or meaningless gestures to command, gesture imitation, gesture discrimination, and novel gesture learning. The results suggested that apraxia associated with CBD is initially induced by a production-execution defect with relative sparing of the movement representations. However, combining neuropsychological and neuroimaging investigations, Peigneux et al. *(145)* found that, in CBD patients, the anterior cingulate cortex is involved when visuospatial attention and conflict monitoring is necessary or when task difficulty, motor output, and recent memory requirements must be combined. However, when apraxia is defined according to a more stringent test of the integrity of the components of the praxic system (measuring the patients' ability to correct their errors on a second attempt), hypometabolism is found in the superior parietal lobule and in the SMA. This demonstrates the importance of parietofrontal circuits in the transformation of sensory input into action. Damage to these systems is likely to produce different types of limb apraxia depending on the injured site, the context in which the movement is performed, and the cognitive demands of the action *(146,147)*.

The superior parietal lobule appears to be crucial in visually guided movements *(148)*, mental transformation of the body in space *(149)*, and elaboration and maintenance of working representation of gestures to perform *(150,151)*. It is also involved in successful integration of internal and external representations to direct action *(152)*. In turn, the SMA is most likely to be involved in transcoding stored space-time representations of movement into limb innervatory patterns *(153)*.

Wenning et al. *(154)* have reported that constructive apraxia, possibly demonstrable as a failure to copy drawings, is reported at the first visit in 64% of pathologically confirmed CBD patients. Since constructive apraxia is unlikely to be an early sign in a patient with an asymmetric parkinsonism, drawing copying might be a useful test to corroborate the CBD diagnosis.

Interestingly, in the same study, two patients with onset of motor symptoms on the left side developed left-sided visuospatial neglect, whereas patients with onset of right motor symptoms developed aphasia. A further pathologically confirmed CBD demonstrating left neglect was reported by Rey et al. *(155)*. More recently, Kleiner-Fisman et al. *(156)* reported a single case study of a professional artist in whom presumed CBD was associated with left hemispatial neglect. It led to a complex alteration of his artistic judgment and production. From a clinical standpoint it should be concluded that in the absence of focal lesions (e.g., of vascular or neoplastic origin), the presence of both ideomotor apraxia and left neglect should give rise to suspicion of CBD.

Following bilateral involvement of the parieto-occipital junction, CBD patients can also show a complete Balint–Holmes syndrome *(157)*, consisting of gaze apraxia (defective visual scanning), optical ataxia (defective visual reaching), impaired visual attention, defective estimation of distance, and impaired depth perception. Mendez *(158)* recently described a patient whose illness began with a slow, rigid gait, abnormal postures of his right hand, and retrocollis. As the disease progressed, he developed prominent visuospatial deficits that, after 8 yr, included a Balint–Holmes syndrome. We have personally observed *(159)* a patient with an opposite disease progression: i.e., beginning with the visuospatial symptoms of the Balint–Holmes syndrome and showing signs and symptoms of basal ganglia involvement only 4 yr after disease onset. Examples of Balint–Holmes syndrome can also be found in early stages of Alzheimer's dementia *(160,161)*. There has been some suggestion that cognitive impairment is a common feature of CBD *(162,163)*. According to Grimes, Lang, and Bergeron *(163)* CBD patients fulfilling classical diagnostic criteria might represent a minority of those with a pathologically confirmed diagnosis. They argue that case series emphasizing motor deficits, originating prevalently from movement disorder clinics, might slight the importance of cognitive impairment in CBD. Such a bias would indeed make the differential diagnosis of a patient presenting with Balint–Holmes syndrome particularly challenging, including besides CBD, Creutzfeld–Jakob disease, multifocal progressive leucoencephalopathy, strokes *(164)*, and a progressive posterior atrophy occurring in isolation *(165–168)*.

DIFFUSE LEWY BODY DISEASE

Dementia with Lewy bodies (DLB) is the second most common type of cognitive degeneration after Alzheimer's disease (AD) *(169)*. Clinically, DLB is characterized by spontaneous parkinsonism and progressive dementia associated with fluctuating cognitive functions, and hallucination *(169)*. Parkinsonism and dementia tend to co-occur. A history of Parkinsonism predating dementia by more than 1 yr might be better designated "Parkinson's disease with dementia." Since publication of the clinical and pathological diagnosis criteria *(169)*, several studies have tried to delineate the neuropsychological features that distinguish DLB disease from AD. A number of them have demonstrated that, compared with AD, visuospatial and visuoconstructive abilities are disproportionately impaired in patients with DLB disease *(170–173)*. Compared with AD patients matched for age, sex, education, and Mini Mental State Examination (MMSE) score, DLB patients perform worse on the Raven Colored Progressive Matrices test and on the picture arrangement, block design, object assembly, and digit symbol substitution subtests of the Wechsler Adult Intelligence Scale–Revised *(173)*. They also perform worse on size discrimination, form discrimination, visual counting, and overlapping figure identification *(174)*.

Mori et al. *(174)* also demonstrated that, in the DLB group, patients with visual hallucinations scored significantly lower on overlapping figure identification than those without, whereas patients with television misidentifications gave significantly lower scores on the size discrimination, form discrimination, and visual counting tasks than those without. The underlying assumption is that specific brain regions are involved in the performance of these tests: the occipital visual association cortex for size discrimination, the occipito-temporal visual association cortex for size discrimination, and the occipito-parietal cortex for visual counting.

Similar results were obtained by Simard, Rikum, and Myran *(175)*. These authors compared the performance on the Benton Judgement Line Orientation Test of patients with DLB and predominant parkinsonism, with DLB and predominant psychosis, and with AD. For this purpose they analyzed errors as resulting from visual attention and visuospatial perception failures. The study did not find significant differences on the total score of the Benton Judgement Line Orientation Test. However, error analysis demonstrated that subjects with DLB and psychosis have more severe visual-perception (VH errors) impairments than subjects with DLB and predominant parkinsonian features, and AD subjects.

These results suggest that defective visual input caused by visual-system damage can result in hallucinations from defective visual processing or abnormal cortical release phenomena *(176)*. Indeed, Imamura et al. *(177)* using positron emission tomography, found that visual hallucinations in DLB patients are associated with relatively preserved metabolism in the right temporoparietal association cortex and severe hypometabolism in the primary and secondary visual cortex.

A practical implication of the disproportionate impairment of DLB patients in visuospatial tasks has been demonstrated by Ala et al. *(178)*. These authors analyzed accuracy in copying the interlocking pentagon item of the MMSE in patients with neuropathologically confirmed DLB and AD. They concluded that in patients with MMSE scores ≥ 13 an inability to accurately copy the pentagons suggests that the diagnosis is more likely DLB than AD with a sensitivity of 88% and a specificity of 59%.

MULTIPLE SYSTEM ATROPHY

Multiple system atrophy (MSA) is a term used to describe a progressive neurological condition incorporating a parkinsonian syndrome (striatonigral degeneration), often accompanied by autonomic failure (Shy–Drager syndrome) or cerebellar and/or pyramidal signs (olivopontocerebellar atrophy—OPCA) *(179,180)*.

Cognitive deterioration is not generally considered to be an integral feature of MSA *(181)*. Indeed, lack of dementia throughout the course of the disease has been proposed as a feature that might help to differentiate between MSA and PD premortem *(182)*.

However, routine neuropsychological assessment often reveals multiple cognitive deficits suggesting a prominent involvement of the frontal lobe *(183)*. MSA patients perform normally on tasks of spatial and pattern recognition, which are sensitive to deficits in patients with AD and medicated PD *(183,184)*. On the contrary, Robbins et al. *(183)* demonstrated that MSA patients are impaired in comparison with matched controls on test of visual memory and learning but in specific and unusual ways. Thus on a matching-to-sample test they were significantly impaired at the simultaneous stage, when no memory was involved, but showed normal delayed matching performance. This particular pattern of deficit is distinct from that reported in PD patients *(184)*. Moreover, on the test of visual learning, unlike PD patients *(184)*, the MSA subjects performed surprisingly well at the more difficult levels of the task but were inefficient at the early stages.

Taken together, this pattern of performance is suggestive of problems in attention and orientation rather than of primary visual learning or memory deficits. Visuospatial contrast thresholds are also unimpaired in MSA, unlike PD patients, who normally exhibit a reduction in contrast sensitivity *(185)*. This finding suggests that reduced contrast sensitivity is related to a dopaminergic pathology, possibly at the level of retinal amacrine cells, which might be affected in PD *(186–188)* but not in MSA *(185)*.

CONCLUSION

Abnormalities of visuospatial functions are common in PD and in atypical parkinsonian disorders. They have been described in several domains of visuospatial ability. In some tasks the alteration can reflect the motor disorders. However, in many instances it is possible to demonstrate that the contribution of motor skills to a task is either minimal or absent. Different disorders have different patterns of impairment. For instance, in CBD, apraxia and optic ataxia are most common, whereas PSP patients show a characteristic impairment in shifting their visual attention downward.

To date, no systematic study of atypical parkinsonian syndromes has been performed using a predefined battery of visuospatial tasks aimed at helping the clinician in the differential diagnosis at disease onset. We would propose that such a battery *(see* Table 1) should at least contain a perceptual task such as the Benton's Judgement of Line Orientation Test *(8)*, a task of visuospatial working memory and a task of visuospatial learning. To examine visuospatial working memory we would propose a visuospatial span task as proposed by Le Bras et al. *(81)*. A computerized maze task *(90)* could be used to test visuospatial learning. The Tower of London task *(189,190)* or one of the several versions of the Tower of Hanoi Test *(191)* could be useful to test visuospatial working memory and some aspects of planning. If administered repeatedly, it can also allow exploration of implicit rule learning, which is typically impaired in PD and in Huntington's disease patients *(192)*. Three-dimensional visual rotation tasks *(97)* appear to be most sensitive to test visuospatial transformation in the imagery domain.

In the clinical setting, we have found it extremely useful to test visuomotor coordination by asking patients to reach for an object that requires precision gripping. Patients with damage to the posterior parietal lobe (as in CBD) show early impairment on this task. A standardization of the procedures for testing visuomotor coordination is likely to improve the sensitivity of this procedure.

To test visuospatial attention in this group of patients we prefer to use visuospatial search tasks. For this purpose, it is important to present the stimuli on a screen in front of the subject and to prepare visual displays that can allow exploration of attentional movements in both the horizontal and the vertical direction. Finally, testing visuospatial functions may be extremely useful in the differential diagnosis of disorders associating parkinsonian features and early cognitive damage. For this purpose, a copying drawing task should be included in the test battery. In this case the motor components cannot be eliminated. However, in most cases it is not difficult to separate them from errors owing to faulty organization of the spatial arrangement of the design to be copied.

Table 1
Visuospatial Test for the Assessment of Parkinsonian Disorders

Test	Reason to Include It in the Visuospatial Assessment
Judgement of Line Orientation *(6)*	Can help differentiate demented from nondemented PD patients.
Copying Drawing Task *(154,178)*	Early impaired in CBD and DLB patients.
Optic Ataxia Assessment (*)	CBD patients are particularly impaired at this task
Tower of London *(76)*	A sensitive task to detect visuospatial working memory deficit in early stages of PD.
Tower of Hanoi *(191,192)*	Comparison of repeated performance at this task allows exploration of implicit rule learning, which is typically impaired after basal ganglia damage.
Wilson-Le Bras test *(81)*	It can measure of the visuospatial span without the motor component involved by the Corsi Block Tapping Test.
Posner test *(45,122,123)*	At this task, PD patients demonstrate defective voluntary control of covert attention. PSP patients, on the contrary, are especially impaired in reflexive orienting.
3D mental rotation *(97)*	PD patients are impaired in 3D mental rotation. Little is known about the performance of atypical parkinsonism patients at this task.

*There is no standardized bedside procedure to administer this task.

SPECIFIC ISSUES THAT CAN BE ADDRESSED BY FUTURE RESEARCH OF VISUOSPATIAL COGNITION IN PARKINSON DISEASE AND IN ATYPICAL PARKINSONIAN DISORDERS

1. What is the role of the colliculus and of the dorsal frontal lobe damage in the visuospatial impairment of PSP patients?
2. To develop a suitable method for assessing attentional movements both in the horizontal and in the vertical direction in a clinical setting.
3. Does unilateral neglect in CBD patients have a different qualitative pattern than in PD patients?
4. Which is the physiological basis of neglect in unilateral PD patients compared with parietal lobe damaged patients?
5. Which is the role of the dopaminergic system in controlling visuospatial exploration in PD patients? Can dopaminergic drugs improve directional attention deficits in PD patients?
6. Is there any difference in depth perception and in reaching performance between PD and atypical parkinsonian syndromes?
7. Can a careful assessment of visuospatial skill help diagnostic accuracy in the early stage of parkinsonian diseases?
8. Is there any role of impairment in size discrimination in determining "freezing" episodes in PD patients?

REFERENCES

1. O' Keefe J, Nadel L. The Hippocampus as a Cognitive Map. New York: Clarendon, 1978.
2. Grüsser OJ. Multimodal structure of the extrapersonal space. In: Hein A, Jeannerod M, eds. Spatially Oriented Behavior. New York: Springer-Verlag, 1987:327–352.
3. Rizzolatti G, Gentilucci M, Matelli M. Selective spatial attention: One centre, one circuit, or many centres? In: Posner MI, Marin OSM, eds. Attention and Performance IX. Hillsdale, NJ: Erlbaum, 1985:251–265.
4. Goodale MA, Milner AD. Separate visual pathways for perception and action. Trends Neurosci 1992;15:20–25.
5. Ungerleider LG, Haxby JV. "What" and "where" in the human brain. Curr Opin Neurobiol 1994;4:157–165.
6. Warrington EK, Rabin P. Perceptual matching in patients with cerebral lesions. Neuropsychologia 1970;8:475–487.
7. Hannay HJ, Varney NR, Benton AL. Visual localization in patients with unilateral disease. J Neurol Neurosurg Psychiatry 1976;39:307–313.
8. Benton AL, Varney NR, Hamsher KD. Visuospatial judgment: a clinical test. Arch Neurol 1978;35:364–367.

9. Boller F, Passafiume D, Keefe NC, Rogers K, Morrow L, Kim Y. Visuospatial impairment in Parkinson's disease: Role of perceptual and motor factors. Arch Neurol 1984;41:485–490.
10. Goldenberg G, Wimmer A, Auff E, Schnaberth G. Impairment of motor planning in patients with Parkinson's disease: evidence from ideomotor apraxia testing. J Neurol Neurosurg Psychiatry 1986;49:1266–1272.
11. Richards M, Cote LJ, Stern Y. The relationship between visuospatial ability and perceptual motor function in Parkinson's disease. J Neurol Neurosurg Psychiatry 1993;56:400–406.
12. Levin BE, Llabre MM, Weiner WJ. Cognitive impairment associated with early Parkinson's disease. Neurology 1989;39:557–561.
13. Levin BE. Spatial cognition in Parkinson disease. Alzheimer Dis Assoc Disord 1990;4:161–170.
14. Montse A, Pere V, Carme J, Francesc V, Eduardo T. Visuospatial deficits in Parkinson's disease assessed by judgment of line orientation test: error analyses and practice effects. J Clin Exp Neuropsychol 2001;23.:592–598.
15. Girotti FS, Soliveri P, Carella F, et al. Dementia and cognitive impairment in Parkinson's disease. Neurology 1988;51:1498–1502.
16. Livingston M, Hubel D. Segregation of form, color, movement, and depth: Anatomy, physiology, and perception. Science 1988;240:740–749.
17. Parker AJ, Cumming BG, Johnston EB, Hurlbert AC. Multiple cues for three-dimensional shape. In: Gazzaniga MS, ed. The Cognitive Neurosciences. Cambridge, MA: MIT Press, 1985:351–364.
18. Gulyas B, Roland PE. Binocular disparity discrimination in human cerebral cortex: functional anatomy by positron emission tomography. Proc Natl Acad Sci USA 1994;91:1239–1243.
19. Ptito A, Zatorre RJ, Petrides M, Frey S, Alivisatos B, Evans AC. Localization and lateralization of stereoscopic processing in the human brain. Neuroreport 1993;4:1155–1158.
20. Fortin A, Ptito A, Faubert J, Ptito M. Cortical areas mediating stereopsis in the human brain: a PET study. Neuroreport 2002;3:895–898.
21. Perenin MT, Vighetto A. Optic ataxia: a specific disruption in visuomotor mechanisms. I. Different aspects of the deficit in reaching for objects. Brain 1988;111(Pt 3):643–647.
22. Bonfiglioli C, De Berti G, Nichelli P, Nicoletti R, Castiello U. Kinematic analysis of the reach to grasp movement in Parkinson's and Huntington's disease subjects. Neuropsychologia 1998;36:1203–1208.
23. Castiello U, Bennett K, Bonfiglioli C, Lim S, Peppard RF. The reach-to-grasp movement in Parkinson's disease: response to a simultaneous perturbation of object position and object size. Exp Brain Res 1999;125:453–462.
24. Fellows SJ, Noth J, Schwarz M. Precision grip and Parkinson's disease. Brain 1998;121:1771–1784.
25. Rearick MP, Stelmach GE, Leis B, Santello M. Coordination and control of forces during multifingered grasping in Parkinson's disease. Exp Neurol 2002;177:428–442.
26. Heilman KM. Neglect and related disorders. In: Heilman KM, ed. Clinical Neuropsychology. New York: Oxford University Press, 1979:268–307.
27. Albert ML. A simple test of visual neglect. Neurology 1973;23:322–326.
28. Gauthier L, Dehaut F, Joannette Y. The Bells Test: A quantitative and qualitative test for visual neglect. Int J Clin Neuropsychool 1989;11:49–54.
29. Mesulam M-M. Principles of Behavioral Neurology. Philadelphia: Davis, 1985.
30. Bradshaw JL, Nettleton NC, Nathan G, Wilson L. Bisecting rods and lines: effects of horizontal and vertical posture on left-side underestimation by normal subjects. Neuropsychologia 1985;23:421–425.
31. Scarisbrick DJ, Tweedy JR, Kuslansky G. Hand preference and performance effects on line bisection. Neuropsychologia 1987;25:695–699.
32. Milner AD, Brechmann M, Pagliarini L. To halve and to halve not: an analysis of line bisection judgements in normal subjects. Neuropsychologia 1992;30:515–526.
33. Ishiai S, Sugishita M, Watabiki S, Nakayama T, Kotera M, Gono S. Improvement of left unilateral spatial neglect in a line extension task. Neurology 1994;44:294–298.
34. Carli M, Evenden JL, Robbins TW. Depletion of unilateral striatal dopamine impairs initiation of contralateral actions and not sensory attention. Nature 1985;313:679–682.
35. Marshall JF, Gotthelf T. Sensory inattention in rats with 6-hydroxydopamine-induced degeneration of ascending dopaminergic neurons: apomorphine-induced reversal of deficits. Exp Neurol 11979;65:398–411.
36. Ljungberg T, Ungerstedt U. Sensory inattention produced by 6-hydroxydopamine-induced degeneration of ascending dopamine neurons in the brain. Exp Neurol 1976;53:585–600.
37. Fleet WS, Valenstein E, Watson RT, Heilman KM. Dopamine agonist therapy for neglect in humans. Neurology 1987;37:1765–1770.
38. Geminiani G, Bottini G, Sterzi R. Dopaminergic stimulation in unilateral neglect. J Neurol Neurosurg Psychiatry 1998;65:344–347.
39. Villardita C, Smirni P, Zappalà G. Visual neglect in Parkinson disease. Arch Neurol 1983;40:737–739.
40. Gauthier L, Gautheir SG, Joannette Y. Visual neglect in left-, right-, and bilateral parkinsonians. J Clin Exp Neuropsychol 1985;7:145 (abstract).

41. Starkstein S, R Leiguarda R, Gershanik O, Berthier M. Neuropsychological disturbances in hemiparkinson's disease. Neurology 1987;37:1762–1764.
42. Ransmayr G, Schmidhuber-Eiler B, Karamath E. Visuoperception and visuospatial and visuorotational performance in Parkinson's disease. J Neurol 1987;235:99–101.
43. Lee AC, Harris JP, Atkinson E, Fowler MS. Evidence from a line bisection task for visuospatial neglect in left hemiparkinson's disease. Vision Res 2001;41:2677–2686.
44. Ebersbach G, Trottenberg T, Hattig H, Schelosky L, Schrag A, Poewe W. Directional bias of initial visual exploration. A symptom of neglect in Parkinson's disease. Brain 1996;119(Pt 1):79–87.
45. Posner MI, Cohen Y, Rafal RD. Neural systems control of spatial orienting. Philos Trans R Soc Lond B Biol Sci 1982;298:187–198.
46. Briand KA, Strallow D, Hening W, Poizner H, Sereno AB. Control of voluntary and reflexive saccades in Parkinson's disease. Exp Brain Res 1999;129:38–48.
47. Crawford T, Henderson L, Kennard C. Abnormalities of nonvisually guided eye movements in Parkinson's disease. Brain 1989;112:1537–1586.
48. Crevits L, De Ridder K. Disturbed striatoprefrontal mediated visual behavior in moderate to severe Parkinsonian patients. J Neurol Neurosurg Psychiatry 1997;63:296–299.
49. O'Sullivan EP, Shaunak LH, Hawken M, Crawford TJ, Kennard C. Abnormalities of predictive saccades in Parkinson's disase. Neuroreport 1997;8:1209–1213.
50. Carl JB, Wurts RH. Asymmetry of saccadic control in patients with hemi-Parkinson's disease. Investigative Ophthalmology and Visual Science 1985;26:258.
51. Kitagawa M, Fukushima J, Tashiro K. Relationship between antisaccades and the clinical symptoms in Parkinson's disease. Neurology 1994;44:2285–2289.
52. Wright MJ, Burns RJ, Geffen GM, Geffen LB. Covert orientation of visual attention in Parkinson's disease: an impairment in the maintenance of attention. Neuropsychologia 1990;28:151–159.
53. Yamada T, Izyuuinn M, Schulzer M, Hirayama K. Covert orienting attention in Parkinson's disease. J Neurol Neurosurg Psychiatry 1990;53:593–596.
54. Bennett KM, Waterman C, Scarpa M, Castiello U. Covert visuospatial attentional mechanisms in Parkinson's disease. Brain 1995;118:153–166.
55. Rafal RD, Posner MI, J.A. W, Friedrich FJ. Cognition and the basal ganglia. Separating mental and motor components of performance in Parkinson's disease. Brain 1984;107:1083–1094.
56. Sharpe MH. Patients with early Parkinson's disease are not impaired on spatial orientating of attention. Cortex 1990;26:515–524.
57. Filoteo JV, Delis DC, Salmon DP, Demadura T, Roman MJ, Shults CW. An examination of the nature of attentional deficits in patients with Parkinson's disease: evidence from a spatial orienting task. J Int Neuropsychol Soc 1997;3 :337–347.
58. Yamaguchi S, Kobayashi S. Contribution of the dopaminergic system to voluntary and automatic orienting of visuospatial attention. J Neurosci 1998;18:1869–1878.
59. Briand KA, Hening W, Poizner H, Sereno AB. Automatic orienting in Parkinson's disease. Neuropsychologia 2001;39:1240–1249.
60. Desimone R, Schein SJ. Visual properties of neurons in area V4 of the macaque: sensitivity to stimulus form. J Neurophysiol 1987;57:835–868.
61. Shiller PH, Lee K. The role of the primate extrastriate area V4 in vision. Science 1991;251:1251–1253.
62. Frassinetti F, Nichelli P, di Pellegrino G. Selective horizontal dysmetropsia following prestriate lesion. Brain 1999;122(Pt 2):339–350.
63. Milner AD, Harvey M. Distortion of size perception in visual spatial neglect. Curr Biol 1995;5:85–89.
64. Harris JP, Atkinson EA, Lee AC, Nithi K, Fowler MS. Hemispace differences in the visual perception of size in left hemiParkinson's disease. Neuropsychologia 2003;41:795–807.
65. Lee AC, Harris JP, Atkinson EA, Fowler MS. Disruption of estimation of body-scaled aperture width in Hemiparkinson's disease. Neuropsychologia 2001;39:1097–1104.
66. Baddeley A. Working Memory. London: Oxford University Press, 1986.
67. Smith EE, J. J. Neuroimaging analyses of human working memory. Proc Natl Acad Sci USA 1998;95:12061–12068.
68. Courtney SM, Petit L, Maisog JM, Ungerleider LG, Haxby JV. An area specialized for spatial working memory in human frontal cortex. Science 1998;279:1347–1351.
69. Milner B. Interhemispheric differences in the localization of psychological processes in man. Br Med Bull 1971;27: 272–277.
70. Orsini A, Fragassi NA, Chiacchio L, Falanga AM, Cocchiaro C, Grossi D. Verbal and spatial memory span in patients with extrapyramidal diseases. Percept Mot Skills 1987;65:555–558.
71. Bradley VA, Welch JL, Dick DJ. Visuospatial working memory in Parkinson's disease. J Neurol Neurosurg Psychiatry 1989;52:1228–1235.

72. Postle BR, Jonides J, Smith EE, Corkin S, Growdon JH. Spatial, but not object, delayed response is impaired in early Parkinson's disease. Neuropsychology 1997;11:171–179.

73. Owen AM, Iddon JL, Hodges JR, Summers BA, Robbins TW. Spatial and non-spatial working memory at different stages of Parkinson's disease. Neuropsychologia 1997;35:519–532.

74. Owen AM, James M, Leigh PN, et al. Fronto-striatal cognitive deficits at different stages of Parkinson's disease. Brain 1992;115(Pt 6):1727–1751.

75. Owen AM, Beksinska M, James M, et al. Visuospatial memory deficits at different stages of Parkinson's disease. Neuropsychologia 1993;31:627–644.

76. Lewis SJ, Cools R, Robbins TW, Dove A, Barker RA, Owen AM. Using executive heterogeneity to explore the nature of working memory deficits in Parkinson's disease. Neuropsychologia 2003;41:645–654.

77. Brown RG, Marsden CD. Dual task performance and processing resources in normal subjects and patients with Parkinson's disease. Brain 1991;114(Pt 1A):215–231.

78. Dalrymple-Alford JC, Kalders AS, Jones RD, Watson RW. A central executive deficit in patients with Parkinson's disease. J Neurol Neurosurg Psychiatry 1994;57:336–367.

79. Fournet N, Moreaud O, Rouliin JL, Naegele B, Pellat J. Working memory functioning in medicated Parkinson's disease patients and the effect of withdrawal of dopaminergic medication. Neuropsychology 2000;14:247–253.

80. Tamura I, Kikuchi S, Otsuki M, Kitagawa M, Tashiro K. Deficits of working memory during mental calculation in patients with Parkinson's disease. J Neurol Sci 2003;209:19–23.

81. Le Bras C, Pillon B, Damier P, Dubois B. At which steps of spatial working memory processing do striatofrontal circuits intervene in humans? Neuropsychologia 1999;37:83–90.

82. Simon SR, Meunier M, Piettre L, Berardi AM, Segebarth CM, Boussaoud D. Spatial attention and memory versus motor preparation: premotor cortex involvement as revealed by fMRI. J Neurophysiol 2002;88:2047–2057.

83. Petrides M, Alivisatos B, Evans AC, Meyer E. Dissociation of human mid-dorsolateral from posterior dorsolateral frontal cortex in memory processing. Proc Natl Acad Sci USA 1993;90:873–877.

84. McCarthy G, Blamire AM, Puce A, et al. Functional magnetic resonance imaging of human prefrontal cortex activation during a spatial working memory task. Proc Natl Acad Sci USA 1994;91:8690–8694.

85. Belger A, Puce A, Krystal JH, Gore JC, Goldman-Rakic P, McCarthy G. Dissociation of mnemonic and perceptual processes during spatial and nonspatial working memory using fMRI. Hum Brain Mapp 1998;6:14–32.

86. Smith ML, Milner B. The role of the right hippocampus in the recall of spatial location. Neuropsychologia 1981;19: 781–793.

87. Pillon B, Ertle S, Deweer B, Sarazin M, Agid Y, Dubois B. Memory for spatial location is affected in Parkinson's disease. Neuropsychologia 1996;34:77–85.

88. Pillon B, Ertle S, Deweer B, Bonnet AM, Vidailhet M, Dubois B. Memory for spatial location in "de novo" parkinsonian patients. Neuropsychologia 1997;35:221–228.

89. Pillon B, Deweer B, Vidailhet M, Bonnet AM, Hahn-Barma V, Dubois B. Is impaired memory for spatial location in Parkinson's disease domain specific or dependent on 'strategic' processes? Neuropsychologia 1998;36:1–9.

90. Wallesch CW, Karnath HO, Papagno C, Zimmermann P, Deuschl G, Lucking CH. Parkinson's disease patient's behaviour in a covered maze learning task. Neuropsychologia 1990;28:839–849.

91. Kosslyn SM. Image and the Brain: The Resolution of the Imagery Debate. CAmbridge, MA: MIT Press, 1996.

92. Le Bihan D, Turner R, Zeffiro TA, Cuenod CA, Jezzard P, Bonnerot V. Activation of human primary visual cortex during visual recall: a magnetic resonance imaging study. Proc Natl Acad Sci U S A 1993;90:11802–11805.

93. Kosslyn SM, Thompson WL, Kim IJ, Alpert NM. Topographical representations of mental images in primary visual cortex. Nature 1995;378:496–498.

94. Cohen MS, Kosslyn SM, Breiter HC, et al. Changes in cortical activity during mental rotation. A mapping study using functional MRI. Brain 1996;119(Pt 1):89–100.

95. Jacobs DH, Shuren J, Bowers D, Heilman KM. Emotional facial imagery, perception, and expression in Parkinson's disease. Neurology 1995;45:1696–1702.

96. Brown RG, Marsden CD. Visuospatial function in Parkinson's disease. Brain 1986;109(Pt 5):987–1002.

97. Lee AC, Harris JP, Calvert JE. Impairments of mental rotation in Parkinson's disease. Neuropsychologia 1998;36:109–114.

98. Bowen B, Hoehn MM, Yahr MD. Parkinsonism: alteration in spatial orientation as determined by route walking task. Neuropsychologia 1972;10:355–361.

99. Buytenhuijs EL, Berger HJ, Van Spaendonck KP, Horstink MW, Borm GF, Cools AR. Memory and learning strategies in patients with Parkinson's disease. Neuropsychologia 1994;32:335–342.

100. Stepankova K, Ruzicka E. Object location learning and non-spatial working memory of patients with Parkinson's disease may be preserved in "real life" situations. Physiol Res 1998;47:377–384.

101. Montgomery P, Silverstein P, Wichmann R, Fleischaker K, Andberg M. Spatial updating in Parkinson's disease. Brain Cogn 1993;23:113–126.

102. Leplow B, Holl D, Zeng L, Herzog A, Behrens K, Mehdorn M. Spatial behaviour is driven by proximal cues even in mildly impaired Parkinson's disease. Neuropsychologia 2002;40:1443–1455.

103. Olton DS, Samuelson RJ. Remmebrance of place passe: spatial memory in rats. J Exp Psychol Anim Behav Proc 1976;2:97–116.
104. Morris RGM. Spatial localization does not require the presence of local cues. Learning and Motivation 1981;12:239–260.
105. Proctor F, Riklan M, Cooper IS, Teuber H-L. Judgement of visual and postural vertical by parkinsnonian patients. Neurology 1964;14:287–293.
106. Danta G, Hilton R. Judgment of the visual vertical and horizontal in patients with Parkinsonism. Neurology 1975;25: 43–47.
107. Della Sala S, Di Lorenzo G, Giordano A, Spinnler H. Is there a specific visuo-spatial impairment in Parkinsonians? J Neurol Neurosurg Psychiatry 1986;49:1258–1265.
108. Direnfeld LK, Albert ML, Volicer L, Langlais PJ, Marquis J, Kaplan E. Parkinson's disease. The possible relationship of laterality to dementia and neurochemical findings. Arch Neurol 1984;41:935–941.
109. Bentin S, Silverberg R, Gordon HW. Asymmetrical cognitive deterioration in demented and Parkinson patients. Cortex 1981;17:533–543.
110. Huber SJ, Freidenberg DL, Shuttleworth EC, Paulson GW, Clapp LE. Neuropsychological similarities in lateralized parkinsonism. Cortex 1989;25:461–470.
111. Riklan M, Stellar S, Reynolds C. The relationship of memory and cognition in Parkinson's disease to lateralisation of motor symptoms. J Neurol Neurosurg Psychiatry 1990;53:359–360.
112. Pillon B, Dubois B, Cusimano G, Bonnet AM, Lhermitte F, Agid Y. Does cognitive impairment in Parkinson's disease result from non-dopaminergic lesions? J Neurol Neurosurg Psychiatry 1989;52:201–206.
113. Saint-Cyr JA, Trepanier LL, Kumar R, Lozano AM, Lang AE. Neuropsychological consequences of chronic bilateral stimulation of the subthalamic nucleus in Parkinson's disease. Brain 2000;123(Pt 10):2091–-108.
114. Rafal RD. Visually guided behavior. In: Litvan I, Agid Y, eds. Progressive Supranuclear Palsy: Clinical and Research Approaches. New York: Oxford University Press, 1992:204–222.
115. Ghika J, Tennis M, Growdon J, Hoffman E, Johnson K. Environment-driven responses in progressive supranuclear palsy. J Neurol Sci 1995;130:104–111.
116. Kimura J, Barnett HJ, Burkhart G. The psychological test pattern in progressive supranuclear palsy. Neuropsychologia 1981;19:301–306.
117. Fisk JD, Goodale MA, Burkhart G, Barnett HJ. Progressive supranuclear palsy: the relationship between ocular motor dysfunction and psychological test performance. Neurology 1982;32:698–705.
118. Soliveri P, Monza D, Paridi D, et al. Cognitive and magnetic resonance imaging aspects of corticobasal degeneration and progressive supranuclear palsy. Neurology 1999;53:502–507.
119. Soliveri P, Monza D, Paridi D, et al. Neuropsychological follow up in patients with Parkinson's disease, striatonigral degenration-type multisystem atrophy, and progressive supranuclear palsy. J Neurol Neurosurg Psychiatry 2000;69:315–318.
120. Esmonde T, Giles E, Gibson M, Hodges JR. Neuropsychological performance, disease severity, and depression in progressive supranuclear palsy. J Neurol 1996;243:638–643.
121. Warrington EK, James M. Visual object and space perception battery. Bury St. Edmonds, UK: Thames Valley Test Co., 1991.
122. Posner MI, Rafal RD, Choate L, Vaughn J. Inhibition of return: Neural basis and function. Cogn Neuropsychol 1985;2:211–228.
123. Rafal RD, Posner MI. Deficits in human visual spatial attention following thalamic lesions. Proc Natl Acad Sci USA 1987;84:7349–7353.
124. Kertzman C, Robinson DL, Litvan I. Effects of physostigmine on spatial attention in patients with progressive supranuclear palsy. Arch Neurol 1990;47:1346–1350.
125. Schiller PH, True SD, Conway JL. Effects of frontal eye field and superior colliculus ablations on eye movements. Science 1979;206:590–592.
126. D'Antona R, Baron J, Samson Y, et al. Subcortical dementia. Frontal cortex hypometabolism detected by positron tomography in patients with progressive supranuclear palsy. Brain 1985;108 (Pt 3):785–799.
127. Posner MI, Walker JA, Friedrich FJ, Rafal RD. Effects of parietal injury on covert orienting of attention. J Neurosci 1984;4:1863–1874.
128. Henik A, Rafal R, Rhodes D. Endogenously generated and vsually guided saccades after lesions of the human frontal eye fields. Soc Neurosc Abstr 1991;17:803.
129. Rafal R, Henik A, Smith J. Exrageniculate contributions toreflex visual orienting in normla humans: A temporal hemified advantage. J Cogn Neurosci 1991;3:323–329.
130. Rafal R, Smith J, Krantz J, Cohen A, Brennan C. Extrageniculate vision in hemianopic humans: saccade inhibition by signals in the blind field. Science 1990;250:118–121.
131. Leiguarda R, Lees AJ, Merello M, Starkstein S, Marsden CD. The nature of apraxia in corticobasal degeneration. J Neurol Neurosurg Psychiatry 1994;57:455–459.
132. Blondel A, Eustache F, Schaeffer S, Marie RM, Lechevalier B, de la Sayette V. Étude clinique et cognitive de l'apraxie dans l'atrophie cortico-basale. Un trouble sélectif du système de production. Rev Neurol (Paris) 1997;153:737–747.

133. Jacobs DH, Adair JC, Macauley B, et al. Apraxia in corticobasal degeneration. Brain Cogn 1999;40:336–354.
134. Merians A, Clark M, Poizner H, et al. Apraxia differs in corticobasal degeneration and left-parietal stroke: A case study. Brain Cogn 1999;40(2):314–335.
135. Otsuki M, Soma Y, Yoshimura N, Tsuji S. Slowly progressive limb-kinetic apraxia. Eur Neurol 1997;37:100–103.
136. Moreaud O, Naegele B, Pellat J. The nature of apraxia in corticobasal degeneration: a case of melokinetic apraxia. Neuropsychiatry Neuropsychol Behav Neurol 1996;9:288–292.
137. Goldenberg G, Wimmer A, Auff E, Schnaberth G. Impairment of motor planning in patients with Parkinson's disease: evidence from ideomotor apraxia testing. J Neurol Neurosurg Psychiatry 1986;49:1266–1272.
138. Watson RT, Fleet WS, Gonzalez-Rothi L, Heilman KM. Apraxia and the supplementary motor area. Arch Neurol 1986;43:787–792.
139. Yamadori A, Osumi Y, Imamura T, Mitani Y. Persistent left unilateral apraxia and a disconnection theory. Behav Neurol 1988;1:11–22.
140. Marchetti C, Della Sala S. On crossed apraxia. Description of a right-handed apraxic patient with right supplementary motor area damage. Cortex 1997;33:341–354.
141. Pause M, Freund HJ. Role of the parietal cortex for sensorimotor transformation. Evidence from clinical observations. Brain Behav Evol 1989;33:136–140.
142. Freund HJ. The parietal lobe as a sensorimotor interface: a perspective from clinical and neuroimaging data. NeuroImage 2001;14(1 Pt 2):S142–S146.
143. De Renzi E, Lucchelli F. Ideational apraxia. Brain 1988;111(Pt 5):1173–1185.
144. Barbieri C, De Renzi E. The executive and ideational components of apraxia. Cortex 1988;24(4):535–534.
145. Peigneux P, Salmon E, Garraux G, et al. Neural and cognitive bases of upper limb apraxia in corticobasal degeneration. Neurology 2001;57:1259–1268.
146. Leiguarda RC, Marsden CD. Limb apraxias: higher-order disorders of sensorimotor integration. Brain 2000;123(Pt 5):860–879.
147. Leiguarda R, Merello M, Balej J. Apraxia in corticobasal degeneration. Adv Neurol 2000;82.
148. Decety J, Perani D, Jeannerod M, et al. Mapping motor representations with positron emission tomography. Nature 1994;371:600–602.
149. Bonda E, Petrides M, Frey S, Evans A. Neural correlates of mental transformations of the body-in-space. Proc Natl Acad Sci USA 1995;92:11180–11184.
150. Sirigu A, Daprati E, Pradat-Diehl P, Franck N, Jeannerod M. Perception of self-generated movement following left parietal lesion. Brain 1999;122(Pt 10):1867–1874.
151. Wolpert DM, Goodbody SJ, Husain M. Maintaining internal representations: the role of the human superior parietal lobe. Nat Neurosci 1998;1:529–533.
152. Andersen RA, Snyder LH, Bradley DC, Xing J. Multimodal representation of space in the posterior parietal cortex and its use in planning movements. Annu Rev Neurosci 1997;20:303–330.
153. Rothi LJ, Ochipa C, Heilman KM. A cognitive neuropsychological model of limb praxis. In: Rothi LJ, Heilman KM, eds. Apraxia: The neuropsychology of action. Hove, UK: Psychology, 1997:29–50.
154. Wenning GK, Litvan I, Jankovic J, et al. Natural history and survival of 14 patients with corticobasal degeneration confirmed at postmortem examination. J Neurol Neurosurg Psychiatry 1998;64:184–189.
155. Rey GJ, Tomer R, Levin BE, Sanchez-Ramos J, Bowen BB, J.H. Psychiatric symptoms, atypical dementia, and left visual field inattention in corticobasal ganglionic degeneration. Mov Disord 1995;10:106–110.
156. Kleiner-Fisman G, Black SE, Lang AE. Neurodegenerative disease and the evolution of art: the effects of presumed corticobasal degeneration in a professional artist. Mov Disord 2003;18:294–302.
157. De Renzi E. Disorders of Space Exploration and Cognition. New York: Wiley, 1982.
158. Mendez MF. Corticobasal ganglionic degeneration with Balint's syndrome. J Neuropsychiatry Clin Neurosci 2000;12:273–275.
159. Leone M, Budriesi C, Molinari MA, Nichelli P. Progressive biparietal atrophy: A case report and a review of clinico-pathological correlations of focal (lobar) atrophy. Neurol Sci 2002;23(suppl):S117.
160. Mendez MF, Turner J, Gilmore GC, Remler B, Tomsak RL. Balint's syndrome in Alzheimer's disease: visuospatial functions. Int J Neurosci 1990;54:339–346.
161. Furey-Kurkjian MI, Pietrini P, Graff-Radford N, et al. Visual variant of Alzheimer disease: Distinctive neurospychological features. Neuropsychology 1996;10:294–300.
162. Bergeron C, Davis A, Lang AE. Corticobasal ganglionic degeneration and progressive supranuclear palsy presenting with cognitive decline. Brain Pathol 1998;8:355–365.
163. Grimes DA, Lang AE, Bergeron CB. Dementia as the most common presentation of cortical-basal ganglionic degeneration. Neurology 1999;53:1969–1974.
164. De Renzi E. Disorders of spatial orientation. In: Frederiks JAM, ed. Handbook of Clinical Neurology, Vol. 45: Clinical Neuropsychology. Amsterdam: Elsevier Science, 1985:405–422.

165. Goethals M, Santens P. Posterior cortical atrophy. Two case reports and a review of the literature. Clin Neurol Neurosurg 2001;103:115–119.
166. Mendez MF. Visuospatial deficits with preserved reading ability in a patient with posterior cortical atrophy. Cortex 2001;37:535–543.
167. Papagno C. Progressive impairment of constructional abilities: a visuospatial sketchpad deficit? Neuropsychologia 2002;40:1858–1867.
168. Suzuki K, Otsuka Y, Endo K, et al. Visuospatial deficits due to impaired visual attention: investigation of two cases of slowly progressive visuospatial impairment. Cortex 2003;39:327–341.
169. McKeith IG, Galasko D, Kosaka K, et al. Consensus guidelines for the clinical and pathologic diagnosis of dementia with Lewy bodies (DLB): report of the consortium on DLB international workshop. Neurology 1996;47:1113–1124.
170. Gnanalingham KK, Byrne EJ, Thornton A. Clock-face drawing to differentiate Lewy body and Alzheimer type dementia syndromes. Lancet 1996;347:696–697.
171. Gnanalingham KK, Byrne EJ, Thornton A, Sambrook MA, Bannister P. Motor and cognitive function in Lewy body dementia: comparison with Alzheimer's and Parkinson's diseases. J Neurol Neurosurg Psychiatry 1997;62:243–252.
172. Walker Z, Allen RL, Shergill S, Katona CL. Neuropsychological performance in Lewy body dementia and Alzheimer's disease. Br J Psychiatry 1997;170:156–158 .
173. Shimomura T, Mori E, Yamashita H, et al. Cognitive loss in dementia with Lewy bodies and Alzheimer disease. Arch Neurol 1998;55:1547–1552.
174. Mori E, Shimomura T, Fujimori M, et al. Visuoperceptual impairment in dementia with Lewy bodies. Arch Neurol 2000;57:489–493.
175. Simard M, van Reekum R, Myran D. Visuospatial impairment in dementia with Lewy bodies and Alzheimer's disease: a process analysis approach. Int J Geriatr Psychiatry 2003;18:387–391.
176. Manford M, Andermann F. Complex visual hallucinations. Clinical and neurobiological insights. Brain 1998;121(Pt 10):1819–1840.
177. Imamura T, Ishii K, Hirono N, et al. Visual hallucinations and regional cerebral metabolism in dementia with Lewy bodies (DLB). Neuroreport 1999;10:1903–1907.
178. Ala TA, Hughes LF, Kyrouac GA, Ghobrial MW, Elble RJ. Pentagon copying is more impaired in dementia with Lewy bodies than in Alzheimer's disease. J Neurol Neurosurg Psychiatry 2001;70:483–488.
179. Quinn N. Multiple system atrophy—the nature of the beast. J Neurol Neurosurg Psychiatry 1989;Special Suppl:78–89.
180. Gilman S, Low PA, Quinn N, et al. Consensus statement on the diagnosis of multiple system atrophy. J Auton Nerv Syst 1998;74:189–192.
181. Litvan I, Bhatia KP, Burn DJ, et al. SIC Task Force appraisal of clinical diagnostic criteria for parkinsonian disorders. Mov Disord 2003;18:467–486.
182. Wenning GK, Ben-Shlomo Y, Hughes A, Daniel SE, Lees A, Quinn NP. What clinical features are most useful to distinguish definite multiple system atrophy from Parkinson's disease? J Neurol Neurosurg Psychiatry 2000;68:434–440.
183. Robbins TW, James M, Lange KW, Owen A, Quinn NP, Marsden CD. Cognitive performance in multiple system atrophy. Brain 1992;115(Pt 1):271–291.
184. Sahakian BJ, Morris RG, Evenden JL, et al. A comparative study of visuospatial memory and learning in Alzheimer-type dementia and Parkinson's disease. Brain 1988;111(Pt 3):695–718.
185. Tebartz van Elst L, Greenlee MW, Foley JM, Lucking CH. Contrast detection, discrimination and adaptation in patients with Parkinson's disease and multiple system atrophy. Brain 1997;120(Pt 12):2219–2228.
186. Bodis-Wollner I. Visual deficits related to dopamine deficiency in experimental animals and Parkinson's disease patients. Trends Neurosci 1990;13:296–302.
187. Haug BA, Kolle RU, Trenkwalder C, Oertel WH, Paulus W. Predominant affection of the blue cone pathway in Parkinson's disease. Brain 1995;118(Pt 3):771–778.
188. Djamgoz MB, Hankins MW, Hirano J, Archer SN. Neurobiology of retinal dopamine in relation to degenerative states of the tissue. Vision Res 1997;37:3509–3529.
189. Shallice T. Specific impairments of planning. Philos Trans R Soc Lond B Biol Sci 1982;298:199–209.
190. Keith Berg W, D. B. The Tower of London spatial problem-solving task: enhancing clinical and research implementation. J Clin Exp Neuropsychol 2002;24:586–604.
191. Goel V, Grafman J. Are the frontal lobes implicated in "planning" functions? Interpreting data from the Tower of Hanoi. Neuropsychologia 1995;33:623–642.
192. Saint-Cyr JA, Taylor AE, Lang AE. Procedural learning and neostriatal dysfunction in man. Brain 1988;111(Pt 4): 941–959.

15

Role of Ocular Motor Assessment in Diagnosis and Research

R. John Leigh and David S. Zee

INTRODUCTION

The clinical evaluation of eye movements can contribute substantially to the diagnosis of parkinsonian disorders, provided the physician performs a proper examination and interprets the findings by referring to a simple scheme of the neurobiology of eye movements *(1)*. Further diagnostic information can often be obtained by recording eye movements, which are more accessible to measurement and analysis than limb movements or gait. A good part of the neurobiological substrate of eye movements has been defined, which makes it possible to attribute disordered properties of eye movements to dysfunction of specific neuronal populations or structures in the brain. In this chapter, first, we review pertinent aspects of the ocular motor examination; second, we highlight some important test paradigms and technical aspects of measuring eye movements; and third, we summarize disorders of ocular motility reported with parkinsonian disorders and diseases affecting the basal ganglia.

CLINICAL EXAMINATION OF EYE MOVEMENTS IN PARKINSONISM

The systematic examination of eye movements is summarized in Table 1. The most useful part of the examination concerns saccades, which are the rapid eye movements by which we voluntarily move our line of sight (direction of gaze). Saccades are perhaps the best understood of all movements both in terms of their dynamic properties and neurobiology *(1–3)*. It is important to differentiate between limited *range* of movement, especially upward, and speed of saccades, especially vertically. Normal elderly subjects show limited upgaze *(4)*, and this may be because of changes in the connective tissues of the orbit *(5)*. Nonetheless, some normal elderly subjects make vertical saccades that have normal velocities, within their restricted range of motion *(6)*. Range of movement is conventionally elicited as the patient attempts to follow the examiner's moving finger, but this does not test saccades. It is important to ask the patient to shift gaze on command between two *stationary* visual targets, displaced horizontally or vertically, such as a pencil tip and the examiner's nose. After each verbal cue (e.g., "look at the pencil; now look at my nose"), note the time taken to initiate the saccade, its speed, and whether it gets the eye on target, or whether further corrective saccades are needed. It is also useful to ask parkinsonian patients to make saccades voluntarily at a rapid pace back and forth between two stationary targets (e.g., a finger from the left and right hand of the examiner. Patients with idiopathic Parkinson's disease (PD) often have difficulty making such self-generated sequences and several saccades, rather than one, are needed for the eye to reach the target (*see* video 1).

From: *Current Clinical Neurology: Atypical Parkinsonian Disorders*
Edited by: I. Litvan © Humana Press Inc., Totowa, NJ

Table 1
Summary of Eye Movement Examination

- Establishment of the range of ocular motility in horizontal and vertical planes
- Fixation stability in central and eccentric gaze (looking for nystagmus or saccades that intrude on steady fixation)
- Horizontal and vertical saccades made voluntarily between two fixed visual targets (noting initiation time, speed, and accuracy)
- Horizontal and vertical pursuit of a smoothly moving target (looking for "catch-up" saccades)
- "Optokinetic nystagmus" induced with horizontal or vertical motion of a hand-held drum or tape
- Ocular alignment during fixation of a distant target, and vergence responses to smooth or stepping motion of targets aligned in the patient's sagittal plane
- The vestibular ocular reflex in response to smooth sinusoidal, or sudden, head rotations in horizontal and vertical planes (looking for corrective saccades that accompany or follow the head rotation)

Another important feature of many parkinsonian disorders is inappropriate saccades that intrude on steady fixation; the most common are small "square-wave jerks" that are most easily appreciated during ophthalmoscopy as to-and-fro movements of the fundus. Smooth pursuit is not usually helpful, because many elderly normal subjects and even some younger subjects may have impaired pursuit that requires catch-up saccades to keep the line of sight on the moving target. Optokinetic stimulation at the bedside may be useful in some patients who have difficulty initiating voluntary saccades (e.g., progressive supranuclear palsy [PSP]); vertical drum motion may induce tonic vertical deviation of the eyes in affected individuals or evoke reflexive "quick phases" of nystagmus. Vergence is also often impaired in normal elderly subjects, and identification of abnormalities may require laboratory assessment.

A NOTE ON LABORATORY METHODS FOR STUDYING EYE MOVEMENTS IN PARKINSONIAN DISORDERS

Perhaps the most important diagnostic contribution to be made by recording eye movements in parkinsonian disorders concerns tests of vertical saccades *(7,8)*. Reliable measurement of horizontal or vertical saccades requires methods with adequate bandwidth (0–150 Hz), sensitivity (0.1°), and linear range (±30°). DC-amplified electro-oculography (EOG) is adequate to signal horizontal eye position and timing at the beginning and end of a saccade, but is unreliable for measuring vertical movements. Infrared methods provide better bandwidth but inferior range to EOG, and also cannot be used to measure vertical movements. The most reliable method is the magnetic search coil which, in our experience, is well tolerated by frail and elderly subjects, and has the added advantage of being calibrated independently of the patient's voluntary range of movements *(1)*. Fast frame-rate video-based techniques are suitable for measuring dynamic properties of horizontal and vertical saccades *(9)*, but their calibration depends on the ability of the patient to look at visual targets, and this may be impaired, for example, in PSP.

Saccades show consistent relationships between their size, speed, and duration *(2,10)*. Thus, the bigger the saccade, the greater its peak velocity and the longer it lasts. Examples of the "main sequence" relationships between peak velocity, duration, and amplitude are provided from normal subjects in Fig. 1; exponential or power-function equations have been used to describe these relationships and define prediction intervals for normal subjects *(2,10,11)*. Deviations of measured eye movements from these relationships indicate either abnormal saccades, or nonsaccadic eye movements. Thus, in Fig. 1, we also provide an example of abnormally slow vertical saccades from a patient with PSP.

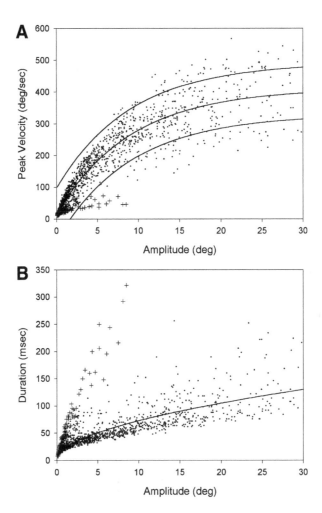

Fig. 1. Plots summarizing important dynamic properties of saccades. (**A**) Plot of peak velocity vs amplitude of vertical saccades. Data points are saccades from 10 normal subjects. The data are fit with an exponential equation; also plotted are the 5% and 95% prediction intervals. The + indicate vertical saccades from a patient with PSP, which lie outside the prediction intervals for normals. (**B**) Plot of duration vs amplitude. The data from 10 normal subjects are fit with a power equation. The + indicate vertical saccades from a patient with PSP, which have greater duration than control subjects.

Aside from measurement of saccadic dynamics, substantial effort has been put into using saccades as a behavioral index of motor programming in basal ganglia and associated cortical disorders *(12)*. Thus, although the frontal and parietal eye fields project directly to the brainstem centers, such as the superior colliculus and pontine nuclei, a second pathway running through the basal ganglia plays an important role, and comprises the caudate, substantia nigra par reticulata (SNpr), subthalamic nucleus, and superior colliculus (Fig. 2). A simplified view of this basal ganglia pathway is that it is composed of two serial, inhibitory links: a caudate-SNpr inhibition, which is only phasically active, and a SNpr-collicular inhibition, which is tonically active *(13)*. If frontal cortex causes caudate neurons to fire, then the SNpr-collicular inhibition is removed and the superior colliculus is able to activate a saccade. In addition, the subthalamic nucleus contains neurons that discharge in relation to saccades and

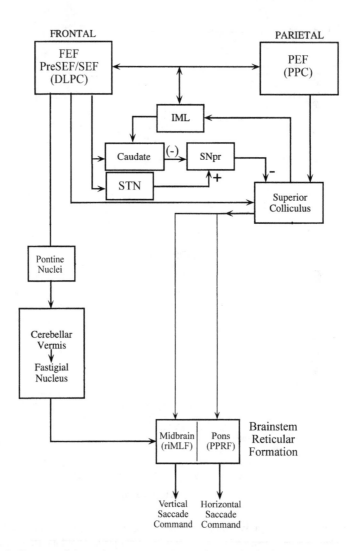

Fig. 2. (**A**) Block diagram of the major structures that project to the brainstem saccade generator (premotor burst neurons in PPRF and riMLF). Also shown are projections from cortical eye fields to superior colliculus. FEF, frontal eye fields; SEF, supplementary eye fields; DLPC, dorsolateral prefrontal cortex; IML, intramedullary lamina of thalamus; PEF, parietal eye fields (LIP); PPC, posterior parietal cortex; SNpr, substantia nigra, pars reticulata.

excites (SNpr), which in turn inhibits the superior colliculus. Animal studies indicate that this pathway appears important for programming of saccades to targets for which there is an expectation of reward *(14,15)*. The caudate nucleus also probably contributes to smooth pursuit *(16)*.

For these reasons, studies of the effects of human diseases affecting basal ganglia have focused on behaviors such as memory-guided or predictive saccades (Fig. 3). Memory-guided saccades are made in darkness several seconds after a visual target has been flashed. Predictive saccades are made in anticipation of a target appearance or jump. In the anti-saccade task, the subject is required to look in the opposite direction (mirror image position) to a visual stimulus. Thus, a reflexive, visually guided saccade must be inhibited and a saccade to an imagined target made instead *(17)*. Such testing is still mainly a research tool, but it has provided insights into the pathogenesis of parkinsonian disorders, as we will mention in discussing each type of disorder.

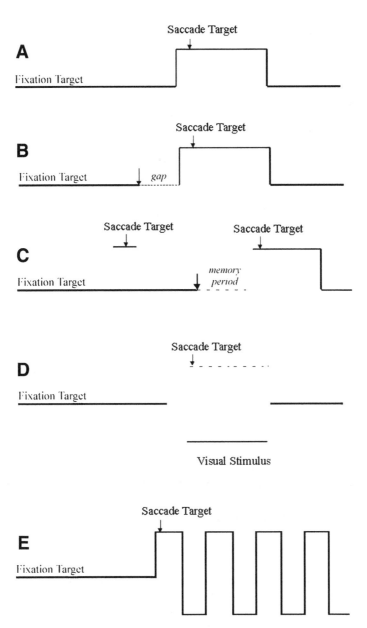

Fig. 3. Schematic summary of stimulus paradigms that have been used to test saccades in Parkinsonian disorders. (**A**) Simultaneous switching of fixation target off and visual target on (overlap paradigm). (**B**) Gap paradigm, in which fixation target is switched off before visual target is switched on. (**C**) Memory target task. The subject views the fixation target during the time that the visual target is flashed and after several seconds (the memory period), the fixation light is switched off and the subject looks toward the remembered location of the target. (**D**) The antisaccade task. The subject is required to look in the opposite direction when the visual stimulus is presented. (**E**) Predictive task. Subject makes saccades to a target that jumps to a predictable location with predictable timing.

IDIOPATHIC PARKINSON'S DISEASE (TABLE 2)

Clinical Findings in PD

Most patients with PD show relatively minor abnormalities at the bedside that may also occur in healthy elderly subjects. For example, steady fixation may be disrupted by saccadic intrusions (square-wave jerks) *(18–20)*, but these are also seen in some normal elderly subjects. Moderate restriction of the range of upward gaze is common in elderly individuals *(4)*, with or without parkinsonism, and has been attributed to changes in the orbital tissues *(5)*. Similarly, smooth pursuit can be impaired in PD but is also abnormal in some healthy normals *(21)*. Convergence insufficiency is common and sometimes symptomatic *(22)*. Patients with PD often have lid lag. Patients with advanced PD may show some slowing of vertical saccades, but PSP should always be considered in such cases.

A characteristic sign in PD is that hypometria becomes more marked when patients are asked to rapidly perform self-paced refixations between two continuously visible targets (e.g., a finger of the examiners right and left hand about 60–80° apart; the normal horizontal ocular motor range is about 45° to either side) (video 1).

Laboratory Findings in PD

Saccades

Saccades in PD usually undershoot the target (i.e., they are hypometric), especially vertically *(20,21)*. Patients may show a "stair-case" of saccades to acquire the target (especially with remembered targets); this "fragmentation" has been interpreted as a robust correction mechanism to compensate for the underlying hypometria *(23)*. It has been possible to investigate the pathogenesis of the hypometria, which becomes more marked when patients are asked to make self-paced refixations between two continuously visible targets. This phenomenon is not simply because of the persistence of the visual targets, because saccades made *in anticipation* of the appearance of a target light at a remembered location are also hypometric *(24,25)*. Patients with PD have difficulty in generating sequences of memory-guided saccades *(26–28)*, whereas saccades made reflexively to novel visual stimuli are normal in size and promptly initiated *(7)*. Furthermore, visually guided adaptation of saccades is preserved whereas memory guided adaptation of saccades is impaired *(29)*. Thus, it appears that PD patients are unable to generate internally guided saccades to accurately shift gaze *(7,30)*. Despite this hypometria, patients can still shift their gaze with a series of saccades to the location of a briefly flashed target; this indicates a retained ability to encode the location of objects in extrapersonal space *(20,24)*.

The reaction time (latency) of saccades made in response to nonpredictable target jumps may be normal or mildly increased *(20,30)*. During self-paced refixations between two visible targets, intersaccadic intervals increase *above* the latency of responses to nonpredictable target jumps *(30,31)* If the fixation light is turned out 100 msec before a target light appears ("gap" paradigm—Fig. 3) PD patients are able to make short-latency (100–130 ms) "express saccades" like normal subjects *(7)*.

The pathophysiology of saccadic disorders in PD is not fully understood. One possible mechanism is via the subthalamic nucleus (Fig. 2), which contains neurons that discharge in relation to saccades. The subthalamic nucleus is hyperactive in PD, and excites the substantia nigra, pars reticulata (SNpr), which in turn inhibits the superior colliculus. It may be that excess activity in SNpr in PD leads to a defect in generation of the more voluntary, internally guided saccades such as those during prediction and to memorized targets. Functional imaging studies have suggested that the basal ganglia are important for processing of temporal information *(32)*, which may be important for generating a regular series of saccades. Furthermore, during predictive visuomanual tracking, there is an underactivity of sensorimotor cortex, but increase in premotor areas, such as pre-SMA (supplementary motor area), which may represent compensation or impaired suppression *(33)*. Finally, PD also affects the dopaminergic

Table 2
Summary of Disordered Eye Movements in Some Basal Ganglia Disorders

Progressive Supranuclear Palsy (PSP)

- Slow vertical saccades, especially down, with a preserved range of movement, may be the first sign of the disorder; later, loss of vertical saccades and quick phases
- Horizontal saccades become slow and hypometric
- Disruption of steady gaze by horizontal saccadic intrusions (square-wave jerks)
- Impaired smooth pursuit, vertically (reduced range) and horizontally (with catch-up saccades)
- Smooth eye-head tracking may be relatively preserved, especially vertically
- Preservation of slow phases of vestibular ocular reflex but quick phases are affected as saccades
- Horizontal disconjugacy suggesting INO
- Loss of convergence
- Ultimately, all eye movements may be lost, but vestibular movements are the last to go
- Eyelid disorders: apraxia of lid opening, lid lag, blepharospasm, inability to suppress a blink to a bright light.

Parkinson's Disease

- Fixation may be disrupted by square-wave jerks
- Hypometria of horizontal and vertical saccades, especially when patients are asked to perform self-paced refixations between two continuously visible targets
- Normal saccadic velocity except in some advanced cases
- Impaired smooth pursuit, horizontally and vertically, owing partly to inadequate catch-up saccades
- Vestibular eye movements normal for natural head movements
- Impaired convergence
- Oculogyric crises
- Lid lag

Huntington's Disease

- Difficulties initiating saccades (without an associated head thrust and blink)
- Difficulties suppressing saccades to novel visual stimuli (especially during the antisaccade task)
- Slow saccades, especially vertically, and in patients with early age of onset
- Impairment of smooth pursuit
- Preservation of VOR and gaze-holding

---

cells within the retina. PD patients have abnormalities of color vision and in detection of spatially and temporally modulated gratings *(34)*.

Smooth Pursuit

Mildly affected PD patients differ little from age-matched control subjects in their smooth-pursuit performance *(21,35)*. During tracking of a target moving in a predictable, sinusoidal pattern, eye speed is less than target speed, leading to catch-up saccades *(20,36)*. In addition, the catch-up saccades are hypometric; thus, the cumulative tracking eye movement is less than that of the target *(35)*. Despite these impairments, the phase relationship between eye and target movement is normal,30 implying a normal predictive smooth tracking strategy. This is in contrast to saccadic tracking of predictive target jumps which, as described earlier, is deficient.

Vestibular Responses

Both caloric and low-frequency rotational vestibular responses, in darkness, may be hypoactive in patients with PD *(37,38)*. However, at higher frequencies of head rotation, and particularly during visual fixation, the vestibular ocular (VOR) reflex adequately compensates for head perturbations, which accounts for the lack of complaint of oscillopsia in patients with PD.

Effects of Disease Course and Treatment

Patients with advanced PD may show greater defects on more demanding tests, such as making memory-guided saccades, and on the anti-saccade tasks (Fig. 3), which requires inhibiting a reflexive saccade, and looking in the opposite direction to the target (its mirror location). In addition, patients with advanced disease may show some slowing of vertical or horizontal saccades.

In general, L-dopa treatment of PD does not seem to improve the ocular motor deficits except for improvement of saccadic accuracy (i.e., saccades become larger) *(36,39)*. Some newly diagnosed patients with idiopathic PD may show improved smooth pursuit after the institution of dopaminergic therapy *(39)*. Memory-guided saccades are reported to be impaired after pallidotomy for PD *(40)*, but improved with subthalamic nucleus stimulation *(41)*, possibly by improving learning abilities in the corticobasal ganglia network *(42)*. Pallidotomy increases saccadic intrusions on steady fixation (square-wave jerks) *(43,44)*.

Toxic Parkinsonism

In patients with parkinsonism owing to methyl-4-phenyl-1,2,3,6-tetrahydropyridine (MPTP) toxicity, saccadic latency is shortened and saccadic accuracy improved by dopaminergic agents; in addition, reflex blepharospasm was improved *(45)*. In monkeys that received MPTP, saccadic abnormalities, including increased latency, increased duration, decreased rate of spontaneous saccades, and inappropriate saccades, were all reversed by dopaminergic therapy *(46,47)*.

PROGRESSIVE SUPRANUCLEAR PALSY

Clinical Features

PSP is a degenerative disease of later life characterized by abnormal vertical saccades; the early appearance of falls, usually within a year of onset, owing to disturbance of tone and posture; difficulties with swallowing and speech; and mental slowing *(48)*. Median survival time is about 6 yr. The disturbance of eye movements is usually present early in the course, but occasionally develops late, or is sometimes not noted by the patient's physicians *(49)*. Patient may complain of blurred vision, double vision, or photophobia *(48)*, and have often been fitted with several different spectacle refractions, without improvement. On direct questioning, it is usually possible to determine that these visual complaints are a result of loss of the ability to voluntarily shift gaze in the vertical plane so that, for example, patients cannot look down to see a plate of food, tie their shoes, or confidently navigate going down the stairs.

The initial ocular motor deficit consists of slowing of vertical saccades and quick phases, either down or up or both *(see* video 2). Sometimes vertical saccades take a curved or oblique trajectory ("round the houses") *(21,50)*. Vertical smooth pursuit is relatively preserved, but of decreased gain *(51)*. Larger targets may elicit greater responses *(52)*, and could be used to evaluate the range of eye movements in patients in whom neck stiffness makes testing of the VOR technically difficult. Similarly, full-field optokinetic stimuli may induce responses that are useful for analysis *(11)*. Combined eye-head tracking may also be relatively spared. As the disease progresses, the range of movements possible with vertical saccades and pursuit declines and eventually no voluntary vertical eye movements are possible. However, the VOR is preserved until late in the disease (although a characteristic rigidity of the neck may make the vertical doll's head maneuver difficult to elicit).

Horizontal eye movements also show characteristic changes: steady fixation is disrupted by square-wave jerks *(11,18,21)*, which are more common than in other parkinsonian disorders. Horizontal saccades are initially hypometric but normal in speed *(see* video 3) *(53)*; as the disease progresses, they also become slow. In some patients, the involvement of horizontal saccades resembles internuclear ophthalmoplegia (INO), although vestibular stimulation may overcome the limitation of adduction *(54)*. Horizontal smooth pursuit appears impaired, in part, because of square-wave jerks. Convergence eye movements are commonly impaired *(55)*. Late in the disease, the ocular motor deficit may progress to a complete ophthalmoplegia. Patients with absent quick phases but intact vestibular eye movements may also show sustained deviation of the eyes in the orbit during body rotation, and if the head is free to move it too may deviate opposite to the direction of body rotation *(56)*.

There are a variety of eyelid abnormalities in PSP: blepharospasm, lid-opening apraxia, eye-closing apraxia, lid retraction, and lid lag *(21)*. Patients typically show an inability to suppress a blink to a bright light—a visual Meyerson's (glabella) sign (*see* video 4) *(57)*. A single patient may have more than one of these abnormalities. Bell's phenomenon is usually absent.

Laboratory Findings in PSP

Saccades

Reliable measurements of saccades in PSP have demonstrated that vertical saccades are slower than horizontal saccades of similar size *(21,58)*. For patients who are able to make only small saccades, it is still possible to determine whether the movements are slowed using an appropriate statistical approach *(59)*. Vertical saccades are generated by "burst neurons" in the midbrain but horizontal saccades are generated by burst neurons in the pons. Thus, the selective involvement of vertical saccades in the early stage of PSP has indicated that the brunt of the disease initially falls on midbrain burst neurons, or their local circuitry (superior colliculus and the adjacent central mesencephalic reticular formation) *(60,61)*.

The latency (reaction time) of horizontal saccades in PSP is prolonged in some patients, but others retain the ability to make short-latency or "express" saccades *(62)*. Patients with PSP also make errors when they are required to look in the opposite direction to a suddenly appearing target (the antisaccade task—Fig. 3). Both the presence of express saccades and errors on the antisaccade task suggest defects in frontal lobe function and, although neuropathological changes there are mild, positron emission scanning indicates profound frontal hypometabolism *(63)*.

Vestibular Eye Movements

Measurements of vestibular eye movements during horizontal rotation, either in darkness, or during fixation of a stationary target, confirms that PSP patients show similar slow-phase responses to normal subjects but quick phases are commonly impaired leading to tonic deviation of the eyes in the contraversive direction in the oribit during rotation in the dark *(51)*.

Smooth-Pursuit, Optokinetic, and Vergence Movements

Smooth pursuit is usually impaired in both horizontal and vertical planes *(21)*. In the vertical plane, no corrective "catch-up" saccades can be made. The combined impairment of vertical saccades and pursuit constitutes voluntary gaze palsy. During large-field, vertical optokinetic stimulation, PSP patients often show tonic deviation of the eyes in the direction of stripe motion, with small or absent resetting quick phases *(11)*. When PSP patients shift their fixation point between distant and near targets, the vergence movement is slowed compared to control subjects *(64)*.

EYE MOVEMENTS IN OTHER DISORDERS CAUSING PARKINSONIAN SYNDROMES: DIFFERENTIATION FROM PSP (TABLE 3)

The clinical challenge often posed to neurologists is to diagnose parkinsonian patients with abnormal eye movements. As noted above, most patients with PD have normal eye movements for their age, whereas as most patients with PSP do not. In fact, a number of other parkinsonian disorders have been reported to produce abnormal eye movements, and it is those disorders that we review in this section, noting features that help to differentiate from PSP.

Table 3
Comparison of Findings in Some Parkinsonian Syndromes

	SWJ During Fixation	Visually Guided Saccades	Laboratory Testing of Saccades
PD	Increased following pallidotomy	Hypometric, when self-generated and especially when instructed to generate successive saccades back and forth at a rapid pace; slow vertically in advanced casedes	Difficulty generating memorized sequences. Advanced cases make errors on antisaccade task
PSP	Markedly increased	Slow; hypometric; initiated with difficulty	Increased errors on antisaccade task
MSA	Increased in some patients	Slow and hypometric in some patients	
CBGD	Increased in some patients	Hypometric and increased latency; deficit more marked in the presence of a visual background	Increased errors on antisaccade task
HD	May be increased	Difficulty with initiation; may be slow and hypometic	Markedly increased errors on antisaccade task; impaired predictive saccade tracking

Conditions that closely mimic PSP, causing slow vertical saccades, horizontal square-wave jerks, dysphagia, and frequent falls, include *multiple infarcts* affecting the basal ganglia, internal capsule, and midbrain (in the distribution of the perforating vessels arising from the proximal portions of the posterior cerebral artery) *(65)*, infiltrative processes such as lymphoma, and paraneoplastic syndromes *(66)*. Disorders causing the dorsal midbrain syndrome, such as tumor and hydrocephalus, can also produce a clinical picture that has some similarities to PSP with vertical-gaze palsy.

Whipple's disease can also closely mimic PSP, with vertical saccadic gaze palsy *(67,68)*. In addition, there may be characteristic "oculomasticatory myorhythmia"— a pendular vergence oscillation with concurrent contractions of the masticatory muscles; occasionally the limb muscles also show rhythmic contractions *(69)*. Whipple's disease can now be diagnosed using polymerase chain reaction (PCR) analysis of involved tissues *(70)*, and can be treated with antibiotics *(71)*.

Pure akinesia is characterized by profound disturbances of speech, handwriting, and gait, so that, for example, affected patients may suffer episodes during which they stand "frozen" for hours on end *(72)*. Tremor, limb rigidity, akinesia, dementia, or responsiveness to levodopa are absent. Such patients may show slow and hypometric vertical saccades. The disorder may be a restricted form of PSP with a longer, more benign course.

Cortical-basal degeneration (CBD) may lead to a defect in range of vertical eye movements but it usually does not cause marked slowing of saccades; instead the defect is an increased saccadic reaction time (latency), which is evident at the bedside *(21,73)*. Hypometria of upward saccades may occur early in the course, and should be differentiated from restricted upward range, which is present in elderly normal subjects. Other occasional findings in CBD include some decrease in horizontal saccade speed in the direction of the more affected limb, and increased distractibility during the antisaccade paradigm (looking at, instead of way from, the visual target). The other features of this degeneration—focal dystonia, ideomotor apraxia, alien hand syndrome, myoclonus, asymmetric akinetic-rigid syndrome with late onset of gait or balance disturbances—are more important in securing the diagnosis *(74,75)*.

Multiple system atrophy (MSA) causes a parkinsonian syndrome with marked autonomic findings. Some patients show slowing of vertical saccades as well as hypometria *(21,76)*, whereas other have cerebellar eye movement findings, including downbeat nystagmus during positional testing *(77)*, impaired smooth ocular and eye-head pursuit.

Dementia with Lewy bodies, which causes parkinsonism and fluctuating dementia with florid visual hallucinations, may be associated with a vertical-gaze paralysis *(78,79)*, but systematic measurements of vertical saccade are not yet available.

Other basal ganglia disorders that have been reported to show features similar to PSP include idiopathic *striopallidodentate calcification (Fahr's disease) (80)*, and autosomal dominant parkinsonism and dementia with *pallido-ponto-nigral degeneration (81)*. Some patients with *Huntington's disease* (HD) may present with vertical saccadic palsy and axial rigidity; this condition is discussed in a later section. Patients with the syndrome of amyotrophic lateral sclerosis (ALS), parkinsonism, and dementia (*Lytico-Bodig*), which is encountered in the inhabitants of the islands of the South Pacific Ocean, including Guam, may show more severe deficits than those with idiopathic PD, including limitation of vertical gaze *(82)*. A variant of ALS has been described, in which slow vertical saccades, gaze-evoked nystagmus, and impaired pursuit were prominent *(83)*. In the French West Indies, a PSP-like syndrome thought to result from neurotoxic alkaloids is associated with ingestion of herbal teas and fruits *(84)*. Slow saccades, with a supranuclear gaze palsy, are also characteristic of *Creutzfeldt–Jakob disease* but usually in both the horizontal and vertical planes *(85)*. Periodic alternating nystagmus, rebound nystagmus, and centripetal nystagmus (slow phases directed eccentrically) on lateral gaze are also characteristic of this condition owing to cerebellar involvement *(85,86)*.

DRUG-INDUCED PARKINSONISM AND OCULOGYRIC CRISIS

Drug intoxications, especially with phenothiazines such as the butyrophenones, may produce a parkinsonian picture with slowing of saccades and an "akinetic mutism" picture. A distinct syndrome is oculogyric crisis, which was once a common feature of postencephalitic parkinsonism, but is now a side effect of drugs, especially neuroleptic agents *(87)*. Oculogyric crises may also rarely be a feature of Wilson's disease *(88)*, and disorders of amino acid metabolism (aromatic L-amino acid decarboxylase deficiency) *(89)*.

A typical oculogyric crisis is ushered in by feelings of fear or depression, which give rise to an obsessive fixation on a thought. The eyes usually deviate upward, and sometimes laterally; they rarely deviate downward. During the period of upward deviation, the movements of the eyes in the upper field of gaze appear nearly normal. Affected patients have great difficulty in looking down, except when they combine a blink and downward saccade. Thus, the ocular disorder may reflect an imbalance of the vertical gaze-holding mechanism (the "neural integrator"). Anticholinergic drugs promptly terminate the thought disorder and ocular deviation, a finding that has led to the suggestion that the disorders of thought and eye movements are linked by a pharmacological imbalance common to both *(87)*. Delayed oculogyric crises have been described after striatocapsular infarction, and with bilateral putaminal hemorrhage *(90)*. Oculogyric crises are distinct from the brief upward ocular deviations that occur in Tourette syndrome *(91)*, Rett syndrome *(92)*, children with benign paroxysmal tonic upgaze *(93)*, and in many patients with tardive dyskinesia *(94)*. In some patients with tardive dyskinesias, however, the upward eye deviations are more sustained and also have the characteristic neuropsychological syndrome of oculogyric crises *(95)*. Episodic brief spells of tonic upgaze have also been reported after bilateral lentiform lesions *(96)*.

HUNTINGTON'S DISEASE

Clinical Findings

HD results from a genetic defect of the IT15 gene ("huntingtin") on chromosome 4, causing increased CAG triplet repeat length. Disturbances of voluntary gaze are common in this disorder *(97–100)*. Initiation of saccades may be difficult with prolonged latencies, especially when the saccade is made to command or in anticipation of a target that is moving in a predictable fashion. An obligatory blink or head turn may be used to start the eye moving (101). Saccades may be slow in the horizontal or vertical plane; this deficit can often be detected early in the disease if eye movements are measured, but may not be evident clinically until late in the course. Longitudinal studies of saccades have documented progressive slowing and prolongation of reaction time (102). Saccades may be slower in patients who become symptomatic at an earlier age, and it has been suggested that such individuals are more likely to have inherited the disease from their father (99).

Fixation is abnormal in some patients with HD because of saccadic intrusions (100). This defect of steady fixation is particularly evident when patients view a textured background. Smooth pursuit may also be impaired with decreased gain, but often is relatively spared compared with saccades. By contrast, gaze holding and the VOR are spared. Late in the disease, rotational stimulation causes the eyes to tonically deviate with few or no quick phases.

Despite the near-ubiquitous finding of abnormal eye movements in HD, some individuals who have been studied at a presymptomatic point in their disease have shown normal eye movements (97,103,104). Thus, routine testing of eye movements cannot be regarded as a reliable method for determining which offspring of affected patients will go on to develop the disease. Some improvement of the eye movement abnormalities in HD has been reported with sulpiride (105).

The paradoxical findings of difficulty in initiating voluntary saccades but with an excess of extraneous saccades during attempted fixation has been further elucidated using special test stimuli (Fig. 3). These have revealed an excessive distractibility in, for example, tasks in which patients are required to look in the opposite direction to a suddenly appearing target (antisaccade task) (106). A second finding is that saccades to visual stimuli are made at normal latency, whereas those made to command are delayed. These findings can be related to the parallel pathways that control the various types of saccadic responses. On the one hand, disease affecting either the frontal lobes or the caudate nucleus, which inhibits the SNpr, may lead to difficulties in initiating voluntary saccades in tasks that require learned or predictive behavior (107). On the other hand, HD also affects the SNpr (108). Since this structure inhibits the superior colliculus (nigro-collicular projection), and so suppresses reflexive saccades to visual stimuli, one might expect excessive distractibility during attempted fixation (107). The slowing of saccades might reflect involvement of saccadic burst neurons (109) but at least some pathologic evidence suggests that disturbance of prenuclear inputs, such as the superior colliculus or frontal eye fields, is responsible (110).

Disorders to be considered in the differential diagnosis of HD include neuroacanthocytosis (111), although abnormal eye movements have not been described as an important feature of this disorder. Dentatorubropallidoluysian atrophy, also called the Haw River syndrome (112), is another CAG triplet repeat disease (B37, chromosome 12) and is characterized by slow saccades but more myoclonus and ataxia than in HD.

OTHER DISORDERS THAT MAY AFFECT THE BASAL GANGLION DISORDERS AND MAY HAVE ABNORMAL EYE MOVEMENTS

Wilson's disease, hepatolenticular degeneration, is an autosomal recessive, inherited disorder of copper metabolism. The defect is in a copper-transporting ATPase with the gene at q14.3 on chromosome 13. CT typically shows hypodense areas, and positron emission tomography (PET) scanning indicates a decreased rate of glucose metabolism in the globus pallidus and putamen. The classic clinical picture is a movement disorder with psychiatric symptoms and associated liver disease. The Kayser–Fleisher ring is typical in the posterior cornea in Descemet's membrane, and some patients may have a sunflower cataract. Ocular motor disorders in Wilson's disease include a distractibility of gaze, with inability to voluntarily fix upon an object unless other, competing, visual stimuli are removed (e.g., fixation of a solitary light in an otherwise dark room) (113). Slow vertical saccades have also been reported in one patient with Wilson's disease (114), but are often normal. A lid-opening apraxia has also been noted *(115)*. Oculogyric crises may occur *(88)*. The eye movements of Wilson's disease, therefore, show some similarities to those described in HD and Alzheimer's disease. The distractibility in both conditions may be owing to involvement of the inhibitory pathways from the basal ganglia to the superior colliculus (Fig. 2).

Ataxia telangiectasia results from a defect on chromosome 11q. Characteristic eye signs include an ocular motor apraxia with hypometria and increased latency, but normal velocity of saccades with head thrusts *(116–119)*. Both vertical and horizontal saccades are affected. Other features are gaze-evoked nystagmus, periodic alternating nystagmus, square-wave jerks, and unusual slow smooth-pursuit-like movements that are used to change gaze voluntarily when saccades are difficult to generate. α-Feto protein levels are usually dramatically elevated.

Niemann–Pick disease (Niemann–Pick type C [2S] disease), usually presents during adolescence with intellectual impairment, ataxia, and dysarthria, and a selective slowing of vertical saccades *(120–122)*. Other eye movements (including horizontal saccades) are normal. Diagonal saccades may show a curved trajectory evident during the clinical examination. A bone marrow examination shows sea blue histiocytes.

Caudate hemorrhage has been associated with ipsilateral gaze preference *(123)*, consistent with experimental dopamine depletion of this structure. Patients with bilateral *lentiform nucleus lesions* show abnormalities of predictive and memory-guided saccades (both internally generated), but visually guided saccades and antisaccades (both triggered by a visual target) are normal *(124)*. It has been suggested that defects in the control of predictive smooth-pursuit eye movements are a feature of striatal damage *(125)*, consistent with demonstration of pursuit projections to the caudate nucleus *(16)*.

Patients with *Gilles de la Tourette syndrome* may show abnormalities such as blepharospasm and eye tics that include involuntary gaze deviations *(91)*. Routine testing of saccades, fixation, and pursuit is normal, but patients show increased latency and decreased peak velocity of antisaccades, as well as impaired sequencing of memory-guided saccades *(126–131)*. The lid abnormalities of Tourette syndrome must be distinguished from benign eye movement tics, which children often outgrow *(132,133)*. Patients with Lesch–Nyhan syndrome—a disorder of purine metabolism—show an impaired ability to make voluntary saccades, errors on the antisaccade task, blepharospasm, and intermittent gaze deviations similar to Tourette syndrome *(134)*.

Patients with *essential blepharospasm* generally show normal eye movements *(135)*, although saccadic latencies may be increased in certain visually guided and memory-guided saccade tests *(136,137)*. Patients with *spasmodic torticollis* may show abnormalities of vestibular function including the torsional VOR *(138,139)*. Whether vestibular abnormalities are the cause or a secondary effect of spasmodic torticollis has not been settled, but affected patients do show changes in their perceptions of the visual vertical and straight ahead *(140)*. Patients with *tardive dyskinesia* may display increased saccade distractibility *(141)*. Patients with active *Sydenham's chorea* are reported to show saccadic hypometria *(142)*. Patients with essential tremor, which may sometimes be confused with PD, have eye movement disorders suggestive of cerebellar dysfunction (impaired pursuit and impaired modulation of the duration of vestibular responses by head orientation) *(143)*.

PROSPECTS FOR EYE MOVEMENTS IN PARKINSONIAN RESEARCH (TABLE 4)

At present, much is known about the neurobiology of eye movements, especially saccades, which can be applied to understanding the pathogenesis of disturbed behavior in a range of movement disorders. It can be expected that the trend of using novel paradigms (such as shown in Fig. 3) along with functional imaging is likely to provide new insights. To the clinical movement disorder specialists, examination of eye movement remains a useful diagnostic tool that will likely become even more important with basic science advances. As more movement disorder specialists incorporate a systematic eye movement examination into their daily routine, not only will diagnostic accuracy

Table 4
Major Issues for Eye Movement Research in Parkinsonian Syndromes

General significance:

Eye movements can contribute to a better understanding of the pathogenesis of parkinsonian disorders, and conversely, the study of patients with parkinsonian disorders can contribute to a better understanding of how the brain controls movement in general and eye movements in particular.

- Many functions are accessible to bedside clinic testing.
- Ease and reliability of eye movement measurement.
- Eye movements, and the stimuli that drive them, are readily quantified.
- Important aspects of the neurobiological substrate of eye movements have been defined.
- Paradigms are readily available that can test brainstem functions as well as the role of eye move ments in prediction, memory, learning, visual search, attention, and reward.

Specific issues that can be addressed by eye movement research

- What is the substrate for frequent saccadic intrusions (square-wave jerks) in PSP and in PD following pallidotomy?
- What is the pathogenesis of selective slowing of vertical saccades early in the course of PSP, and what accounts for the curved trajectories of saccades?
- Why do patients with PSP smoothly track a large visual target better than a small one?
- What is the role of the basal ganglia in generation of pursuit eye movements?
- Why do PD patients have difficulty generating voluntary saccades between visible targets without an external cue (such as an auditory prompt)?
- What are the effects of deep brain stimulation on the full range of saccadic and pursuit dynamics?
- Why do head thrusts and a blinks facilitate the generation of saccades in patients with HD?
- What is the neurobiological basis for ocular motor tics?
- What is the role of the basal ganglia in ocular motor learning?

increase, but there will be more insights into the pathophysiology of the ocular motor disturbances in parkinsonian disorders and how they respond to treatment.

ACKNOWLEDGMENTS

Dr. Leigh is supported by the Office of Research and Development, Medical Research Service, Department of Veterans Affairs; NIH grant EY06717; Evenor Armington Fund. Dr. Zee is support by NIH grant EY01849 and the Robert M. and Annetta J. Coffelt endowment for PSP research.

VIDEO LEGENDS

Video 1: Voluntary saccades in Parkinson's disease. During the initial part of the clip, the patient is verbally instructed to look between two visual targets (a pen and the camera); some mild hypometria is evident. Subsequently, the patient is instructed to make self-generate saccades between two stationary targets about 60–80° apart; hypometria becomes much more marked, as well as some delayed in initiation.

Video 2: Vertical saccades in PSP. The patient is looking between two stationary targets about 40° apart in the vertical plane. The movements are slow, but carry the eyes to their targets. Their trajectories are slightly oblique or curved with a horizontal correction at the end ("round the houses") *(50)*.

Video 3: Horizontal saccades in PSP. The patient is looking between two stationary targets separated about 60° in the horizontal plane. Horizontal saccades are faster than vertical saccades (Video 2), but tend to be hypometric.

Video 4: Light-induced blink response in a patient with PSP. This was tested by flashing a penlight repetitively into one eye at 1–2 Hz, as he viewed a distant target with both eyes. Unlike normals, or patients with PD, no habituation occurred.

REFERENCES

1. Leigh RJ, Zee DS. The neurology of eye movements. New York: Oxford University Press, 1999.
2. Becker W. Metrics. In: Wutz RH, Goldberg ME, eds. The Neurobiology of Saccadic Eye Movements. Amsterdam: Elsevier, 1989: 13–67.
3. Scudder CA, Kaneko CS, Fuchs AF. The brainstem burst generator for saccadic eye movements: a modern synthesis. Exp Brain Res 2002; 142(4):439–462.
4. Chamberlain W. Restriction of upward gaze with advancing age. Am J Ophthalmol 1971;71:341–346.
5. Demer JL. Pivotal role of orbital connective tissues in binocular alignment and strabismus. Invest Ophthalmol Vis Sci 2004;45(3):729–738.
6. Huaman AG, Sharpe JA. Vertical saccades in senescence. Invest Ophthalmol Vis Sci 1993;34:2588–2595.
7. Vidailhet M, Rivaud S, Gouider-Khouja N, Bonnet A, Gaymard B, Agid Y, et al. Eye movements in parkinsonian syndromes. Ann Neurol 1994;35:420–426.
8. Bhidayasiri R, Riley DE, Somers JT, Lerner AJ, Buttner-Ennever JA, Leigh RJ. Pathophysiology of slow vertical saccades in progressive supranuclear palsy. Neurology 2001;57(11):2070–2077.
9. DiScenna AO, Das VE, Zivotofsky AZ, Seidman SH, Leigh RJ. Evaluation of a video tracking device for measurement of horizontal and vertical eye rotations during locomotion. J Neurosci Methods 1995;58:89–94.
10. Lebedev S, Van Gelder P, Tsui WH. Square-root relation between main saccade parameters. Invest Ophthalmol Vis Sci 1996;37:2750–2758.
11. Garbutt S, Riley DE, Kumar AN, Han U, Harwood MR, Leigh RJ. Abnormalities of optokinetic nystagmus in progressive supranuclear palsy, J Neurosurg Psychiatry 2004, in press.
12. Pierrot-Deseilligny C, Ploner CJ, Muri RM, Gaymard B, Rivaud-Pechoux S. Effects of cortical lesions on saccadic: eye movements in humans. Ann N Y Acad Sci 2002;956:216–229.
13. Hikosaka O, Takikawa Y, Kawagoe R. Role of the basal ganglia in the control of purposive saccadic eye movements. Physiol Rev 2000;80(3):953–978.
14. Itoh H, Nakahara H, Hikosaka O, Kawagoe R, Takikawa Y, Aihara K. Correlation of primate caudate neural activity and saccade parameters in reward-oriented behavior. J Neurophysiol 2003;89:1774–1783.
15. Sato M, Hikosaka O. Role of primate substantia nigra pars reticulata in reward-oriented saccadic eye movement. J Neurosci 2002;22(6):2363–2373.
16. Cui D, Yan Y, Lynch J. Pursuit subregion of the frontal eye field projects to the caudate nucleus in monkeys. J Neurophysiol 2003;89:2678–2684.
17. Crawford TJ, Bennett D, Lekwuwa G, Shaunak S, Deakin JF. Cognition and the inhibitory control of saccades in schizophrenia and Parkinson's disease. Prog Brain Res 2002;140:449–466.
18. Rascol O, Sabatini U, Simonetta-Moreau M, Montastruc JL, Rascol A, Clanet M. Square wave jerks in Parkinsonian syndromes. J Neurol Neurosurg Psychiatry 1991;54:599–602.
19. O'Sullivan JD, Maruff P, Tyler P, Peppard RF, McNeill P, Currie J. Unilateral pallidotomy for Parkinson's disease disrupts ocular fixation. J Clin Neurosci 2003;10(2):181–185.
20. White OB, Saint-Cyr JA, Tomlinson RD, Sharpe J. Ocular motor deficits in Parkinson's disease. II: Control of saccadic and smooth pursuit systems. Brain 1983;106:571–587.
21. Rottach KG, Riley DE, DiScenna AO, Zivotofsky AZ, Leigh RJ. Dynamic properties of horizontal and vertical eye movements in parkinsonian syndromes. Ann Neurol 1996;39:368–377.
22. Repka MX, Claro MC, Loupe DN, Reich S. Ocular motility in Parkinson's disease. Pediatr Ophthalmol Strabismus 1996;33:144–147.
23. Kimmig H, Haussmann K, Mergner T, Lucking CH. What is pathological with gaze shift fragmentation in Parkinson's disease? J Neurol 2002;249(6):683–692.
24. Crawford T, Goodrich S, Henderson L, Kennard C. Predictive responses in Parkinson's disease: Manual key presses and saccadic eye movements to regular stimulus events. J Neurol Neurosurg Psychiatry 1989;52:1033–1042.
25. Lueck CJ, Crawford TJ, Henderson L, Van Gisbergen JA, Duysens J, Kennard C. Saccadic eye movements in Parkinson's disease: II. Remembered saccades - towards a unified hypothesis? Quart J Exp Psychol 1992;45A:211–233.
26. Nakamura T, Bronstein AM, Lueck CJ, Marsden CD, Rudge P. Vestibular, cervical and visual remembered saccades in Parkinson's disease. Brain 1994;117:1423–1432.
27. Vermersch AI, Rivaud S, Vidailhet M, Bonnet A, Gaymard B, Agid Y, et al. Sequences of memory-guided saccades in Parkinson's disease. Ann Neurol 1994;35:487–490.
28. Kimmig H, Haussmann K, Mergner T, Lucking CH. What is pathological with gaze shift fragmentation in Parkinson's disease? J Neurol 2002;249(6):683–692.

29. MacAskill MR, Anderson TJ, Jones RD. Saccadic adaptation in neurological disorders. Prog Brain Res 2002;140: 417–431.
30. Bronstein AM, Kennard C. Predictive ocular motor control in Parkinson's disease. Brain 1985;108:925–940.
31. Ventre J, Zee DS, Papageorgiou H, Reich S. Abnormalities of predictive saccades in hemi-parkinson's disease. Brain 1992;115:1147–1165.
32. Nenadic I, Gaser C, Volz H, Rammsayer T, Hager F, Sauer H. Processing of temporal information and the basal ganglia: new evidence from fMRI. Exp Brain Res 2003;148:238–246.
33. Turner R, Grafton S, McIntosh A, DeLong M, Hoffman J. The functional anatomy of parkinsonian bradykinesia. Neuroimage 2003;19:163–179.
34. Djamgoz M, Hankins M, Hirano J, Archer S. Neurobiology of retinal dopamine in relation to degenerative states of the tissue. Vision Res 1997;37:3509–3529. 1997.
35. Waterston JA, Barnes GR, Grealy MA, Collins S. Abnormalities of smooth eye and head movement control in Parkinson's disease. Ann Neurology 1996;39:749–760.
36. Rascol O, Clanet M, Montastruc JL, Simonetta M, Soulier-Esteve MJ, Doyon B, et al. Abnormal ocular movements in Parkinson's disease. Evidence for involvement of dopaminergic systems. Brain 1989;112:1193–1214.
37. White OW, Saint-Cyr JA, Sharpe JA. Ocular motor deficits in Parkinson's disease. I. The horizontal vestibulo-ocular reflex and its regulation. Brain 1983;106:555–570.
38. Reichert WH, Doolittle J, McDowell FH. Vestibular dysfunction in Parkinson's disease. Neurology 1982;32:1133–1138.
39. Gibson JM, Pimlott R, Kennard C. Ocular motor and manual tracking in Parkinson's disease and the effect of treatment. J Neurol Neurosurg Psychiatry 1987;50:853–860.
40. Blekher T, Siemers E, Abel LA, Yee RD. Eye movements in Parkinson's disease: before and after pallidotomy. Invest Ophthalmol Vis Sci 2000;41(8):2177–2183.
41. Rivaud-Pechoux S, Vermersch AI, Gaymard B, Ploner CJ, Bejjani BP, Damier P, et al. Improvement of memory guided saccades in parkinsonian patients by high frequency subthalamic nucleus stimulation. J Neurol Neurosurg Psychiatry 2000;68(3):381–384.
42. Carbon M, Ghilardi M, Feigin A, Fukuda M, Silvestri G, Mentis M, et al. Learning networks in health and Parkinson's disease: reproducibility and treatment effects. Hum Brain Mapp 2003;19:197–211.
43. O'Sullivan JD, Maruff P, Tyler P, Peppard RF, McNeill P, Currie J. Unilateral pallidotomy for Parkinson's disease disrupts ocular fixation. J Clin Neurosci 2003;10(2):181–185.
44. Averbuch-Heller L, Stahl JS, Hlavin ML, Leigh RJ. Square wave jerks induced by pallidotomy in parkinsonian patients. Neurology 1999;52:185–188.
45. Hotson JR, Langston EB, Langston JW. Saccade responses to dopamine in human MTPT-induced parkinsonism. Ann Neurol 1986;20:456–463.
46. Schultz W, Romo R, Scarnati E, Sundstrom E, Jonsson G, Studer A. Saccadic reaction times, eye-arm coordination and spontaneous eye movements in normal and MTPT-treated monkeys. Exp Brain Res 1989;78:253–267.
47. Brooks BA, Fuchs AF, Finochio D. Saccadic eye movement deficits in the MTPT monkey model of Parkinson's disease. Brain Res 1986;383:402–407.
48. Nath U, Ben-Shlomo Y, Thomson R, Lees A, Burn D. Clinical features and natural history of progressive supranuclear palsy. A clinical cohort study. Neurology 2003;60:910–916.
49. Davis PH, Bergeron C, McLachlan DR. Atypical presentation of progressive supranuclear palsy. Ann Neurol 1985;17:337–343.
50. Quinn N. The "round the houses" sign in progressive supranuclear palsy. Ann Neurol 2003;40:951.
51. Das V, Leigh R. Visual-vestibular interaction in progressive supranuclear palsy. Vision Res 2000;40:2077–2081.
52. Seemungal B, Faldon M, Revesz T, Lees A, Zee D, Bronstein A. Influence of target size on vertical gaze palsy in a pathologically proven case of progressive supranuclear palsy. Mov Disord 2003;18:818–822.
53. Bhidayasiri R, Riley DE, Somers JT, Lerner AJ, Buttner-Ennever JA, Leigh RJ. Pathophysiology of slow vertical saccades in progressive supranuclear palsy. Neurology 2001;57(11):2070–2077.
54. Mastaglia FL, Grainger KMR. Internuclear ophthalmoplegia in progressive supranuclear palsy. J Neurol Sci 1975;25:303–308.
55. Kitthaweesin K, Riley DE, Leigh RJ. Vergence disorders in progressive supranuclear palsy. Ann N Y Acad Sci 2002;956:504–507.
56. Jenkyn LR, Walsh DB, Walsh BT, Culver CM, Reeves AG. The nuchocephalic reflex. J Neurosurg Psychiatry 1975;38:561–566.
57. Kuniyoshi S, Riley DE, Zee DS, Reich SG, Whitney C, Leigh RJ. Distinguishing progressive supranuclear palsy from other forms of Parkinson's disease: evaluation of new signs. Ann N Y Acad Sci 2002;956:484–486.
58. Bhidayasiri R, Riley DE, Somers JT, Lerner AJ, Buttner-Ennever JA, Leigh RJ. Pathophysiology of slow vertical saccades in progressive supranuclear palsy. Neurology 2001;57(11):2070–2077.
59. Garbutt S, Harwood M, Kumar A, Han Y, Leigh R. Evaluating small eye movements in patients with saccadic palsies. Ann NY Acad Soc 2003;1004:337–346.

60. Bhidayasiri R, Plant GT, Leigh RJ. A hypothetical scheme for the brainstem control of vertical gaze. Neurology 2000;54(10):1985–1993.

61. Bhidayasiri R, Riley DE, Somers JT, Lerner AJ, Buttner-Ennever JA, Leigh RJ. Pathophysiology of slow vertical saccades in progressive supranuclear palsy. Neurology 2001;57(11):2070–2077.

62. Pierrot-Deseilligny C, Rivaud S, Fournier E, Agid Y. Lateral visually-guided saccades in progressive supranuclear palsy. Brain 1989;112:471–487.

63. Goffinet AM, DeVolder AG, Gillian C, Rectem D, Bol A, Michel C et al. Positron tomography demonstrates frontal lobe hypometabolism in progressive supranuclear palsy. Ann Neurol 1989;25:131–139.

64. Kitthaweesin K, Riley DE, Leigh RJ. Vergence disorders in progressive supranuclear palsy. Ann N Y Acad Sci 2002;956:504–507.

65. Moses HI, Zee DS. Multi-infarct PSP. Neurology 1987;37:1819.

66. Bhidayasiri R, Plant GT, Leigh RJ. A hypothetical scheme for the brainstem control of vertical gaze. Neurology 2000;54(10):1985–1993.

67. Averbuch-Heller L, Paulson G, Daroff R, Leigh R. Whipple's disease mimicking progressive supranuclear palsy: the diagnostic value of eye movement recording. J Neurol Neurosurg Psychiatry 1999;66:532–535.

68. Knox DL, Green WR, Troncosa JC, Yardley JH, Hsu J, Zee DS. Cerebral ocular Whipple's disease: a 62 year-old odyssey from death to diagnosis. Neurology 1995;45:617–-625.

69. Schwartz MA, Selhorst JB, Ochs AL, Beck RW, Campbell WW, Harris JK, et al. Oculomasticatory myorhythmia: a unique movement disorder occurring in Whipple's disease. Ann Neurol 1986;20:677–683.

70. Lowsky R, Archer GL, Fyles G, Minden M, Curtis J, Messner H, et al. Diagnosis of Whipple's disease by molecular analysis of peripheral blood. N Engl J Med 1994;331:1343–1346.

71. Fleming JL, Wiesner RH, Shorter RG. Whipple's disease: clinical, biochemical, and histopathological features and assessment of treatment in 29 patients. Mayo Clin Proc 1988;63:539–551.

72. Riley DE, Fogt N, Leigh RJ. The syndrome of "pure akinesia" and its relationship to progressive supranuclear palsy. Neurology 1994;44:1025–1029.

73. Vidailhet M, Rivaud-Pechoux S. Eye movement disorders in corticobasal degeneration. Adv Neurol 2000;82:161–167.

74. Riley DE, Lang AE, Lewis A, Resch L, Ashby P, Hornykiewicz O et al. Cortical-basal ganglionic degeneration. Neurology 1990;40:1203–1212.

75. Gibb WRG, Luthert PJ, Marsden CD. Corticobasal degeneration. Brain 1989;112:1171–1192.

76. Bhidayasiri R, Riley DE, Somers JT, Lerner AJ, Buttner-Ennever JA, Leigh RJ. Pathophysiology of slow vertical saccades in progressive supranuclear palsy. Neurology 2001;57(11):2070–2077.

77. Bertholon P, Bronstein A, Davies R, Rudge P, Thilo K. Positional down beating nystagmus in 50 patients: cerebellar disorders and possible anterior semicircular canalithiasis. J Neurol Neurosurg Psychiatry 2002;72:366–372.

78. Brett F, Henson C, Staunton H. Familial diffuse Lewy body disease, eye movement abnormalities, and distribution of pathology. Arch Neurol 2003;59:464–467.

79. de Bruin VM, Lees AJ, Daniel SE. Diffuse Lewy body disease presenting with supranuclear gaze palsy, parkinsonism, and dementia: a case report. Mov Disord 1992;7:355–358.

80. Saver JL, Liu GT, Charness ME. Idiopathic striopallidodentate calcification with prominent supranuclear abnormality of eye movement. J Neuro-ophthalmology 1994;14:29–33.

81. Wszolek ZK, Pfeiffer RF, Bhatt MH, Schelper RL, Cordes M, Snow BJ, et al. Rapidly progressive autosomal dominant parkinsonism and dementia with pallido-ponto-nigral degeneration. Ann Neurol 1992;32:312–320.

82. Lepore FE, Steele JC, Cox TA, Tillson G, Calne DB, Duvoisin RC, et al. Supranuclear disturbances of ocular motility in Lytico-Bodig. Neurology 1988;38:1849–1853.

83. Averbuch-Heller L, Helmchen C, Horn AKE, Leigh RJ, Büttner-Ennever JA. Slow vertical saccades in motor neuron disease: correlation of structure and function. Ann Neurol 1998;44:641–648.

84. Caparros-Lefebvre D, Sergeant N, Lees A, Camuzat A, Daniel S, Lannuzel A, et al. Guadeloupean parkinsonism: a cluster of progressive supranuclear palsy-like tauopathy. Brain 2002;125:801–811.

85. Grant MP, Cohen M, Petersen RB, Halmagyi GM, McDougall A, Tusa RJ, et al. Abnormal eye movements in Creutzfeldt–Jakob disease. Ann Neurology 1993;34:192–197.

86. Helmchen C, Büttner U. Centripetal nystagmus in a case of Creutzfeldt–Jakob disease. Neuro-ophthalmology 1995;15:187–192.

87. Leigh RJ, Foley JM, Remler BF, Civil RH. Oculogyric crisis: a syndrome of thought disorder and ocular deviation. Ann Neurol 1987;22:13–17.

88. Lees A, Kim Y, Lyoo C. Oculogyric crisis as an initial manifestation of Wilson's disease. Neurology 1999;52:1714–1715.

89. Swoboda K, Hyland K, Goldstein D, Kuban K, Arnold L, Holmes C, et al. Clinical and therapeutic observations in aromatic L-amino decarboxylase deficiency. Neurology 1999;53:1205–1211.

90. Liu GT, Carrazana EJ, Macklis JD, Mikati MA. Delayed oculogyric crises associated with striatocapsular infarction. J Clin Neuro-ophthalmol 1991;11:198–201.

91. Frankel M, Cummings JL. Neuro-ophthalmic abnormalities in Tourette's syndrome. Functional and anatomical implications. Neurology 1984;34:359–361.

92. FitzGerald PM, Jankovic J, Glaze DG, Schultz R, Percy AK. Extrapyramidal involvement in Rett's syndrome. Neurology 1990;40:293–295.

93. Hoyt CS, Mousel DK. Transient supranuclear disturbances of gaze in healthy neonates. Am J Ophthalmol 1980;89: 708–713.

94. FitzGerald PM, Jankovic J. Tardive oculogyric crisis. Neurology 1989;39:1434–1437.

95. Sachdev P. Tardive and chronically recurrent oculogyric crises. Mov Disord 1993;8:93–97.

96. Kim JS, Kim HK, Im JH, Lee MC. Oculogyric crisis and abnormal magnetic resonance imaging signals in bilateral lentiform nuclei. Mov Disord 1996;11:756–758.

97. Collewijn H, Went LN, Tamminga EP, Vegter-Van der Vlis M. Oculomotor defects in patients with Huntington's disease and their offspring. J Neurol Sci 1988;86:307–320.

98. Lasker AG, Zee DS. Ocular motor abnormalities in Huntington's disease. Vision Res 1997;37:3639-3645.

99. Lasker AG, Zee DS, Hain TC, Folstein SE, Singer HS. Saccades in Huntington's disease: initiation defects and distractability. Neurology 1987;37:364–370.

100. Leigh RJ, Newman SA, Folstein SE, Lasker AG, Jensen BA. Abnormal ocular motor control in Huntington's disease. Neurology 1983;33:1268–1275.

101. Zangemeister WH, Mueller-Jensen A. The coordination of gaze movements in Huntington's disease. Neuro-ophthalmology 1985;5:193–206.

102. Rubin AJ, King WM, Reinbold KA, Shoulson I. Quantitative longitudinal assessment of saccades in Huntington's disease. J Clin Neuro-opthalmol 1993;13:59–66.

103. Kirkwood SC, Siemers E, Bond C, Conneally PM, Christian JC, Foroud T. Confirmation of subtle motor changes among presymptomatic carriers of the Huntington disease gene. Arch Neurol 2000;57(7):1040–1044.

104. Rothlind JC, Brandt J, Zee D, Codori AM, Folstein S. Verbal memory and oculomotor control are unimpaired in asymptomatic adults with the genetic marker for Huntington's disease. Arch Neurol 1993;50:799–802.

105. Reveley MA, Dursun SM, Andrews H. Improvement of abnormal saccadic eye movements in Huntington's disease by sulpiride: a case study. Journal of Psychopharmacology 1994;8:262–265.

106. Lasker AG, Zee DS, Hain TC, Folstein SE, Singer HS. Saccades in Huntington's disease: initiation defects and distractibility. Neurology 1987;37:364–370.

107. Hikosaka O, Takikawa Y, Kawagoe R. Role of the basal ganglia in the control of purposive saccadic eye movements. Physiol Rev 2000;80(3):953–978.

108. Oyanagi K, Takeda S, Takahashi H, Ohama E, Ikuta F. A quantitative investigation of the substantia nigra in Huntington's disease. Ann Neurol 1989;26:13–19.

109. Koeppen AH. The nucleus pontis centralis caudalis in Huntington's disease. J Neurol Sci 1989;91:129–141.

110. Leigh RJ, Parhad IM, Clark AW, Buettner-Ennever JA, Folstein SE. Brainstem findings in Huntington's disease. J Neurol Sci 1985;71:247–256.

111. Rinne JO, Daniel SE, Scaravilli F, Pires M, Harding AE, Marsden CD. The neuropathological features of neuroacanthocytosis. Mov Disord 1994;9:297–304.

112. Burke JR, Wingfield MS, Lewis KE, Roses AD, Lee JE, Hulette C, et al. The haw river syndrome: dentatorubro-pallidoluysian atrophy (DRPLA) in an African-American family. Nat Genet 1994;7:521–524.

113. Lennox G, Jones R. Gaze distractibility in Wilson's disease. Ann Neurol 1989;25:415–417.

114. Kirkham TH, Kamin DF. Slow saccadic eye movements in Wilson's disease. J Neurol Neurosurg Psychiatry 1974;37:191–194.

115. Keane JR. Lid-opening apraxia in Wilson's disease. J Clin Neuro-ophthalmol 1988;8:31–33.

116. Lewis RF. Ocular motor apraxia and ataxia-telangiectasia. Arch Neurol 2001;58(8):1312.

117. Lewis RF, Crawford TO. Ocular motor abnormalities in ataxia telangiectasia. Neurology 1998;50(Suppl).

118. Lewis RF, Crawford TO. Slow target-directed eye movements in ataxia-telangiectasia. Invest Ophthalmol Vis Sci 2002;43(3):686–691.

119. Stell R, Bronstein AM, Plant GT, Harding AE. Ataxia telangiectasia: a reappraisal of the ocular motor features and their value in the diagnosis of atypical cases. Mov Disord 1989;4:320–329.

120. Rottach KG, von Maydell RD, Das VE, Zivotofsky AZ, DiScenna AO, Gordon JL, et al. Evidence for independent feed-back control of horizontal and vertical saccades from Niemann–Pick type C disease. Vision Res 1997;37:3627–3638.

121. Garbutt S, Harris CM. Abnormal vertical optokinetic nystagmus in infants and children. Br J Ophthalmol 2000;84(5):451–455.

122. Higgins JJ, Patterson MC, Dambrosia JM, Pikus AT, Pentchev PG, Sato S, et al. A clinical staging classification for type C Niemann–Pick disease. Neurology 1992;42:2286–2290.

123. Stein RW, Kase CS, Hier DB, Caplan LR, Mohr JP. Caudate hemorrhage. Neurology 1984;34:1549–1554.

124. Vermersch AI, RM M, Rivaud S, Vidailhet M, Gaymard B, Agid Y, et al. Saccade disturbances after bilateral lentiform nucleus lesions in humans. J Neurol Neurosurg Psychiatry 1996;60:179–184.

125. Lekwuwa GU, Barnes GR. Cerebral control of eye movements. II. Timing of anticipatory eye movements, predictive pursuit and phase errors in focal cerebral lesions. Brain 1996;119:491–505.
126. Dursun SM, Burke JG, Reveley MA. Antisaccade eye movement abnormalities in Tourette syndrome: evidence for cortico-striatal network dysfunction? J Psychopharmacol 2000;14(1):37–39.
127. LeVasseur AL, Flanagan JR, Riopelle RJ, Munoz DP. Control of volitional and reflexive saccades in Tourette's syndrome. Brain 2001;124(Pt 10):2045–2058.
128. Mostofsky SH, Lasker AG, Singer HS, Denckla MB, Zee DS. Oculomotor abnormalities in boys with Tourette syndrome with and without ADHD. J Am Acad Child Adolesc Psychiatry 2001;40(12):1464–1472.
129. Munoz DP, Le Vasseur AL, Flanagan JR. Control of volitional and reflexive saccades in Tourette's syndrome. Prog Brain Res 2002;140:467–481.
130. Narita AS, Shawkat FS, Lask B, Taylor DS, Harris CM. Eye movement abnormalities in a case of Tourette syndrome. Dev Med Child Neurol 1997;39:270–273.
131. Straube A, Mennicken J-B, Riedel M, Eggert T, Müller N. Saccades in Gilles de la Tourette's syndrome. Movement Disorders 1997;12:536–546.
132. Binyon S, Prendergast M. Eye-movement tics in children. Dev Med Child Neurol 1991;33:343–355.
133. Shawkat FS, Harris CM, Jacobs M, Taylor D, Brett EM. Eye movement tics. Brit J Ophthalmol 1992;76:697–699.
134. Jinnah HA, Lewis RF, Visser JE, Eddey GE, Barabas G, Harris JC. Ocular motor dysfunction in Lesch–Nyhan disease. Pediatr Neurol 2001;24(3):200–204.
135. Demer JL, Holds JB, Hovis LA. Ocular movements in essential blepharospasm. Am J Ophthalmol 1990;110:674–682.
136. Aramideh M, Bour LJ, Koelman JHTM, Speelman JD, Ongerboer de Visser BW. Abnormal eye movements in blepharospasm and involuntary levator palpebrae inhibition. Brain 1994;117:1457–1474.
137. Bollen E, Van Exel E, van der Velde EA, Buytels P, Bastiaanse J, van Dijk JG. Saccadic eye movements in idiopathic blepharospasm. Movement Disorders 1996;11:678–682.
138. Averbuch-Heller L, Rottach KG, Zivotofsky AZ, Suarez JI, Pettee AD, Remler BF et al. Torsional eye movements in patients with skew deviation and spasmodic torticollis: responses to static and dynamic head roll. Neurology 1997;48:506–514.
139. Stell R, Bronstein AM, Marsden CD. Vestibulo-ocular abnormalites in spasmodic torticollis before and after botulinum toxin injections. J Neurol Neurosurg Psychiatry 1989;52:57–62.
140. Anastasopoulos D, Nasios G, Psilas K, Mergner T, Maurer C, Lücking C-H. What is straight ahead to a patient with torticollis? Brain 1998;121:91–101.
141. Thaker GK, Nguyen JA, Tamminga CA. Increased saccadic distractibility in tardive dyskinesia: functional evidence for subcortical GABA dysfunction. Biol Psychiatry 1989;25:49–59.
142. Cardosa F, Eduardo C, Silva AP, Mota CCC. Chorea in fifty consecutive patients with rheumatic fever. Mov Disord 1997;12:701–703.
143. Helmchen C, Hagenow A, Miesner J, Sprenger A, Rambold H, Wenzelburger R et al. Eye movement abnormalities in essential tremor may indicate cerebellar dysfunction. Brain 2003;126:1319–1392.

16

Characterizing and Assessing Speech and Language Disturbances

Carol Frattali and Joseph R. Duffy

INTRODUCTION

Speech and language disturbances in atypical parkinsonian disorders often present as initial symptoms or prominent neurobehavioral sequelae that worsen as the disease progresses. These disorders, even in their early stages, can have profound effects on communicative functioning and, by extension, psychosocial well-being. In the face of neurodegenerative disease, the downward course of the ability to communicate mirrors a loss considered elemental to the human condition; it unavoidably robs the individual of a primary mode of expression of thoughts and ideas and, in its most severe form, basic needs.

We draw a distinction between *speech* and *language* for purposes of clarity throughout this chapter. These terms, sometimes used interchangeably or in combination by clinicians and researchers, can be defined and distinguished in a hierarchical representational framework *(1)*:

- Language represents high-order cortico-cortical and cortical-subcortical network activity as a component of cognitive-linguistic processes. These processes represent thoughts, feelings, and emotions that generate intent to communicate. They are next converted to verbal symbols that follow psycholinguistic rules (e.g., phonology, morphology, syntax, semantics, pragmatics) as ordered meaningfully by propositional elements (units of meaning). Language processes can be divided broadly as those that link thought (meaning) to word forms (lexical-semantic) and those that sequence words and word endings to convey relationships among words (syntactic) *(2)*. In its disordered state, a breakdown of language, either at lexical-semantic or syntactic process levels, is called aphasia.
- Speech represents cortical-subcortical and brain stem activity via neuromuscular and central and peripheral nervous system activity involving two processes: motor speech programming and neuromuscular execution. In motor speech programming, selection and organization of sensorimotor plans activate the speech musculature at appropriate coarticulated times, durations, and intensities. During speech production, the neuromuscular transmissions that involve respiration, phonation, resonation, articulation, and prosody generate muscle contractions and finely coordinated movements of oral/motor structures that generate an identifiable acoustic signal. In their disordered states, breakdowns of motor speech programming and related neuromuscular activity are known as apraxia (nonverbal orofacial or buccofacial apraxia, apraxia of speech) and dysarthria respectively.

Overview of Neuroanatomical Correlates

If approached from the perspective of classical neuroanatomical correlates, damage to portions of the auditory and visual association areas of the cortex can result in comprehension deficits of the spoken or written word. Damage to Wernicke's area (Brodmann area 22), in the posterior portion of

From: *Current Clinical Neurology: Atypical Parkinsonian Disorders*
Edited by: I. Litvan © Humana Press Inc., Totowa, NJ

the superior temporal gyrus of the dominant hemisphere, can result in a type of aphasia generally called Wernicke's aphasia. Wernicke's aphasia is marked by reduced comprehension and fluent but often paragrammatic verbal output characterized by word or nonword substitutions (paraphasias) sometimes to the extent of producing fluent streams of non-English or neologistic jargon. In contrast, damage to Broca's area (Brodmann areas 44–45), in the third convolution or inferior gyrus of the frontal lobe of the dominant hemisphere can result in a type of aphasia generally called Broca's aphasia. Broca's aphasia, in contrast to Wernicke's aphasia, is marked by relatively spared comprehension but sparse, effortful, nonfluent, and agrammatic verbal output. Along the parameters of fluency, comprehension, repetition, and naming, other classic aphasia syndromes have been identified including conduction, transcortical motor, transcortical sensory, and global aphasia.

The nondominant hemisphere is also increasingly implicated in its role in language functions, particularly for global and thematic processing of narratives, pragmatics (relation between language behavior and context in which it is used or interpreted), and prosody (elements of speech melody, rate, stress, juncture, and duration) of language, and inferencing, coherence, and topic maintenance during discourse processing and production (3,4).

Skilled motor programs for control of the larynx, lips, mouth, respiratory system, and other accessory muscles of articulation are thought to be initiated from Broca's area. Damage to this area, or within other parts of the left hemisphere's network of structures involved in the planning and programming of speech, results in apraxia of speech. Once these programs are activated via the premotor zone of Broca's area, thus mediating orofacial and speech praxis, the facial and laryngeal regions of the motor cortex (bilaterally) activate the speech musculature for actual emission of sound. The neural substrates of neuromuscular execution originate in the primary motor cortex (Brodmann area 4) with pathways descending either directly or indirectly via the pyramidal or extrapyramidal tracts. The pyramidal tract consists of upper motoneurons in the cerebral cortex with axons coursing through the pyramidal tract in the medulla and terminating on anterior horn cells or interneurons in the spinal cord. The pyramidal tract is composed of the corticospinal tract and the corticobulbar tract that influences cranial nerve activity. Types of dysarthria that could result (e.g., spastic dysarthria) would have features of spasticity, increased muscle stretch reflexes, and clonus. In contrast, damage to lower motoneurons from spinal and cranial nerves results in loss of voluntary and reflex responses of muscles. The result would be hypotonia and absence of muscle stretch reflexes. Paralysis and atrophy would occur, with the early stages of atrophy resulting in fibrillations and fasciculations. Dysarthrias with damage to lower motoneurons would have characteristics of flaccidity (e.g., flaccid dysarthria) (5). Other pathways that, if interrupted, would result in dysarthria, include extrapyramidal (coursing through structures of the basal ganglia) and cerebellar motor pathways, which could result in hyperkinetic or hypokinetic components following extrapyramidal damage, or ataxic dysarthria following cerebellar damage (see Appendix A for descriptions of aphasia syndromes, apraxias, and dysarthria types; Appendix B for case descriptions and test stimuli used for audio samples of speech and language disorders that accompany this chapter).

With advances in neuroimaging techniques, a dynamic systems rather than localization view of speech and language functions is being adopted. Neuroimaging findings have shown that language processing extends beyond the classical perisylvian region containing Broca's and Wernicke's areas and depends on many neural sites linked as systems. For example, both left temporal and prefrontal/premotor cortices have been found to be activated by language processing, and do so selectively. Neuroimaging studies have also shown that structures in the basal ganglia, thalamus, and supplementary motor area are engaged in language processing (6). Adding to the evidence of functional connectivity, a recent study suggests that the anatomical and functional organization of the human auditory cortical system points to multiple, parallel, hierarchically organized processing pathways involving temporal, parietal, and frontal cortices (7). Computational mapping methods, which can combine probabilistic maps of cytoarchitectonically defined regions with functional imaging data, hold promise for further elucidating brain region specialization. For example, Horwitz et al. *(8)*. found that BA 45, not BA 44, is activated by oral or signed language production, implicating BA 45 as the part of Broca's area that is fundamental to the modality-independent aspects of language generation.

Overview of Clinical Assessment Procedures

In order to clinically assess or scientifically examine aspects of speech and language, the clinician or researcher employs a battery of instrumental and behavioral tests or experimental tasks that tap both isolated and integrated components of speech and language. This approach is intended to determine relative strengths and weaknesses necessary for differential diagnosis, and to assess the consequential effects of specific disturbances on functional communication in daily life contexts. Therefore, a clinical battery is best composed of diagnostic instruments that measure the fine-grained features of speech or language, and functional measures of communication that address speech or language as an integrative construct in the context of daily life activities. In line with contemporary models of health and disability that encompass both biophysical and psychosocial aspects of medical intervention (e.g., World Health Organization International Classification of Functioning, Disability and Health; *see* ref. *9*). Clinicians and researchers are also extending clinical measurement to aspects of general wellness or quality of life in order to determine the effect of an impairment or activity limitation on social participation, autonomy, and self-worth.

Specific to language, behavioral measurement (online automated tasks that capture aspects of processing or production as they occur in real time; standardized paper-and-pencil tests) typically includes assessment of aspects of spontaneous speech, comprehension of oral and written language, repetition of words and phrases of increasing length, naming of objects and actions, and writing. Assessment of these parameters allows differential diagnosis of aphasia, either as a classical syndrome or as a constellation of deficits that point to specific neuropathological processes.

Assessment of speech typically is conducted via a combination of perceptual, acoustic, and physiologic methods *(1)*. Perceptual methods are based primarily on auditory-perceptual attributes that allow clinical differential diagnosis. Acoustic methods contribute to acoustic quantification and description of clinically perceived impaired speech and confirm perceptual judgments of, for example, slow speech rate, breathy or tremulous voice quality, vocal pitch and loudness variations, hypernasal resonance, and imprecise articulation. Their ability to make visible and quantify the speech signal can be used as baseline data or as an index of stability or change. Physiologic methods focus on characterizing the movements of speech structures and respiratory function, muscle contractions that generate movement, temporal parameters and relationships among central and peripheral neural activity and biomechanical activity, and temporal relationships among active CNS (central nervous system) structures during the planning and execution of speech (for comprehensive reviews of assessment methods, *see* ref. *1* for motor speech disorders; refs. *10* and *11* for aphasia and related neurologic language disorders; refs. *4* and *12* for right-hemisphere communication disorders; ref. *13* for functional communication and psychosocial consequences of neurologic communication disorders).

Our purposes here are to characterize the atypical Parkinsonian disorders of corticobasal degeneration (CBD), progressive supranuclear palsy (PSP), multiple systems atrophy (MSA), and dementia with Lewy Body disease (DLB) from the perspectives of speech and language. For each diagnostic group, we: (a) describe the neuroanatomical correlates of speech and language disorders, (b) identify their clinically common and differentiating features on the bases of clinical assessment and clinical research findings, and (c) offer some clinical management suggestions. We end by suggesting some directions for future research. Table 1 abstracts the common and distinctive features of speech and language disturbances across diagnostic groups.

Table 1
Common and Differentiating Features of Speech and Language by Diagnostic Group

Feature	CBD	PSP	MSA	Dementia with Lewy Bodies
Speech				
Oral/motor programming (praxis)	Presence of nonverbal orofacial apraxia or apraxia of speech is commonly reported. Apraxia of speech often presents concurrently with orofacial apraxia, whereas orofacial apraxia may occur singly.	Nonverbal orofacial apraxia or apraxia of speech is atypical.	Rare	Rare
Neuromuscular Execution	Dysarthria is commonly reported with primarily hypokinetic and spastic features. Dysarthria severity has not been found to correlate with disease duration.	Dysarthria is commonly reported with primarily hypokinetic and spastic components. Ataxic and hyperkinetic features are less common.	Dysarthria is very common, with hypokinetic predominating in MSA-P, and ataxic predominating in MSA-C. Spastic, hyperkinetic, and flaccid types may also occur.	Dysarthria (hypokinetic) probably common, but not early in course of disease.
Language	Aphasia present in approximately one third to one half of cases, of mild to moderate severity, and characterized primarily by anomic or non-fluent features. Yes/no reversals may be present. Predominantly receptive aphasic disturbances are atypical.	Classic aphasias are atypical. Dynamic aphasia is a common presenting feature. Slowed information processing, reduced verbal fluency, and word retrieval deficit may also be present.	Aphasia not expected. Dementia, when present, can affect communication ability.	Aphasia is uncommon/rare as an isolated or dominant deficit. Semantic deficits often present but embedded within other cognitive impairments (e.g., visuoperceptual, working memory and attention deficits, fluctuating attention).

CORTICOBASAL DEGENERATION

CBD, a rare neurodegenerative multisystem disorder of insidious onset, is typically described and characterized by its asymmetric motor signs of limb function abnormalities. We report on the nature, frequency, and severity of speech and language disturbances (*see* Chapters 18–21).

Neuroanatomical Correlates

A striking feature of CBD is the asymmetry with which the disease presents. Its progressive nature eventually involves extensive and bilateral damage to cortical and basal ganglionic structures. Both the asymmetry and involvement of cerebral cortex and basal ganglia influence motor speech and language disturbances, which increase in severity as the disease progresses. A structural magnetic resonance imaging (MRI) study of 25 patients with CBD *(14)* found that this series of cases presented almost exclusively with asymmetric posterior frontal and parietal atrophy, which explains the prevalence of motor speech and language disorders owing to perisylvian area involvement. In addition, postmortem studies of basal ganglia abnormalities explain a prevalent finding of hypokinetic features of dysarthria resulting from damage to the extrapyramidal tract (the reader is referred to Chapter 4 for further information regarding neuroanatomical correlates of CBD, PSP, MSA, and Dementia with Lewy bodies).

Speech Disturbances

Dysarthria in CBD is commonly reported *(15–18)*, but with variable dysarthria types including hypokinetic and spastic features primarily and a wide frequency range from 29% to 93%. In their comprehensive review of the literature, Lehman Blake et al. *(18)* found descriptions of speech or language characteristics in 60 of 66 papers characterizing the features of CBD, representing 457 cases. Across these studies, motor speech disorders were identified in 55% of the cases, with dysarthria reported in 42% of the cases, nonverbal oral apraxia reported in 4% of the cases, and apraxia of speech reported in 3.9% of the cases.

Among group studies, Riley et al. *(15)* documented the presence of dysarthria in about half of their 15 cases followed. Wenning and colleagues *(16)* found dysarthria in 29% of their sample during the first visit (on average 3 [–1.9] yr after onset of symptoms, and 75% of their sample during the last visit (on average 6.1 [–2.0] after onset of symptoms). In the Wenning et al. study, speech abnormalities were variably described as slurred ($n = 9$), dysphonic ($n = 5$), mute ($n = 5$), aphonic ($n = 4$), unintelligible ($n = 4$), echolalic (i.e., compulsive and unsolicited complete or partial repetition of other's utterances) ($n = 2$), or palilalic (i.e., compulsive word and phase repetitions with increased rate usually during spontaneous speech) ($n = 1$), suggesting that identification of speech characteristics also extended to language abnormalities (i.e., echolalia, and possibly mutism). Frattali and Sonies *(17)* found dysarthria in 13 (93%) of their sample of 14 cases, therefore documenting dysarthria as a prominent feature of CBD, even in the relatively early phases of disease progression (mean disease duration = 3.5 yr). Using the dysarthria classifications of Darley, Aronson, and Brown *(19)*, dysarthria varied in both type and severity. Of the 13 cases, the majority had mild symptoms, with 7 patients presenting with mild symptoms, 5 with moderate symptoms, and only 1 case with severe symptoms. Five patients (35.7%) had hypokinetic dysarthria, three patients (21.4%) had mixed dysarthria with predominant hypokinetic features, two patients (14.3%) had mixed dysarthria with predominant hyperkinetic features, two patients (14.3%) had mixed dysarthria with predominant spastic features, and one patient (7.1%) had spastic dysarthria. It should be noted that 57% of this clinical sample displayed hypokinetic features of dysarthria—features that characterize the dysarthria of patients with parkinsonism resulting from extrapyramidal damage. This finding provides one explanation for the misdiagnoses of CBD for Parkinson's disease (PD), particularly in early stages. Type or severity of dysarthria did not correlate with duration of disease. Apraxia was also prevalent in this sample, which was assessed in 13 patients. Of this sample, six patients (46%) had orofacial apraxia and five patients (38%) had combined orofacial apraxia and apraxia of speech. Of interest was that none of the patients had apraxia of speech in the absence of orofacial apraxia, but orofacial apraxia presented singly in nearly 50% of this clinical sample. In the most severe cases of oral apraxia, two patients (15.3%) could not voluntarily open their mouths, pucker their lips, or even volitionally perform activities automatic to oral movements (e.g., taking pills, drinking, or eating). The severity of orofacial apraxia for these patients resulted in mechanical interference during their modified barium swallow study procedures. When instructed to look straight ahead, hold bolus in mouth momentarily, and swallow, both patients unintentionally opened their mouths with subsequent loss of bolus from the oral cavity, commenting, "I tried as hard as I could," or "My mouth would not cooperate."

Lehman Blake et al. *(18)*, in their study of 13 autopsy-confirmed cases of CBD, found dysarthria and apraxia of speech in 31% and 38% of their sample, respectively. Of the patients with apraxia of speech, two exhibited nonverbal oral apraxia. Of the patients with dysarthria, dysarthria type was typically mixed, with either spastic or hypokinetic features present in all cases. Lehman Blake and colleagues further found that speech and/or language difficulties were either the first sign, or among the first signs of CBD in 6 (46%) of the 13 patients.

In another study of dysarthria and orofacial apraxia in CBD *(20)*, 9 of the 10 patients followed were mildly dysarthric on the bases of results from administration of the *Frenchay Dysarthria Assessment (21)*. Severity of dysarthria, as assessed by an intelligibility score, correlated with global severity but not with duration of disease. Voluntary movement of the tongue and lips were impaired in all patients. Orofacial apraxia was present in the same nine patients. The apraxia scores, however, did not correlate with the severity of dysarthria, suggesting independent underlying mechanisms. The study concluded that the presence of dysarthria and orofacial apraxia is more frequent in CBD than usually reported.

One study used discriminant analysis to sensitively characterize the variability of dysarthria in 20 patients with atypical parkinsonism *(22)*, resulting in classifications among the three types of hypokinetic, spastic, or ataxic dysarthria for the seven patients with CBD.

An atypical example of a patient with CBD who presented with isolated speech deficits for several years before other symptoms emerged is found in the literature. Bergeron et al. *(23)* described an unusual presentation in a case with an isolated speech disturbance for 5 yr before developing the more typical features of CBD. The most severe neuroanatomical changes were observed in the left motor cortex and adjacent Broca's area.

Language Disturbances

Aphasia, though included in accounts of the clinical syndrome of CBD, has neither been well described in the literature nor sufficiently studied to determine its clinical frequency, behavioral features, and neuropathological correlates *(24)*. For example, Rinne et al. *(25)* reported language disturbances to be uncommon in CBD whereas Wenning et al. *(16)* reported one-third of their 14 patients to have aphasia.

Because of their suspected underreporting in the literature, Frattali et al. *(26)* attempted to systematically identify and characterize the language deficits of CBD. Based on performance on the *Western Aphasia Battery* (WAB) *(27)* and related language and cognitive measures, 53% of the 15 patients studied had identifiable aphasia syndromes, including anomic, Broca's, and transcortical motor aphasias. WAB aphasia quotients (100 being normal) ranged from 56.3 to 89.8 (mean = 87.2 ± 12.2) suggesting the presence of mildly to moderately severe aphasia among the cases studied. As aphasia quotients decreased, indicating increasing severity, aphasia classifications changed on an index of fluency, from fluent anomic to nonfluent Broca's or transcortical motor aphasia. None of the patients with aphasia showed predominant receptive aphasic disturbances, suggesting a predominance of frontal involvement. Corroborating these findings, Lehman Blake et al. *(18)* found aphasia to be present in 7 (54%) of the 13 patients with autopsy-confirmed CBD studied, with aphasia type most often characterized as nonfluent (i.e., agrammatic, telegraphic, reduced phrase length) or anomic.

Recently, a unique behavioral feature of language disturbance, termed yes/no reversals, has been described in CBD among other neurodegenerative diseases *(28)*. For this phenomenon, a patient verbalizes or gestures 'yes' when meaning no, or vice versa, when responding to queries during social discourse. Though not a distinguishable feature of CBD, the prospective arm of this study found its presence in 11 of 34 patients (32%) or nearly one-third of those with CBD (i.e., met the modified diagnostic criteria of Lang et al., ref. *29*). Of those who presented with yes/no reversals and for whom MRI data were available ($N = 10$), 7 had left-hemisphere involvement, suggesting a prominent role of the left hemisphere in this lexically related cognitive sign. Although the phenomenon was dissociated from features of aphasia, correlations of yes/no reversals with frontal lobe functions suggested that higher-order mental disruptions (i.e., mental flexibility and inhibitory control) interacting with motor programming disruptions were associated with the phenomenon.

Consistent with the findings of unusual case presentations depending on lesion topography in CBD *(23)*, an atypical case of progressive sensory aphasia resulting from CBD is found in the literature *(30)*. This patient showed progressive sensory aphasia as an initial symptom, then developed "total aphasia" within 6 yr and finally severe dementia. Neuropathological correlates were found in the cerebral cortex, with the superior and transverse temporal gyri most severely affected, and subsequently in the inferior frontal gyrus. Degeneration of the subcortical gray matter was most severe in the substantia nigra, and it was moderate to mild in the ventral part of the thalamus, globus pallidus, and striatum. A subsequent survey of 28 pathologically evaluated cases of CBD revealed two similar cases, both of which began with progressive aphasia and presented cortical degeneration in the superior temporal gyrus. Also in the literature is a case report of a patient with CBD whose initial symptom was progressive nonfluent aphasia, with the distribution of her cortical lesion at autopsy accentuated in the frontal language-related area *(31)*. In summary, progressive aphasia, either fluent or nonfluent, should be considered among the initial symptoms in CBD.

Clinical Management

The likelihood that speech and language disorders will become prominent features in CBD is high, with the late-stage results severely compromising interpersonal communication. Given this profile, periods of speech-language treatment regimens for the purposes of maintaining functional communication are warranted. Intervention should be tailored to the various stages of decline, beginning with instruction of compensatory strategies (e.g., pacing and overarticulation to improve speech intelligibility, instruction of communication partners to rephrase questions requiring simpler or shorter responses, increasing the salience and structure of context during interactions, and reducing ambient noise in the patient's environments to minimize distractions), proceeding to use of augmentative communication systems (e.g., picture boards, portable voice amplifiers) tailored to the functional use of the patient, and use of multimodality cues to enhance communication (e.g., say it, show it, draw it, point it out). In late stages, the speech-language pathologist can serve as a facilitator to determine what residual communication skills can be used by the patient and can tailor these skills to allow communication of strong preferences or basic need.

PROGRESSIVE SUPRANUCLEAR PALSY

PSP is a multisystem neurodegenerative disease that commonly presents with dysarthria among its early features. Using the Litvan et al. criteria *(32)*, probable PSP is diagnosed on the bases of parkinsonism with age at onset over 40 yr, supranuclear vertical gaze palsy, postural instability in the first year of illness, late mild dementia, and poor or absent response to L-dopa, in the absence of other diseases that could explain the signs and symptoms.

Neuroanatomical Correlates

PSP is differentiated neuropathologically from CBD by its limited cortical pathology, less common white matter pathology, and more common distribution of tract degeneration affecting the corticospinal tract *(33)*. In a recent review of 24 cases *(14)*, MRI studies demonstrated symmetrical cerebral atrophy in 19 patients (79.2%), midbrain atrophy in 22 cases (91.7%) (accounting for the atypical hyperextended head positioning found in this clinical population), and a slight increase in signal intensity in the periaqueductal region (consistent with cell loss and gliosis) in 16 patients

(66.7%). Because of progressive and selective neuronal loss in the subcortical gray nuclei and brainstem, the neural pathways controlling oral sensorimotor function are affected in PSP.

Speech Disturbances

Sonies *(34)* conducted a systematic investigation of speech in 22 patients with a confirmed diagnosis of PSP. The patients, (12 males, 10 females) ranged in age from 52 to 77 yr with a mean duration of illness of 41.14 mo. Seventeen patients (71%) were found to have one or more abnormal speech symptoms. The most common symptom was imprecise articulation evident in 50% of the patients. In frequency, this symptom was followed by reduced ability to sustain phonation and reduced voice volume in eight patients (36.4%), hypernasality in seven patients (31.8%), slowed rate of speaking in five patients (22.7%), hoarseness, reduced variation in intonation (monotone), and slow alternating motion rate in four patients (18.2%), rapid rate of speech and strained/strangled voice quality in three patients (13.6%), aphonia in three patients (13.6%), and harsh voice quality, unintelligible speech, and uncontrolled vocal bursts in two patients (9.1%). Sonies reported that these characteristics can be categorized into both hypokinetic and hyperkinetic classifications of dysarthria, with many combined characteristics suggesting mixed dysarthrias in this study sample. Also suggested among the characteristics reported are features of spastic and ataxic dysarthrias.

Kluin et al. *(35)* also found a high frequency of dysarthria in PSP, consisting of prominent hypokinetic and spastic components with less prominent ataxic components. In the 14 patients studied, all had hypokinetic and spastic components of dysarthria. Nine patients had ataxic components. When compared with neuropathological findings, the severity of hypokinetic features correlated significantly with the degree of neuronal loss and gliosis in the substantia nigra pars compacta and pars reticulata, but not in the subthalamic nucleus, striatum, or globus pallidus. The severity of spastic and ataxic components did not correlate significantly with neuropathological changes in the frontal cortex or cerebellum. In an earlier study of 44 patients with PSP *(36)*, all were found to have dysarthria with variable degrees of spasticity, hypokinesia, and ataxia. Twenty-eight patients had all three components, and 16 patients had only two components. Twenty-two patients (50%) had predominantly spastic components, 15 (34%) had predominantly hypokinetic components, and 6 (14%) had predominantly ataxic components. Stuttering also occurred in nine patient (20%) and palilalia in five (11%). The finding of mixed dysarthria with a combination of spastic, hypokinetic, and ataxic components was considered important to diagnosis and coincided with the neuropathologic changes found in PSP.

Consistent with the findings of Kluin et al. *(35)*, Auzou et al. *(22)* found that the seven patients with PSP all had hypokinetic dysarthria. Also noted were the speech abnormalities of palilalia and repetitive speech phenomena in case studies *(37,38)*.

Among atypical presentations, a case study of a patient with atypical PSP reports the presence of progressive apraxia of speech and nonverbal oral apraxia, along with progressive nonfluent aphasia *(39)*. This patient showed progressive changes reflecting left- greater than right-cerebral-hemisphere dysfunction with a more widespread cortical pathology than is typical of PSP, found at autopsy.

Language Disturbances

Though classical language disturbances are uncommon in PSP, dynamic aphasia can be a common presenting symptom (*see* Appendix A for description). For example, a study of three cases found presenting symptoms as difficulty with language output *(40)*. Behavioral testing showed considerable impairment on a range of single-word tasks requiring active initiation and search strategies (letter and category fluency, sentence completion), and on a test of narrative language production. In contrast, naming from pictures and verbal descriptions, as well as word and sentence comprehension, were largely intact. Esmonde et al. concluded that selective involvement of cognitive processes critical for planning and initiating language output may occur in some patients with PSP. This presentation resembles the phenomenon of verbal adynamia or dynamic aphasia seen in patients with frontal lobe damage. The deficit is thought to reflect frontal deafferentation secondary to interruption of frontostriatal feedback loops.

As mentioned above, a case study of a patient with atypical PSP also reported the presence of progressive nonfluent aphasia and subsequent dementia *(39)*. SPECT (single photon emission computed tomography) scans showed progressive changes reflecting left > right cerebral hemisphere dysfunction with hypoperfusion in the left temporal > frontal > parietal cortex. Neuropathological examination revealed findings characteristics of PSP but with more widespread cortical pathology. Thus, PSP can present clinically as an atypical dementing syndrome dominated by progressive nonfluent aphasia and apraxia of speech.

Among characteristic language or related cognitive features of PSP, Bak and Hodges *(41)* include general slowness of information processing, deficits in focused and divided attention, impaired initiation (a symptom of dynamic aphasia), grossly reduced verbal fluency, and memory impairment affecting active recall *(41)* Word retrieval deficit has also been reported by Gurd and Hodges *(42)*. Two cases of PSP demonstrated word-finding difficulties associated with pervasive problems in word retrieval. The deficit was also found to be less amenable to cue facilitation than that found in word retrieval deficits associated with PD. Reduced frontal perfusion was found in one of the two cases.

Clinical Management

As in the management of other progressive neurological diseases, educating communication partners to facilitate interactions, and offering compensatory strategies to maintain functional communication over time, which changes in need and method as the disease progresses, become important aspects of clinical intervention. For those PSP patients with dynamic aphasia, it is helpful for communication partners to explicitly lead the patient into conversations by asking direct questions that are weighted toward the concrete and personal rather than abstract, and to increase the salience of context during interactions. If processing is slowed, it is helpful to allow extra time (without interruption) for the patient to process and respond. Verifying receipt of the message conveyed before proceeding in an interaction is also helpful.

For dysarthria, clinical interventions can include the use of pacing methods to slow rate of speech, and the use of pausing, chunking streams of speech into units, and, in severe, cases, a one-word-at-a-time approach. If hypophonia is present, frequent cues to increase loudness, and use of voice amplifiers and other augmentative communication devices/systems may be warranted as tailored to the abilities of the patient.

MULTIPLE SYSTEM ATROPHY

MSA is an uncommon, sporadic (nonfamilial), and distinct neurodegenerative condition that is characterized by varying combinations of parkinsonism, cerebellar ataxia, spasticity, and autonomic dysfunction *(43)*. Its onset is usually in the sixth to seventh decade, with a duration range of 1–18 yr and median survival of about 9 yr *(44,45)*. Recognizing MSA as distinct from PD is important because prognosis, counseling, and treatment of the communication problems of people with PD and MSA differ.

MSA is a plural disorder, with three previously recognized subtypes that include Shy–Drager syndrome, sporadic olivopontocerebellar atrophy (OPCA), and striatonigral degeneration. A recent consensus statement on MSA *(45)* recommended replacing these subtype designations with MSA-P if parkinsonian features predominate, and MSA-C if cerebellar features predominate. Because the literature contains references to both subtyping schemes, both will be used here when applicable.

Neuroanatomical Correlates

The range of neuroanatomic involvement in MSA includes neuronal loss and gliosis in the basal ganglia (neostriatum), substantia nigra, cerebellum, inferior olives, middle cerebellar peduncles, basis pontine nuclei, intermediolateral and anterior horn cells, and corticospinal tracts. Some investigations have reported cerebral atrophy, especially in the frontal lobes *(46–49)*. In light of the motor speech disorders that can occur, it is reasonable to assume that the corticobulbar tracts can also be involved.

The predominant loci of nerve cell loss vary across the MSA subtypes, but with overlap, and they are associated with the prominent but overlapping clinical features, including speech and language findings. Thus, in striatonigral degeneration (MSA-P) nerve cell loss and gliosis predominate in the neostriatum and substantia nigra; parkinsonian features, including hypokinetic dysarthria, are prominent and beneficial response to levodopa is limited because striatal neurons containing dopamine receptors are lost. In OPCA (MSA-C), there may be prominent involvement of the cerebellum, explaining clinical cerebellar features, including ataxic dysarthria. In Shy–Drager syndrome, early and prominent dysautonomia (including orthostatic hypotension, incontinence, reduced respiration, and impotence) stems from loss of preganglionic sympathetic neurons in the intermediolateral horns; because the substantia nigra, striatum, cerebellum, and corticospinal tracts are also affected, parkinsonism (possibly including hypokinetic dysarthria) with suboptimal response to levodopa, ataxia (possibly including ataxic dysarthria), and spasticity (possibly including spastic dysarthria) may also be evident *(50,51)*.

Speech Disturbances

A review of clinical studies suggest that apraxia of speech (AOS) is rarely, if ever, associated with MSA. For example, in Duffy's *(1)* review of etiologies for 107 quasirandomly selected cases with AOS, in which 16% of the cases had degenerative neurologic disease, no patient had a diagnosis of MSA or any of its subtypes. And, in a review of 61 patients with AOS associated with degenerative neurologic disease, in only 1 patient was MSA (vs PSP) considered a diagnostic possibility *(52)*. Relatedly, Leiguardia et al. *(53)* found no evidence of limb, nonverbal oral or respiratory apraxia in 10 patients with MSA.

In contrast, dysarthria is common, sometimes occurring in 100% of patients in series unselected for dysarthria *(54)*. It tends to emerge relatively early (median onset within the first 2 yr) in the course of the disease, generally earlier than in PD, and on average the dysarthrias of MSA are believed to be more severe than in PD *(55–57)*. Müller et al. *(55)* reported severe (i.e., unintelligible) speech impairment in 60% of their 15 MSA patients at the time of their last clinic visit (a median of 5 mo before death).

The types of dysarthria generally correlate with other neuromotor signs of MSA, and the dysarthria type is most often mixed. MSA, including each of its subtypes, accounted for about 8% of all mixed dysarthrias attributable to degenerative neurologic disease in a series of patients reviewed by Duffy *(1)*. Kluin et al. *(54)* evaluated 46 patients with MSA, unselected for type of speech disorder. All had dysarthria with combinations of hypokinetic, ataxic, and spastic types. Seventy percent had all three types, 28% had two types, and one patient had only ataxic dysarthria. The hypokinetic component predominated in 48%, the ataxic component in 35%, and the spastic component in 11%. The presence in MSA of dysarthria types other than hypokinetic is important to differential diagnosis. For example, because untreated PD is associated only with hypokinetic dysarthria, recognizing another dysarthria type or a mixed dysarthria can help distinguish PD from MSA or other degenerative neurologic diseases.

The most comprehensive study of dysarthria in a MSA subtype is that by Linebaugh *(58)*, who reviewed 80 cases with a diagnosis of Shy–Drager syndrome seen at the Mayo Clinic over a 14-yr period. Forty-four percent had dysarthria, 43% ataxic dysarthria, 31% hypokinetic dysarthria, and 26% mixed dysarthrias. The mixed dysarthrias included hypokinetic-ataxic, ataxic-spastic, and spastic-ataxic-hypokinetic.

The dysarthrias associated with OPCA (MSA-C) have received little study. Gilman and Kluin *(59)* examined three patients with OPCA who had clinical signs of cerebellar involvement plus corticobulbar findings suggestive of spasticity (e.g., pseudobulbar affect, active gag reflex, slow facial movements). The primary speech findings were consistent with mixed ataxic-spastic dysarthria, but some had stridor, which would suggest a flaccid component. Hartman and O'Neill *(60)* discussed a man with a clinical diagnosis of OPCA whose predominant deviant speech characteristics were consistent with a mixed flaccid–spastic dysarthria (stuttering-like dysfluencies were also apparent, possibly reflecting a reemergence of developmental stuttering.). Palatal myoclonus, technically a hyperkinetic dysarthria if apparent in speech, has been noted as variably present in OPCA *(61)*. Because features of parkinsonism can occur in OPCA, hypokinetic dysarthria should also be expected in some cases. It thus appears that a variety of dysarthria types are possible. Considering the areas of the motor system that are commonly affected, ataxic, spastic, hypokinetic, and flaccid dysarthria, singly or in combination, are the common expected types.

The dysarthrias associated with striatonigral degeneration (MSA-P) have not been studied systematically, but dysarthria is probably common. Hypokinetic dysarthria is the most common expected type, but hyperkinetic and perhaps spastic dysarthria would seem possible based on the common loci of pathology.

Stridor can be present in as many as one-third of people with MSA *(44)*. It can be associated with severe upper-airway obstruction and death, and nasal continuous positive airway pressure or tracheostomy is often recommended to treat it. It is manifest as excessive snoring and sleep apnea, and sometimes is evident as audible inspiration just before speech is initiated, or at phrase boundaries during ongoing speech. Inhalatory stridor associated with various combinations of spastic, ataxic, and hypokinetic dysarthria is probably uncommon in degenerative diseases other than MSA. The cause of the stridor is some matter of debate. It is commonly thought to reflect abductor laryngeal paresis or paralysis, particularly in the posterior cricoarytenoid muscles with pathology in the nucleus ambiguous *(62)*, but more recent evidence suggests that laryngeal dystonia may be the cause *(63,64)*. Relatedly, cervical and limb dystonia are not uncommon in untreated patients with MSA-P, and levodopa-induced neck and face dystonia can also occur *(65)*.

Language Disturbances

To our knowledge, aphasia has not been reported and, in fact, focal aphasia is considered one exclusionary criterion for MSA diagnosis *(45)*. Dementia is considered to be a variably evident deficit *(61)*, perhaps present to a mild–moderate degree in about one-fifth of patients *(44)*. When present, nonaphasic cognitive deficits can influence an affected individual's communication abilities.

Clinical Management

In MSA, management efforts focus primarily on the dysarthrias. Their emphasis may be on: (a) improving physiologic support for speech to improve speech intelligibility, (b) compensatory strategies to improve the intelligibility or comprehensibility of speech, or (c) developing alternative or augmentative means of communication. In general, such approaches are effective in improving communication ability (*see* ref. 66, for a review of data on treatment effectiveness). Such management is often staged during the course of the disease, with early efforts aimed at improving speech or maintaining intelligibility, and later efforts aimed at developing augmentative or alternative means of communication. If the dysarthria is hypokinetic or predominantly hypokinetic, the patient may benefit from Lee Silverman Voice Treatment (LSVT), a program involving vigorous vocal exercise that has been shown to be effective for the dysarthria associated with PD (*see* ref. 67, for a comprehensive review). If individuals undergo tracheotomy for stridor/sleep apnea, a number of prosthetic devices are available to permit vocalization or the generation of artificial voice.

DEMENTIA WITH LEWY BODIES

DLB is a clinically identifiable dementing illness that often includes parkinsonian features *(68)*. The average ages at onset is 75 yr, and mean survival is about 3.5 yr, with a range of 1–20 yr *(69)*. The central feature of DLB is progressively disabling dementia, but its core features, of which two out of three are necessary for a "probable" diagnosis, include fluctuating cognition, visual hallucinations, and motor signs of parkinsonism. Additional problems that may support the diagnosis include falls, syncope, loss of consciousness, delusions and hallucinations (auditory, olfactory, tactile), and sensitivity to neuroleptic medications *(70)*. At its end stage profound dementia and parkinsonism may be present *(70)*. Speech and language deficits may be present in DLB but they do not contribute to differential diagnosis of the condition.

Neuroanatomical Correlates

The neuropathology of DLB is complex. This brief discussion will emphasize the loci of pathology because of their direct relevance to clinical features, particularly speech and language deficits.

Pathologic abnormalities are found in the neocortex, limbic cortex, subcortical nuclei, and brainstem, but brainstem or cortical Lewy bodies (LBs) are the only features that must be present for a pathologic diagnosis *(70)*. Spongioform changes and some pathologic features of Alzheimer's disease (AD) may also be present. Limbic and neocortical LBs are logically related to neuropsychiatric and cognitive signs and symptoms. LBs in spinal cord sympathetic neurons and dorsal vagal nuclei may be linked to autonomic failure and dysphagia (and some aspects of dysarthria), respectively *(69,70)*.

On neuroimaging, in contrast to findings in AD, people with DLB have relative preservation of medial temporal structures, including the hippocampus. In comparison to AD, DLB is associated with greater occipital hypoperfusion and greater compromise in the nigrostriatal pathways *(69)*.

Speech Disturbances

Müller et al. *(55)* examined the evolution of dysarthria and dysphagia in 14 patients with pathologically confirmed DLB. Dysarthria was present in 72%. Dysarthria and dysphagia onset were not early in DLB (median onset was 42 and 43 mo, respectively), but were typically earlier than in PD. Dysarthria was said to be predominantly hypophonic/monotonous in 70%. Severe speech impairment at the last clinical visit (~ 5 mo before death) was present in 29%. McKeith et al. *(70)* note that motor features of parkinsonism are typically mild but can include hypophonic speech. In general, hypokinetic dysarthria is the primary and perhaps only neurologic motor speech disturbance expected in DLB.

Language Disturbances

Language impairments, particularly aphasia, are not among the signs or symptoms included in clinical criteria for the diagnosis of DLB, and only infrequently are they mentioned in case descriptions. Only one single case study *(71)* has documented primary progressive aphasia as the initial presentation (and only sign for 6 yr) in a patient who eventually developed visual hallucinations and parkinsonism; the pathology was that of DLB and AD. A few additional case descriptions have made reference to the presence of aphasia, or signs suggestive of aphasia, such as difficulty with word recall and retrieval and sentence completion *(72,73)*, but the language deficits in each case were vaguely described and appeared to be part of widespread cognitive and personality changes.

Deficits within the language domain probably are not uncommon but they likely are most often embedded within a constellation of other cognitive impairments. For example, in a study of people with AD and DLB, matched in age and severity of cognitive impairment, Lambon Ralph et al. *(74)* found both groups to have semantic memory deficits as reflected in a graded naming test, picture naming, spoken word to picture matching, semantic association, a category sorting test, and a word and letter fluency test. In comparison to the AD group, the DLB group had more severe semantic deficits for pictures than words, as well as visuoperceptual deficits. The authors concluded that patients with DLB have a generalized dementia that affects many different domains of performance, including semantic abilities.

Although impairment of cognitive functions in DLB appears broad, cognitive reaction time, attention, fluctuations of attention, working memory, and (particularly) visuoperceptive abilities are often noteworthy and, on average, are more impaired in DLB than AD *(75–78)*. McKeith et al. *(70)* note that prominent memory impairment may not be evident early in DLB, but that with disease progression deficits in memory, language, and other cognitive skills frequently overlap with those seen in AD.

Clinical Management

If hypokinetic dysarthria is present, and cognitive deficits not severe, LSVT may help improve loudness and intelligibility. Otherwise listener and speaker strategies must be considered to maximize comprehensibility (e.g., amplifier, pacing board, reduce noise, intelligibility breakdown repair strategies). If visuoperceptual deficits are prominent, increased emphasis is placed on the verbal (and other nonvisual) modality to enhance comprehension. It is important to work with significant others to identify strategies to maximize communication (e.g., how best to provide verbal input, how best to ask or make confirmatory statements to clarify needs and wants). With the exception of the complication of visuoperceptual deficits, these strategies would probably be common to those often used for people with AD.

DIRECTIONS FOR FUTURE RESEARCH

Directions for future research point strongly toward the need to develop both specific and combined behavioral, pharmacotherapeutic, or neurostimulation interventions that might slow, arrest, or even reverse the progression of the speech and language manifestations of atypical parkinsonian disorders (*see* Table 2 for summary). For example, cholinergic stimulation using centrally active cholinesterase inhibitors may be beneficial in improving cognitive or linguistic performance in the early stages of disease progression. Transcranial magnetic stimulation (TMS) can also be used to investigate the excitability of motor cortices in neurodegenerative diseases, thus providing important information having pathophysiological and clinical relevance. For example, TMS can be used to study the effects of drugs and surgery thus introducing the possibility of monitoring the action of treatment of movement disorders (including dysarthria) on cortical excitability *(79)*. As medical treatments become available for atypical parkinsonian conditions, their effects on speech and language abilities need to be established. Relative to motor speech abilities, for example, medical interventions that may improve limb motor deficits may or may not have a positive effect on speech.

The epidemiology of speech and language disorders must also evolve to a more accurate science. This calls for the development of explicit clinical diagnostic criteria for sensitively and differentially characterizing the features of these disorders and the relative influence of each on communication ability. Currently, comparisons across natural history studies suffer from variability in their assessment methods and descriptions of the various features that constitute dysarthria, apraxia, or aphasia. A second limitation across studies is small sample size. Therefore, multi-institution studies, using consistent and agreed-upon taxonomies in characterizing speech and language functions, and consistent methods in assessing these functions, could increase our understanding of the pathogeneses of these diseases. A solid foundation for such a taxonomy for speech functions has already been established by the extensive work of Darley, Aronson, and Brown *(19)*; any effort to develop explicit criteria for differentiating the dysarthrias should begin with their seminal work.

The efficacy of various approaches to management of communication disorders, including how approaches to management may be influenced by some of the unique characteristics of these diseases (e.g., limb apraxia, visual deficits, deficits of attention) will need to be determined. Also to be determined are the best way to stage management during the course of these conditions. For example, when should management attempt to improve impairment (e.g., LSVT) vs work to compensate for deficits?

Of future interest will also be the combined effects of disease progression and aging, with a normative databank created against which to compare various dimensions of performance. These comparisons may help to parse out the effects of the disease thus increasing clinical management precision. Neuroimaging studies should investigate the effects of neuronal loss from the perspective of studying neural networks and functional connectivity. The methods of probabilistic computational mapping and structural equation modeling will assist with hypothesis-driven studies that can eluci-

Table 2
Summary of Future Research Directions

Study Type	Example
Drug Effect	Cholinergic stimulation to improve cognitive and linguistic skills in the early stages of disease progression.
Neurostimulation	TMS to investigate the effects of surgery and drugs on cortical excitability and their relationship to changes in speech.
Medical Intervention	Nerve growth implantation and relative effects on motor speech abilities.
Epidemiology	Development of explicit clinical diagnostic criteria and an agreed-upon taxonomy for characterizing speech and language disorders.
Treatment Efficacy	Conventional and new behavioral approaches to speech or language management as influenced by unique disease characteristics (e.g., limb apraxia, visual deficits, attention deficit).
Natural History	Development of normative databank to determined combined effects of disease progression and aging.
Neuroimaging	Investigations of the effects of neuronal loss from the perspective of functional connectivity, and their relationships with specific speech and language disturbances.
Genetic	Identification of gene abnormalities to assist in early diagnosis and increase the effectiveness of preventive therapies. Establish the relationships between specific genetic findings and speech and language manifestations.

date links between neural breakdowns and behavioral effects *(8)*. Finally genetic studies designed to identify gene abnormalities may assist in reducing the incidence and prevalence of atypical parkinsonian disorders and can assist in their early diagnosis and increase the effectiveness of preventive therapies.

ACKNOWLEDGMENTS

The authors would like to thank Yun Kyeong Kang for expert assistance in manuscript and audio samples preparation.

REFERENCES

1. Duffy JR. Motor Speech Disorders: Substrates, Differential Diagnosis, and Management. St. Louis: Mosby, 1995.
2. Mesulam M-M. Principles of Behavioral and Cognitive Neurology. New York: Oxford University Press, 2000.
3. Beeman M, Chiarello C, eds. Right Hemisphere Language Comprehension: Perspectives from Cognitive Neuroscience. Erlbaum: Mahwah, NJ, 1998.
4. Tompkins CA. Right Hemisphere Communication Disorders: Theory and Management. San Diego: Singular, 1995.
5. Gilman S, Newman SW, Manter JT, Gatz AJ. Essentials of clinical neuroanatomy and neurophysiology. 6 ed. Philadelphia: F.A. Davis Company, 1996.
6. Damasio A, Damasio H. Aphasia and the neural basis of language. In: Mesulam M-M, ed. Principles of Behavioral and Cognitive Neurology. New York: Oxford University Press, 2000:294–315.
7. Scott S, Johnsrude J. The neuroanatomical and functional organization of speech perception. TRENDS in Neurosciences 2003;26(2):100–107.
8. Horwitz B, Amunts K, Bhattacharyya R, et al., Activation of Broca's area during the production of spoken and signed language: a combined cytoarchitectonic mapping and PET analysis. Neuropsychologia 2003;41(14):1868–1876.
9. World Health Organization, International Classification of Functioning, Disability and Health (ICF). Geneva, Switzerland: WHO, 2001.
10. LaPointe LL, ed. Aphasia and Related Neurogenic Language Disorder, 3rd ed., New York: Thieme, is still in press.
11. Davis G. Aphasiology: Disorders and Clinical Practice. Boston: Allyn & Bacon, 2000.
12. Myers PS. Right Hemisphere Damage: Disorders of Communication and Cognition. 1999, San Diego: Singular, 1999.
13. Worrall LW, Frattali C, eds. Neurogenic Communication Disorders: A Functional Approach. New York: Thieme, 2000.
14. Savoiardo M, Grisoli M, Girotti F. Magnetic resonance imaging in CBD, related atypical parkinsonian disorders, and dementias. In: Litvan I, Goetz C, Lang AE, eds. Advance in Neurology, Corticobasal Degeneration and Related Disorders, vol. 82. Philadelphia: Lippincott Williams & Wilkins, 2000:197–208.
15. Riley DE, Lang AE, Lewis A, et al., Cortical-basal ganglionic degeneration. Neurology 1990;40:1203–1212.
16. Wenning G, Litvan I, Jankovic J, et al. Natural history and survival of 14 patients with autopsy-confirmed corticobasal degeneration. J Neurol Neurosurg Psychiatry 1998;64:184–189.
17. Frattali CM, Sonies BC. Speech and swallowing disturbances in corticobasal degeneration. In: Litvan I, Goetz CG, Lang AE, eds. Advances in Neurology, Corticobasal Degeneration and Related Disorders, vol. 82. Philadelphia: Lippincott Williamas & Wilkins, 2000:153–160.
18. Lehman Blake M, Duffy JR, Boeve BF, et al., Speech and language disorders associated with corticalbasal degeneration. J Med Speech Lang Pathol 2003;11:131–146.
19. Darley FL, Aronson AE, Brown JR. Motor Speech Disorders. Philadelphia: Saunders, 1975.
20. Ozsancak C, Auzou P, Hannequin D. Dysarthria and orofacial apraxia in cortical degeneration. Mov Disord 2000;15(5):905–910.
21. Enderby P. Frenchay Dysarthria Assessment. San Diego: College-Hill, 1986.
22. Auzou P, Ozsancak C, Jan M, et al., Evaluation of motor speech function to diagnose different types of dysarthria. Rev Neurol (Paris) 2000;156(1):47–52.
23. Bergeron C, Pollanen M, Weyer L, et al. Unusual clinical presentations of cortical basal ganglionic degeneration. Ann Neurol 1996;40(6):893–900.
24. Black SE. Aphasia in corticobasal degeneration. In: Litvan I, Goetz CG, Lang AE, eds. Corticobasal degeneration and related disorders. Philadelphia: Lippincott Williams & Wilkins, 2000:123–133.
25. Rinne J, Lee M, P. Thompson PD, Marsden C. Corticobasal degeneration. A Clinical study of 36 cases. Brain 1994;117:1183–1196.
26. Frattali CM, Grafman J, Patronas N, Makhlouf MS, Litvan I. Language disturbances in corticobasal degeneration. Neurology 2000;54(4)990–992.
27. Kertesz A. Western Aphasia Battery. Test Manual. San Antonio, TX: Psychological Corporation, 1982.
28. Frattali CM, Duffy JR, Litvan I, et al., Yes/no reversals as neurobehavioral sequela: a disorder of language, praxis or inhibitory control? Eur J Neurol 2003;10:103–106.

29. Lang AE, Riley DE, BergeronC. Cortical-basal ganglionic degeneration. In: Calne DB, ed. Neurodegenerative Diseases. Philadelphia: Saunders, 1994:877–894.

30. Ikeda K, Akiyama H, Iritana S, et al. Corticobasal degeneration with primary progressive aphasia and accentuated cortical lesion in superior temporal gyrus: Case report and review. Acta Neuropathol 1996;92(5):534–539.

31. Mimura M, Oda T, Tsuchiya K, et al. Corticobasal degeneration presenting with nonfluent primary progressive aphasia: A clinicopathological study. J Neurol Sci 2001;183:19–26.

32. Litvan I, Agid Y, Jankovic J, et al. Accuracy of clinical criteria for the diagnosis of progressive supranuclear palsy (Steele–Richardson–Olszewski syndrome). Neurology 1996:46:922–930.

33. Dickson DW, Liu WK, Rsiezak-Reding H, Yen SH. Neuropathologic and molecular considerations. In: Litvan I, Goetz CG, Lang AE, eds. Advances in Neurology, Corticobasal Degeneration and Related Disorders, vol. 82. Philadelphia: Lippincott Williams & Wilkins, 2000:9–27.

34. Sonies B. Swallowing and speech disturbances. In: Litvan I, Agid Y, eds. Progressive Supranuclear Palsy: Clinical and Research Approaches. New York: Oxford University Press, 1992:240–253.

35. Kluin KJ, Gilman S, Foster NL, et al. Neuropathological correlates of dysarthria in progressive supranuclear palsy. Arch Neurol 2001;58:265–269.

36. Kluin KJ, Foster NL, Berent S, Gilman S. Perceptual analysis of speech disorders in progressive supranuclear palsy. Neurology 1993;43:563–566.

37. Benke T, Butterworth B. Palilalia and repetitive speech: Two case studies. Brain Lang 2001;78:62–81.

38. Benke T, Hohenstein C, Poewe W, Butterworth B. Repetitive speech phenomena in Parkinson's disease. J Neurol Neurosurg Psychiatry 2000:63:319–325.

39. Boeve B, Dickenson D, Duffy JR, et al. Progressive nonfluent aphasia and subsequent aphasic dementia associated with atypical progressive supranuclear palsy pathology. Eur Neurol 2003;49(2):72–78.

40. Esmonde T, Giles E, Xuereb J, Hodges J. Progressive supranuclear palsy presenting with dynamic aphasia. J Neurol Neurosurg Psychiatry 1996;60:403–410.

41. Bak TH, Hodges JR. The neuropsychology of progressive supranuclear palsy. Neurocase, 1998;4:89–94.

42. Gurd JM, Hodges JR. Word-retrieval in two cases of progressive supranuclear palsy. Behav Neurol 1997;10:31–41.

43. The Consensus Committee of the American Autonomic Society and the American Academy of Neurology, Consensus statement on the definition of orthostatic hypotention, pure autonomic failure, and multiple system atrophy. Neurology 1996;46(5):1470.

44. Bower JH. Multiple system atrophy. In: Adler CH Ahlskog JE, eds. Parkinson's Disease and Movement Disorders: Diagnosis and Treatment Guidelines for the Practicing Physician. Totowa, NJ: Humana, 2000.

45. Gilman S, Low PA, Quinn N, et al. Consensus statement on the diagnosis of multiple system atrophy. J Neurol Sci 1999;163:94–98.

46. Konagaya M, Konagaya Y, Sakai M, et al. Progressive cerebral atrophy in multiple system atrophy. J Neurol Sci 2002;195:123–127.

47. Naka H, Ohshita T, Maruta Y, et al. Characteristic MRI findings in multiple system atrophy: comparison of the three subtypes. Neuroradiology 2002;44:204–209.

48. Su M, Yoshida Y, Hirata, Y, et al. Primary involvement of the motor area in association with the nigrostriatal pathway in multiple system atrophy: neuropathological and morphometric evaluations. Acta Neuropathol 2001;101:57–64.

49. Watanabe H, Saito Y, Terao S, et al. Progression and prognosis in multiple system atrophy: an analysis of 230 Japanese patients. Brain 2002;125:1070–1083.

50. Dewey RB. Clinical features of Parkinson's disease. In: Adler CH, Ahlskog JE, eds. Parkinson's Disease and Movement Disorders: Diagnosis and Treatment Guidelines for the Practicing Physician. Totowa, NJ: Humana Press, 2000.

51. Fahn S, Przedborski S. Parkinsonism. In: Rowland L, ed. Merritt's Neurology, Philadelphia: Lippincott Williams & Wilkins, 2000.

52. Duffy JR. Progressive apraxia of speech: A retrospective study. Paper presented at the Conference on Motor Speech. Williamsburg, VA, 2002.

53. Leiguardia RC, Pramstaller PP, Merello M, et al. Apraxia in Parkinson's disease, progressive supranuclear palsy, multiple system atrophy and neuroleptic-induced parkinsonism. Brain 1997;120:75–90.

54. Kluin K, Gilman S, Lohman M, Junck L. Characteristics of the dysarthria of multiple system atrophy. Arch Neurol 1996;53:545–548.

55. Müller J, Wenning GK, Verny M, et al. Progression of dysarthria and dysphasia in postmortem-confirmed parkinsonian disorders. Arch Neurol 2001;58:259–264.

56. Quinn N. Multiple system atrophy: the nature of the beast [review]. J Neurol Neurosurg Psychiatry 1989;52(Suppl): 78–89.

57. Wenning G, Ben-Shlomo Y, Hughes A, et al. What clinical features are most useful to distinguish definite multiple atrophy from Parkinson's disease? J Neurol Neurosurg Psychiatry 2000;68:434–440.

58. Linebaugh CW. The dysarthria of Shy–Drager syndrome. J Speech Hear Disord 1979;44:55–60.

59. Gilman, S. and D. Kluin, Perceptual analysis of speech disorders in Friedreich disease and olivopontocerebellar atrophy. In: Bloedel JR, Dichgans J, Precht W, eds. Cerebellar Functions, New York: Springer-Verlag, 1984.

60. Hartman DE, O'Neil BP. Progressive dysfluency, dysphagia, dysarthria: a case of olivopontocerebellar atrophy. In: Yorkston KM, Beukelman DR, eds. Recent Advances in Dysarthria. Boston: College-Hill, 1989.

61. Duvoisin RC. The olivopontocerebellar atrophies. In: Marsden CD, Fahn S, eds. Movement Disorders 2. Boston: Butterworth, 1987.

62. Bannister R, Gibson W, Michael L, Oppenheimer DR. Laryngeal abductor paralysis in multiple system atrophy; a report on three necropsied cases, with observations on the laryngeal muscles and the nuclei ambigui. Brain 1981;104:351–368.

63. Benarroche EE, Schmeichel AM, Parisi JE. Preservation of branchiomotor neurons of the nucleus ambiguus in multiple system atrophy. Neurology 2003;60:115–117.

64. Isono S, Shiba K, Yamaguchi M, et al. Pathogenesis of laryngeal narrowing in patients with multiple system atrophy. J Physiol 2001;536:237–249.

65. Boesch S, Wenning GK, Ransmayr G, Poewe W. Dystonia in multiple system atrophy. J Neurol Neurosurg Psychiatry 2002;72:300–303.

66. Yorkston KM. Treatment efficacy: dysarthria. J Speech Hear Res 1996;39:S46–S57.

67. Fox CM, Morrison CE, Ramig LO, Sapir S. Current perspectives on the Lee Silverman Voice Treatment (LSVT) for individuals with idiopathic Parkinson disease. Am J Speech Lang Pathol 2002;11:111–123.

68. Small S, Mayeux R. Alzheimer disease and related dementias. In: Rowland LP, ed. Merritt's Neurology. Philadelphia: Lippincott Williams & Wilkins, 2000.

69. Barber R, Panikkar A, McKeith IG. Dementia with Lewy bodies: diagnosis and management. Int J Geriatr Psychiatry 2001;16:S12–S18.

70. McKeith I, Galasko D, Kosaka K, et al. Consensus guidelines for the clinical and pathological diagnosis of dementia with Lewy bodies (DLB); report of the consortium on DLB international workshop. Neurology 1996;47:1113–1124.

71. Caselli R, Beach TG, Sue LI, et al., Progressive aphasia with Lewy bodies. Dement Geriatr Cogn Disord 2002;14:55–58.

72. Galvin JE, Lee SL, Perry A, et al., Familial dementia with Lewy bodies: clinicopathologic analysis of two kindreds. Neurology 2002;59:1079–1082.

73. Tsuang DW, Dalan AM, Eugenio CJ, et al., Familial dementia with Lewy bodies: a clinical and neuropathological study of 2 families. Arch Neurol 2002;59:1162–1630.

74. Lambon Ralph MA, Powell J, Howard D, et al., Semantic memory is impaired in both dementia with Lewy bodies and dementia of Alzheimer's type: a comparative neuropsychological study and literature review. J Neurol Neurosurg Psychiatry 2001;70:149–156.

75. Ballard C, O'Brien J, Gray A, et al., Attention and fluctuating attention in patients with dementia with Lewy bodies and Alzheimer disease. Arch Neurol 2001;58:997–982.

76. Calderon J, Perry RJ, Erzinclioglu SW, et al., Perception, attention, and working memory are disproportionately impaired in dementia with Lewy bodies compared to Alzheimer's disease. J Neurol Neurosurg Psychiatry 2001;70:157–164.

77. Galasko D. Lewy bodies and dementia. Curr Neurol Neurosci Rep 2001;1:435–441.

78. Mori E, Shimomura T, Fujimori M, et al., Visuoperceptual impairment in dementia with Lewy bodies. Arch Neurol 2000;57:489–493.

79. Priori A, Berardelli A. Transcranial brain stimulation in movement disorders. In: . Pascual-Leone A, Davey NJ, Rothwell J, Wassermann EM, Puri BK, eds. Handbook of Transcranial Magnetic Stimulation. London, Arnold, 2002.

80. Gernsbacher MA. Handbook of Psycholinguistics. San Diego: Academic, 1994.

81. Damasio H, Damasio AR. Lesion Analysis in Neuropsychology. New York: Oxford University Press, 1989.

82. Alexander MP. Disorders of language after frontal lobe injury: Evidence for the neural mechanisms of assembling language. In: Stuss DT, Knight RT, eds. Principles of Frontal Lobe Function. New York: Oxford University Press, 2002:159–167.

83. Luria A. The working brain. New York: Basic Books, 1973.

84. Luria AR, Tsevkosva LS. Towards the mechanism of "dynamic aphasia." Acta Neurol Psychiatrica Belg 1967;67:1045–1067.

85. Tognolo G, Vignolo LA. Brain lesions associated with oral apraxia in stroke patients: A clinico-neuroradiological investigation with the CT scan. Neuropsychologia 1980;18(3):257–272.

86. Helm-Estabrooks N. Test of oral and limb apraxia, normed edition. Chicago: Riverside, 1992.

87. Darley F, Aronson AE, Brown JR. Differential diagnostic patterns of dysarthria. J Speech Hear Res 1969;12:246–269.

88. Benson DF. Aphasia, alexia, and agraphia. New York: Churchill Livingstone, 1979.

Appendix A
Descriptions of Classic Aphasia Syndromes[b], Apraxias, and Dysarthria Types

Type of Speech or Language Disturbance	Classical Neuroanatomical Correlates	Clinical Features
Aphasias: Broca's	Primarily posterior aspects of the third frontal convolution and adjacent inferior aspects of the precentral gyrus of the dominant hemisphere (80).	Major disturbance in speech production with sparse, halting speech, often misarticulated, frequently missing function words (articles, conjunctions, pronouns, prepositions, auxiliary verbs) and bound morphemesi (80). Connected speech is often described as telegraphic or agrammatic, with relatively spared auditory comprehension (11). Verbal problems often reflect a concomitant apraxia of speech. Repetition of spoken words and phrases and confrontation naming are also impaired. Writing is impaired with written errors resembling verbal production errors qualitatively. Reading comprehension is deficient to a degree that generally parallels auditory comprehension.
Wernicke's	Posterior portion of the superior temporal gryus and possible adjacent cortex of the dominant hemisphere (80).	Major disturbance in auditory comprehension, fluent speech with disturbances of the sounds and structures of words (phonemic, morphological and semantic paraphasias, including neologisms) (80). Often described as press of speech (must often be stopped as conversation is continuous). Defective repetition of words and phrases, both reading and writing are usually disturbed.
Global	Large portion of the perisylvian association cortex in distribution of middle cerebral artery of the dominant hemisphere (80).	Disruption of all language-processing components (80). Some patients may speak noncommunicatively with verbal stereotypes (e.g., dee, dee, dee, down the hatch), although they may be alert and aware of their surroundings, and often express feeling and thoughts through facial, vocal, and manual gestures (11).
Anomic	Wide range of lesion patterns, both focal and diffuse. Linked to large left-hemisphere lesions or focal lesions of connections between the left temporal and parietal cortex (81). Also inferior parietal lobe lesions (80).	Disturbance in the production of single words, most marked for common nouns and variable comprehension problems (80). Presence of fluent, grammatically coherent utterances weakened in communicative power by a word retrieval deficit. Utterances are vacuous with indefinite nouns and pronouns filling in for substantive words.
Transcortical Motor	Continual debate, however, lesion localization thought to be mid- and upper premotor cortex around or including the supplementary motor area. Disruptions of white matter tracts deep to Broca's area (80). Lesions also described in the left lateral frontal lobe, variably anterior and superior to Broca's area (82).	Disturbance of spontaneous speech similar to Broca's aphasia with relatively preserved repetition (80). Verbal output is nonfluent with relatively spared visual and auditory comprehension.

Transcortical Sensory	Disturbance in single-word comprehension with relatively intact repetition (80). Also, fluent verbal output with poorer auditory and visual comprehension. Echolalia (patient repeats a question instead of answering it) is prominent feature of this syndrome.	Associated with lesions of the left inferior parieto-temporo-occipital area, however localization remains controversial (81). Also, disruptions of white matter tracts connecting parietal lobe to temporal lobe or in portions of the inferior parietal lobe (80).
Conduction	Disturbance of repetition and spontaneous phonemic paraphasias (80). No significant difficulty in comprehension of normal conversation.	Lesion in the arcuate fasciculus and/or cortico-cortical connections between temporal and frontal lobes (80). Also, damage to the insula, contiguous auditory cortex, and underlying white matter of the left hemisphere (81).
Dynamic aphasia	Cardinal features of reduction in spontaneous speech with lack of initiation, limitations in the amount and range of narrative expression, and loss of verbal fluency. Articulation and speech motor programming remain intact, however language is impoverished with decreases in propositions and length and complexity of response. Singly described as a disturbance of complex, open-ended sentence assembly (82–84).	Frontal deafferentation secondary to interruption of frontostriatal feedback loops (40).Lesions in dorsolateral (BA 8, 9, 10, 46), with particular emphasis on posterior portion of the second frontal convolution.
Apraxias: Orofacial or Buccofacial Apraxia	Disturbances in purposeful, learned movement of the oral/respiratory structures despite intact strength of the peripheral speech musculature (1,86).	Frontal and central (rolandic) opercula, adjacent portions of the first temporal convolution, and the anterior portion of the insula (85).
Apraxia of Speech	An articulatory disorder marked by difficulty in programming the positioning of the speech muscles and sequencing the muscle movements for volitional production of phonemes (1).	Brodmann area 44 or third frontal convolution (Broca's area), premotor and supplementary motor areas of the frontal lobe of dominant hemisphere. Also the parietal lobe somatosensory cortex and supramarginal gyrus play a role in motor speech planning and programming. The insula has also been implicated (1).
Dysarthrias: Flaccid	Weakness and hypotonia are the underlying neuromuscular deficits that explain most of the speech characteristics (1). Most deviant features (listed in order from most to least severe) include hypernasality[a], imprecise consonants, breathiness[a], monopitch, nasal emission[a], audible inspiration[a], harsh voice quality, short phrases[a], and monoloudness (87).	Damage to lower motor neurons or motor units of cranial or spinal nerves that innervate speech muscles (1).
Spastic	Salient effects of upper motor neuron lesions on speech movements include spasticity, weakness, reduced range of movement, and slowness of movement (1). Most deviant features encountered (in order from	Damage to the direct (pyramidal) and indirect (extra-pyramidal and cerebellar) activation pathways (upper motor neurons) bilaterally (1).

Appendix A (*continued*)

Type of Speech or Language Disturbance	Classical Neuroanatomical Correlates	Clinical Features
		least to most severe) are imprecise consonants[a], monopitch, reduced prosodic stress, harshness[a], monoloudness, low pitch[a], slow rate[a], hypernasality, strained-strangled quality, short phrases[a], distorted vowels, pitch breaks[a], breathy voice, excess and equal prosodic stress (87).
Hyperkinetic	Usually associated with dysfunction of the basal ganglia control circuit, but may also be related to involvement of the cerebellar control circuit or other portions of the extrapyramidal system (1).	Characteristics can be manifest in the respiratory, phonatory, resonatory, and articulatory levels of speech, and prosody is often prominently affected. Deviant speech characteristics reflect the effects on speech of abnormal rhythmic or irregular and unpredictable, rapid or slow involuntary movements (1). Most deviant features encountered (listed in order from most to least severe) are imprecise consonants, prolonged intervals[a], variable rate[a], monopitch, harsh voice quality, inappropriate silences[a], distorted vowels, excess loudness variations[a], prolonged phonemes[a], monoloudness, short phrases, irregular articulatory breakdowns, excess and equal stress, hypernasality, reduced stress, strained-strangled quality, sudden forced inspiration or expiration[a], voice stoppages[a], transient breathiness[a] (87).
Hypokinetic	Damage to basal ganglia control circuit (1).	Characteristics are most evidence in voice, articulation, and prosody. The effects of rigidity, reduced force and range of movement, and slow individual and sometimes fast repetitive movements seem to account for many of its deviant speech characteristics (1). Most deviant features encountered (listed in order from most to least severe) are monopitch[a], reduced stress[a], monoloudness[a], imprecise consonants, inappropriate silences[a], short rushes of speech[a], harsh voice quality, breathy voice, low pitch, variable rate[a], increased rate in segments[a], increase of rate overall[a], repeated phonemes[a] (87).
Ataxic	Damage to the cerebellar control circuit, most frequently to the lateral hemispheres or vermis (1).	Deficits are most evident in articulation and prosody. Incoordination and reduced muscle tone appear responsible for the slowness of movement and inaccuracy in the force, range, timing, and direction of speech movements (1). Most deviant features encountered (listed from most to least severe) are imprecise consonants, excess and equal stress[a], irregular articulatory breakdowns[a], distorted vowels[a], harsh voice quality, prolonged phonemes[a], prolonged intervals, monopitch, monoloudness, slow rate, excess loudness variations[a], and voice tremor (87).

[a]Tend to be distinctive features or more severely impaired than in any other single dysarthria (1).

[b]Classifiable in only about half of the cases of aphasia seen routinely in a clinical practice (88). Advances in neuroimaging technologies reduce the utility of clinical assessment for lesion localization.

Appendix B
Case Descriptions and Text Stimuli Used to Elicit Audio-Recorded Speech and Language Samples

Case no.	Age	Gender	Medical Diagnosis	Speech or Language Disturbances	Notes
Speech Disturbances					
1	65	F	Indeterminate corticobulbar dysfunction	Spastic dysarthria	2-yr history of progressive speech and swallowing difficulty
2	57	M	Olivopontocerebellar atrophy	Ataxic dysarthria	1.5-yr history of progressive incoordination and speech difficulty
3	73	M	Multiple System Atrophy	hypokinetic dysarthria	10-yr history of nonspeech signs and symptoms of MSA. 2-yr history of progressive speech difficulty.
4	75	M	Corticobasal Degeneration	Apraxia of speech; mixed hypolinetic-spastic and possible ataxic aysarthria	2.5-yr history of progressive speech disturbance; evidence of only equivocal aphasia.
5	70	M	Progressive Supranuclear Palsy	Hypokinetic dysarthria	Prominent characteristic of excessive rate of speech.
Language Disturbances					
6	63	F	Corticobasal Degeneration	Broca's aphasia and co-occurring apraxia of speech	Characteristics of language deficit include agrammatism and repetition deficit.
7	38	F	Primary Progressive Aphasia; possible CBD	Anomic aphasia	Characteristics of language deficit include fluent verbal output with vacuous content, impaired confrontation naming of objects, and impaired auditory comprehension.
8	72	F	Corticobasal Degeneration	Nonfluent aphasia close in features to transcortical motor aphasia, with co-occurring mixed dysarthria	Characteristics of language deficit include nonfluent verbal output, dysnomia, impaired auditory comprehension for sequential commands, and perserveration, with relatively spared repetition.
9	58	F	Corticobasal Degeneration	Tangential discourse with impaired topic maintenance, with co-occurring features of fluent aphasia	Characteristics of languate deficits include semantic paraphasia and perserveration.
10	68	F	Corticobasal Degeneration	Dynamic aphasia	Characteristics of language include reduced initiation, low propositionality, reduced verbal fluency, and yes/no reversals.

Picture description used for Case no. 4 was the Cookie Theft Scene from the *Boston Diagnostic Aphasia Examination*; all other picture descriptions were elicited from the Picnic Scene from the *Western Aphasia Battery*. (Case numbers are linked to .wav files on accompanying DVD.)

TEST STIMULI FOR AUDIOTAPED SAMPLES

Grandfather Passage

You wish to know all about your grandfather. Well, he is nearly 93 years old, yet he still thinks as swiftly as ever. He dresses himself in an old black frock coat, usually several buttons missing. A long beard clings to his chin, giving those who observe him a pronounced feeling of the utmost respect. Twice each day he plays skillfully and with zest upon a small organ. Except in the winter when the snow or ice prevents, he slowly takes a short walk in the open air each day. We have often urged him to walk more and smoke less, but he always answers, Banana Oil! Grandfather likes to be modern in his language.

Test Stimuli used for Picture descriptions:

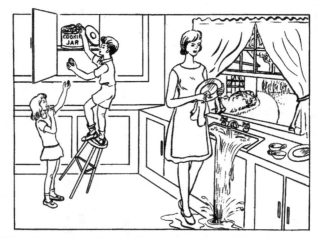

Source: Cookie Theft Picture from Boston Diagnostic Aphasia Exam in *The Assessment of Aphasia and related Disorders* (second edition) by Goodglass, H & Kaplan, E., 1983, Philadelphia: Lea & Febiger. Reproduced with permission.

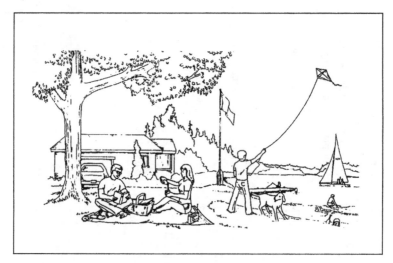

Source: Picnic scene picture from *Western Aphasia Battery* by Kertesz, A., 1982, by The Psychological Corporation, a Harcourt Assessment Company. Reproduced with permission. All rights reserved.

17

Quality of Life Assessment in Atypical Parkinsonian Disorders

Anette Schrag and Caroline E. Selai

INTRODUCTION

The atypical parkinsonian disorders are chronic progressive conditions, which not only shorten life expectancy but affect many aspects of patients' and their carers' lives. No curative treatment for these disorders is available, and management of these patients largely has to concentrate on amelioration of symptoms, such as falls, immobility, autonomic features or dysphagia, activities of daily living and (in)dependence, and patients' social and emotional well-being; in short, the improvement of patients' quality of life. Assessment of patients with atypical parkinsonism has concentrated on objective measures such as mortality and clinical evaluation of impairment and physical functioning, supplemented by laboratory test results. However, a large literature shows that patients' own assessments of their health, their preferences, and their views regarding health often differ significantly from physicians' objective assessments (1). Where possible, treatment decisions should focus on health outcomes of value to the individual patient.

Scales to measure Hr-QoL, fully psychometrically tested and validated, are now used in a number of clinical and research contexts. Some types of Hr-QoL scale yield information that, combined with economic data, can be used to assess the cost benefit of health interventions and to inform decisions about the allocation of scarce health care resources. There are currently no validated measures to assess Hr-QoL in patients with atypical parkinsonian disorders.

This chapter starts with a general overview of some of the conceptual and methodological issues relating to the measurement of subjective health assessment and Hr-QoL. Section two gives an overview of Hr-QoL instruments that have been used in Parkinson's disease (PD) and the impact of PD on Hr-QoL. The third section addresses what is known about the Hr-QoL of patients with atypical parkinsonism, in particular multiple system atrophy (MSA) and progressive supranculear palsy (PSP). The chapter concludes with some comments about future research in this area.

HEALTH-RELATED QUALITY OF LIFE: CONCEPTUAL AND METHODOLOGICAL ISSUES

What Is Quality of Life?

Although the definition of this somewhat elusive term is still occasionally discussed in the literature, there is general consensus on some fundamental points. First, although the phrases "quality of

From: *Current Clinical Neurology: Atypical Parkinsonian Disorders*
Edited by: I. Litvan © Humana Press Inc., Totowa, NJ

life," "health-related quality of life," and health status are used somewhat interchangeably, there is broad agreement that, in the medical context, Hr-QoL should be regarded as a multidimensional construct *(2)*, comprising physical, psychological, and social well-being. Within these three broad dimensions, most Hr-QoL scales have items on physical health and functioning, activities of daily living, mental health (e.g., perceived stigma, anxiety, depression), social activities, family relationships, and cognitive functioning. Because of these multiple factors, it has been argued that although it may be helpful to derive a summary index of Hr-QoL, the different aspects of Hr-QoL as measured by the scale domains should also be presented separately in order to better understand the precise impact of interventions *(3)*.

Second, since quality of life is highly subjective, any appraisal of Hr-QoL should rely, where possible, on the perception of the individual patient. Many groups of patients cannot, however, assess their own Hr-QoL, e.g., those with severe dementia, and there is a growing literature on the use of proxy ratings.

Third, no quality of life instrument can comprehensively cover all aspects of Hr-QoL. Although some scales attempt to comprehensively assess all aspects of Hr-QoL, such instruments are often lengthy and burdensome and so are not feasible in clinical practice, particularly where patients have disabling conditions. Therefore, most measures focus on a limited number of specific aspects of Hr-QoL. The choice of instrument will be determined by the precise aim of the study.

Finally, in order to provide meaningful data for research and clinical practice, Hr-QoL measures need to be carefully developed and validated and there is now a large literature on the validation and psychometric properties that need to be demonstrated before the scientific community will accept that an instrument has been shown to be appropriately validated. Before considering psychometric testing in more detail, it is useful to consider next why Hr-QoL might be measured.

Why Assess Health-Related Quality of Life?

Though Hr-QoL measures have been developed for a number of reasons, two basic aspects of health care underlie most of the questions that Hr-QoL appraisals set out to answer: outcome of treatment and cost. As discussed above, Hr-QoL has emerged as an important outcome that incorporates patients' views of their health. Also, since no country in the world can *afford* to do all that it is technically possible to do to improve the health of its citizens, the need has arisen for some system of setting priorities. The assessment of the Hr-QoL of patients with atypical parkinsonian disorders will become increasingly important if and when new drug treatments and other therapies for these disorders are developed. Trials will need to address the benefit of therapeutic interventions and measure change of symptoms in relation to Hr-QoL.

HEALTH-RELATED QUALITY OF LIFE MEASURES: DEVELOPMENT AND VALIDATION

All clinical assessment measures need to be shown to be valid and reliable. In addition, self-completed measures for patients with a disabling disease need to be short and feasible. Instrument developers must test the psychometric properties of a new instrument, which is a labor-intensive exercise, involving a series of studies to obtain data on the performance of the measure in different situations. For a comprehensive review of the statistical procedures, see Streiner and Norman *(4)*. In brief, *validity* is how well the instrument measures what it purports to measure. There are various statistical procedures for testing different aspects of an instrument's validity. The terminology is somewhat confusing but Streiner and Norman provide a useful guide to the various types (e.g., *face* validity, *construct* validity, *criterion* validity, *concurrent* validity, and *predictive* validity). *Reliability* assesses whether the same measurement can be obtained on other occasions and concerns the amount of error inherent in any measurement. Two basic tests are the *internal consistency* of a test, measured by coefficient alpha, and *test–retest* reliability where scores taken on two occasions are compared. *Sensi-*

tivity or *responsiveness to change* is concerned with how sensitive the measure is to detecting clinically relevant changes in Hr-QoL. This is important for monitoring benefits of treatment. Newer methods that allow further improvement of scales include Rasch analysis and Item Response Theory, a discussion of which is beyond the scope of this chapter.

This psychometric testing has not uniformly been conducted with all instruments, particularly older instruments.

Types of Hr-QoL Measures

There is no "gold standard" for measuring Hr-QoL and there is a wide range of instruments available, or in development. The categories of Hr-QoL measures have been comprehensively reviewed elsewhere *(5)*. In brief, *generic* instruments cover a broad range of Hr-QoL domains in a single instrument. Their chief advantage is in facilitating comparisons among different disease groups. *Disease-specific* instruments reduce patient burden by including only relevant items for a particular illness but their main disadvantage is the lack of comparability of results with those from other disease groups. *Health profiles* provide separate scores for each of the dimensions of Hr-QoL, whereas a *health index*, a type of generic instrument, gives a single summary score, usually from 0 (death) to 1 (perfect health). A further category, developed within the economic tradition, is that of *utility* measures, which are based on preferences for health states. Preference weighted measures are required when the focus is on *society* as a whole and the societal allocation of scarce resources. The choice of measure will depend upon the goal of the study.

Preference-Based Outcome Measures

Preference-based outcome measures are a particular type of measure used in economic analyses, such as cost-utility analyses. Cost-utility analysis is a technique that uses the quality adjusted life year (QALY) as an outcome measure. For its calculation, the QALY requires well-being or Hr-QoL to be expressed as a single index score. The three most commonly used preference measurement techniques are visual analog scales, time trade-off, and standard gamble. A review of the literature on the use of Hr-QoL life data in economic studies is beyond the scope of this chapter, but interested readers can consult a series of chapters on this topic in ref. *6*. As treatments for atypical parkinsonisan disorders become available, they will undoubtedly be subject to economic appraisal and robust, prospectively collected Hr-QOL data will be important for the calculation of QALYs and for other economic analyses.

Which Outcome Measure to Use?

The choice of instrument depends on the purpose of the study. A common recommendation is to include both disease-specific and generic measures in an investigation. The generic measure facilitates comparisons of the target group with the normal population and/or other patient groups whereas the disease-specific instrument provides more sensitivity and is therefore usually more responsive to change in health status. If pharmaco-economic evaluation or a comparison of two or more treatment options is the aim of the study, incorporation of an additional utility measure is recommended. In atypical parkinsonism no disease-specific instruments are available to date but disease-specific instruments for MSA and PSP are currently being developed.

HEALTH-RELATED QUALITY OF LIFE IN PARKINSON'S DISEASE

Health-Related Quality of Life Instruments Used in Parkinson's Disease

A number of studies have assessed Hr-QoL in idiopathic PD. The authors of the first of these studies used generic instruments including the Sickness Impact Profile (SIP) *(7)*, the Nottingham Health Profile (NHP) *(8)*, the Medical Outcomes Short Form (SF 36) *(9)*, and EQ-5D *(10)*. These measures were shown to be valid to varying degrees. However, the older instruments, such as the SIP and the NHP have been criticized for their content and their psychometric properties. For example, the NHP is skewed toward the severe end of disability and worse functional status and is therefore less likely to capture subtle changes in early stages of disease. The questions in the SIP have been felt to be offensive to patients by some *(11)*, and the SF 36 may have limited feasibility and validity in patients with parkinsonism *(12)*. However, the SF 36, a widely used Hr-QoL instrument, which has been translated in several languages and been validated for use in many cultures, enables comparisons across cultures and disease groups. The EQ-5D has also been shown to be valid in patients with PD *(12)*, and its brevity of five questions and a visual analog scale is an advantage in disabled patients. In addition, its summary index yields a utility score that can be used in pharmaco-economic analyses. The EQ-5D has also been translation into many languages.

More recently, PD-specific Hr-QoL measures have been developed. Table 1 briefly describes the PD-specific Hr-QoL measures, showing the scale domains. All of the PD-specific instruments have been shown to have good psychometric properties, but only the Parkinson's Disease Questionnaire (PDQ 39; ref. *13*) and the Parkinson's Disease Quality of Life Questionnaire (PDQL; ref. *14*) have been validated by researchers independent of the developers *(15)*. The PDQ 39 is the most widely used Hr-QoL instrument in Parkinson's disease. It has been translated in several languages, and has been shown to be valid, reliable and sensitive to change. An abbreviated format, the PDQ 8, which has been shown to have comparable validity *(16)*, is also available. Although PDQ 39 has been validated in some cultures, including Britain, the United States, Spain, France, China, and Japan, its validity in other cultures needs to be established. The PDQL is similar to the PDQ 39 in content and format, but includes some questions that are missing in the PDQ 39, e.g., on sexuality. It has been validated in The Netherlands and Britain, but it has not been translated into other languages and no validation studies in other cultures are currently available. Its psychometric properties are less well tested than those of the PDQ 39 and some issues such as self-care, role functions, and close relationships are not addressed *(15)*. The Parkinson's Impact Scale (PIMS) was developed to identify the major problems in patients' lives in a clinical setting. It is based on consensus rather than testing in a patient sample and its content validity has been criticized *(15)*. However, it is the only instrument that distinguishes between on and off periods and has been reported to be valid, reliable, and sensitive to change *(17)*. The Parkinson's Disease Quality of Life Scale (PDQUALIF) includes questions on fatigue and driving ability, concentrates on the nonmotor symptoms of Parkinson's disease, and has more emphasis on social functioning than other scales *(18)*. The Parkinson's Disease Symptom Inventory (PDSI; ref. *19*) has a larger number of questions (51 items) and asks patients to indicate the frequency as well as the distress caused by each item. There is also a German questionnaire, the ParkinsonLebensqualität (PQL), which has been psychometrically tested in a German population *(20)*. The differences between some of these scales are discussed in an excellent review by Marinus et al. *(15)*.

Finally, a number of measures that assess only the psychosocial aspects of Hr-QoL, excluding items relating to physical impairment, have recently been developed and validated *(21,22)*. The choice of instrument in each setting will be guided by the differences between the content of the questionnaires, published data on the psychometric testing, and, if relevant to the study, the availability of translations and cultural adaptation. For specific interventions different aspects of Hr-QoL will be important and as no instrument can be both completely comprehensive and feasible, the selection of the instrument will be based on the particular aim of the study. As discussed above, whereas generic instruments can be used in patients with Parkinson's disease, PD-specific instruments are likely to be more valid, sensitive, and responsive to change.

Table 1
Disease-Specific Hr-QoL Measures Developed for Parkinson's Disease

PD-Specific Measure	Number of Items	Domains of Hr-QoL Covered by Scale	Reference
Parkinson' Disease Questionnaire 39-item version (PDQ-39)	39	mobility, activities of daily living, emotional well-being, stigma, social support, cognition, communications, bodily discomfort	Peto et al. 1995 (13)
Parkinson' Disease Questionnaire 8-item version (PDQ-8)	8	mobility, activities of daily living, emotional well-being, stigma, social support, cognition, communications, bodily discomfort™	Peto et al. 1998 (16)
Parkinson' Disease Quality of Life Questionnaire (PDQL)	37	Parkinsonian symptoms, systemic symptoms, emotional functioning, social functioning	De Boer et al. 1996 (14)
Parkinson's Impact Scale (PIMS)	10	Work, finance, leisure, safety, travel, self, feel, family, friend, sexuality; differentiates between on- and off-states	Schulzer et al. 2002 (17)
Parkinson's Disease Quality of Life Scale (PDQUALIF)	33	Social/role function, self-image/sexuality, sleep, outlook, physical function, independence, urinary function, global HrQoL	Welsh et al. 2003 (18)
Parkinson's Disease Symptom Inventory (PDSI)	51	Frequency and distress of symptoms; further analysis on scoring ongoing	Hogan et al. 1999 (19)
Fragebogen Parkinson LebensQualität (PLQ)	44	Depression, physical achievement, leisure, concentration, social integration, insecurity, restlessness, activity limitation, anxiety	Van den Berg, 1998 (20)

THE IMPACT OF PARKINSONISM ON HEALTH-RELATED QUALITY OF LIFE

Parkinson's Disease

The only parkinsonian disorder that has been assessed in detail with regard to Hr-Qol is PD. Studies on Hr-QoL of patients with PD have improved our understanding of subjectively experienced difficulties associated with this disease, and we now have a clearer understanding of what aspects of Hr-QoL are most important to patients with PD. A full review of the expanding Hr-QoL literature in PD is beyond the scope of this chapter. However, it has consistently been found that all areas of Hr-QoL are affected by PD, not merely the physical impairment or functioning *(23,25,26)*. The main areas of impairment in PD are in physical functioning, emotional reactions, social isolation, and energy. Other domains of impairment of Hr-QoL in PD, include bodily discomfort/pain, self-image, cognitive function, communication, sleep, role function, and sexual function *(23,25–27)*. It has also become clear that in PD, it is not primarily disease severity and presence of the symptoms of PD that determine Hr-QoL, but the disability associated with these symptoms and, more than any other factor, the presence and severity of depression *(24,25,28)*. Further symptoms, which have also been found to be highly relevant to Hr-QoL of patients with PD, are postural instability and falls, impaired cognition, and insomnia. Other factors, including motor complications of treatment, may also be associated with poorer Hr-QoL in subgroups of patients, but this association is no longer significant once other important factors such as depression and disability due to parkinsonism are accounted for.

Potentially Important Quality-of-Life Issues in Atypical Parkinsonian Disorders

A wide range of symptoms are likely to be associated with impaired Hr-QoL in atypical parkinsonian disorders, including the cardinal features of parkinsonism, nonmotor symptoms such as sexual and autonomic dysfunction, postural instability and falls, cognitive impairment, and visual disturbances.

Some analogies can usefully be drawn from Hr-QoL studies in PD. The degree of disability in atypical parkinsonism is at least as great as in PD and depression occurs in all atypical parkinsonian disorders *(29,30)*. It is therefore likely that these factors are also important in atypical parkinsonian disorders. However, these are likely not to be the only difficulties encountered by patients with atypical parkinsonism in whom, frequently, many systems are affected. The impact of features such as greater autonomic dysfunction, higher rate of falls, behavioral changes, or cognitive impairment, will depend on the type of atypical parkinsonism. In addition, the shortened life expectancy, greater disability, lack of response to treatment, associated nonmotor features, cognitive impairment, and behavioral disturbances in atypical parkinsonian disorders will all impact on patients' subjective evaluation of their Hr-QoL. On the other hand, symptoms that occur less frequently in atypical parkinsonism than in PD, such as tremor, hallucinations, dyskinesias, and motor fluctuations, are likely to be of lesser importance to the Hr-QoL in patients with atypical parkinsonian disorders.

All of these symptoms may lead to increased dependence on others, a diminished sense of autonomy and self-image *(31)*, impairment of role functioning, emotional disturbances, fear of social stigma associated with physical symptoms, and impairment of social functioning. Table 2 gives examples of features of atypical parkinsonism, domains of Hr-QoL, which can be affected, and demographic and psycho-social variables, which may influence Hr-QoL in patients with atypical parkinsonism.

Multiple System Atrophy (MSA) and Progressive Supranuclear Palsy (PSP)

We have recently undertaken in-depth interviews with patients with MSA and PSP and their carers, and conducted a large survey on issues relevant to patients with atypical parkinsonian disorders, with the aim of developing disease-specific Hr-QoL questionnaires for patients with MSA and PSP. There was considerable overlap in reported areas of health-related quality of life issues relevant to patients with PSP and MSA, but also some differences.

Table 2
Examples of Factors Relevant to Hr-Qol in Atypical Parkinsonian Disorders

Domains of HR-QoL That May Be Affected	Features of Atypical Parkinsonian Disorders	Demographic Variables	Psychosocial Variables
Physical function, e.g., mobility, bodily discomfort, bladder problems	Motor symptoms	Age	Personal, e.g., coping strategies, personal attitudes, expectation of optimism
Activites of daily living, e.g., self-care, communication, difficulties eating, reading difficulties	Speech impairment	Gender	Social and environmental, e.g., social support, health care resource circumstances, e.g., family or in nursing home
Psychological, e.g., stigma, self-image, depression, isolation, fear of future	Autonomic dysfunction	Socioeconomic class	
Social, e.g., family life, social interaction, dependence on others	Visual impairment	Area of residence	
Role functioning, e.g., emotional, physical	Sexual dysfunction		
	Insomnia		
	Cognitive impairment, including bradyphrenia, executive dysfunction, retrieval difficulties, apraxia, neglect		
	Affect, e.g., depression, anxiety		
	Behavioral disturbances, e.g., apathy, disinhibition		

The main presentations of MSA, which include autonomic dysfunction and cerebellar symptoms in addition to parkinsonism, were reflected in our preliminary Hr-QoL interviews. Patients with MSA reported difficulties with bladder and autonomic dysfunction among their most common and severe problems, which were not reported as commonly by patients with PSP, or those with PD *(32)*. Lack of coordination, which was also more commonly reported in MSA patients than in PSP patients, is likely to reflect not only parkinsonism but also cerebellar dysfunction, which also results in "difficulty walking" and "balance problems." The reported items "transferring from lying down to sitting" or "difficulty standing up without support" may reflect orthostatic hypotension in addition to bradykinesia. Other issues more often rated as important by patients with MSA such as "worrying about the family," "worrying about the future," or "change of role within the family" may reflect the younger age group affected by MSA. Although these issues can also be important to patients with PSP, other items were rated as more important by patients with PSP.

Problems commonly reported in PSP but rare in Parkinson's disease or MSA include early postural impairment and falls, visual impairment owing to supranuclear gaze palsy, eyelid apraxia or photophobia, clinically relevant cognitive impairment, personality change, swallowing difficulties, and speech disturbances *(33)*. In addition, patients with PSP may develop neuropsychiatric complications, including apathy, inhibition, and depression *(29,30)*. From the patients' point of view, these issues are also particular problems, although apathy and personality change were less problematic from the patients than from the carers' point of view *(34)*.

In patients with MSA as well as PSP, difficulties beyond those of physical and mental symptoms of the disease were rated as important. Patients in both groups not only reported difficulties in daily activities but patients with MSA reported being anxious and worried about the future, had experienced loss of self-esteem and confidence, felt ignored or that nobody could understand their difficulties. Patients with PSP reported difficulties in showing their emotions, frustration and isolation, difficulties in communication, and worrying about others' reactions. Without doubt, the impact on the emotional and social aspects of Hr-QoL goes beyond that of physical impairment and disability in both disorders.

Other Parkinsonian Disorders

For other atypical parkinsonism such as corticobasal degeneration there are currently no data available on Hr-QoL. However, it is likely that, as in the other atypical parkinsonian disorders, there is considerable overlap of Hr-QoL issues, but that some features specific to this syndrome are also particularly relevant to their Hr-QoL, e.g., loss of hand function owing to alien limb, and impairment of activities of daily living because of apraxia. Other features important to PSP or MSA, such as bladder dysfunction or visual disturbances, are likely to have less impact in this patient group.

CARER BURDEN

It is not only the lives of patients that are severely affected by the chronic progressive disease course, by decreased life expectancy, and by the multiple consequences of atypical parkinsonian disorders; the lives of each family member and, particularly their carers, are also affected. It is likely that atypical parkinsonian disorders affect carers' physical functioning (e.g., caring affecting the carer's own health), emotional well-being (e.g., response to change in role, feelings of hopelessness and depression), and social functioning (limitations on social life), but no studies to date have assessed the different aspects of caregiver burden in these disorders. However, one study investigated the correlates and determinants of carer burden in PSP *(35)*. In this study, the impact of PSP on carers increased with advancing disease severity and disability. Interestingly, this was most pronounced in the first 18 mo after diagnosis, but carer burden plateaued after this initial increase. The presence of affective and behavioral problems such as depression and aggression was associated with greater carer burden, and women reported greater carer burden then men, even when disease severity and behavioral disturbances were accounted for. The overall degree of carer burden appeared similar to that reported in carers of patients with Alzheimer's disease.

CONCLUSION

The assessment of Hr-QoL in patients with atypical parkinsonian disorders is important for clinical research, surveys, and clinical trials. Since there is no cure, the management and current treatment of these chronic, disabling disorders is aimed at improving patients' subjective Hr-QoL. The impact of these disorders on an individual is complex, comprising multiple aspects of physical, cognitive, emotional, and social functioning. The patient's rating of their own Hr-QoL may vary considerably from their physician's assessment. The valid and reliable assessment of patient-rated health status and Hr-QoL will become even more relevant as treatments for these disorders become available and the benefits of treatment need to be rigorously assessed. Generic Hr-QoL instruments can be used, but their validity and feasibility in patients with atypical parkinsonism is not known. PD-specific Hr-QoL instruments, although incorporating a number of features of relevance to atypical parkinsonism, have not been validated in any of the atypical parkinsonian disorders and are likely to lack some of the salient features. The particular manifestations of each of the atypical parkinsonian disorders, e.g., the specific cognitive impairments in PSP or the autonomic features in MSA together with the features of parkinsonism, are not adequately reflected in any of these instruments. Hr-QoL instruments specifically for patients with MSA and PSP and for their carers are currently being developed.

FUTURE RESEARCH

Little information is available on the impact of atypical parkinsonism on specific domains of Hr-QoL. Our starting point must be to ask the patients what factors are most important to their Hr-QoL. It is anticipated that, analogous to the clinical presentations, some aspects of Hr-QoL, such as mobility, will be common to all of these disorders, whereas specific aspects will be associated with particular disorders, e.g., bladder function in patients with MSA. Identifying the most important aspect of Hr-QoL in these disorders, from the patient's perspective, will assist in the management of these patients and will inform debate about the provision of health care resources. Finally, but perhaps most importantly, if and when symptomatic treatments for these disorders become available, their efficacy and relevance can be assessed by arguably the most important outcome measure: the effect on patients' Hr-QoL as rated by the patients themselves.

MAJOR QUESTIONS FOR FUTURE RESEARCH

- What aspects of Hr-QOL are important in atypical parkinsonian disorders, as judged by the patients themselves?
- Which instruments are most useful to assess Hr-QoL in atypical parkinsonian disorders?
- Which areas of Hr-QoL are most affected in each of the atypical parkinsonian disorders and what are the implications for the allocation of health care resources?
- Which demographic, clinical, and environmental factors have the greatest influence on patients's subjective Hr-QoL?
- What is the effect of potential symptomatic treatments for atypical parkinsonian disorders on patients' Hr-QoL as rated by the patients themselves?

REFERENCES

1. Slevin ML, Plant H, Lynch D, Drinkwater J, Gregory WM. Who should measure quality of life, the doctor or the patient? Br J Cancer 1988;57:109–112.
2. Spilker B, Revicki DA. Taxonomy of quality of life. In: Spilker B, ed. Quality of Life and Pharmacoeconomics in Clinical Trials, 2nd ed. Philadelphia: Lippincott-Raven, 1996:25–31.
3. McDowell I, Newell C. Measuring Health: A Guide to Rating Scales and Questionnaires. New York: Oxford University Press, 1987.
4. Streiner,DL, Norman GR. Health Measurement Scales: A Practical Guide to Their Development and Use, 2nd ed. Oxford: Oxford Medical Publications, 1995.

5. Brooks RG. Health Status Measurement: A Perspective on Change. Philadelphia: Macmillan, 1995.

6. Spilker B, ed. Quality of Life and Pharmacoeconomics in Clinical Trials, 2nd ed. Philadelphia: Lippincott-Raven, 1996.

7. Bergner M, Bobbitt RA, Carter WB, et al. The Sickness Impact Profile: development and final revision of a health status measure. Med Care 1981;19:787–805.

8. Hunt SM, McEwen J, McKenna SP. Measuring health stats: a new tool for clinicians and epidemiologists. J Royal Coll Gen Pract 1985;35:185–188.

9. Ware JE, Sherbourne CD. The MOS 36-item short form health survey (SF 36). I. Conceptual framework and item selection. Med Care 1992;30:473–483.

10. EuroQoL Group. EuroQoL: a new facility for the measurement of health-related quality of life. Health Policy 1990;16:199–208.

11. Mitchell JD, O'Brien MR. Quality of life in motor neurone disease—towards a more practical assessment tool? J Neurol Neurosurg Psychiatry. 2003;74:287–288.

12. Schrag A, Selai C, Jahanshahi M, Quinn NP. The EQ-5D—a generic quality of life measure—is a useful instrument to measure quality of life in patients with Parkinson's disease. J Neurol Neurosurg Psychiatry 2000;69:67–73

13. Peto V, Jenkinson C, Fitzpatrick R, Greenhall R. The development and validation of a short measure of functioning and well being for individuals with Parkinson's disease. Qual Life Res 1995;4:241–248.

14. de Boer AG, Wijker W, Speelman JD, de Haes JC . Quality of life in patients with Parkinson's disease: development of a questionnaire. J Neurol Neurosurg Psychiatry 1996;61:70–74.

15. Marinus J, Ramaker C, van Hilten JJ, Stiggelbout AM. Health related quality of life in Parkinson's disease: a systematic review of disease specific instruments. J Neurol Neurosurg Psychiatry 2002;72:241–248.

16. Peto V, Jenkinson C, Fitzpatrick R. PDQ-39: a review of the development, validation and application of a Parkinson's disease quality of life questionnaire and its associated measures. J Neurol 1998;245(Suppl 1):S10–S14.

17. Schulzer M, Mak E, Calne SM. The psychometric properties of the Parkinson's Impact Scale (PIMS) as a measure of quality of life in Parkinson's disease. Parkinsonism Relat Disord 2003;9:291–294.

18. Welsh M, McDermott MP, Holloway RG, Plumb S, Pfeiffer R, Hubble J, The Parkinson Study Group development and testing of the Parkinson's Disease Quality of Life Scale. Mov Disord 2003;18:637–645.

19. Hogan T, Grimaldi R, Dingemanse J, Martin M, Lyons K, Koller W. The Parkinson's disease symptom inventory (PDSI): a comprehensive and sensitive instrument to measure disease symptoms and treatment side-effects. Parkinsonism Relat Disord 1999;5:93–98.

20. Van den Berg M. Leben mit Parkinson: Entwicklung und psychometrische Testung des Fragenbogens PLQ. Neurol Rehabil 1998;4:221–226.

21. Marinus J, Visser M, Martinez-Martin P, van Hilten JJ, Stiggelbout AM. Questionnaire for patients with Parkinson's disease: the SCOPA-PS. J Clin Epidemiol 2003;56:61–67.

22. Spliethoff-Kamminga NGA, Zwinderman AH, Springer MP, Roos RAC. Psychosocial problems in Parkinson's disease: evaluation of a disease-specific questionnaire. Mov Disord 2003;18: 503–509.

23. Schrag A, Jahanshahi M, Quinn N. How does Parkinson's disease affect quality of life? A comparison with quality of life in the general population. Mov Disord 2000;15:1112–1118.

24. Schrag A, Jahanshahi M, Quinn N.What contributes to quality of life in patients with Parkinson's disease? J Neurol Neurosurg Psychiatry 2000;69:308–312.

25. Karlsen KH, Larsen JP, Tandberg E, Maland JG. Quality of life measurements in patients with Parkinson's disease: a community-based study. Eur J Neurol 1998;5:443–450.

26. Kuopio AM, Marttila RJ, Helenius H, Toivonen M, Rinne UK. The quality of life in Parkinson's disease. Mov Disord 2000;15:216–223.

27. Damiano AM, McGrath MM, Willian MK, et al. Evaluation of a measurement strategy for Parkinson's disease: assessing patient health-related quality of life. Qual Life Res 2000;9:87–100.

28. Global Parkinson's Disease Survey Steering Committee. Factors impacting on quality of life in Parkinson's disease: results from an international survey. Mov Disord 2002;17:60–67.

29. Litvan I, Mega MS, Cummings JL, Fairbanks L. Neuropsychiatric aspects of progressive supranuclear palsy. Neurology 1996;47:1184–1189.

30. Aarsland D, Litvan I, Larsen JP. Neuropsychiatric symptoms of patients with progressive supranuclear palsy and Parkinson's disease. J Neuropsychiatry Clin Neurosci 2001;13:42–49.

31. Fitzsimmons B, Bunting LK. Parkinson's disease—quality of life issues. Nurs Clin North Am 1993;28:807–818

32. Fitzpatrick R, Peto V, Jenkinson C, Greenhall R, Hyman N. Health-related quality of life in Parkinson's disease: a study of outpatient clinic attenders. Mov Disord 1997;12:916–922.

33. Nath U, Ben-Shlomo Y, Thomson RG, Lees AJ, Burn DJ. Clinical features and natural history of progressive supranuclear palsy: a clinical cohort study. Neurology 2003;60:910–916.

34. Schrag A, Selai D, Davis J, Lees A, Jahanshahi M, Quinn N. Health-related quality of life in patients with progressive supranuclear palsy (PSP). Mov Disord 2003;18:1464–1469.

35. Uttl B, Santacruz P, Litvan I, Grafman J. Caregiving in progressive supranuclear palsy. Neurology 1998;51:1303–1309.

18

Progressive Supranuclear Palsy

Irene Litvan

INTRODUCTION

Progressive supranuclear palsy (PSP) is the most common atypical neurodegenerative parkinsonian disorder *(1,2)*. It was first described as a discrete clinicopathological entity by Steele et al. *(3)* in 1964 (Fig. 1), but there are several previous clinical descriptions of patients who may have had this disease (*see* Chapter 2). Clinically, PSP typically presents at middle-to-late age with progressive unexplained prominent postural instability with falls, supranuclear vertical gaze palsy, pseudobulbar palsy, levodopa-unresponsive parkinsonism, and frontal cognitive disturbances *(3–5)*. Neuropathologically, PSP is characterized by the presence of neurofibrillary tangles in neurons and glia in specific basal ganglia and brainstem areas *(6)* (Fig.2). Neurofibrillary tangles are abnormal aggregates of tau protein that are also the main pathologic feature in corticobasal degeneration (CBD), Pick's disease, frontotemporal dementia with parkinsonism associated to chromosome 17 abnormalities (FTDP-17), and Alzheimer's disease (AD). Hence, as all these disorders, PSP is considered a "tauopathy" (*see* also Chapter 4).

CLINICAL FEATURES AND DIFFERENTIAL DIAGNOSIS

The most important features that characterize and differentiate PSP from other disorders are presented in Table 1 and described in more detail in the subheading that follows.

Postural Instability and Falls

Postural instability manifested as nonexplained and unexpected falls or tendency to falls is the most frequent symptom presentation in PSP *(7–14)*. In the National Institutes of Neurological Disorders and Stroke (NINDS) study *(10)*, 96% of 24 PSP patients had gait disorder and postural instability (83% history of falls) at the first visit to a specialized neurology center, which generally occurred 3–3.5 yr after symptom onset. Falls usually occur backward in PSP, but they can occur in any direction *(7,10)* (described by a patient in the video-PSP). The presence of nonexplained and unexpected falls within the first year of symptom onset is in fact one of the required criteria for the diagnosis of PSP when using the NINDS–Society for PSP (SPSP) diagnostic criteria (Table 2). PSP is the most likely diagnosis when unexplained postural instability and falls occur within the first year of symptom onset, but after that, multiple system atrophy (MSA) is equally possible. When postural instability and falls are the only features of the disease and an abnormal response to the postural reflex may be the only abnormality in patient's examination, diagnostic problems are frequent.

From: *Current Clinical Neurology: Atypical Parkinsonian Disorders*
Edited by: I. Litvan © Humana Press Inc., Totowa, NJ

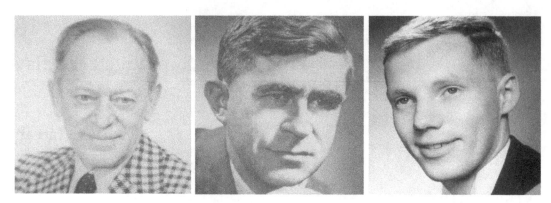

Fig. 1. (*Left*) Neurologist J. Clifford Richardson (1909–1986) realized that a set of patients evaluated since 1955 in Toronto had an unusual combination of symptoms that seemed to correspond to a disease he was unaware of. (*Middle*) pathologist Jerry Olszewski (1913–1964) described in detail the pathological findings of seven cases that came to autopsy. (*Right*) John C. Steele (1934) joined the neurology residency in 1961 and investigated with Dr. Richardson the clinical features and progression of these patients during the following 2 yr. From Progressive Supranuclear Palsy: Clinical and Research Approaches, edited by Irene Litvan and Yves Agid, copyright 1992 by Oxford University Press, Inc. Used by permission of Oxford University Press, Inc.

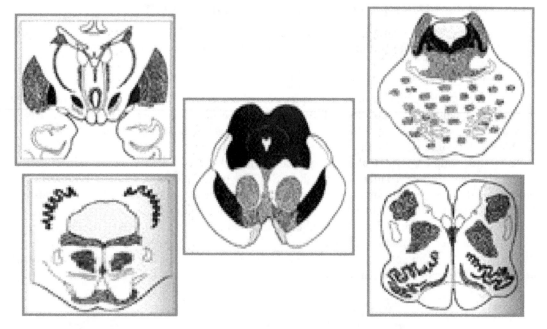

Fig. 2. Pattern of lesions found in the nine cases reported by Prof. Olszewski in 1963 and published in *Archives of Neurology* in 1964 *(3)*, with permission.

Table 1
Comparison of Features of Various Atypical Parkinsonian Neurodegenerative Disorders

Characteristics	PSP	MSA	CBD Lateralized Phenotype	CBD Dementia Phenotype	DLB
Progression	Rapid	Rapid	Rapid	Rapid	Rapid
Postural Instability/Falls	Initial	Early	Present (late unless limbs are initially affected)	Late usually	Early
Parkinsonism	Symmetric/Axial Distal	Asymmetric/Distal /Distal	Asymmetric	Bilateral	Asymmetric
Levodopa response	Initial? ⇒ Absent	1/3 of cases	Absent	Absent?	Variable
Cognitive disturbances (Severe)	Early/Frontal	Frontal Mild (Severe)	Lateralized[a]	Early/Frontal	Early/Frontal (Severe)/Cortical
Psychiatric disturbances	Apathy, disinhibition	Depression	Depression	Apathy	Hallucinations, Delusions
Myoclonus	Absent	Distal	Present	Present	Present
Dystonia (retrocollis)	Axial Limbs	Axial (antecollis)	Asymmetric	Bilateral?	Late
Contracture	Late	Late	Early	Late?	Late?
Saccades latency	Normal	Normal	Impaired vertical and horizontal	?	?
Saccades speed	Slow vertical ⇒ horizontal	Normal	Normal	?	?
Pyramidal signs	Late (Bilateral)	Present (Bilateral)	Unilateral (Bilateral	Bilateral	Late, bilateral
Cerebellar signs	Absent in limbs, but wide gait	Present	Absent	Absent	Absent
Dysautonomia	Absent	Initial, severe	Absent	Absent	Present
Gait	Ataxic (wide-step)	Ataxic small-step	Apraxic/ small-step	Small-step	Apraxic/

[a]Lateralized cognitive disturbances: sensory or visual neglect, ideomotor apraxia, aphasia, or alien limb syndrome. Cortical disturbances: memory, aphasia, apraxia, and agnosia. PSP, progressive supranuclear palsy; MSA, multiple system atrophy; CBD, corticobasal degeneration; DLB, dementia with Lewy bodies.

Diagnostic certainty only increases with the appearance of telltale signs. Instability and falls in MSA are usually present when patients already exhibit autonomic disturbances. Early instability or falls may also rarely develop early in patients with CBD when symptoms initially occur in lower extremities, but examination shows unilateral features *(15)*. Falls are not an early feature in Parkinson's disease (PD), but they may occur early in dementia with Lewy bodies (DLB) and usually associate to cognitive disturbances.

Table 2
Revised NINDS–SPSP Consensus Criteria for Clinical Diagnosis

Definite PSP: Clinically probable or possible PSP and histologically typical PSP

Clinically Definite PSP

Step 1 Mandatory Inclusion Criteria:
1. Gradually progressive disorder with onset at age 40 or later *and*
2. *Vertical supranuclear ophthalmoparesis* (either moderate to severe upward or any downward gaze abnormalities) *and*
3. *Prominent postural instability with falls (or tendency to falls) in the first year of symptom onset*

Clinically Probable PSP

Step 1 Mandatory Inclusion Criteria:
1. Gradually progressive disorder with onset at age 40 or later and *either:*
2a. *Vertical supranuclear ophthalmoparesis* (either moderate to severe upward- or any downward-gaze abnormalities) *or*
2b. Slowing of vertical saccades and prominent postural instability with *falls (or tendency to falls) in the first year* of symptom onset

For Both Clinically Definite and Clinically Probable PSP

Step 2 Mandatory Exclusion Criteria:
1. History compatible with encephalitis lethargica
2. Alien hand syndrome, cortical sensory deficits, focal frontal or temporoparietal atrophy
3. Hallucinations or delusions unrelated to dopaminergic therapy
4. Cortical dementia of Alzheimer's type (severe amnesia and aphasia or agnosia, NINCDS–ADRDA criteria)
5. Prominent cerebellar symptomatology or unexplained dysautonomia (early, prominent inconti nence, impotence, or symptomatic postural hypotension)
6. Severe asymmetry of parkinsonian signs (bradykinesia)
7. Neuroradiologic evidence of relevant structural abnormality (basal ganglia or brainstem infarcts, lobar atrophy)
8. Whipple's disease, confirmed by polymerase chain reaction, if indicated

Clinically Possible PSP

To be defined

Ocular Motor Abnormalities

Supranuclear vertical gaze palsy allows the diagnosis of PSP to be made and distinguishes it from all other related disorders such as CBD, MSA, PD, and DLB (*see* video-PSP and Chapter 15). However, vertical supranuclear gaze palsy is rarely (8%) present at symptom onset; it usually takes 3–4 yr for it to develop *(10)*. Vertical supranuclear gaze palsy, moderate or severe postural instability, and falls during the first year after onset of symptoms classified the NINDS sample with 9% error using logistic regression analysis *(16)*. Although supranuclear gaze palsy is key in diagnosing PSP, it may occasionally be present in patients with DLB, arteriosclerotic pseudoparkinsonism, MSA, Creutzfeldt–Jakob disease, Whipple's disease, or CBD.

Symptom progression is usually very helpful to differentiate these disorders. Whereas in PSP the vertical supranuclear gaze palsy precedes the development of the horizontal gaze palsy, in CBD the supranuclear gaze palsy, when present, usually affects both horizontal and vertical gaze and is usually preceded by ocular motor apraxia (*see* video-oculomotor apraxia Chapter 1). Both downward- and upward-gaze palsy can be observed in PSP, but the upward-gaze palsy needs to be differentiated from the limitation of upward gaze observed in elderly patients.

Slowing of vertical saccades (rapid eye movement between two stimuli not letting the eyeball movement be seen) usually precedes the development of the supranuclear vertical gaze palsy and allows an earlier diagnosis of the disease *(4)* *(see* video-slowing of saccades). In fact, marked slowing of vertical saccades should point toward the diagnosis of PSP. The saccades in CBD may have an increased latency but normal speed, and are similarly affected in the vertical and horizontal plane, whereas in MSA, the saccades have normal speed and latency. Similarly, note that the vertical saccades of elders with upward-gaze limitation are of normal speed.

Blink rate usually becomes profoundly sparse in PSP, although often diminished in PD and MSA. The combination of rare blinking, facial dystonia, and gaze abnormalities leads to the development of a particular "staring and nonblinking faces." Eyelid apraxia (a difficulty or slowness with opening or closing the eyelids accompanied by compensatory elevation of the eyebrows and frontalis overactivity giving a furrowed brow) or blepharospasm (a forceful contraction of orbicularis oculi squeezing the eyes shut and making the eyebrows descend) are also features observed in PSP *(14,17,18)*, but they hardly help in the diagnosis as they may be observed in other parkinsonian disorders (i.e., CBD).

Behavioral and Cognitive Frontal Features

Florid frontal lobe symptomatology (impaired abstract thought, decreased verbal fluency) including motor perseveration and frontal behavioral disturbances, primarily apathy, but also disinhibition, depression, and anxiety, usually manifests at early stages in PSP, whereas it is typically less evident or manifests later in the other parkinsonian disorders *(19–25)*. Apathy, but not depression, is frequently observed in patients with PSP and may be the initial symptom *(24)*. Almost all PSP patients examined neuropsychologically demonstrate an early and prominent executive dysfunction that includes difficulty with planning, problem solving, concept formation, and social cognition. Moreover, executive dysfunction may be the presenting symptom in some PSP patients and is a frequent feature throughout the disease.

In PD and MSA, in contrast to PSP, frontal lobe features are usually mild, and revealed only on detailed neuropsychological testing *(26)*. Because patients with PSP usually exhibit early frontal lobe cognitive and/or behavioral disturbances, they occasionally are confused with patients with Pick's disease or AD. However in PSP, "cortical" dementia is rare or only mild.

Extrapyramidal Signs

PSP patients usually exhibit axial more than limb muscle involvement *(10,27)* *(see* video-PSP). In the NINDS study, at the first visit to a specialized neurology center, 88% had bilateral bradykinesia; 63% a predominant akinetic-rigid disease course, and 63% axial rigidity *(10)*. An absent, poor, or waning response to levodopa is a characteristic feature defining the atypical parkinsonian disorders *(see* Chapter 1) and is a feature of PSP. For practical purposes, all PD patients have a good or excellent response to dopaminergic agents given in appropriate doses for an adequate period of time. If they do not respond, they almost certainly do not have PD. A few PSP patients show a moderate transient response from dopaminergic agents, but most do not. Indeed, this may be because many PSP patients have little or no limb parkinsonism to respond to. In addition, PSP patients uncommonly develop levodopa-induced involuntary movements and if they do, they usually develop dystonia (i.e., blepharospasm). The disproportionate retrocollis that used to be thought of as characteristic of PSP is infrequently observed, but other types of dystonia such as oromandibular, blepharospasm, and more rarely limb dystonia, have been reported *(18)*. In those cases dopaminergic medication should be cautiously reduced or discontinued to rule out the possibility of treatment-induced symptoms.

Speech, Swallowing, and Other Neurological Features

Patients with PSP may also present prominent early, or severe, speech and swallowing difficulties, but these features may also be present in CBD. PSP patients classically have a hypokinetic-spastic dysarthria (*see* video-PSP, and also Chapter 16). Speech perseveration, where whole words or phrases are repeated, and anomia, but not true aphasia may be observed in PSP.

Swallowing disturbances occur early in PSP. PD rarely causes early dysphagia, and even later in the disease, severe dysphagia is more common in PSP and MSA. Severe early sialorrhoea may be observed in PSP, but is rarely observed early in PD. Drooling of saliva and the voluntary down-gaze palsy causing food to fall from the fork may lead to the reported "sloppy tie or shirt sign."

Even at early stages of the disease, PSP patients may have difficulty judging the amount of food they can swallow and tend to take oversize mouthfuls or overstuff their mouths when eating (*see* video-PSP). This type of change in eating behavior is infrequent in patients with other atypical parkinsonian disorders or PD.

Pyramidal signs, usually bilateral, are features that present later in PSP than in MSA or CBD. About one-third of patients with PSP and one-half of those with MSA and CBD develop pyramidal signs. In these disorders, it may be hard to differentiate a Babinski sign from a "striatal" toe owing to dystonia.

Early or late insomnia and difficulties in maintaining sleep have all been reported in this disorder, but REM sleep behavioral abnormalities are infrequently reported. Sleep disturbances are thought to be a result of abnormalities in sleep patterns and in motor function.

In general, symptoms and signs apparent early in the course of PSP progress steadily. Most PSP patients eventually require a wheelchair and a feeding tube, and speech may become unintelligible, palilalic, or mute. Goetz et al. reported that these three milestones (wheelchair, unintelligible speech, and feeding tube) occur rapidly in PSP and can be monitored with standardized rating scales *(28)*. In their study, 88% of the sample (50 patients) met at least one of the three milestones, but the need for nasogastric tube was never the first. The median time from symptom onset to the first key motor impairment was 48 mo; gait disturbances occurred at a median symptom duration of 57 mo, and unintelligible speech at 71 mo. As a composite end point, speech and gait accounted for 98% of this sample first key motor impairment. These indices could be used as outcome measures in clinical trials to assess how interventions alter anticipated disease progression *(29)*.

DIAGNOSTIC DIFFICULTIES AND DIAGNOSTIC ACCURACY

In the tertiary referral setting, the diagnosis of a patient consulting with a history of early falls and visual disturbances can be obvious, however, the diagnosis of PSP may be challenging at early disease stages when the clinician is not familiar with the condition or does not have a high index of suspicion. This is particularly true since, as discussed, individual clinical features of PSP may occur in other parkinsonian or dementia disorders, and telltale signs may present in midstages of the disease. It can be particularly difficult to distinguish PSP from PD during the first 2–3 yr from symptom onset if patients with PSP do not yet clearly exhibit postural instability or ophthalmoplegia, and when they may still show a levodopa response. This presentation is infrequent, but the presence of only axial or additional symmetric limb signs at onset should raise suspicion that the diagnosis of PD may be incorrect. Patients with PD, DLB, or CBD usually have asymmetric signs. In patients with isolated asymmetric parkinsonism that does not respond to levodopa, the development of increased latency of horizontal saccades, ideomotor apraxia, cortical sensory signs, visual neglect, severe dystonia, or myoclonus should suggest a diagnosis of CBD. In the presence of severe autonomic signs (e.g., impotence, incontinence, syncope, or presyncope) or cerebellar disturbances with normal cognition and behavior, MSA should be considered. However, one should recognize that urinary symptoms, rarely incontinence but not retention, can also occur in PSP.

Neuropathologic and clinical criteria for the diagnosis of PSP have been standardized and validated and are widely accepted *(4,6,30)*. Both possible and probable NINDS–SPSP criteria were shown to have a high specificity and positive predictive value in an independent study sample *(30)*. Such specific criteria are ideal for genetic studies, clinical drug trials, and analytic epidemiologic studies. Because of their high specificity, the probable NINDS–SPSP criteria was renamed as clinically definite and the possible NINDS–SPSP as clinically probable criteria (Table 2). Criteria for clinically possible PSP are being developed and will require validation. The newly developed possible criteria should have a higher sensitivity but will still maintain relatively preserved specificity so it could be used for descriptive epidemiologic studies as well as clinical practice.

In addition to the difficulty in diagnosing PSP because of nonspecific features, PSP may infrequently be associated with unusual traits. There are reports of neuropathologically confirmed cases of PSP without ophthalmoplegia or with dementia or akinesia as the only presenting symptoms, or with unilateral dystonia and apraxia or with motor aphasia and speech apraxia *(31–35)*. One should consider that PSP is an unlikely diagnosis when symptoms develop before age 40 or last longer than 20 yr, because none of these characteristics have been reported in neuropathologically confirmed cases of PSP.

EPIDEMIOLOGIC ASPECTS

The incidence of PSP is closer to 10% of PD *(36)*, making it much more common than previously recognized. Early crude incidence rates of PSP ranged from 0.3 to 0.4 per 100,000 per year *(37)*, but an incidence study of PSP and all types of parkinsonism in Olmsted County, Minnesota, from 1976 to 1990 *(1,36)* found a crude incidence rate for PSP of 1.1 per 100,000 per year, which increased from 1.7 cases per 100,000 per year at age 50–59 years to 14.7 per 100,000 per year at ages 80–99 yr *(1)*. It is thought that these figures are higher because of better methodological case finding and increased recognition of the disorder by neurologists and non-neurologists *(1)*. Similarly, the earlier underestimated prevalence of 1.39 per 100,000 *(38)* has been found to be 6.0–6.4/100,000 in two population-based prevalence studies using currently accepted diagnostic criteria for PSP conducted in the United Kingdom *(2,39)*.

The natural history of PSP, as evaluated by surveying a large sample of caregivers of living and deceased patients with PSP *(12)* and by retrospectively evaluating the medical records of a small sample of autopsy-confirmed cases *(40)*, found that onset of falls during the first year, early dysphagia, and incontinence predicted a shorter survival time. Similar predictors of survival were identified in a recently published record-based study of 187 PSP patients of which 33% were examined by the investigators, but none of those who died during follow-up underwent autopsy confirmation *(14)*. These investigators found that classification as probable PSP according to the NINDS–SPSP criteria was associated with a poorer survival. In particular, they found that onset of falls, speech problems, or diplopia within 1 yr and swallowing problems within 2 yr, were associated with a worse prognosis.

NEUROPATHOLOGY

Neuropathologically, PSP is characterized by abundant neurofibrillary tangles and/or neuropil threads particularly in the striatum, pallidum, subthalamic nucleus, substantia nigra, oculomotor complex, periaqueductal gray, superior colliculi, basis pontis, dentate nucleus, and prefrontal cortex *(see* Fig. 2). Neuronal loss and gliosis are variable *(see* Chapter 4) *(6,41)*. Pathological tau in PSP is composed of aggregated four-repeat (E10+) isoforms that accumulate as abnormal filamentous lesions in cells and glia in subcortical and cortical areas *(42,43)*. In the normal adult human brain, there are six different tau isoforms with different microtubule-binding domains and the ratio of tau isoforms with three- (3-R) and four-repeat (4-R) microtubule binding domains is 1:1. In AD, there is amyloid deposition and the six tau isoforms aggregate mainly in neurons, but the 1:1 ratio is maintained. By contrast, in PSP and CBD, there is no amyloid deposition and tau aggregates in neurons and glia mainly as a 4-R isoform, altering the 3-R:4-R ratio *(6,44–46)*.

Neurochemical studies indicate that the degenerative process in PSP involves dopaminergic neurons that innervate the striatum and form the nigrostriatal dopamine system, as well as cholinergic and GABAergic efferent neurons in the striatum and other basal ganglionic and brain stem nuclei, thereby explaining the lack or transient nature of the levodopa response *(47–51)*.

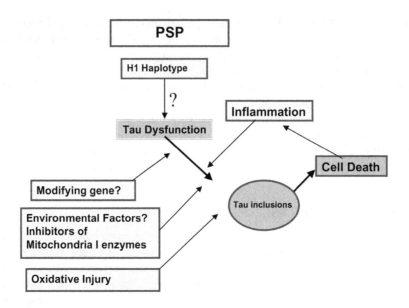

Fig. 3. Hypothesized pathways to neurodegeneration in PSP. Genetic, toxins, oxidative injury, and inflammation are thought to contribute to neurodegeneration in this disease.

ETIOPATHOGENESIS

The cause of PSP is unknown but it is hypothesized that genetic and/or environmental factors contribute to its development *(52,53)* (Fig. 3). Environmental and genetic factors have also been linked to other neurodegenerative disorders.

Genetic

PSP is associated with a specific form of the tau gene (H1 tau haplotype) *(5,54,55)* (*see* Chapters 5 and 9). However, since the H1/H1 genotype is present in approx 90% of patients with this disorder, and also in approx 60% of healthy Caucasians, it is unclear whether inheritance of the H1/H1 tau genotype represents a predisposition to develop PSP (requiring other environmental or genetic factors), or whether a relatively rare mutation with low penetrance (rather than an inherited susceptibility variant) could contribute to the abnormal tau aggregation present in this disorder.

CBD is also associated with the inheritance of the H1 haplotype *(54,55)*. The observation that coding and splice-site mutations in the tau gene cause FTDP-17 demonstrates that tau dysfunction is sufficient to induce neurodegeneration *(44,56–58)*. The parallels between FTDP-17 and PSP/CBD also include the fact that there are FTDP-17 patients with defined tau mutations (e.g., P-301, N279K) who share many clinical and pathologic features with PSP and CBD *(59–61)* such as selective deposition of 4-R tau. However, because highly penetrant tau mutations are not found in PSP and CBD, it is likely that other genetic or environmental factors contribute to the development of these disorders. Litvan et al. recently showed in a pilot study that H1 haplotype dosage does not influence age of onset, severity, or survival of PSP patients *(5)* in contrast to what is observed with ApoEε4 in AD. It is likely that differential environmental or genetic factors may lead to different cell vulnerability, phenotypes, and rate of disease progression observed in PSP patients. Whether the rarely reported familial cases of PSP *(62,63)* are owing to unidentified FTDP-17 mutations or they are a result of non-tau mutated genes, is currently the subject of investigation.

Oxidative Injury

Several laboratories have suggested that mitochondrial abnormalities *(64–66)* and lipid peroxidation may play a role in the neurodegeneration occurring in PSP *(67–71)*. Albers et al. measured tissue malondialdehyde (MDA) levels in the subthalamic nucleus and cerebellum from brain tissue of 11 PSP and 11 age-matched control cases using sensitive HPLC techniques, and found a significant MDA increase in the subthalamic nucleus, but not in the cerebellum, of the PSP patients *(69)*. Significant increases (+36%) were also found in tissue MDA levels in the superior frontal cortex of 14 PSP patients as compared with controls, and significant decreases (–39%) were also found in the α-ketoglutarate dehydrogenase complex/glutamate dehydrogenase ratio *(70)*. Increased oxidation has been also found in the substantia nigra of PSP patients. These findings suggest that lipid peroxidation may explain regionally specific neurodegeneration in PSP. Further, Odetti et al. *(71)* showed that lipoperoxidation is selectively involved in PSP and hypothesized that intraneuronal accumulation of toxic aldehydes may hamper tau degradation leading to abnormal aggregation. It is likely that irrespective of the primary cause of PSP, the onset of oxidative stress is a common mechanism by which neuronal death occurs, and one that contributes to disease progression.

Inflammation

Inflammation is thought to play a role in the etiopathogenesis of PSP because of strong evidence that in PSP there is activated glia *(72–76)* and that there may be augmented complement activation in the brain (higher CSF levels of C4 in PSP compared to controls and PD) *(77)*. Moreover, active glial involvement in PSP is as (or more) severe than that found in AD *(54)*. Inflammation has also been demonstrated in other neurodegenerative disorders. In AD, activation of the complement cascade and accumulation and activation of microglia *(78,79)* have also been reported. Although there is limited information about a decreased inflammatory reaction after treatment with antiinflammatory medication in autopsy-confirmed AD cases *(79,80)*, several epidemiologic studies have shown that antiinflammatory agents may delay the onset and slow the progression of AD *(81–83)*.

Environmental/Occupational Factors

Only a few case-control studies have been conducted in PSP and the findings reported have limited value because of the small sample size of the studies. Two case-control studies from the same institution resulted in conflicting conclusions on the role of education as a risk factor for PSP *(38,84)*. The authors attributed this disparity to methodologic differences in control selection *(84)*. The possibility that lower educational attainment may be a proxy for poor early-life nutrition or exposure to neurotoxic substances or that alternatively, subtle cognitive changes of PSP begin early in life so as to impair intellectual or educational motivation, have been hypothesized *(84)*. Davis et al. found that cases of PSP had a significantly higher educational level than controls in two of three categories tested (odds ratio [OR] 3.1 for completing high school, and 2.9 for completing college, $p < 0.05$) *(38)*, whereas Golbe et al. found that patients with PSP were less likely to have completed at least 12 yr of school (OR = 0.35) *(84)*.

On the other hand, recent studies in the French West Indies suggest that environmental factors may be relevant for developing PSP. Caparros-Lefebvre et al. *(85)* reported an unusually high frequency of patients with an atypical parkinsonian syndrome (postural instability with early falls, L-dopa unresponsiveness, prominent frontal lobe dysfunction, and pseudo-bulbar palsy) over the past 5 yr in the French West Indies. This new focus of atypical parkinsonism has been linked to exposure to tropical plants containing mitochondrial complex I inhibitors (quinolines [TIQ], acetogenins, rotenoids). In an initial case-control study, Caparros-Lefebvre et al. *(86)* reported an association with consumption of tropical fruits (pawpaw) or herbal teas (boldo) in 31 patients with PSP and 30 patients with atypical parkinsonism compared to controls (OR = 4.35). More recently, the authors reported that from 220 patients consecutively evaluated at the Guadeloupe University Hospital, they found 58 with probable PSP, 96 with undetermined parkinsonism, 50 with PD, 15 with ALS and parkinsonism, and 1 with probable MSA. This cluster of cases seem to have a tauopathy closely related to PSP. Neuropathological examination of three patients who died and were homozygous for the H1 tau haplotype showed an accumulation of four-repeat tau proteins predominating in the midbrain (85). There is evidence that TIQs are potentially neurotoxic (87,88). Injections of TIQs have caused parkinsonism in mice (89–91) and in primates (92–94). In addition, cellular studies showed that TIQs exert a direct toxicity to dopaminergic neurons through inhibition of complex I enzymes, a mitochondrial mechanism similar to that of 1-methyl-4-phenyl-1,2,3,6-tetrahydropyridine (MPTP) or rotenone exposure (95,96). It is unlikely that PSP patients seen in the United States or Europe are past consumers of the tropical fruits and herbal teas that have been linked to PSP in Guadeloupe. However, TIQs have been found in foods that are common in the Western diet, specifically, in cheese, milk, eggs, cocoa, and bananas (97,98). Although the amounts of TIQs in these foods vary, they may accumulate in the brain over many years (97). There have also been reports of other toxins causing atypical parkinsonism. There is some evidence of an environmental effect in Lytico–Bodig disease (99) and ecological correlations support the cycad hypothesis (100,101).

Environmental exposure to organic solvents has also been reported in patients with PSP (102,103). Petroleum waste ingestion has been linked to parkinsonism in a 20-yr-old man (104). N-Hexane has been shown to induce parkinsonism in rats (105), and was linked to parkinsonism in a 49-yr-old Italian leather worker (106). Although PSP patients were not found to have an association with any occupation or toxin exposure in the two previous case-control studies (38,84), these studies were not powered to test this hypothesis.

A possible role for traumatic brain injury (TBI) as a risk factor in the development of 4R-tauopathies such as PSP is supported by several observations. First, it is well known that repetitive TBI induces the formation of neurofibrillary tangles (107), which are found in PSP. Second, post-traumatic parkinsonism may occur following cumulative head trauma in contact sports and infrequently after a single severe closed head injury (108,109). However, it is unclear whether TBI should be considered a risk factor in the pathogenesis of PD (110). Third, several epidemiologic studies have demonstrated that TBI is a risk factor for developing another tauopathy, AD (111–113), although controversy exists over the extent to which TBI and genetics contribute to the development of AD. A recent large cross-sectional multicenter study of first-degree relatives of AD patients suggest that the influence of TBI on developing AD is greater among persons lacking APOE-ε4 compared with those having one or two ε4 alleles (113). These findings were confirmed in a retrospective study that evaluated two autopsy-confirmed cohorts of patients with AD with known APOE-ε4 genotype (114). On the other hand, two recent large European prospective clinical epidemiologic studies suggest that a history of TBI, with or without an association with APOEε4, is not a risk factor for developing AD (115,116), although major or many TBIs may increase the risk of cognitive decline (117). Finally, a large number of experimental animal studies support the role of TBI in the onset or progression of AD. Regrettably, a previous epidemiologic study in PSP had limited power to study this issue but note that it found high ORs for boxing (4.0), TBI with loss of consciousness (2.4), and TBI with memory loss (1.8), although none of them reach statistical significance (38).

Davis et al. found that heavy coffee drinking (>5 cups/d) and cigarette smoking were inversely associated with PSP, but that the results of their case-control study were statistically insignificant (38). Vanacore et al. found no difference in tobacco use between PSP cases and controls (118). The number of cases in both PSP studies, however, was small (50,55). Risk factors that occur with low frequency in the population may not be detected, thus resulting in type II error. These findings contrast with those in PD. An analysis from the Honolulu-Asia Aging Study based on a large sample size suggest that midlife coffee consumption is significantly inversely associated with PD independent of the effect of tobacco use (119). Similarly, a significant inverse association between heavy coffee drinking (>5 cups/d) before or at age 40 yr and PD (120) and that tobacco use is inversely associated with PD, has been tested in several studies (121).

The role of hypertension (HTN) in PSP remains controversial. Dubinsky and Jankovic proposed a "vascular" etiology for some of the cases diagnosed as clinical PSP *(122)*. They found that 19/58 PSP patients (32.8%) had radiological evidence of cortical, subcortical, or brainstem strokes, compared with 25/426 (5.9%) of PD patients ($p < 0.001$). The same group of investigators (123) found that 30/128 (23.3%) of PSP patients satisfied the criteria for vascular PSP. However, there have been few autopsy-confirmed cases of exclusively vascular PSP. Frequently, PSP associates with strokes or other neurodegenerative diseases *(124)*. Two studies looked at the presence of presymptomatic HTN in patients with PSP *(125,126)*. Ghika et al. excluded clear-cut cases of vascular parkinsonism by omitting cases with obvious multilacunar state on computed tomography (CT) or magnetic resonance imaging (MRI), severe hypertensive leukoencephalopathy, Binswanger disease, pseudo-PSP owing to small vessel disease, and vascular dementia. They found that the prevalence of presymptomatic HTN in patients with clinically diagnosed PSP was 34/42 (81%). Because the vascular cases were excluded, they proposed that HTN may be the first symptom of PSP, arising from degeneration of adrenergic nuclei in the brainstem. However, Fabbrini et al. *(125)*, and a previous case-control study conducted by Davis et al. *(38)*, found no increased frequency of HTN in PSP patients. Further studies are needed to evaluate whether HTN is simply acting as a risk factor for vascular parkinsonism.

Whether the factors discussed provide a clue for the pathogenesis of 4R-tauopathies, are applicable to a possible protective mechanism, or whether the epidemiologic data support the notion that different risks factors may be associated with different groups of neurodegenerative disorders, needs to be further investigated. Although the literature on PSP is definitely limited, it is reasonable to consider that there may be different risk factors for PSP than for the other neurodegenerative parkinsonian disorders.

NOSOLOGY

PSP and CBD have much in common from a clinical, pathologic, and genetic perspective *(16,44,45)*. Besides both being sporadic 4-R tauopathies, they both may present with frontal cognitive disturbances, parkinsonism not responding to levodopa therapy, ocular motor, and speech and swallowing disturbances *(16,127)*. The similarities between PSP and CBD have led investigators to question whether the two disorders are distinct nosologic entities or different phenotypes of the same disorder *(128)*. Recently validated neuropathologic diagnostic criteria *(129)* emphasize the presence of tau-immunoreactive lesions in neurons, glia, and cell processes in these disorders and also provide good differentiation between PSP and CBD *(129)*. For further details on the discussion of the nosology of PSP and its relationship with CBD and other disorders, the reader is remitted to Chapters 8 and 9.

LABORATORY

There are no laboratory markers for the diagnosis of PSP but ocular motor studies, electrophysiological studies, MRI, magnetic resonance spectroscopy, and positron emission tomography (PET) scans may be helpful to support the diagnosis or exclude other disorders. In general the sensitivity and specificity of these techniques in distinguishing patients with clinically equivocal or early PSP from other conditions has not been assessed. For this reason this techniques are not yet considered standard diagnostic tools in PSP. The availability and cost of some of these tools also limits their use to research settings for the foreseeable future.

Ocular Motor Studies

Electrooculographic recording may help distinguish PSP patients from other parkinsonian disorders at an early stage *(130)*. There is slight or no saccade impairment in PD and MSA patients with parkinsonism (i.e., those with no cerebellar signs). PSP patients have decreased horizontal saccade amplitude and velocity but normal latency, whereas opposite results are observed in CBD patients. The antisaccade task (looking in the direction opposite to a visual stimulus), which correlates well with frontal lobe dysfunction, is reported to be markedly impaired in patients with PSP, although it may also be impaired in patients with AD. A pilot study suggest that longitudinal electrooculographic studies may help distinguish patients with PSP from those with CBD *(131)*. For further details on the role of electrooculographic studies in the diagnosis of PSP, see Chapter 15.

Neuroimaging

Structural Imaging Changes

CT, as well as MRI, may at some stage in the disease show definite atrophy of the midbrain and of the region around the third ventricle in more than half of PSP patients *(132–135)* (Figs. 4 A,B). Thinning of the quadrigeminal plate, particularly in its superior part, better seen in sagittal MRI sections, has been shown to support a diagnosis of PSP (Fig. 4C). Minimal signal abnormalities in the periaqueductal region could also be seen in proton density MRI (Fig. 4D). Although CT or MRI of the brain are generally of little help in establishing the diagnosis of PSP, they can aid in ruling out other diagnoses (e.g., CBD when asymmetric atrophy may be present in the parietal area, or MSA when there may be atrophy of the pons, middle cerebellar peduncles, and cerebellum or altered signal intensity in the putamen; it may also be used to rule out multiinfarct states, hydrocephalus, or tumors). See also Chapter 25 for further details on the role of MRI studies in the diagnosis of PSP.

Functional Imaging

Magnetic resonance spectroscopy imaging detects different patterns of cortical and subcortical involvement in PSP, CBD, and PD. PSP patients, compared with controls, have reduced NA/Cre in the brainstem, centrum semiovale, frontal and precentral cortex, and reduced NA/Cho in the lentiform nucleus. On the other hand, CBD patients, compared with control subjects, have reduced NA/Cre in the centrum semiovale, and reduced NA/Cho in the lentiform nucleus and parietal cortex. Although significant group differences can be found using this technique, magnetic resonance spectroscopy is not helpful to differentiate between individual patients.

[18]F-Fluorodeoxyglucose PET scans and [123]IMP–single photon emission computed tomography (SPECT) blood flow studies have both shown marked reduction in frontal and striatal metabolism in PSP. Frontal hypometabolism in PSP is secondary to deafferentation and cortical pathology. However, this finding is not specific to PSP. PET measures of striatal dopamine D_2 receptor density using [76]Br-bromospiperone, or ^{11}C-raclopride are also significantly reduced in most PSP patients, but again, these findings are not specific to PSP. Hypometabolism of glucose in the frontal cortex, and decreased ^{18}F-fluorodopa uptake in the presynaptic nigrostriatal dopaminergic system (with similar reduction in both putamen and caudate) have also been shown by PET in PSP patients. *See* Chapters 26 and 27 for further details on the role of functional neuroimaging studies in the diagnosis of PSP.

Behavioral and Neuropsychological Evaluations

When evaluated with a series of neuropsychological tests that included the Wisconsin Card Sorting Test, Trail Making Tests, Tower of Hanoi, fluency test, the Similarity and Picture Arrangement subtests of the WAIS–R (Wechsler Adult Intelligence Scale–Revised), motor series of Luria, or imitation behavior, almost all PSP patients examined demonstrate an early and prominent difficulty executive dysfunction *(19,20,22,23,26,136)* Similarly, the use of the Neuropsychiatric Inventory helps identify the apathy these patients usually manifest *(24)*. Identification of these deficits is helpful for the diagnosis and for the management of these patients. A lack of benefit from levodopa therapy and the presence of severe frontal cognitive and/or behavioral deficits help support the diagnosis of PSP and differentiate this disorder from related disorders as shown in Fig. 5. Consideration of both, patients' response to levodopa and identified deficits in neuropsychological testing not only improves clinicians' diagnostic accuracy but helps us manage these two important aspects of the disease. *See* Chapters 11–14 for details on the role of neuropsychological studies in the diagnosis of this patient population.

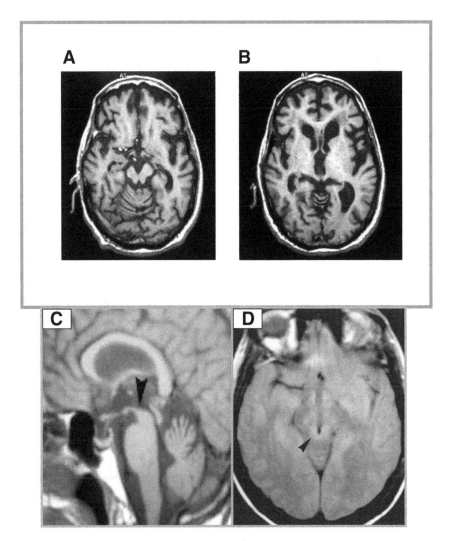

Fig. 4. MRI abnormalities in PSP. Midbrain atrophy (**A,C**), dilation of third ventricle (**B**), and an increased signal intensity in the periaqueduct gray matter in T2 (**D**) are the changes typically observed in PSP. Midbrain atrophy measured by an anteroposterior (AP) diameter equal or less than 13.4 mm *(135) or* an AP diameter equal or less than 17 mm in addition to dilation of third ventricle *(132)* have been proposed as radiologic features that help distinguish PSP from related parkinsonian disorders, particularly PD and MSA.

Neurophysiological Studies

PSP patients have both slowed movement and information processing. Their cognitive slowness can be evaluated with complex reaction time tasks or with cognitive evoked potentials. Event-related brain potentials recorded while PSP patients perform an Oddball task show a normal N1 component but dramatically increased latencies and decreased amplitudes of the P2 and P300 components *(137)*. The remarkably delayed latencies found in PSP have not been reported in any other type of dementia. These findings are different from those reported in CBD *(138,139)*.

Polysomnographic studies show a diminished total sleep time, an increase in awakenings, and progressive loss of REM sleep. These disturbances can be attributed to degeneration of brainstem structures crucial to generate normal sleep patterns, such as the pontine tegmentum, characteristically involved in PSP.

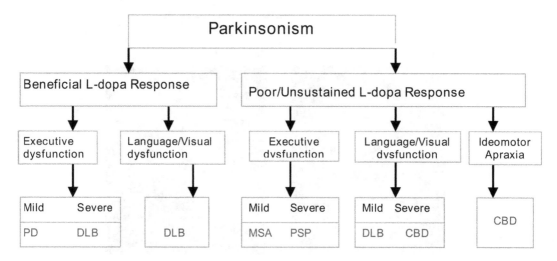

Fig. 5. Levodopa responsiveness and cognitive patterns. A lack of response to levodopa and a severe executive dysfunction supports the diagnosis of PSP.

Brainstem auditory evoked potentials are normal in PSP, however other neurophysiological measures of brainstem function are abnormal, reflecting the widespread pathological alteration in the pons and mesencephalon in these patients. Whereas the blink reflex to an electrical stimulus is normal, there is an absence of the orbicularis oculi response in patients with PSP exhibiting a mentalis response to electrical stimulation of the median nerve. This finding differentiates PSP patients from those with PD, MSA, and CBD, all of them presenting simultaneous responses of the orbicularis oculi and mentalis muscles after median nerve electrical stimulation (140). The startle response in which brainstem circuits are also implicated has been found to be markedly altered in PSP, but generally normal in PD and MSA. Valls-Sole et al. recently developed a functional method for studying the startle circuit consisting of the administration of the startling stimulus with a go signal in a reaction time task paradigm (140). The rapid habituation to the motor response that normally follows the delivery of a startling stimulus and that markedly limits the practical value of this test in the laboratory is dramatically reduced in this manner (114).

Urinary incontinence is not infrequent in PSP and anal sphincter electromyogram (EMG) has been found abnormal in about 40% of patients, with findings indicative of denervation (141). Similar findings are encountered in MSA but not in PD. See Chapter 24 for further details on the role of electrophysiological studies in the diagnosis of this patient population.

MANAGEMENT

General Considerations

At present there are no effective therapies that could slow or completely resolve patients' symptoms, however, state-of-the-art management should include the palliative treatment of patients's symptoms at the different stages of the disease, as well as providing education and support to the patient and their caregivers. In our clinical experience, both contribute to the improvement of the quality of life of patients and caregivers and help delay institutionalization. Informed patients are usually eager to participate in research and should be provided with the latest information.

Neurotransmitter Replacement

Neurotransmitter replacement therapeutic approaches have thus far failed in PSP because of the widespread involvement of dopaminergic and non-dopaminergic neurotransmitter systems

(GABAergic striatal interneurons, cholinoceptive striatal interneurons, cholinergic brainstem, and opioid striatal neurons) *(142)*. Case studies and our clinical experience show no significant improvement with levodopa. Similar findings are observed in double-blind placebo-controlled studies with dopamine agonists (e.g., bromocriptine, pergolide including newer dopaminergic agonists such as ropinirole or pramipexole) *(143,144)*. Although dopaminergic replacement therapies are usually only transiently and/or mildly effective, they should be tried when patients have parkinsonism since lack of sustained and/or marked benefit from levodopa therapy effectively rules out PD, and may also support the diagnosis of PSP (or other atypical parkinsonism). Future studies should evaluate the effects of selective D1 agonists since D1 receptors are relatively preserved in PSP.

Several randomized, double-blind controlled trials using cholinergic agents (physostigmine; RS-86; donepezil) showed similar mild or no efficacy *(145–148)*. However, as PSP patients' mental status and gait may worsen on anticholinergic drugs, these drugs should generally be avoided unless needed to treat particular symptoms *(142)*. Despite reported noradrenergic deficits in PSP *(149)*, these agents failed to benefit patients. Although PSP patients were reported to have some minor improvement in motor performance after the administration of idazoxan *(150)*, they failed to respond to efaroxan, a more potent noradrenergic agent *(151)*.

Palliative Measures

The combination of frontal lobe-type disturbances (impulsivity, unawareness, disinhibition) and postural instability may result in significant difficulty in the management of patients with PSP who, misjudging their disability, are exposed to a higher than necessary risk of falling. Palliative therapeutic approaches used in practice are listed in Table 3 and rehabilitation approaches are detailed in Chapter 29. Future studies should systematically evaluate whether symptomatic palliative therapies (e.g., speech therapy, physical therapy) improve the quality of life or survival of PSP patients (e.g., by preventing aspiration).

A small number of PSP patients have been subjected to pallidotomy, without significant benefit. At present, there is no evidence that pallidotomy or any other surgical procedure helps PSP patients.

Future Therapies

The development of biologic therapies for PSP requires additional pathogenetic studies. Recently developed four-repeat tau-transgenic animal models resembling PSP will likely accelerate efforts to discover more effective therapies (*see* Chapter 5). Given the recent progress that has been made in understanding the significance of tau in the development of neurodegeneration, it would seem likely that the most promising approaches are those that aim at preventing the abnormal aggregation of microtubule-associated protein tau. Future drug design should explore the use of agents that prevent tau aggregation such as oligonucleotides or peptide nucleic acids that inhibit the splicing of tau E10 or the translation of E10+ mRNA, and thus the generation of four-repeat tau isoforms, *(152)*. Alternatively, microtubule stabilizers such as Taxol derivatives may turn out to be promising therapeutic approaches.

Additional potential biologic therapeutic targets include free radical scavengers, enhancers of cell metabolism, and anti-inflammatory agents (nonsteroidals) that cross the blood brain barrier. Agents that could block microglial activation such as minocyclin may prove to be of therapeutic value.

Similarly, because in PSP the principal neuronal types affected are dopaminergic, cholinergic, and GABAergic, neurotrophic factors that promote the growth, survival, and differentiation of these cells or small molecules having nerve growthlike activity may end up being beneficial. However, potentially useful proteins, such as growth factors, cannot be administered systemically or in the ventricles since they have peripheral and central side effects and do not cross the blood brain barrier. Moreover, high levels of growth factors in the cerebrospinal fluid (CSF) can lead to side effects associated with circulating growth factors. On the other hand direct intraparenchymal administration of proteins into

Table 3
Management Approach: Palliative Treatments

Feature	Palliative Approach
Gait Instability/Falls	Physical therapy, weighted walkers
Speech disturbances	Speech therapy, communication devices
Dysphagia	Thickeners, percutaneus endoscopic grastostomy (PEG)
Blepharospasm, levator inhibition and other dystonias	Botulinum toxin (except antecollis)
Tearing, light sensitivity	Natural tears, dark glasses
Depression	Antidepressants; support therapy
Emotional incontinence	Antidepressants
Drooling	Anticholinergics (use cautiously!)
Patient and family support	Social services; support therapy; lay associations: (caregiver burden) Society for PSP, Inc. Suite 515, Woodholme Medical Building, 1838 Greene Tree Road, Baltimore, MD 21208, http://www.psp.org/); *and* the PSP (Europe) Association (The Old Rectory, Wappenhan, Towcester NN12 8SQ, UK, http://www.ion.ucl.ac.uk/~hmorris/contact.htm)

the lenticular nuclei by acute and/or chronic infusions may provide a means of delivery. Preliminary results of a double-blind, placebo-controlled pilot study in a single patient using a chronic intraparenchymal administration of GDNF/placebo (one side each) by convection-enhanced delivery recently conducted at the NINDS did not seem as promising as expected (personal communication). Alternative approaches to chronically deliver therapeutic growth factors that might slow down or halt the degeneration process in PSP include the administration of therapeutic genes to the disease-affected regions of the brain. Newly developed transgenic tau animal models will allow us to explore these alternatives as well as whether the administration of viral vectors by convection-enhanced delivery may improve the spread of vector particles in the brain resulting in more uniform transgene expression.

CONCLUSION AND FUTURE DIRECTIONS

Knowledgeable physicians can easily diagnose PSP when the disease presents with its classical features, but at early disease stages or when it presents with atypical features, the hunted biologic markers are expected to be of assistance. Palliative treatment rather than neurotransmitter replacement therapies are being used in clinical practice, whereas coordinated research efforts to find the cause and cure for this devastating disease remain crucial (Box). It is conceivable that therapeutic strategies aimed at limiting free radical production, oxidative stress, inflammation, and/or tau aggregation, may slow the advance of PSP. The availability of recently developed four-repeat tau-animal models resembling PSP will likely accelerate the translation of research from bench to bedside. It is hoped that as a result of these efforts, investigators will identify biologic markers to diagnose PSP at earlier stages and will develop biologic therapies that could prevent the abnormal aggregation of tau and prolong neuronal survival, which in turn will slow or stop the disease progression.

LEGEND TO VIDEOTAPE

PSP: Brief history and exam of a patient with the disorder. Falls, speech and visual disturbances are the major problems reported. Severe limitation in the range of ocular motor movements affects voluntary gaze, saccades, and OKNs. Motor disturbances affect axial (gait, neck) more than limb muscles (tapping). There is an impaired postural reflex with the backward pull test. The patient would have fallen, unless aided by the examiner.

FUTURE RESEARCH DIRECTIONS FOR PSP

Continue the search for:

- Diagnostic criteria for possible PSP that will increase the sensitivity in the diagnosis of this disease.
- Biologic markers of the disease that will improve the diagnostic accuracy.
- Cause(s) for PSP (case-control and genetic studies) that will help in turn to find appropriate biologic therapies.
- Improved transgenic animal models of the disease that will help to test therapies.
- Refined biologic therapies that will slow or stop disease progression.

REFERENCES

1. Bower JH, Maraganore DM, McDonnell SK, Rocca WA. Incidence of progressive supranuclear palsy and multiple system atrophy in Olmsted County, Minnesota, 1976 to 1990. Neurology 1997;49(5):1284–1288.
2. Schrag A, Ben-Shlomo Y, Quinn NP. Prevalence of progressive supranuclear palsy and multiple system atrophy: a cross-sectional study. Lancet 1999;354(9192):1771–1775.
3. Steele JC, Richardson JC, Olszewski J. Progressive supranuclear palsy. Arch Neurol 1964;10:333–359.
4. Litvan I, Agid Y, Calne D, Campbell G, Dubois B, Duvoisin RC, et al. Clinical research criteria for the diagnosis of progressive supranuclear palsy (Steele–Richardson–Olszewski syndrome): report of the NINDS–SPSP international workshop. Neurology 1996;47(1):1–9.
5. Houlden H, Baker M, Morris HR, MacDonald N, Pickering-Brown S, Adamson J, et al. Corticobasal degeneration and progressive supranuclear palsy share a common tau haplotype. Neurology 2001;56(12):1702–1706.
6. Hauw JJ, Daniel SE, Dickson D, Horoupian DS, Jellinger K, Lantos PL, et al. Preliminary NINDS neuropathologic criteria for Steele–Richardson–Olszewski syndrome (progressive supranuclear palsy). Neurology 1994;44(11):2015–2019.
7. Maher ER, Lees AJ. The clinical features and natural history of the Steele–Richardson–Olszewski syndrome (progressive supranuclear palsy). Neurology 1986;36(7):1005–1008.
8. Walsh JS, Welch HG, Larson EB. Survival of outpatients with Alzheimer-type dementia. Ann Intern Med 1990;113(6):429-434.
9. Tolosa E, Valldeoriola F, Marti MJ. Clinical diagnosis and diagnostic criteria of progressive supranuclear palsy (Steele–Richardson–Olszewski syndrome). J Neural Transm Suppl 1994;42:15–31.
10. Litvan I, Mangone CA, McKee A, Verny M, Parsa A, Jellinger K, et al. Natural history of progressive supranuclear palsy (Steele–Richardson–Olszewski syndrome) and clinical predictors of survival: a clinicopathological study. J Neurol Neurosurg Psychiatry 1996;60(6):615–620.
11. Verny M, Jellinger KA, Hauw JJ, Bancher C, Litvan I, Agid Y. Progressive supranuclear palsy: a clinicopathological study of 21 cases. Acta Neuropathol 1996;91(4):427–431.
12. Santacruz P, Uttl B, Litvan I, Grafman J. Progressive supranuclear palsy: a survey of the disease course. Neurology 1998;50(6):1637-1647.
13. Wenning GK, Ebersbach G, Verny M, Chaudhuri KR, Jellinger K, McKee A, et al. Progression of falls in postmortem-confirmed parkinsonian disorders. Mov Disord 1999;14(6):947-950.
14. Nath U, Ben-Shlomo Y, Thomson RG, Lees AJ, Burn DJ. Clinical features and natural history of progressive supranuclear palsy: A clinical cohort study. Neurology 2003;60(6):910–916.
15. Litvan I, Grimes DA, Lang AE, Jankovic J, McKee A, Verny M, et al. Clinical features differentiating patients with postmortem confirmed progressive supranuclear palsy and corticobasal degeneration. J Neurol 1999;246 Suppl 2:II1–II5.
16. Litvan I, Campbell G, Mangone CA, Verny M, McKee A, Chaudhuri KR, et al. Which clinical features differentiate progressive supranuclear palsy (Steele–Richardson–Olszewski syndrome) from related disorders? A clinicopathological study. Brain 1997;120(Pt 1):65–74.
17. Collins SJ, Ahlskog JE, Parisi JE, Maraganore DM. Progressive supranuclear palsy: neuropathologically based diagnostic clinical criteria. J Neurol Neurosurg Psychiatry 1995;58(2):167–173.
18. Barclay CL, Lang AE. Dystonia in progressive supranuclear palsy. J Neurol Neurosurg Psychiatry 1997;62(4):352–356.
19. Pillon B, Dubois B, Lhermitte F, Agid Y. Heterogeneity of cognitive impairment in progressive supranuclear palsy, Parkinson's disease, and Alzheimer's disease. Neurology 1986;36(9):1179–1185.

20. Grafman J, Litvan I, Gomez C, Chase TN. Frontal lobe function in progressive supranuclear palsy. Arch Neurol 1990;47(5):553–558.

21. Grafman J, Weingartner H, Newhouse PA, Thompson K, Lalonde F, Litvan I, et al. Implicit learning in patients with Alzheimer's disease. Pharmacopsychiatry 1990;23(2):94–101.

22. Pillon B, Dubois B, Ploska A, Agid Y. Severity and specificity of cognitive impairment in Alzheimer's, Huntington's, and Parkinson's diseases and progressive supranuclear palsy. Neurology 1991;41(5):634–643.

23. Pillon B, Deweer B, Michon A, Malapani C, Agid Y, Dubois B. Are explicit memory disorders of progressive supranuclear palsy related to damage to striatofrontal circuits? Comparison with Alzheimer's, Parkinson's, and Huntington's diseases. Neurology 1994;44(7):1264–1270.

24. Litvan I, Mega MS, Cummings JL, Fairbanks L. Neuropsychiatric aspects of progressive supranuclear palsy. Neurology 1996;47(5):1184–1189.

25. Litvan I, Paulsen JS, Mega MS, Cummings JL. Neuropsychiatric assessment of patients with hyperkinetic and hypokinetic movement disorders. Arch Neurol 1998;55(10):1313–1319.

26. Robbins TW, James M, Owen AM, Lange KW, Lees AJ, Leigh PN, et al. Cognitive deficits in progressive supranuclear palsy, Parkinson's disease, and multiple system atrophy in tests sensitive to frontal lobe dysfunction. J Neurol Neurosurg Psychiatry 1994;57(1):79–88.

27. Verny M, Duyckaerts C, Agid Y, Hauw JJ. The significance of cortical pathology in progressive supranuclear palsy. Clinico-pathological data in 10 cases. Brain 1996;119(Pt 4):1123–1136.

28. Goetz CG, Leurgans S, Lang AE, Litvan I. Progression of gait, speech and swallowing deficits in progressive supranuclear palsy. Neurology 2003;60(6):917–922.

29. Siderowf A, Quinn NP. Progressive supranuclear palsy: setting the scene for therapeutic trials. Neurology 2003;60(6):892–893.

30. Lopez OL, Litvan I, Catt KE, Stowe R, Klunk W, Kaufer DI, et al. Accuracy of four clinical diagnostic criteria for the diagnosis of neurodegenerative dementias. Neurology 1999;53(6):1292–1299.

31. Davis PH, Bergeron C, McLachlan DR. Atypical presentation of progressive supranuclear palsy. Ann Neurol 1985;17(4):337–343.

32. Matsuo H, Takashima H, Kishikawa M, Kinoshita I, Mori M, Tsujihata M, et al. Pure akinesia: an atypical manifestation of progressive supranuclear palsy. J Neurol Neurosurg Psychiatry 1991;54(5):397–400.

33. Daniel SE, de Bruin VM, Lees AJ. The clinical and pathological spectrum of Steele–Richardson–Olszewski syndrome (progressive supranuclear palsy): a reappraisal. Brain 1995;118(Pt 3):759–770.

34. Bergeron C, Pollanen MS, Weyer L, Lang AE. Cortical degeneration in progressive supranuclear palsy. A comparison with cortical-basal ganglionic degeneration. J Neuropathol Exp Neurol 1997;56(6):726–734.

35. Boeve B, Dickson D, Duffy J, Bartleson J, Trenerry M, Petersen R. Progressive nonfluent aphasia and subsequent aphasic dementia associated with atypical progressive supranuclear palsy pathology. Eur Neurol 2003;49(2):72–78.

36. Bower JH, Maraganore DM, McDonnell SK, Rocca WA. Incidence and distribution of parkinsonism in Olmsted County, Minnesota, 1976–1990. Neurology 1999;52(6):1214–1220.

37. Mastaglia FL, Grainger K, Kee F, Sadka M, Lefroy R. Progressive supranuclear palsy (the Steele–Richarson–Olszewski syndrome) clinical and electrophysiological observations in eleven cases. Proc Aust Assoc Neurol 1973;10:35–44.

38. Davis PH, Golbe LI, Duvoisin RC, Schoenberg BS. Risk factors for progressive supranuclear palsy. Neurology 1988;38(10):1546–1552.

39. Nath U, Ben-Shlomo Y, Thomson RG, Morris HR, Wood NW, Lees AJ, et al. The prevalence of progressive supranuclear palsy (Steele–Richardson–Olszewski syndrome) in the UK. Brain 2001;124(Pt 7):1438–1449.

40. Gilman S, Low P, Quinn N, Albanese A, Ben-Shlomo Y, Fowler C, et al. Consensus statement on the diagnosis of multiple system atrophy. American Autonomic Society and American Academy of Neurology. Clin Auton Res 1998;8(6):359–362.

41. Litvan I, Hauw JJ, Bartko JJ, Lantos PL, Daniel SE, Horoupian DS, et al. Validity and reliability of the preliminary NINDS neuropathologic criteria for progressive supranuclear palsy and related disorders. J Neuropathol Exp Neurol 1996;55(1):97–105.

42. Mailliot C, Sergeant N, Bussiere T, Caillet-Boudin ML, Delacourte A, Buee L. Phosphorylation of specific sets of tau isoforms reflects different neurofibrillary degeneration processes. FEBS Lett 1998;433(3):201–204.

43. Buee L, Delacourte A. Comparative biochemistry of tau in progressive supranuclear palsy, corticobasal degeneration, FTDP-17 and Pick's disease. Brain Pathol 1999;9(4):681–693.

44. Goedert M, Crowther RA, Spillantini MG. Tau mutations cause frontotemporal dementias. Neuron 1998;21(5):955–958.

45. Sergeant N, Wattez A, Delacourte A. Neurofibrillary degeneration in progressive supranuclear palsy and corticobasal degeneration: tau pathologies with exclusively "exon 10" isoforms. J Neurochem 1999;72(3):1243–1249.

46. Chambers CB, Lee JM, Troncoso JC, Reich S, Muma NA. Overexpression of four-repeat tau mRNA isoforms in progressive supranuclear palsy but not in Alzheimer's disease. Ann Neurol 1999;46(3):325–332.

47. Ruberg M, Javoy-Agid F, Hirsch E, Scatton B, R LH, Hauw JJ, et al. Dopaminergic and cholinergic lesions in progressive supranuclear palsy. Ann Neurol 1985;18(5):523–529.

48. Agid Y, Javoy-Agid F, Ruberg M, Pillon B, Dubois B, Duyckaerts C, et al. Progressive supranuclear palsy: anatomoclinical and biochemical considerations. Adv Neurol 1987;45:191–206.

49. Hirsch EC, Graybiel AM, Duyckaerts C, Javoy-Agid F. Neuronal loss in the pedunculopontine tegmental nucleus in Parkinson disease and in progressive supranuclear palsy. Proc Natl Acad Sci U S A 1987;84(16):5976–5980.

50. Javoy-Agid F. Cholinergic and peptidergic systems in PSP. J Neural Transm Suppl 1994;42:205–218.

51. Kasashima S, Oda Y. Cholinergic neuronal loss in the basal forebrain and mesopontine tegmentum of progressive supranuclear palsy and corticobasal degeneration. Acta Neuropathol (Berl) 2003;105(2):117–124.

52. Frattali CM, Grafman J, Patronas N, Makhlouf F, Litvan I. Language disturbances in corticobasal degeneration. Neurology 2000;54(4):990–992.

53. Golbe L. Progressive supranuclear palsy in the molecular age. Lancet 2000;356:870–871.

54. Baker M, Litvan I, Houlden H, Adamson J, Dickson D, Perez-Tur J, et al. Association of an extended haplotype in the tau gene with progressive supranuclear palsy. Hum Mol Genet 1999;8(4):711–715.

55. Di Maria E, Tabaton M, Vigo T, Abbruzzese G, Bellone E, Donati C, et al. Corticobasal degeneration shares a common genetic background with progressive supranuclear palsy. Ann Neurol 2000;47(3):374–377.

56. D'Souza I, Poorkaj P, Hong M, Nochlin D, Lee VM, Bird TD, et al. Missense and silent tau gene mutations cause frontotemporal dementia with parkinsonism-chromosome 17 type, by affecting multiple alternative RNA splicing regulatory elements. Proc Natl Acad Sci USA 1999;96(10):5598–5603.

57. Iijima M, Tabira T, Poorkaj P, Schellenberg GD, Trojanowski JQ, Lee VM, et al. A distinct familial presenile dementia with a novel missense mutation in the tau gene. Neuroreport 1999;10(3):497–501.

58. Grover A, Houlden H, Baker M, Adamson J, Lewis J, Prihar G, et al. 5' splice site mutations in tau associated with the inherited dementia FTDP-17 affect a stem-loop structure that regulates alternative splicing of exon 10. J Biol Chem 1999;274(21):15134–15143.

59. Bird TD, Nochlin D, Poorkaj P, Cherrier M, Kaye J, Payami H, et al. A clinical pathological comparison of three families with frontotemporal dementia and identical mutations in the tau gene (P301L). Brain 1999;122(Pt 4):741–756.

60. Bugiani O, Murrell JR, Giaccone G, Hasegawa M, Ghigo G, Tabaton M, et al. Frontotemporal dementia and corticobasal degeneration in a family with a P301S mutation in tau. J Neuropathol Exp Neurol 1999;58(6):667–677.

61. van Swieten JC, Stevens M, Rosso SM, Rizzu P, Joosse M, de Koning I, et al. Phenotypic variation in hereditary frontotemporal dementia with tau mutations. Ann Neurol 1999;46(4):617–626.

62. Rojo A, Pernaute RS, Fontan A, Ruiz PG, Honnorat J, Lynch T, et al. Clinical genetics of familial progressive supranuclear palsy. Brain 1999;122(Pt 7):1233–1245.

63. Morris HR, Katzenschlager R, Janssen JC, Brown JM, Ozansoy M, Quinn N, et al. Sequence analysis of tau in familial and sporadic progressive supranuclear palsy. J Neurol Neurosurg Psychiatry 2002;72(3):388–390.

64. Swerdlow RH, Golbe LI, Parks JK, Cassarino DS, Binder DR, Grawey AE, et al. Mitochondrial dysfunction in cybrid lines expressing mitochondrial genes from patients with progressive supranuclear palsy. J Neurochem 2000;75(4):1681-1684.

65. Albers DS, Beal MF. Mitochondrial dysfunction in progressive supranuclear palsy. Neurochem Int 2002;40(6):559–564.

66. Di Monte DA, Harati Y, Jankovic J, Sandy MS, Jewell SA, Langston JW. Muscle mitochondrial ATP production in progressive supranuclear palsy. J Neurochem 1994;62(4):1631–1634.

67. Jenner P, Dexter DT, Sian J, Schapira AH, Marsden CD. Oxidative stress as a cause of nigral cell death in Parkinson's disease and incidental Lewy body disease. The Royal Kings and Queens Parkinson's Disease Research Group. Ann Neurol 1992;32(Suppl):S82–S87.

68. Jenner P. Oxidative stress in Parkinson's disease and other neurodegenerative disorders. Pathol Biol (Paris) 1996;44(1):57–64.

69. Albers DS, Augood SJ, Martin DM, Standaert DG, Vonsattel JP, Beal MF. Evidence for oxidative stress in the subthalamic nucleus in progressive supranuclear palsy. J Neurochem 1999;73(2):881–884.

70. Albers DS, Augood SJ, Park LC, Browne SE, Martin DM, Adamson J, et al. Frontal lobe dysfunction in progressive supranuclear palsy: evidence for oxidative stress and mitochondrial impairment. J Neurochem 2000;74(2):878–881.

71. Odetti P, Garibaldi S, Norese R, Angelini G, Marinelli L, Valentini S, et al. Lipoperoxidation is selectively involved in progressive supranuclear palsy. J Neuropathol Exp Neurol 2000;59(5):393–397.

72. Ferrer I, Blanco R, Carmona M, Puig B. Phosphorylated mitogen-activated protein kinase (MAPK/ERK-P), protein kinase of 38 kDa (p38-P), stress-activated protein kinase (SAPK/JNK-P), and calcium/calmodulin-dependent kinase II (CaM kinase II) are differentially expressed in tau deposits in neurons and glial cells in tauopathies. J Neural Transm 2001;108(12):1397–1415.

73. Ferrer I, Blanco R, Carmona M, Ribera R, Goutan E, Puig B, et al. Phosphorylated map kinase (ERK1, ERK2) expression is associated with early tau deposition in neurones and glial cells, but not with increased nuclear DNA vulnerability and cell death, in Alzheimer disease, Pick's disease, progressive supranuclear palsy and corticobasal degeneration. Brain Pathol 2001;11(2):144–158.

74. Drache B, Diehl GE, Beyreuther K, Perlmutter LS, Konig G. Bcl-xl-specific antibody labels activated microglia associated with Alzheimer's disease and other pathological states. J Neurosci Res 1997;47(1):98–108.

75. Lippa CF, Flanders KC, Kim ES, Croul S. TGF-beta receptors-I and -II immunoexpression in Alzheimer's disease: a comparison with aging and progressive supranuclear palsy. Neurobiol Aging 1998;19(6):527–533.
76. Lippa CF, Smith TW, Flanders KC. Transforming growth factor-beta: neuronal and glial expression in CNS degenerative diseases. Neurodegeneration 1995;4(4):425–432.
77. Uchihara T, Mitani K, Mori H, Kondo H, Yamada M, Ikeda K. Abnormal cytoskeletal pathology peculiar to corticobasal degeneration is different from that of Alzheimer's disease or progressive supranuclear palsy. Acta Neuropathol (Berl) 1994;88(4):379–383.
78. McGeer PL, Rogers J. Anti-inflammatory agents as a therapeutic approach to Alzheimer's disease. Neurology 1992;42(2):447–449.
79. Halliday G, Robinson SR, Shepherd C, Kril J. Alzheimer's disease and inflammation: a review of cellular and therapeutic mechanisms. Clin Exp Pharmacol Physiol 2000;27(1–2):1–8.
80. Mackenzie IR. Anti-inflammatory drugs and Alzheimer-type pathology in aging. Neurology 2000;54(3):732–734.
81. Arima K, Murayama S, Oyanagi S, Akashi T, Inose T. Presenile dementia with progressive supranuclear palsy tangles and Pick bodies: an unusual degenerative disorder involving the cerebral cortex, cerebral nuclei, and brain stem nuclei. Acta Neuropathol (Berl) 1992;84(2):128–134.
82. Imran MB, Kawashima R, Awata S, Sato K, Kinomura S, Ono S, et al. Parametric mapping of cerebral blood flow deficits in Alzheimer's disease: a SPECT study using HMPAO and image standardization technique. J Nucl Med 1999;40(2):244–249.
83. McGeer PL, Schulzer M, McGeer EG. Arthritis and anti-inflammatory agents as possible protective factors for Alzheimer's disease: a review of 17 epidemiologic studies. Neurology 1996;47(2):425–432.
84. Golbe LI, Rubin RS, Cody RP, Belsh JM, Duvoisin RC, Grosmann C, et al. Follow-up study of risk factors in progressive supranuclear palsy. Neurology 1996;47(1):148–154.
85. Caparros-Lefebvre D, Sergeant N, Lees A, Camuzat A, Daniel S, Lannuzel A, et al. Guadeloupean parkinsonism: a cluster of progressive supranuclear palsy-like tauopathy. Brain 2002;125(Pt 4):801–811.
86. Caparros-Lefebvre D, Elbaz A. Possible relation of atypical parkinsonism in the French West Indies with consumption of tropical plants: a case-control study. Caribbean Parkinsonism Study Group. Lancet 1999;354(9175):281–286.
87. Kikuchi T, Tottori K, Uwahodo Y, Hirose T, Miwa T, Oshiro Y, et al. 7-(4-[4-(2,3-Dichlorophenyl)-1-piperazinyl]butyloxy)-3,4-dihydro-2(1H)-qui nolinone (OPC-14597), a new putative antipsychotic drug with both presynaptic dopamine autoreceptor agonistic activity and postsynaptic D2 receptor antagonistic activity. J Pharmacol Exp Ther 1995;274(1):329–336.
88. Soto-Otero R, Mendez-Alvarez E, Hermida-Ameijeiras A, Munoz-Patino AM, Labandeira-Garcia JL. Autoxidation and neurotoxicity of 6-hydroxydopamine in the presence of some antioxidants: potential implication in relation to the pathogenesis of Parkinson's disease. J Neurochem 2000;74(4):1605–1612.
89. Kotake Y, Tasaki Y, Makino Yea. 1-Benzyl-1,2,3,4-Tetrahydroisoquinoline as a parkinsonism-inducing agent: a novel endogenous amine in mouse brain and parkinsonian CSF. J Neurochem 1995;65:2633–2638.
90. Kawai H, Makino Y, Hirobe M, Ohta S. Novel Endogenous 1,2,3,4-tetrahydroisoquinoline derivative: uptake by dopamine transporter and activity to induce parkinsonism. J Neurochem 1998;70:745–751.
91. Tasaki Y, Makino Y, Ohta S, Hirobe M. 1-Methyl-1,2,3,4-tetrahydroisoquioline, decreasing in 1-methyl-4-phenyl-1,2,3,6-tetrahydropyridine-treated mouse, prevents parkinsonims-like behavior abnormalities. J Neurochemi 1991;57:1940–1943.
92. Kotake T, Yoshida M, Ogawa Mea. Chronic Administration of 1-benzyl-1,2,3,4-tetrahydroisoquinoline, an endogenous amine in the brain, induces parkinsonism in a primate. Neuroscience Letters 1996;217:69–71.
93. Nagatsu T, Yoshida M. An edogenous substance of the brain, tetrahydroisoquinoline, produces parkinsonism in primates with decreased dopamine, tyrosine hydroxylase and biopterin in the nigrostriatal regions. Neurosci Lett. 1988;87:178–182.
94. Yoshida M, Niwa T, Nagatsu T. Parkinsonism in monkeys produced by chronic administration of an endogenous substance of the brain, tetrahydroisoquinolone: the behavioral and biochemical changes. Neuroscie Lett. 1990;119:109–113.
95. Lannuzel A, Michel PP, Abaul MJ, Caparros-Lefebvre D, Ruberg M. Neurotoxic effects of alkaloids from Annona muricata (sour-sop) on dopaminergic neurons: potential role in etiology of atypical parkinsonism in French West Indies. Mov Disord 2000;13(Suppl 3):28 [Abstract].
96. Friedrich MJ. Pesticide study aids Parkinson research. JAMA 1999;282:2200.
97. Makino Y, Ohta S, Tachikawa O, Hirobe M. Presence of Tetrahydroisoquinoline and 1-Methyl-Tetrahydro-Isoquinoline in Foods: Compounds Related to Parkinson's Disease. Life Sciences 1988;43:373–378.
98. Niwa T, Takeda N, Sasaoka T, Kaneda T, hashizume Y, Yoshizumi H, Tatematsu A, et al. Detection of tetrahydroisoquinoline in parkinsonian brain as an endogenous amine by use of gas chromatography-mass spectrometry. J Chromatogr 1989;491:397–403.
99. Spencer PS, Kisby GE, Ross SM, Roy DN, Hugon J, Ludolph AC, et al. Guam ALS-PDC: possible causes. Science 1993;262(5135):825–826.
100. Zhang ZX, Anderson DW, Mantel N, Roman GC. Motor neuron disease on Guam: geographic and familial occurrence, 1956–85. Acta Neurol Scand 1996;94(1):51–59.

101. Zhang ZX, Anderson DW, Mantel N. Geographic patterns of parkinsonism-dementia complex on Guam, 1956 through 1985. Arch Neurol 1990;47(10):1069–1074.
102. McCrank E. PSP risk factors. Neurology 1990;40(10):1637.
103. McCrank E, Rabheru K. Four cases of progressive supranuclear palsy in patients exposed to organic solvents. Can J Psychiatry 1989;34(9):934–936.
104. Tetrud J, Langston J, Irwin I, Snow B. Parkinsonism caused by petroleum waste ingestion. Neurology 1994;44: 1051–1054.
105. Pezzoli G, Ricciardi S, Masotto C, Mariani CB, Carenzi A. n-Hexane induces parkinsonism in rodents. Brain Res 1990;531(1-2):355–357.
106. Pezzoli G, Barbieri S, Ferrante C, Zecchinelli A, Foa V. Parkinsonism due to n-hexane exposure [letter]. Lancet 1989;2(8667):874.
107. Geddes JF, Vowles GH, Nicoll JA, Revesz T. Neuronal cytoskeletal changes are an early consequence of repetitive head injury. Acta Neuropathol (Berl) 1999;98:171–178.
108. Bhatt M, Desai J, Mankodi A, Elias M, Wadia N. Posttraumatic akinetic-rigid syndrome resembling Parkinson's disease: a report on three patients. Mov Disord 2000;15(2):313–317.
109. Goetz CG, Pappert EJ. Trauma and movement disorders. Neurol Clin 1992;10(4):907–919.
110. Gomez-Tortosa E, Newell K, Irizarry MC, Albert M, Growdon JH, Hyman BT. Clinical and quantitative pathologic correlates of dementia with Lewy bodies. Neurology 1999;53(6):1284–1291.
111. O'Meara ES, Kukull WA, Sheppard L, Bowen JD, McCormick WC, Teri L, et al. Head injury and risk of Alzheimer's disease by apolipoprotein E genotype. Am J Epidemiol 1997;146:373–384.
112. Nemetz PN, Leibson C, Naessens JM, Beard M, Kokmen E, Annegers JF, et al. Traumatic brain injury and time to onset of Alzheimer's disease: a population-based study. Am J Epidemiol 1999;149:32–40.
113. Guo Z, Cupples LA, Kurz A, Auerbach SH, Volicer L, Chui H, et al. Head injury and the risk of AD in the MIRAGE study. Neurology 2000;54:1316–1323.
114. Kofler M, Muller J, Wenning GK, Reggiani L, Hollosi P, Bosch S, et al. The auditory startle reaction in parkinsonian disorders. Mov Disord 2001;16(1):62–71.
115. Mehta KM, Ott A, Kalmijn S, Slooter AJ, vanDuijn CM, Hofman A, et al. Head trauma and risk of dementia and Alzheimer's disease: the Rotterdam Study. Neurology 1999;53:1959–1962.
116. Launer LJ, Andersen K, Dewey ME, Letenneur L, Ott A, Amaducci LA, et al. Rates and risk factors for dementia and Alzheimer's disease: results from EURODEM pooled analyses. EURODEM Incidence Research Group and Work Groups. European Studies of Dementia. Neurology 1999;52:78–84.
117. Luukinen H, Viramo P, Koski K, Laippala P, Kivela SL. Head injuries and cognitive decline among older adults—a population-based study. Neurology 1999;52:557–562.
118. Vanacore N, Bonifati V, Fabbrini G, Colosimo C, Marconi R, Nicholl D, et al. Smoking habits in multiple system atrophy and progressive supranuclear palsy. European Study Group on Atypical Parkinsonisms. Neurology 2000;54(1):114–119.
119. Fujii C, Harado S, Ohkoshi N, Hayashi A, Yoshizawa K. Cross-cultural traits for personality of patients with Parkinson's disease in Japan. Am J Med Genet 2000;96:1–3.
120. Nefzger M, Quadfasel F, Karl V. A retrospective study of smoking in parkinson's disease. Am J Epidemiol 1968;88:149–158.
121. Morens D, Grandinetti A, Reed D, White L, Ross G. Cigarette smoking and protection from Parkinson's disease: false association or etiologic clue? Neurology 1995;45:1041–1051.
122. Dubinsky RM, Jankovic J. Progressive supranuclear palsy and a multi-infarct state. Neurology 1987;37(4):570–576.
123. Winikates J, Jankovic J. Vascular progressive supranuclear palsy. J Neural Transm Suppl 1994;42:189–201.
124. Gearing M, Olson DA, Watts RL, Mirra SS. Progressive supranuclear palsy: neuropathologic and clinical heterogeneity. Neurology 1994;44(6):1015–1024.
125. Fabbrini G, Vanacore N, Bonifati V, Colosimo C, Meco G. Presymptomatic hypertension in progressive supranuclear palsy. Study Group on Atypical Parkinsonisms [letter]. Arch Neurol 1998;55(8):1153–1155.
126. Ghika J, Bogousslavsky J. Presymptomatic hypertension is a major feature in the diagnosis of progressive supranuclear palsy. Arch Neurol 1997;54(9):1104–1108.
127. Litvan I, Agid Y, Jankovic J, Goetz C, Brandel JP, Lai EC, et al. Accuracy of clinical criteria for the diagnosis of progressive supranuclear palsy (Steele–Richardson–Olszewski syndrome). Neurology 1996;46(4):922–930.
128. Boeve BF, Lang AE, Litvan I. Corticobasal degeneration and its relationship to progressive supranuclear palsy and frontotemporal dementia. Ann Neurol 2003;54(Suppl 5):S15–S19.
129. Boeve BF, Maraganore DM, Parisi JE, Ivnik RJ, Westmoreland BF, Dickson DW, et al. Corticobasal degeneration and frontotemporal dementia presentations in a kindred with nonspecific histopathology. Dement Geriatr Cogn Disord 2002;13(2):80–90.
130. Vidailhet M, Rivaud S, Gouider-Khouja N, Pillon B, Bonnet AM, Gaymard B, et al. Eye movements in parkinsonian syndromes. Ann Neurol 1994;35(4):420–426.

131. Rivaud-Pechoux S, Vidailhet M, Gallouedec G, Litvan I, Gaymard B, Pierrot-Deseilligny C. Longitudinal ocular motor study in corticobasal degeneration and progressive supranuclear palsy. Neurology 2000;54(5):1029–1032.

132. Schrag A, Good CD, Miszkiel K, Morris HR, Mathias CJ, Lees AJ, et al. Differentiation of atypical parkinsonian syndromes with routine MRI. Neurology 2000;54(3):697–702.

133. Yekhlef F, Ballan G, Macia F, Delmer O, Sourgen C, Tison F. Routine MRI for the differential diagnosis of Parkinson's disease, MSA, PSP, and CBD. J Neural Transm 2003;110(2):151–169.

134. Savoiardo M. Differential diagnosis of Parkinson's disease and atypical parkinsonian disorders by magnetic resonance imaging. Neurol Sci 2003;24(Suppl 1):S35–S37.

135. Warmuth-Metz M, Naumann M, Csoti I, Solymosi L. Measurement of the midbrain diameter on routine magnetic resonance imaging: a simple and accurate method of differentiating between Parkinson disease and progressive supranuclear palsy. Arch Neurol 2001;58(7):1076–1079.

136. Pillon B, Dubois B, Agid Y. Testing cognition may contribute to the diagnosis of movement disorders. Neurology 1996;46:329–334.

137. Johnson R, Jr., Litvan I, Grafman J. Progressive supranuclear palsy: altered sensory processing leads to degraded cognition. Neurology 1991;41(8):1257–1262.

138. Takeda M, Tachibana H, Okuda B, Kawabata K, Sugita M. Electrophysiological comparison between corticobasal degeneration and progressive supranuclear palsy. Clin Neurol Neurosurg 1998;100(2):94–98.

139. Okuda B, Tachibana H, Takeda M, Kawabata K, Sugita M. Asymmetric changes in somatosensory evoked potentials correlate with limb apraxia in corticobasal degeneration. Acta Neurol Scand 1998;97(6):409–412.

140. Valls-Sole J. Neurophysiological characterization of parkinsonian syndromes. Neurophysiol Clin 2000;30(6):352–367.

141. Valldeoriola F, Valls-Sole J, Tolosa ES, Marti MJ. Striated anal sphincter denervation in patients with progressive supranuclear palsy. Mov Disord 1995;10(5):550–555.

142. Litvan I, Blesa R, Clark K, Nichelli P, Atack JR, Mouradian MM, et al. Pharmacological evaluation of the cholinergic system in progressive supranuclear palsy. Ann Neurol 1994;36(1):55–61.

143. Kompoliti K, Goetz CG, Litvan I, Jellinger K, Verny M. Pharmacological therapy in progressive supranuclear palsy. Arch Neurol 1998;55(8):1099–1102.

144. Weiner WJ, Minagar A, Shulman LM. Pramipexole in progressive supranuclear palsy. Neurology 1999;52(4):873–874.

145. Litvan I, Gomez C, Atack JR, Gillespie M, Kask AM, Mouradian MM, et al. Physostigmine treatment of progressive supranuclear palsy. Ann Neurol 1989;26(3):404–407.

146. Foster NL, Aldrich MS, Bluemlein L, White RF, Berent S. Failure of cholinergic agonist RS-86 to improve cognition and movement in PSP despite effects on sleep. Neurology 1989;39(2 Pt 1):257–261.

147. Frattali CM, Sonies BC, Chi-Fishman G, Litvan I. Effects of physostigmine on swallowing and oral motor functions in patients with progressive supranuclear palsy: a pilot study. Dysphagia 1999;14(3):165–168.

148. Litvan I, Phipps M, Pharr VL, Hallett M, Grafman J, Salazar A. Randomized placebo-controlled trial of donepezil in patients with progressive supranuclear palsy. Neurology 2001;57(3):467–473.

149. Pascual J, Berciano J, Gonzalez AM, Grijalba B, Figols J, Pazos A. Autoradiographic demonstration of loss of alpha 2-adrenoceptors in progressive supranuclear palsy: preliminary report. J Neurol Sci 1993;114(2):165–169.

150. Ghika J, Tennis M, Hoffman E, Schoenfeld D, Growdon J. Idazoxan treatment in progressive supranuclear palsy. Neurology 1991;41(7):986–991.

151. Rascol O, Sieradzan K, Peyro-Saint-Paul H, Thalamas C, Brefel-Courbon C, Senard JM, et al. Efaroxan, an alpha-2 antagonist, in the treatment of progressive supranuclear palsy. Mov Disord 1998;13(4):673–676.

152. Litvan I, Dickson DW, Buttner-Ennever JA, Delacourte A, Hutton M, Dubois B, et al. Research goals in progressive supranuclear palsy. First International Brainstorming Conference on PSP. Mov Disord 2000;15(3):446–458.

153. Steele JC. Introduction. In: Litvan I, Agid A, eds. Progressive Supranuclear Palsy: Clinical and Research Aspects. New York: Oxford University Press, 1992:3–14.

19

Corticobasal Degeneration

The Syndrome and the Disease

Bradley F. Boeve

INTRODUCTION

In 1967, Rebeiz, Kolodny, and Richardson described three patients with a progressive asymmetric akinetic-rigid syndrome and apraxia and labeled these cases as "corticodentatonigral degeneration with neuronal achromasia" *(1,2)*. Additional reports on this disorder were almost nonexistent until the early 1990s. Over the past 10 yr, interest in this disorder has increased markedly. The nomenclature has also undergone evolution. The core clinical features that have been considered characteristic of the disorder include progressive asymmetric rigidity and apraxia, with other findings suggesting additional cortical (e.g., alien limb phenomena, cortical sensory loss, myoclonus, mirror movements) and basal ganglionic (e.g., bradykinesia, dystonia, tremor) dysfunction.

The characteristic findings at autopsy have been asymmetric cortical atrophy, which is typically maximal in the frontoparietal regions, basal ganglia degeneration, and nigral degeneration. Microscopically, swollen neurons that do not stain with conventional hematoxylin/eosin (so-called ballooned, achromatic neurons) are found in the cortex. Abnormal accumulations of the microtubule-associated tau protein are found in both neurons and glia.

In this chapter, the concepts and data relating to the corticobasal syndrome and corticobasal degeneration as presented in a recent review *(3)* are expanded.

NOMENCLATURE

The terminology relating to corticobasal degeneration (CBD) has been confusing. The following terms have been used: *corticodentatonigral degeneration with neuronal achromasia (1,2)*, *corticonigral degeneration* (CND) *(4)*, *cortical-basal ganglionic degeneration* (CBGD) *(5)*, *corticobasal ganglionic degeneration* (CBGD) *(6)*, and *corticobasal degeneration* (CBD) *(7)*. Analyses from several academic centers have shown that the constellation of clinical features originally considered characteristic of this disorder can be seen in several non-CBD disorders, leading others to suggest syndromic terms such as *corticobasal syndrome (3)*, *corticobasal degeneration syndrome (8)*, *Pick complex (9)*, *progressive asymmetric rigidity and apraxia* (PARA) *syndrome (10)*, and *asymmetric cortical degeneration syndrome–perceptual-motor type (11)*. Consensus on the terminology has not been established. In this review, the term *corticobasal syndrome* (and abbreviation CBS) will be used to characterize the constellation of clinical features initially considered characteristic of corticobasal degeneration, and the term *corticobasal degeneration* (and abbreviation CBD) will be used for the histopathologic disorder.

From: *Current Clinical Neurology: Atypical Parkinsonian Disorders*
Edited by: I. Litvan © Humana Press Inc., Totowa, NJ

DEMOGRAPHICS AND EPIDEMIOLOGY

Like many other neurodegenerative disorders, symptoms usually begin insidiously in the sixth to eighth decade and gradually progress over 3–15 yr until death. Males and females are equally affected. A defining characteristic of the CBS is asymmetric limb findings, but there does not appear to be any predilection to the right or left side. A relatively high frequency of coexisting autoimmune diseases was noted in one series *(12)*. This is a sporadic disorder, although there are rare reports of a similarly affected relative *(13)*.

The incidence and prevalence of the CBS and CBD are not known. Bower et al. did not identify any case of CBS or CBD in their analysis of parkinsonism in Olmsted County, Minnesota *(14)*. However, in a review of the autopsy records of the Mayo Clinic from 1970 to 2000, two residents of Olmsted County, Minnesota, were found to have CBD pathology, with one exhibiting the CBS and the other exhibiting dementia of the Alzheimer type (B. Boeve, unpublished data). As of 2003, we are following 11 patients with the CBS in the Mayo Alzheimer's Disease Research Center who reside in the state of Minnesota. Considering there are approx 5 million residents in the state, a minimum prevalence estimate is at least 2 per million (B. Boeve, unpublished data). The rarity of the CBS and CBD will make more definitive incidence and prevalence estimates difficult.

CLINICAL FEATURES OF THE CORTICOBASAL SYNDROME

Details regarding the specific clinical features of the CBS can be found in several sources *(3,5,10,12,15–17)*.

Progressive Asymmetric Rigidity and Apraxia

The core clinical features are progressive asymmetric rigidity and apraxia. Symptoms typically begin in one limb, with no apparent predilection for the right or left side. Patients describe their limb as "clumsy," "incoordinated," or "stiff." On examination the limb is mildly to severely rigid, and sometimes adopts a dystonic posture. Features of both rigidity (i.e., velocity-independent increased tone) and spasticity (i.e., velocity-dependent increased tone) can be present in the affected limbs. Alternating motion rates are markedly reduced. The affected limb often becomes profoundly apraxic. Initially, the clumsiness and breakdown of complex coordinated movements may represent limb-kinetic apraxia. However, this is difficult to completely distinguish from the effects of basal ganglia dysfunction including rigidity, bradykinesia, and dystonia. Later, clear features of ideomotor apraxia develop with the inability to correctly perform or imitate gestures and simple activities. When asked to perform these activities or gestures with an involved hand, patients often glare at the limb in question and visibly struggle. With time, the limb becomes completely useless, and other limbs become similarly affected. Typically, progressive asymmetric rigidity and apraxia is present in one of the upper limbs for at least 2 yr, then either the ipsilateral lower limb or contralateral upper limb becomes involved, eventually leading to severe generalized disability several years later. Less commonly, a lower limb is affected first, or progression occurs rapidly over many months.

Apraxia and rigidity have undegone further study. Leiguarda et al. evaluated buccofacial, ideomotor, and ideational praxis in 10 patients with the CBS *(18)*. Their findings suggested that ideomotor apraxia was the most common type of apraxia in the CBS, and likely reflected dysfunction of the supplementary motor area. Those who had coexisting ideational apraxia correlated with global cognitive impairment, which suggested additional parietal or more diffuse cortical dysfunction *(18)*. Caselli et al. compared detailed kinematic data in several patients with the CBS, including one case who had CBD at autopsy and another who had Alzheimer's disease (AD) *(19)*. Severe abnormalities in temporal and spatial control, motor programming, and intermanual symmetry were present regardless of the presence or absence of dementia or specific histology *(19)*. Boeve et al. studied two siblings with a familial neurodegenerative disorder associated with nonspecific histopathology, in which one brother exhibited the CBS during life whereas the other had classic frontotemporal dementia

(FTD) features *(20)*. The case with the CBS features had no significant degenerative changes in the basal ganglia and substantia nigra, suggesting that extrapyramidal dysfunction can exist in the absence of appreciable pathology in the nigrostriatal system *(20)*. Hence, additional clinical, radiologic, and pathologic studies are necessary to better define the anatomic substrates underlying apraxia and rigidity in the CBS.

Alien Limb Phenomenon

The alien limb phenomenon is an intriguing feature in the CBS. Patients often describe their affected limb as "alien," "uncontrollable," or "having a mind of its own," and often label the limb as "it" when describing the limb's behavior. The movements are spontaneous and minimally affected by mental effort, sometimes requiring restraint by the contralateral limb. This phenomenon often lasts a few months to a few years before progressive rigidity or dystonia supercedes.

There has been debate as to what constitutes true alien behavior from pseudoathetosis owing to cortical sensory loss to simple levitation of a limb *(21–25)*. This phenomenon likely relates to pathology in the supplementary motor area and the efferent/afferent connections.

Cortical Sensory Loss

Cortical sensory loss is often manifested symptomatically as "numbness" or "tingling." Impaired joint position sense, impaired two-point discrimination, agraphasthesia, and astereognosis in the setting of intact primary sensory modalities are all evidence of cortical sensory loss. This likely relates to pathology in somotosensory cortex ± thalamus.

Myoclonus

Myoclonus, if present, usually begins distally in one upper limb and may spread proximally. The frequency and amplitude of myoclonic jerks typically increase with tactile stimulation (i.e., stimulus-sensitive myoclonus) and action (i.e., action myoclonus). Recent electrophysiologic studies suggest that the myoclonus in this disorder results from enhanced direct sensory input to cortical motor areas. Typically, a peripheral stimulus inducing myoclonic jerks is not associated with an enhanced somatosensory evoked potential (SSEP) and the latency from stimulus to jerk is brief, just sufficient to have reached the cortex and returned to the periphery (i.e., ~ 40 ms in the upper limb). These features are distinct from most other forms of cortical reflex myoclonus (which is associated with enlarged SSEPs and a longer stimulus-to-jerk latency) *(26,27)*.

Mirror Movements

Mirror movements are present if the opposite limb involuntary performs the same activity as the one being examined. Mirror movements are often suppressible, but when the individual is distracted and rechallenged with the same maneuver several minutes later, they will recur. Patients also frequently demonstrate overflow movements on the same side of the body, whereby attempted movement in an arm or leg causes additional movement in the ipsilateral limb, including elevation, mirroring, etc. Mirror movements have been associated with the alien hand syndrome *(28)*, although many patients have them without alien limb features. Mirror movements are often found on examination but are rarely symptomatic.

Dystonia

Dystonic posturing of a limb is a common early manifestation, usually affecting one upper limb. Frequently, the posturing of the hand takes on a "fisted" appearance, although hyperextension of one or more fingers may occur. Initially, dystonia may only be evident during walking or reaching. In those with symptoms beginning in a lower limb, the foot is often tonically inverted, and ambulation is severely limited. Pain often but not always accompanies dystonia. The "fisted hand sign" may represent one of the most specific clinical features for underlying CBD in the CBS (Rippon et al., unpublished data).

Tremor

Tremor is another common presenting feature, and patients typically describe the affected extremity as "jerky." A postural and action tremor often evolves to a more jerky tremor and then to myoclonus. Unlike the tremor of Parkinson's disease (PD), which is most prominent at rest and dampens with action, the tremor is amplified with activity and minimal at rest. A classical 4- to 6-Hz parkinsonian rest tremor is rarely, if ever, evident in this disorder.

Lack of Levodopa Response

There are no published cases in which a significant and sustained clinical improvement has occurred with levodopa therapy *(29)*. Many regard the lack of objective improvement during therapy with at least 750 mg of daily levodopa (divided doses, on an empty stomach) as a diagnostic feature of the disorder (realizing that other akinetic-rigid syndromes fail to respond to levodopa as well).

Dementia

Clinically significant dementia is not a typical early finding in patients with the CBS, but impairment in one or more cognitive domains is often present. However, it should be emphasized that the absence of early clinically significant dementia relates largely to the application of diagnostic criteria that have attempted to exclude other disorders such as AD and Lewy body dementia. In fact, as discussed below, although the pathology of CBD may be the most common cause of the CBS, some studies have found that it presents more commonly as a dementia syndrome *(30)*.

Yes/No Reversals

A very intriguing feature in the CBS (as well as other disorders) is the tendency for patients to shake their head and respond "yes" when they actually mean "no," and vice versa *(31)*. Whereas some patients and relatives describe this phenomenon spontaneously, this often requires specific questioning by the clinician. Relatives and friends of affected patients tend to repeat their questions, or ask "do you really mean yes or no?" and thus this issue can significantly affect communication in some patients. This phenomenon is likely due to frontosubcortical dysfunction, in which mental flexibility and inhibitory control is impaired *(31)*.

Focal or Lateralized Cognitive Features

Aphasia (which is typically nonfluent) *(32)*, ideomotor apraxia, hemineglect, etc., are lateralized cognitive features that are as frequent as the motor features. Apraxia of speech and/or nonverbal oral apraxia are quite common; in fact, one published case presented with speech apraxia and did not develop other "typical" features until at least 5 yr later *(33)*. Although rarely symptomatic, patients often demonstrate constructional dyspraxia on drawing tasks, particularly if the parietal lobe of the nondominant hemisphere is sufficiently affected. Other nondominant parietal lobe findings such as hemineglect and poor spatial orientation can also occur, which often are symptomatic in activities of daily living. Apraxic agraphia may result if the homologous region of the dominant hemisphere is dysfunctional. The lack of these findings being noted in the CBD literature probably stems from clinicians not including assessment of visuospatial/visuoperceptual functioning and neglect *(11,16)*.

Neuropsychiatric Features

Depression, obsessive-compulsive symptomatology, and "frontal" behavioral disturbances can occur in the CBS syndrome *(34,35)*. Visual hallucinations and delusions are very rare. The presence of visual hallucinations in the setting of cognitive impairment and/or parkinsonism may therefore favor a diagnosis of Lewy body disease rather than CBD *(36,37)*.

Ocular Motor Apraxia

Ocular motor apraxia occurs to some degree in almost every patient *(17)*. This includes difficulty initiating saccades and voluntary gaze, but pursuit and optokinetic nystagmus are typically preserved. In contrast to patients with progressive supranuclear palsy (PSP), those with the CBS have normal speed and amplitude of the saccades. On the other hand, eventually patients may develop supranuclear gaze paresis that can be indistinguishable from that seen in PSP. Eyelid opening/closing apraxia is also frequent.

Other Findings

Several other less specific findings may also occur. Frontal release signs, hypokinetic dysarthria, asymmetric hyperreflexia, and/or extensor toe responses also occur with some frequency. Postural instability is very common later in the disease and may be related to gait apraxia, bilateral lowerlimb parkinsonian, dystonia, or less frequently vestibular involvement. If balance problems are present at an early stage, they are usually secondary to lower-limb involvement at onset. Appendicular ataxia, chorea, and blepharospasm are infrequent manifestations. Dysphagia begins insidiously in the later stages of the disease in contrast to what usually occurs in PSP, and as in that disorder eventually leads to aspiration pneumonia and death in most instances.

DIAGNOSTIC CRITERIA

Four sets of clinical diagnostic criteria have been published *(3,5,38,39)* (Tables 1-4). The criteria by Maraganore et al., Lang et al., and Kumar et al. are similar to other sets of criteria (e.g., AD, ref. *40*, PSP, ref. *41*; etc.) in which those clinical features that are thought to best predict underlying CBD are listed and qualified. Yet, several investigators have shown considerable clinicopathologic heterogeneity in patients clinically suspected to have CBD *(42–44)*. The criteria proposed by Boeve et al. takes this heterogeneity into account and lists the clinical features for the *syndrome*, which is conceptually similar to the syndromes of frontotemporal dementia, progressive nonfluent aphasia, and semantic dementia *(45)*. None of these sets of criteria have been rigorously validated, and refinements are likely to be necessary.

Consensus was reached for the neuropathologic criteria for the diagnosis of CBD *(46)*. The core features are listed in Table 5. A critical point is that appropriate staining techniques (i.e., Gallyas silver staining, immunocytochemistry with tau, and phospho-neurofilament or α-B-crystallin), should be performed in appropriate cases, particularly in those with dementia and/or parkinsonism where no significant Alzheimer or Lewy body pathology is found. More details on the neuropathologic findings in CBD are discussed below.

FINDINGS ON ANCILLARY TESTING

Many of the diagnostic studies available for evaluating brain disease have been studied in the CBS and CBD, and like so many other facets of the syndrome and the disorder, the findings are difficult to interpret. Most of the literature on the laboratory, neuropsychologic, electrophysiologic, and radiologic findings in CBD have involved patients with clinically diagnosed CBD (i.e., the CBS) but without pathologic confirmation. Since a considerable proportion of patients with the CBS (approx 50% in one series—see subheading Diagnostic Accuracy) have a non-CBD disorder underlying their symptoms, one must view the findings described below consistent with the CBS but as yet unproven for the disorder of CBD.

Laboratory Findings

Routine blood, urine, and cerebrospinal fluid (CSF) tests are typically normal. Recent studies indicate that the tau haplotype in CBD is similar to that in PSP *(47)*. Elevation of tau in the CSF has also been identified in CBD patients *(48)*. Whether the tau haplotype or CSF tau level improves antemortem diagnostic accuracy requires further study.

Table 1
Clinical Diagnosis of Corticobasal Degeneration: Criteria of Maraganore et al.

Clinically Possible CBD:

No identifiable cause (e.g., tumor, infarct), at least three of the following:

- **P**rogressive course
- **A**symmetric distribution   "PARA" syndrome
- **R**igidity
- **A**praxia

Clinically Probable CBD:

All four of clinically possible criteria, no identifiable cause, at least two of the following:

- Focal or asymmetric appendicular dystonia
- Focal or asymmetric appendicular myoclonus
- Focal or asymmetric appendicular postural/action tremor
- Lack of levodopa response

Clinically Definite CBD:

Meets criteria for clinically probable CBD, at least one of the following:

- Alien limb phenomenon
- Cortical sensory loss
- Mirror movements

Supportive findings:

- Asymmetric amplitude on EEG
- Focal or asymmetric frontoparietal atrophy on CT or MRI
- Focal or asymmetric frontoparietal ± basal ganglia hypoperfusion on SPECT
- Focal or asymmetric frontoparietal ± basal ganglia hypometabolism on PET

From ref. *38*.

Table 2
Clinical Diagnosis of Corticobasal Degeneration: Criteria of Lang et al.

Inclusion criteria:

- Rigidity plus one cortical sign (apraxia, cortical sensory loss, or alien limb phenomenon)
          or
- Asymmetric rigidity, dystonia, and focal reflex myoclonus

Qualifications of clinical features:

- Rigidity: easily detectable without reinforcement
- Apraxia: more than simple use of limb as object; clear absence of cognitive or motor deficit sufficient to explain disturbance
- Cortical sensory loss: preserved primary sensation; asymmetric
- Alien limb phenomenon: more than simple levitation
- Dystonia: focal in limb; present at rest at onset
- Myoclonus: reflex myoclonus spreads beyond stimulated digits

Exclusion criteria:

- Early dementia
- Early vertical-gaze palsy
- Rest tremor
- Severe autonomic disturbances
- Sustained responsiveness to levodopa
- Lesions on imaging studies indicating another pathologic process is responsible

From ref. *5*.

Table 3
Clinical Diagnosis of Corticobasal Degeneration: Criteria of Kumar et al.

Core features:

- Chronic progressive course
- Asymmetric at onset (includes speech dyspraxia, dysphasia)
  Presence of:
- "Higher" cortical dysfunction (apraxia, cortical sensory loss, or alien limb) and
- Movement disorders (akinetic-rigid syndrome resistant to levodopa, and limb dystonia or spontaneous and reflex focal myoclonus)

Qualifications of clinical features:

Same as criteria of Lang et al.

Exclusion criteria:

Same as criteria of Lang et al.

From ref. *39*.

Table 4
Proposed Criteria for the Diagnosis of the Corticobasal Syndrome

Core Features:

- Insidious onset and progressive course
- No identifiable cause (e.g., tumor, infarct)
- Cortical dysfunction as reflected by at least one of the following:
  - focal or asymmetric ideomotor apraxia
  - alien limb phenomenon
  - cortical sensory loss
  - visual or sensory hemineglect
  - constructional apraxia
  - focal or asymmetric myoclonus
  - apraxia of speech/nonfluent aphasia
- Extrapyramidal dysfunction as reflected by at least one of the following:
  - Focal or asymmetric appendicular rigidity lacking prominent and sustained levodopa response
  - Focal or asymmetric appendicular dystonia

Supportive Investigations:

- Variable degrees of focal or lateralized cognitive dysfunction, with relative preservation of learning and memory, on neuropsychometric testing
- Focal or asymmetric atrophy on CT or MRI, typically maximal in parietofrontal cortex
- Focal or asymmetric hypoperfusion on SPECT and hypometabolism on PET, typically maximal in parietofrontal cortex ± basal ganglia ± thalamus

From ref. *3*.

Table 5
Office of Rare Diseases Neuropathologic Criteria for the Diagnosis of Corticobasal Degeneration

Core Features:

- Focal cortical neuronal loss, most often in frontal, parietal, and/or temporal regions
- Substantia nigra neuronal loss
- Gallyas/tau-positive neuronal and glial lesions, especially astrocytic plaques and threads, in both white matter and gray matter, most often in superior frontal gyrus, superior parietal gyrus, pre- and postcentral gyri, and striatum

Supportive Features:

- Cortical atrophy, often with superficial spongiosis
- Ballooned neurons, usually numerous in atrophic cortices
- Tau-positive oligodendroglial coiled bodies

Adapted from ref. *46*.

Neuropsychological Findings

Neuropsychometric testing typically shows impairment in those domains subserved by frontal/ frontostriatal and parietal cognitive networks: attention/concentration, executive functions, verbal fluency, praxis, and visuospatial functioning *(49,50)*. The profile of impairment depends in part on which cerebral hemisphere is maximally affected. Performance on tests of learning and memory tends to be mildly impaired if impaired at all. Alternative diagnoses, particularly AD, should be considered if performance on delayed recall and recognition measures are markedly abnormal.

It should be noted that the few published reports on the neuropsychological findings in CBD have involved clinically but not pathologically diagnosed cases, thus these patients had the CBS and may or may not have had underlying CBD. Since the diagnosis of CBS is based on the constellation of clinical features, which reflects the topography of dysfunction in the frontostriatal and parietal neural networks, the findings on neuropsychological testing should mirror this topography. Thus, the neuropsychological findings noted above should be considered typical of the CBS but not be considered diagnostic of underlying CBD.

Electrophysiologic Findings

Findings on electroencephalography (EEG) have varied from normal to marked dysrhythmic and delta slowing *(51,52)*. Asymmetric amplitudes of background alpha activity and sleep spindles have been reported in the CBS *(20)*.

The electrophysiologic aspects of myoclonus in cases of presumed CBD have been discussed in detail elsewhere *(26,27)*, including the short reflex latency and reduced inhibition following magnetic stimulation over the cortex *(53)*. Although there is at least one case of pathologically proven CBD who had a longer latency more typical of cortical reflex myoclonus, other cases of CBS with a long latency form of reflex myoclonus that have been studied have demonstrated other pathologies at postmortem (e.g., Pick's disease, AD, and motor neuron inclusion body dementia). In contrast, to date, the few cases coming to autopsy in which the short latency form was present in life have had the pathology of CBD *(3)*. These findings may be the most specific antemortem predictor of underlying CBD identified thus far; however, many more cases need to be studied with clinical, electrophysiological, and pathological correlation.

Magnetic Resonance Imaging Findings

The purpose of performing a computed tomography (CT) or magnetic resonance imaging (MRI) scan of the brain is to exclude a structural lesion such as a tumor, abscess, hematoma, or infarct. In the absence of these lesions, some findings can be supportive of the diagnosis of CBS, such as asymmetric cortical atrophy, especially frontoparietal, with the more prominent atrophy existing contralateral to the side most severely affected clinically *(54–59)* (Fig. 1). The lateral ventricle in the maximally affected cerebral hemisphere can also be slightly larger than opposite one. Asymmetric atrophy in the cerebral peduncles may be present *(5)* (Fig. 2). Other reported MRI findings in the CBS include atrophy of the middle or posterior segment of the corpus callosum *(60)* (Fig. 3), hyperintense signal changes lateral to the putamen *(54,56,61)* (Fig. 4), atrophy of the putamen *(61)*, and subtle hyperintense subcortical signal changes in motor ± somatosensory cortex *(62,63)* (Fig. 5). These are often subtle findings and their presence or absence should not alter the clinical diagnosis of the CBS. Importantly, the majority of cases in which these MRI findings were identified have not had CBD verified postmortem. In the only series of patients with the CBS associated with CBD pathology, CBS associated with non-CBD pathology, and CBD pathology associated with non-CBS clinical features, none of these MRI findings were found to be adequately sensitive or specific for CBD–the disease *(64)*.

Progressive parietal ± frontal atrophy (Fig. 6) and thinning of the middle and posterior portion of the corpus callosum (Fig. 7) often occurs on serial MRI scans in patients with the CBS. Some patients present with a focal cortical degeneration syndrome such as frontotemporal dementia (Fig. 8), progressive aphasia, or posterior cortical atrophy (Fig. 9) and subsequently develop CBS findings.

We have also observed several atypical MRI findings in the CBS and CBD. Focal hyperintense subcortical signal changes can evolve (Figs. 10–12). The hazy or hyperintense signal changes may reflect gliosis and/or secondary demyelination. Some patients have minimal cortical atrophy, and despite unequivocal clinical progression, progressive atrophy is difficult to appreciate, although ventricular dilatation may be evident (Fig. 13). Increased signal along the parietofrontal cortical ribbon can be seen in patients with Creutzfeldt–Jakob disease who present with the CBS (Fig. 14).

Functional Neuroimaging Findings

Asymmetric hypoperfusion on single photon emission computed tomography (SPECT) and asymmetric hypometabolism on positron emission tomography (PET) involving the parietofrontal cortex ± basal ganglia have been reported *(65–71)* (Fig. 15). Imaging of the nigrostriatal dopamine system typically demonstrates a reduction of striatal tracer uptake greater contralateral to the clinically most affected side. Unlike PD, uptake in the caudate is generally reduced to the same extent as in the putamen. However, these findings are not specific for CBD–the disease *(72)*.

In summary, although the electrophysiologic findings in myoclonus and association of a specific tau haplotype and increased CSF tau are promising, there are no antemortem features or biologic markers identified to date that definitively distinguishes CBD from the CBD mimickers.

NEUROPATHOLOGIC FINDINGS

Consensus criteria for the pathologic diagnosis of CBD have recently been published *(46)* (Table 5).

Macroscopic

Asymmetric parietofrontal or frontotemporal cortical atrophy (Fig. 16), and pallor of the substantia nigra, are the typical macroscopic pathologic findings. Some individuals with typical clinical and microscopic findings do not have appreciable cortical atrophy, however.

Microscopic

Neuronal loss, gliosis, and superficial spongiosus are prominent in the maximally affected cortical gyri. Immunocytochemistry with tau as well as phosphorylated neurofilament or αB-crystallin is imperitive when characterizing cases with possible CBD. The pathologic features of CBD–the disease include tau-positive (tau+) astrocytic plaques and tau+ threadlike lesions in gray and white

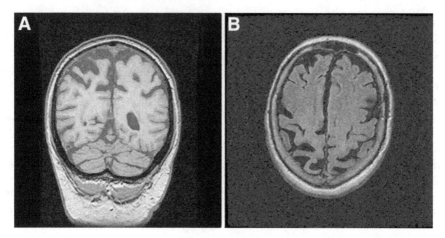

Fig.1. Coronal T1-weighted (**A**) and axial FLAIR (**B**) MR images in a patient with the corticobasal syndrome. Note the asymmetric parietal cortical atrophy, more evident in the right hemisphere in this patient.

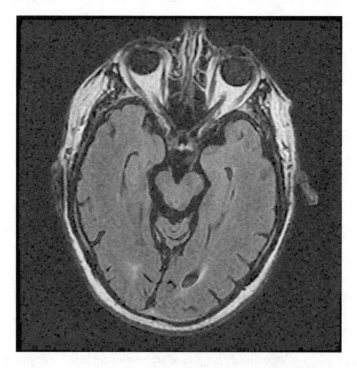

Fig. 2. Axial FLAIR MR image in a patient with the corticobasal syndrome, showing asymmetric atrophy of the cerebral peduncles.

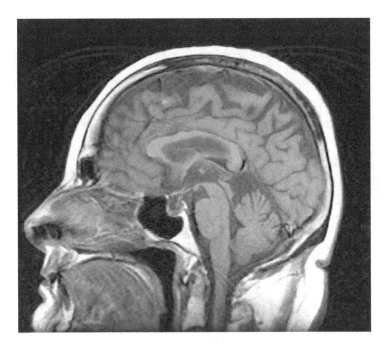

Fig. 3. Midsagittal T1-weighted MR image in a patient with the corticobasal syndrome, showing thinning of the corpus callosum where the projections between the parietal cortices traverse.

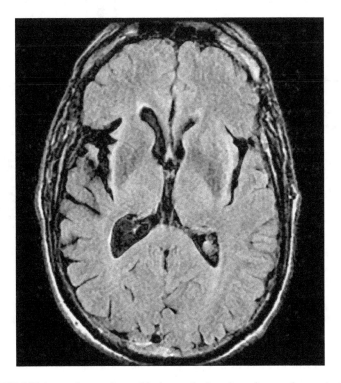

Fig. 4. Axial FLAIR MR image in a patient with the corticobasal syndrome, demonstrating the rare finding of increased signal lateral to the putamen.

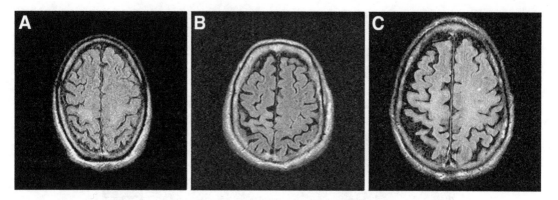

Fig. 5. Axial FLAIR MR images of three patients with the corticobasal syndrome, showing subtle, hazy increased signal in the subcortical posterior frontal/parietal white matter. The signal changes are asymmetric in **B** and **C**, but quite symmetric in **A** despite strikingly asymmetric clinical findings in all three patients.

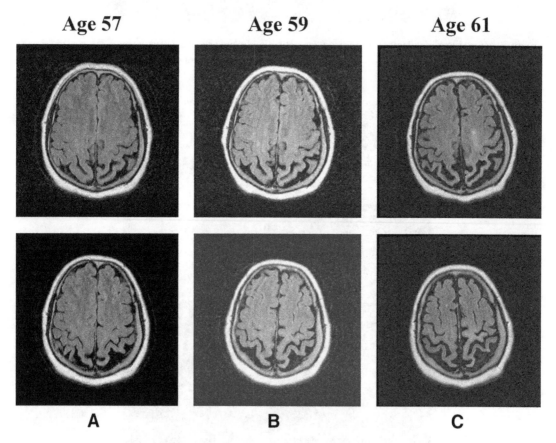

Fig. 6. Serial axial FLAIR MR images in a patient with the corticobasal syndrome. By age 61 (images in column **C**), she had also developed features of the Balint's syndrome.

Age 64   **Age 66**

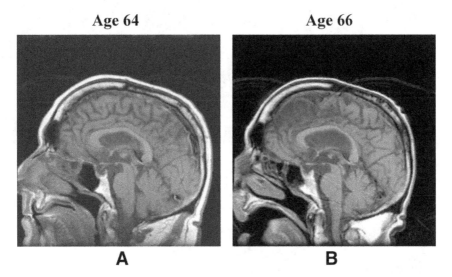

Fig. 7. Serial midsagittal MR images in a patient with the corticobasal syndrome. Note the progressive thinning of the posterior aspect of the corpus callosum (but sparing the splenium) and mild ventricular dilatation. The decreased signal along the mesial frontal region in B reflects evolving atrophy in this region.

Age 79   **Age 81**   **Age 82**

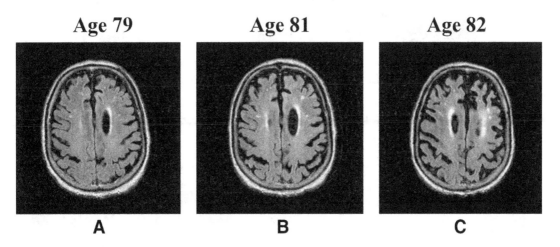

Fig. 8. Serial axial FLAIR MR images in a patient with features of frontotemporal dementia at age 79 (**A**), which then evolves to include nonfluent aphasia at age 81 (**B**) and corticobasal syndrome findings at age 82 (**C**).

matter, most often in superior frontal gyrus, superior parietal gyrus, pre- and postcentral gyri, and striatum (Fig. 17). Tau+ oligodendroglial coiled bodies are also common (Fig. 18). While achromatic, ballooned neurons that are immunoreactive to phosphorylated neurofilament or αB-crystallin are typically present in CBD (Fig. 19), their absence does not preclude the diagnosis of CBD if the appropriate tau+ lesions are present. These criteria have been validated (Litvan et al., in preparation).

These pathological features are indistinguishable from those in frontotemporal dementia and parkinsonism linked to chromosome 17 (FTDP-17) *(46)*. Thus, knowledge about the family history and molecular genetics is necessary to adequately classify cases with CBD-type pathology.

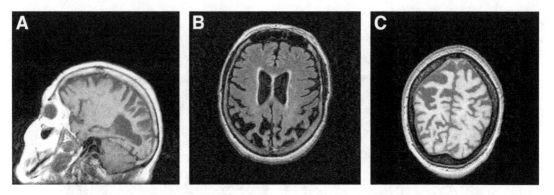

Fig. 9. Sagittal T1-weighted (**A**), axial FLAIR (**B**), and coronal T1-weighted (**C**) MR images in a patient who presented with the posterior cortical atrophy syndrome (i.e., Balint's syndrome, Gerstmann's syndrome, etc.) and subsequently developed classic corticobasal syndrome features.

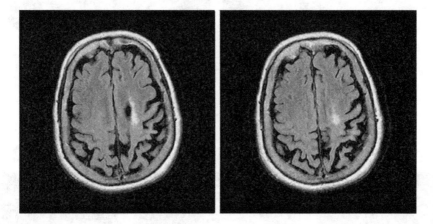

Fig. 10. Axial FLAIR MR images in a patient with the corticobasal syndrome, showing focal increased signal in the left posterior frontal white matter. Autopsy revealed corticobasal degeneration with significant tau-positive glial pathology in this region.

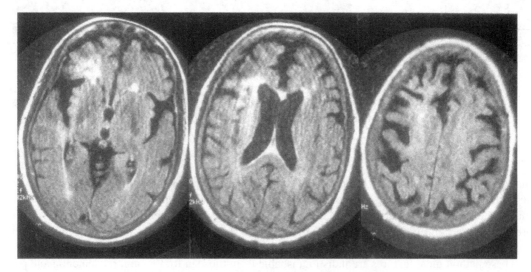

Fig. 11. Axial FLAIR MR images in a patient with the corticobasal syndrome, showing focal increased signal in the right frontal > parietal white matter. Autopsy revealed corticobasal degeneration with significant tau-positive glial pathology in this region.

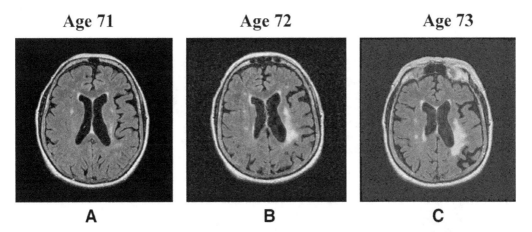

Fig. 12. Serial axial FLAIR MR images in a patient with the corticobasal syndrome, showing progressive focal increased signal evolving in the periventricular and subcortical white matter of the left parietal region.

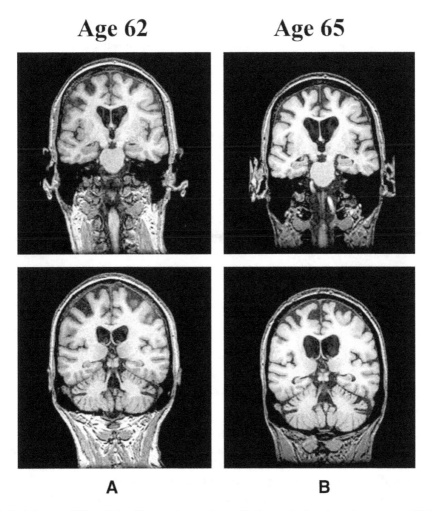

Fig. 13. Serial coronal T1-weighted images in a patient with the corticobasal syndrome at age 62 (**A**) and age 65 (**B**). Despite striking progression in her asymmetric CBS findings, note the rather mild and minimally progressive cerebral cortical atrophy over the frontal convexities. Mild progressive ventricular dilatation is evident, but the hippocampi do not appear significantly atrophic. This patient had progressive supranuclear palsy at autopsy.

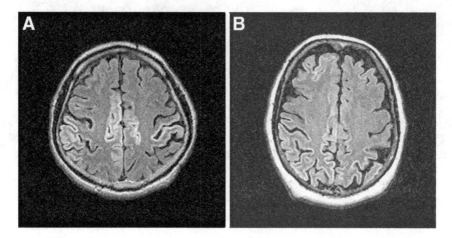

Fig. 14. Axial FLAIR MR images in two patients with the corticobasal syndrome. The patient in **A** has had a 3-yr course and is still alive, whereas the patient in **B** died after a 14-mo course. Note the striking increased signal along the cortical ribbon in the posterior frontal/parietal regions in both patients. Autopsy in patient B revealed Creutzfeldt–Jakob disease.

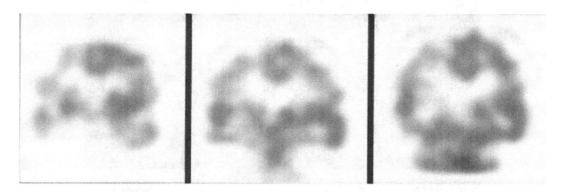

Fig. 15. Coronal single photon emission computed tomography (SPECT) images in a patient with the corticobasal syndrome. Note the hypoperfusion in the right frontoparietal > temporal cortex as well as basal ganglia and thalamus. Autopsy confirmed corticobasal degeneration in this patient.

CLINICAL FEATURES OF CORTICOBASAL DEGENERATION: THE DISEASE

There are few reports in which the clinical features in pathologically proven CBD have been characterized. Caselli et al. found subtle differences in kinematic abnormalities in a pathologically proven case of CBD compared to a patient with CBS who had AD pathology *(19)*. The speech and language abnormalities associated with pathologically confirmed CBD have recently been described *(73)*. Symptoms and signs of speech or language dysfunction were among the presenting features in over half of the patients in this series. Among these 13 cases, the features included dysarthria (*n* = 4; hypokinetic, spastic, ataxic, and mixed forms), apraxia of speech (*n* = 5), and aphasia (*n* = 7; fluent, nonfluent, and mixed forms). Hence, speech and language dysfunction is common in CBD, and the findings include variable degrees of dysarthria, apraxia of speech, and aphasia *(73)*.

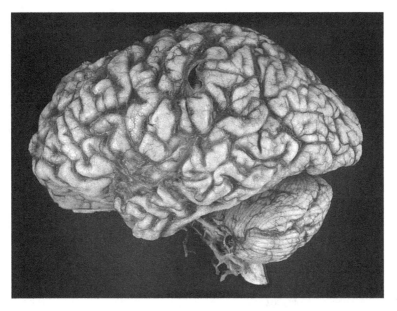

Fig. 16. Photograph of the brain of a patient with corticobasal degeneration who had exhibited classic corticobasal syndrome features antemortem. Note the cortical atrophy is maximal in the posterior frontal and parietal region. Courtesy Joseph E. Parisi, MD, Mayo Clinic, Rochester, Minnesota.

Fig. 17. Photomicrograph of parietal cortex with tau immunocytochemistry (×20) in a patient with corticobasal degeneration. Note the tau-positive threads and clusters of tau-positive astrocytes ("astrocytic plaques") typical of CBD. Courtesy Joseph E. Parisi, MD, Mayo Clinic, Rochester, Minnesota.

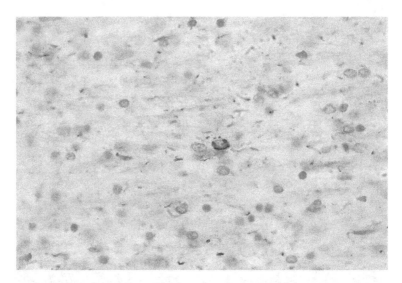

Fig. 18. Photomicrograph of subcortical frontal white matter with tau immunocytochemistry (x60) in a patient with corticobasal degeneration. Note the coiled or comma-shaped appearance of the inclusion characteristic of an "oligodendroglial coiled body." Courtesy Joseph E. Parisi, MD, Mayo Clinic, Rochester, Minnesota.

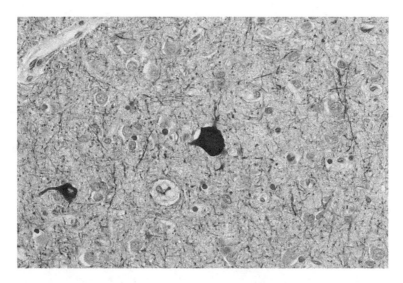

Fig. 19. Photomicrograph of parietal cortex with phosphorylated-neurofilament immunocytochemistry (×60) in a patient with corticobasal degeneration. Note the intense staining in a "ballooned" neuron typical of CBD. Courtesy Joseph E. Parisi, MD, Mayo Clinic, Rochester, Minnesota.

Table 6

Pathologic Diagnoses in 36 Consecutive Autopsied Cases at the Mayo Clinic With the Corticobasal Syndrome

Diagnosis	No. of cases
Corticobasal degeneration	18
Progressive supranuclear palsy	6
Alzheimer's disease	4
Creutzfeldt–Jakob disease	3
Nonspecific degenerative changes	3
Pick's disease	1
Combined Alzheimer's disease/Pick's disease	1

Table 7

Clinical Diagnoses in 32 Consecutive Autopsied Cases at the Mayo Clinic With Pathologically Proven CBD

Initial Clinical Diagnosis		Final Clinical Diagnosis
10	Corticobasal degeneration	18	Corticobasal degeneration
6	Atypical Parkinson's disease	7	Progressive supranuclear palsy
6	Dementia/Alzheimer's disease	4	Primary progressive aphasia
4	Primary progressive aphasia	1	Alzheimer's disease
2	Progressive supranuclear palsy	1	Dementia with Lewy bodies
1	Dementia with Lewy bodies	1	Marchiafava–Bignami disease
1	Marchiafava–Bignami disease		
1	Multiple sclerosis		
1	Stroke		

The disorder of CBD can also present as several clinical syndromes. In addition to the CBS, the reported focal/asymmetric cortical degeneration syndromes associated with CBD pathology include frontotemporal dementia (74–77), a progressive aphasia syndrome (fluent and nonfluent subtypes) (76–81), and posterior cortical atrophy (with some or all features of the Balint's syndrome) (82). Some patients have been diagnosed antemortem as probable AD (30, 77). In fact, dementia was the most common presentation of CBD in one series (30). Many patients have had clinical findings indistinguishable from PSP (44,83–88). One patient presented with apraxia of speech and subsequently developed more typical CBD features (33). Another presented with obsessive-compulsive features and visual inattention (89). Hence, from the clinicopathologic perspective, CBD is a heterogeneous disorder.

CLINICOPATHOLOGIC HETEROGENEITY

Although the early literature on CBD suggested it was a distinct clinicopathologic entity, numerous case reports and small series clearly indicates considerable clinicopathologic heterogeneity in the CBS and CBD–the disease. An updated review of this heterogeneity from one institution (43,90) is shown in Tables 6 and 7. Thus, the following disorders can underlie the CBS: CBD, AD, Pick's disease, PSP, dementia lacking distinctive histopathology, and Creutzfeldt–Jakob disease (43), as well as dementia with Lewy bodies (91), motor neuron inclusion body dementia (92), and neurofilament inclusion body dementia (93). As noted above, CBD can present clinically as the CBS, dementia (not otherwise specified), primary progressive aphasia, frontotemporal dementia, posterior cortical atro-

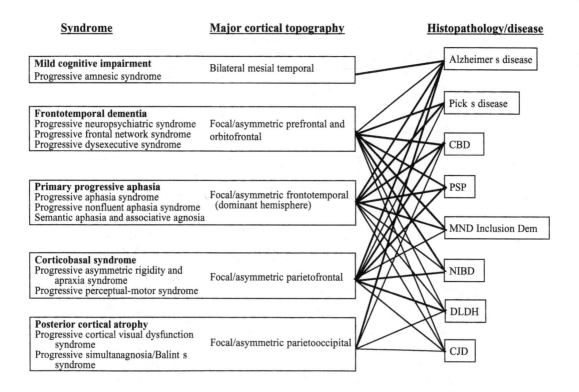

Fig. 20. Note the close syndrome-topography association for each syndrome, but the variable associated histopathologies for each syndrome. Darker lines signify associations that occur more frequently. Abbreviations: CBD, corticobasal degeneration; CJD, Creutzfeldt-Jacob disease; DLB, dementia with Lewy bodies; DLDH, dementia lacking distinctive histopathology; MND Inclusion Dem, motor neuron disease inclusion dementia; NIBD, neurofilament inclusion body dementia; PSP, progressive supranuclear palsy. Adapted from ref. *99.*

phy, and progressive speech apraxia. Some patients often present with one of these focal cortical degeneration syndromes and subsequently develop features overlapping with one or more syndromes *(8,9).* Hence, it is now clear that in the CBS—like in the other focal/asymmetric cortical degeneration syndromes *(11,94,95)*—the clinical presentation and progression of symptoms reflect the topographic distribution of histopathology more so than the specific underlying disease. Furthermore, CBD has a variable pattern of cerebral cortical pathology, and the topographic distribution of pathology dictates the clinical presentation. A summary of the clinicopathologic correlations in the focal/asymmetric cortical degeneration syndromes is shown in Fig. 20. As therapies are developed that specifically target amyloid, tau, prion protein, synuclein, etc., pathophysiology, particularly if any such therapies have toxic side effects, improving the diagnostic accuracy of patients with the CBS and other focal/ asymmetric cortical degeneration syndromes will become increasingly important.

DIAGNOSTIC ACCURACY

The clinicopathologic heterogeneity in CBS and CBD has led to relatively poor sensitivity and specificity for the diagnosis of CBD. As shown in Tables 6 and 7, among 36 consecutive patients with clinically suspected CBD (i.e., the CBS) who underwent autopsy, only half were found to have underlying CBD (specificity of the CBS for CBD = 50%). Furthermore, among 32 patients with pathologically proven CBD, only 18 exhibited the CBS (sensitivity of the CBS for CBD = 56%). Other investigators found high sensitivity but low specificity in the clinical diagnosis of CBD *(96).* This poor sensitivity and specificity has clearly stymied research in this area. However, if one views the disorders as they relate to the putative dysfunctional protein, the specificity of the CBS for the tauopathies (considering AD as an amyloidopathy for this calculation) is 69%. Since some therapies that affect tau pathophysiology may have efficacy for any of the tauopathies, delineation of the specific histopathologic disorder may not be as important determining whether patients have a tauopathy underlying their symptoms. Clearly, biomarkers that are more sensitive and specific for CBD as well as the other tauopathies are needed.

PATHOPHYSIOLOGY

Several lines of evidence point toward dysfunction in microtubule-associated tau as a primary factor in the pathogenesis of CBD. The inclusions in glia and neurons are immunoreactive to tau *(46)*. The pathology of CBD has been associated with mutations in tau *(97)*. Transgenic mice with the P301L mutation have exhibited clinical and neuropathologic findings similar to humans *(98)*. Hyperphosphorylation of tau disrupts binding to microtubules. Further characterization of the cascade of events involved in tau dysfunction and neurodegeneration will be critical to ultimately develop therapy.

MANAGEMENT

Since no therapy yet exists for CBD that affects the neurodegenerative process, management must be tailored toward symptoms. Pharmacotherapy directed toward parkinsonism has been disappointing *(29)*. Levodopa, dopamine agonists, and baclofen tend to have little effect on rigidity, spasticity, bradykinesia, or tremor. However, levodopa should be titrated upward as tolerated to at least 750 mg per day in divided doses on an empty stomach to provide an adequate trial. Some patients have noted significant improvement in parkinsonism but this rarely persists beyond several months. In those who do improve dramatically with levodopa therapy, one must question whether CBD is the underlying disorder, as levodopa-refractory parkinsonism is considered by many to be a characteristic feature of the CBS and CBD. Anticholinergic agents rarely improve dystonia, and their use is limited by side effects. Botulinum toxin can alleviate pain owing to focal dystonia. Central pain has been rare, but some patients have responded to gabapentin. Tremor may respond initially to propranolol or primidone, but their effects wane with progression of the disorder. Clonazepam and/or gabapentin may reduce myoclonus in some cases. Although intuitively one would not consider any of the cholinesterase inhibitors to be beneficial in this disorder, we have seen rare cases who note improvement in psychomotor speed, concentration, and problem-solving abilities with donepezil, rivastigmine, or galantamine. Vitamin E and other antioxidant agents have been tried in hopes of delaying progression of the disorder, but there is no evidence yet supporting a disease-altering effect.

Because of the poor response to pharmacotherapy, the mainstay of management is therefore physical, occupational, and speech therapies. A home assessment by an occupational therapist can aid in determining which changes could be made to facilitate functional independence (e.g., replacing rotating doorknobs with handles; attaching specially formed pads around the handles of eating utensils and toothbrushes; purchasing clothing with velcro instead of buttons or laces, etc.). Passive range of motion (ROM) exercises minimize development of contractures, and all caregivers should be instructed to provide passive ROM exercises daily. In those who develop dystonic flexion of the hand musculature to form a "fisted hand," the fingernails can become imbedded in the palmar tissue leading to cellulitis and even osteomyelitis of the hand. One can avoid this by clipping the fingernails periodically, and by placing a rolled-up washcloth or hand towel in the palm of the hand. All patients experience gait impairment at some point during their illness. A walker with handbrakes can improve ambulation for some patients. Wheelchair and handicap priviledges are warranted in essentially every patient. Use of a bedside commode is also worthwhile. Apraxia is often the most debilitating feature of the disorder, and this feature can complicate one's ability to operate a wheelchair or motorized scooter. However, many patients are able to learn to operate these devices and use them effectively for months or years. We have seen a few patients whose "useless hand" was "made useful" by employing constraint-induced movement therapy. Some third-party payers have denied coverage for these devices and therapies, which is very unfortunate as any element of functional improvement and independence is important for these patients. Speech therapy and communication devices can optimize communication when dysarthria, apraxia of speech, or aphasia is present. Therapists also counsel patients and families on swallowing maneuvers and food additives to minimize aspiration when dysphagia occurs. Feeding gastrostomy should be discussed with all patients, although many decide not to undergo this procedure.

Some patients with the CBS develop elements of other focal cortical degeneration syndromes, such that features of frontotemporal dementia (FTD), primary progressive aphasia (PPA), posterior cortical atrophy (PCA), or some combination of these can evolve. Also, patients who present with one of these syndromes can develop features of the CBS. Management of many of these non-CBS syndromes is discussed elsewhere *(99)*.

Other treatable comorbid illnesses must also be considered, most notably infections (e.g., pneumonia and urinary tract infections), psychiatric disorders, and sleep disorders. Although psychotic features rarely occur in the CBS, depression evolves in essentially every patient, likely owing in part to the preserved insight that is also characteristic of the disorder. Sleep disorders such as obstructive sleep apnea, central sleep apnea, restless legs syndrome, periodic limb movement disorder, etc. occur with some frequency in the CBS, and treatment can improve quality of life *(100)*. REM sleep behavior disorder is very rare in the CBS; in fact if it is present, one must suspect some contribution of synucleinopathy pathology *(101)*. Despite the difficulties of manipulating the headgear as part of nasal continuous positive airway pressure (CPAP) therapy owing to the limb apraxia, CPAP therapy for obstructive sleep apnea can be tolerated and used effectively in many patients. Patients and caregivers eventually require assistance in maintaining optimal care, which can be provided either through home health care or in a skilled nursing facility.

FUTURE DIRECTIONS

Clearly, with the CBS being no more than 60% sensitive and specific for CBD–the disease, further research in improving the antemortem diagnosis of CBD is necessary. No consensus yet exists for the diagnosis of the CBS. Further characterization of the natural history of patients with the CBS involving serial assessments of clinical, laboratory, neuropsychologic, and radiologic features is very important, as this information will be necessary to design future drug trials, particularly if agents active against tau pathophysiology are developed. Debate continues regarding whether CBD and PSP are variants of the same pathophysiologic process or distinctly separate disorders, and this warrants clarification. Additional studies on the rare kindreds with the clinical features of CBS *(20,102)* and/or pathologic features of CBD *(13)*, whether associated with mutations in tau (i.e., FTDP-17) or not, may offer key insights as other genes impacting tau pathophysiology have yet to be identified. Finally, patients and their families should be encouraged to access sources of information and support as well as participate in research.

MAJOR ISSUES TO BE STUDIED IN THE FUTURE:

- Establish consensus criteria for the diagnosis of the CBS.
- Identify which clinical, laboratory, neuropsychologic, and neuroradiologic features are most predictive of underlying CBD in the CBS.
- Characterize the natural history of clinical, laboratory, neuropsychologic, and neuroradiologic findings in patients with the CBS to design future drug trials.
- Determine if CBD and PSP are distinct disorders or variants of the same pathophysiologic process.
- Identify kindreds with familial CBS and/or CBD.
- Identify genetic mechanisms involved in CBS and CBD pathogenesis.

WEBSITES

The Association for Frontotemporal Dementias Corticobasal Degeneration
http://www.ftd-picks.org/?p=diseases/corticobasaldegeneration
Caregivers Guide to Cortical Basal Ganglionic Degeneration (CBGD)
http://www.tornadodesign.com/cbgd/

NINDS Corticobasal Degeneration Information Page
http://www.ninds.nih.gov/health_and_medical/disorders/cortico_doc.htm

WEMOVE - Corticobasal Degeneration
http://www.wemove.org/cbd.html

Parkinson's Institute on Corticobasal Degeneration
http://www.parkinsonsinstitute.org/movement_disorders/corticobasal.html

ACKNOWLEDGMENTS

Supported by grants AG06786, AG16574, and AG17216 from the National Institute on Aging.

This author thanks his many colleagues for their ongoing support and collaborations in CBD research, and particularly extends his appreciation to the patients and their families for participating in research on CBD.

REFERENCES

1. Rebeiz J, Kolodny E, Richardson E. Corticodentatonigral degeneration with neuronal achromasia: a progressive disorder of late adult life. Trans Am Neurol Assoc 1967;92:23–26.
2. Rebeiz J, Kolodny E, Richardson E. Corticodentatonigral degeneration with neuronal achromasia. Arch Neurol 1968;18:20–33.
3. Boeve B, Lang A, Litvan I. Corticobasal degeneration and its relationship to progressive supranuclear palsy and frontotemporal dementia. Ann Neurol 2003;54:S15–S19.
4. Lippa C, Smith T, Fontneau N. Corticonigral degeneration with neuronal achromasia: a clinicopathologic study of two cases. J Neurol Sci 1990;98:301–310.
5. Lang A, Riley D, Bergeron C. Cortical-basal ganglionic degeneration. In: Calne D, ed. Neurodegenerative Diseases. Philadelphia: Saunders, 1994:877–894.
6. Riley D, Lang A. Corticobasal ganglionic degeneration (CBGD): further observations in six additional cases. Neurology 1988;38(Supp 1):360.
7. Gibb W, Luthert P, Marsden C. Corticobasal degeneration. Brain 1989;112:1171–1192.
8. Kertesz A, Martinez-Lage P, Davidson W, Munoz DG. The corticobasal degeneration syndrome overlaps progressive aphasia and frontotemporal dementia. Neurology 2000;55(9):1368–1375.
9. Kertesz A, Davidson W, Munoz D. Clinical and pathological overlap between frontotemporal dementia, primary progressive aphasia and corticobasal degeneration: the Pick complex. Dement Geriatr Cogn Disord 1999;10(Suppl 1):46–49.
10. Boeve B. Corticobasal Degeneration. In: Adler C, Ahlskog J, eds. Parkinson's Disease and Movement Disorders: Diagnosis and Treatment Guidelines for the Practicing Physician. Totawa, NJ: Humana, 2000:253–261.
11. Caselli R. Focal and asymmetric cortical degeneration syndromes. The Neurologist 1995;1:1–19.
12. Riley D, Lang A, Lewis A, Resch L, Ashby P, Hornykiewicz O, et al. Cortical-basal ganglionic degeneration. Neurology 1990;40:1203–1212.
13. Boeve B, Parisi J, Dickson D, Baker M, Hutton M, Wszolek Z, et al. Familial dementia/parkinsonism/motor neuron disease with corticobasal degeneration pathology but absence of a tau mutation. Neurobiol Aging 2002;23:S269.
14. Bower J, Maraganore D, McDonnell S, Rocca W. Incidence and distribution of parkinsonism in Olmsted County, Minnesota, 1976-1990. Neurology 1999;52:1214–1220.
15. Rinne J, Lee M, Thompson P, Marsden C. Corticobasal degeneration: a clinical study of 36 cases. Brain 1994;117:1183–1196.
16. Wenning G, Litvan I, Jankovic J, Granata R, Mangone C, McKee A, et al. Natural history and survival of 14 patients with corticobasal degeneration confirmed at postmortem examination. J Neurol Neurosurg Psychiatry 1998;64:184–189.
17. Litvan I, Goetz C, Lang A, eds. Corticobasal Degeneration and Related Disorders. Phildelphia: Lippincott, Williams & Wilkins, 2000.
18. Leiguarda R, Lees A, Merello M, Starkstein S, Marsden C. The nature of apraxia in corticobasal degeneration. J Neurol Neurosurg Psychiatry 1994;57:455–459.

19. Caselli R, Stelmach G, Caviness J, Timmann D, Royer T, Boeve B, et al. A kinematic study of progressive apraxia with and without dementia. Mov Disord 1999;14:276–287.

20. Boeve BF, Maraganore DM, Parisi JE, Ivnik RJ, Westmoreland BF, Dickson DW, et al. Corticobasal degeneration and frontotemporal dementia presentations in a kindred with nonspecific histopathology. Dem Geriatr Cog Disord 2002;13(2):80–90.

21. Ball J, Lantos P, Jackson M, Marsden C, Scadding J, Rossor M. Alien hand sign in association with Alzheimer's histopathology. J Neurol Neurosurg Psychiatry 1993;56:1020–1023.

22. Doody R, Jankovic J. The alien hand and related signs. J Neurol Neurosurg Psychiatry 1992;55:806–810.

23. Feinberg T, Schindler R, Flanagan N, Haber L. Two alien hand syndromes. Neurology 1992;42:19–24.

24. Gasquoine P. Alien hand sign. J Clin Exp Neuropsychol 1993;15:653–667.

25. Goldberg G, Bloom K. The alien hand sign: localization, lateralization and recovery. Am J Phys Med & Rehabil 1990;69:228–238.

26. Thompson P, Day B, Rothwell J, Brown P, Britton T, Marsden C. The myoclonus in corticobasal degeneration: evidence for two forms of cortical reflex myoclonus. Brain 1994;117:1197–1207.

27. Thompson PD, Shibasaki H. Myoclonus in corticobasal degeneration and other neurodegenerations. Adv Neurol 2000;82:69–81.

28. Gottlieb D, Robb K, Day B. Mirror movements in the alien hand syndrome. Am J Phys Med Rehabil 1992;71:297–300.

29. Kompoliti K, Goetz C, Boeve B, Maraganore D, Ahlskog J, Marsden C, et al. Clinical presentation and pharmacological therapy in corticobasal degeneration. Arch Neurol 1998;55:957–961.

30. Grimes DA, Lang AE, Bergeron CB. Dementia as the most common presentation of cortical-basal ganglionic degeneration. Neurology 1999;53(9):1969–1974.

31. Frattali C, Duffy J, Litvan I, Patsalides A, Grafman J. Yes/no reversals as neurobehavioral sequela: a disorder of language, praxis, or inhibitory control? Eur J Neurol 2003;10:103–106.

32. Frattali CM, Grafman J, Patronas N, Makhlouf F, Litvan I. Language disturbances in corticobasal degeneration. Neurology. 2000;54(4):990–992.

33. Lang A. Cortical basal ganglionic degeneration presenting with "progressive loss of speech output and orofacial dyspraxia." J Neurol Neurosurg Psychiatry 1992;55:1101.

34. Litvan I, Cummings J, Mega M. Neuropsychiatric features of corticobasal degeneration. J Neurol Neurosurg Psychiat 1998;65:717–721.

35. Cummings J, Litvan I. Neuropsychiatric aspects of corticobasal degeneration. In: Litvan I, Goetz C, Lang A, eds. Corticobasal Degeneration and Related Disorders. Philadelphia: Lippincott Williams & Wilkins, 2000, 147–152.

36. McKeith IG, Galasko D, Kosaka K, Perry EK, Dickson DW, Hansen LA, et al. Consensus guidelines for the clinical and pathologic diagnosis of dementia with Lewy bodies (DLB): report of the consortium on DLB international workshop. Neurology 1996;47(5):1113–1124.

37. Geda Y, Boeve B, Parisi J, Dickson D, Maraganore D, Ahlskog J, et al. Neuropsychiatric features in 20 cases of pathologically-diagnosed corticobasal degeneration. Mov Disord 2000;15(Suppl 3):229.

38. Maraganore D, Ahlskog J, Petersen R. Progressive asymmetric rigidity with apraxia: a distinct clinical entity [abstract]. Mov Disord 1992;7(Supp 1):80.

39. Kumar R, Bergeron C, Pollanen M, Lang A. Cortical-basal ganglionic degeneration. In: Jankovic J, Tolosa E, eds. Parkinson's Disease and Movement Disorders, 3rd ed. Baltimore: Williams & Wilkins, 1998:297–316.

40. McKhann G, Drachman D, Folstein M, Katzman R, Price D, Stadlan E. Clinical diagnosis of Alzheimer's disease: report of the NINCDS–ADRDA work group under the auspices of the Department of Health and Human Services Task Force on Alzheimer's disease. Neurology 1984;34:939–944.

41. Litvan I, Agid Y, Calne D, et al. Clinical research criteria for the diagnosis of progressive supranuclear palsy (Steele–Richardson–Olszewski syndrome): report of the NINDS–SPSP International Workshop. Neurology 1996;47:1–9.

42. Movement Disorders Symposium on Cortical-Basal Ganglionic Degeneration and Other Asymmetric Cortical Degeneration Syndromes. Mov Disord 1996;11:346–357.

43. Boeve BF, Maraganore DM, Parisi JE, Ahlskog JE, Graff-Radford N, Caselli RJ, et al. Pathologic heterogeneity in clinically diagnosed corticobasal degeneration. Neurology 1999;53(4):795–800.

44. Schneider J, Watts R, Gearing M, Brewer R, Mirra S. Corticobasal degeneration: neuropathologic and clinical heterogeneity. Neurology 1997;48:959–969.

45. Neary D, Snowden J, Gustafson L, Passant U, Stuss D, Black S, et al. Frontotemporal lobar degeneration: a consensus on clinical diagnostic criteria. Neurology 1998;51:1546–1554.

46. Dickson D, Bergeron C, Chin S, Duyckaerts C, Horoupian D, Ikeda K, et al. Office of Rare Diseases neuropathologic criteria for corticobasal degeneration. J Neuropathol Exp Neurol 2002;61:935–946.

47. Houlden H, Baker M, Morris H, MacDonald N, Pickering-Brown S, Adamson J, et al. Corticobasal degeneration and progressive supranuclear palsy share a common tau haplotype. Neurology 2001;56:1702–1706.

48. Urakami K, Wada K, Arai H, Sasaki H, Kanai M, Shoji M, et al. Diagnostic significance of tau protein in cerebrospinal fluid from patients with corticobasal degeneration or progressive supranuclear palsy. J Neurol Sci 2001;183:95–98.

49. Pillon B, Blin J, Vidailhet M, Deweer B, Sirigu A, Dubois B, et al. The neuropsychological pattern of corticobasal degeneration: comparison with progressive supranuclear palsy and Alzheimer's disease. Neurology 1995;45:1477–1483.
50. Massman P, Kreiter K, Jankovic J, Doody R. Neuropsychological functioning in cortical-basal ganglionic degeneration: differentiation from Alzheimer's disease. Neurology 1996;46:720–726.
51. Westmoreland B, Boeve B, Maraganore D, Ahlskog J. The EEG in cortical-basal ganglionic degeneration. Mov Disord 1996;11:352.
52. Westmoreland B, Boeve B, Parisi J, Dickson D, Maraganore D, Ahlskog J, et al. Electroencephalographic findings in clinically- and/or pathologically-diagnosed corticobasal degeneration. Mov Disord 2000;15(Suppl 3):229.
53. Strafella A, Ashby P, Lang A. Reflex myoclonus in cortical-basal ganglionic degeneration involves a transcortical pathway. Mov Disord 1997;12:360–369.
54. Hauser RA, Murtaugh FR, Akhter K, Gold M, Olanow CW. Magnetic resonance imaging of corticobasal degeneration. J Neuroimaging 1996;6(4):222–226.
55. Ballan G, Tison F, Dousset V, Vidailhet M, Agid Y, Henry P. Study of cortical atrophy with magnetic resonance imaging in corticobasal degeneration. Rev Neurolog 1998;154(3):224–227.
56. Frasson E, Moretto G, Beltramello A, Smania N, Pampanin M, Stegagno C, et al. Neuropsychological and neuroimaging correlates in corticobasal degeneration. Ital J Neurol Sci 1998;19(5):321–328.
57. Soliveri P, Monza D, Paridi D, Radice D, Grisoli M, Testa D, et al. Cognitive and magnetic resonance imaging aspects of corticobasal degeneration and progressive supranuclear palsy. Neurology 1999;53(3):502–507.
58. Schrag A, Good CD, Miszkiel K, Morris HR, Mathias CJ, Lees AJ, et al. Differentiation of atypical parkinsonian syndromes with routine MRI. Neurology 2000;54(3):697–702.
59. Savoiardo M, Grisoli M, Girotti F. Magnetic resonance imaging in CBD, related atypical parkinsonian disorders, and dementias. Adv Neurol 2000;82:197–208.
60. Yamauchi H, Fukuyama H, Nagahama Y, Katsumi Y, Dong Y, Hayashi T, et al. Atrophy of the corpus callosum, cortical hypometabolism, and cognitive impairment in corticobasal degeneration. Arch Neurol 1998;55(5):609–614.
61. Macia F, Yekhlef F, Ballan G, Delmer O, Tison F. T2-hyperintense lateral rim and hypointense putamen are typical but not exclusive of multiple system atrophy. Arch Neurol 2001;58:1024–1026.
62. Winkelmann J, Auer DP, Lechner C, Elbel G, Trenkwalder C. Magnetic resonance imaging findings in corticobasal degeneration. Mov Disord 1999;14(4):669–673.
63. Doi T, Iwasa K, Makifuchi T, Takamori M. White matter hyperintensities on MRI in a patient with corticobasal degeneration. Acta Neurol Scand 1999;99(3):199–201.
64. Josephs K, Tang-Wai D, Boeve B, Knopman D, Dickson D, Parisi J, et al. Clinicopathologic and imaging correlates in corticobasal degeneration. Neurology 2002;58:A132.
65. Sawle G, Brooks D, Marsden C, Frackowiak R. Corticobasal degeneration: a unique pattern of regional cortical oxygen hypometabolism and striatal fluorodopa uptake demonstrated by positron emission tomography. Brain 1991;114:541–556.
66. Blin J, Vidailhet M-J, Pillon B, Dubois B, Feve J-R, Agid Y. Corticobasal degeneration: decreased and asymmetrical glucose consumption as studied with PET. Mov Disord 1992;4:348–354.
67. Brooks DJ. Functional imaging studies in corticobasal degeneration. Adv Neurol 2000;82:209–215.
68. Okuda B, Tachibana H, Kawabata K, Takeda M, Sugita M. Comparison of brain perfusion in corticobasal degeneration and Alzheimer's disease. Dem Geriatr Cog Disord 2001;12(3):226–231.
69. Pirker W, Asenbaum S, Bencsits G, Prayer D, Gerschlager W, Deecke L, et al. beta-CIT SPECT in multiple system atrophy, progressive supranuclear palsy, and corticobasal degeneration. Mov Disord 2000;15(6):1158–1167.
70. Okuda B, Tachibana H, Kawabata K, Takeda M, Sugita M. Cerebral blood flow in corticobasal degeneration and progressive supranuclear palsy. Alz Dis Assoc Disord 2000;14(1):46–52.
71. Zhang L, Murata Y, Ishida R, Saitoh Y, Mizusawa H, Shibuya H. Differentiating between progressive supranuclear palsy and corticobasal degeneration by brain perfusion SPET. Nucl Med Commun 2001;22(7):767–772.
72. Hauser M, Mullan B, Boeve B, Maraganore D, Ahlskog J, Parisi J, et al. SPECT findings in clinically- and/or pathologically-diagnosed corticobasal degeneration. Mov Disord 2000;15(Suppl 3):221.
73. Lehman M, Duffy J, Boeve B, Parisi J, Dickson D, Maraganore D, et al. Speech and language disorders associated with corticobasal degeneration. J Med Speech Lang Dis 2003;11:131–146.
74. Lerner A, Friedland R, Riley D, Whitehouse P, Lanska D, Vick N, et al. Dementia with pathological findings of cortical-basal ganglionic degeneration. Ann Neurol 1992;32:271.
75. Lennox G, Jackson M, Lowe J. Corticobasal degeneration manifesting as a frontal lobe dementia. Ann Neurol 1994;36:273–274.
76. Boeve B, Maraganore D, Parisi J, Ahlskog J, Graff-Radford N, Muenter M, et al. Clinical heterogeneity in patients with pathologically diagnosed cortical-basal ganglionic degeneration. Mov Disord 1996;11:351–352.
77. Boeve B, Parisi J, Maraganore D, Ahlskog J, Caselli R, Graff-Radford N, et al. Clinicopathologic heterogeneity in clinically- and/or pathologically-diagnosed cortical-basal ganglionic degeneration. J Neurol Sci 1997;150:S109–S110.
78. Lippa C, Cohen R, Smith T, Drachman D. Primary progressive aphasia with focal neuronal achromasia. Neurology 1991;41:882–886.

79. Arima K, Uesugi H, Fujita I, Sakurai Y, Oyanagi S, Andoh S, et al. Corticonigral degeneration with neuronal achromasia presenting with primary progressive aphasia: ultrastructural and immunocytochemical studies. J Neurol Sci 1994;127:186–197.

80. Ikeda K, Akiyama H, Iritani S, Kase K, Arai T, Niizato K, et al. Corticobasal degeneration with primary progressive aphasia and accentuated cortical lesion in superior temporal gyrus: case report and review. Acta Neuropathol 1996;92:534–539.

81. Sakurai Y, Hashida H, Uesugi H, Arima K, Murayama S, Bando M, et al. A clinical profile of corticobasal degeneration presenting as primary progressive aphasia. European Neurology 1996;36(3):134–137.

82. Tang-Wai D, Josephs K, Boeve B, Dickson D, Parisi J, Petersen R. Pathologically confirmed corticobasal degeneration presenting with visuospatial dysfunction. Neurology 2003;61:1134–1135.

83. Boeve B, Maraganore D, Parisi J, Ahlskog J, Muenter M, Graff-Radford N, et al. Disorders mimicking the "classical" clinical syndrome of cortical-basal ganglionic degeneration: report of nine cases. Movement Disorders 1996;11:351.

84. Davis P, Bergeron C, McLachlan D. Atypical presentation of progressive supranuclear palsy. Ann Neurol 1985;17:337–343.

85. Ford B, Fahn S. 60-year-old woman with parkinsonism and unilateral dystonia. Mov Disord 1996;11:355–356.

86. Gearing M, Olson D, Watts R, Mirra S. Progressive supranuclear palsy: neuropathologic and clinical heterogeneity. Neurology 1994;44:1015–1024.

87. Saint-Hilaire M-H, Handler J, McKee A, Feldman R. Clinical overlap between corticobasal ganglionic degeneration and progressive supranuclear palsy. Mov Disord 1996;11:356.

88. Scully R, Mark E, McNeely W, McNeely B. Case records of the Massachusetts General Hospital (Case 46-1993). N Engl J Med 1993;329:1560–1567.

89. Rey GJ, Tomer R, Levin BE, Sanchez-Ramos J, Bowen B, Bruce JH. Psychiatric symptoms, atypical dementia, and left visual field inattention in corticobasal ganglionic degeneration. Mov Disord 1995;10(1):106–110.

90. Boeve B, Parisi J, Dickson D, Maraganore D, Ahlskog J, Graff-Radford N, et al. Demographic and clinical findings in 20 cases of pathologically-diagnosed corticobasal degeneration. Mov Disord 2000;15(Suppl 3):228.

91. Horoupian D, Wasserstein P. Alzheimer's disease pathology in motor cortex in dementia with Lewy bodies clinically mimicking corticobasal degeneration. Acta Neuropathol 1999;98:317–322.

92. Grimes DA, Bergeron CB, Lang AE. Motor neuron disease-inclusion dementia presenting as cortical-basal ganglionic degeneration. Mov Disord 1999;14(4):674–680.

93. Josephs K, Holton J, Rossor M, Braendgaard H, Ozawa T, Fox N, et al. Neurofilament inclusion body disease: a new proteinopathy? Brain 2003;126:2291–2303.

94. Caselli RJ. Asymmetric cortical degeneration syndromes. Curr Opin Neurol 1996;9(4):276–280.

95. Caselli R. Asymmetric cortical degeneration syndromes: clinicopathologic considerations. Mov Disord 1996;11:347–348.

96. Litvan I, Agid Y, Goetz C, et al. Accuracy of the clinical diagnosis of corticobasal degeneration: a clinicopathological study. Neurology 1997;48:119–125.

97. Reed L, Wszolek Z, Hutton M. Phenotypic correlations in FTDP-17. Neurobiol Aging 2001;22:89–107.

98. Lewis J, McGowan E, Rockwood J, Melrose H, Nacharaju P, Van Slegtenhorst M, et al. Neurofibrillary tangles, amyotrophy and progressive motor disturbance in mice expressing mutant (P301L) tau protein. Nat Genet 2000;25(4):402–405.

99. Boeve B. Diagnosis and management of the non-alzheimer dementias. In: Noseworthy JW, ed. Neurologic Therapeutics. London: Martin Dunitz, 2003:2826–2854.

100. Boeve B, Silber M. Sleep disorders and dementia and related degenerative disorders. In: Carney PR, Berry RB, Geyer J, eds. Sleep Medicine. Philadelphia: Lippincott Williams & Wilkins, 2003, in press.

101. Boeve B, Silber M, Ferman T, Lucas J, Parisi J. Association of REM sleep behavior disorder and neurodegenerative disease may reflect an underlying synucleinopathy. Mov Disord 2001;16:622–630.

102. Bugiani O, Murrell JR, Giaccone G, Hasegawa M, Ghigo G, Tabaton M, et al. Frontotemporal dementia and corticobasal degeneration in a family with a P301S mutation in tau. J Neuropathol Exp Neurol 1999;58(6):667–677.

20

Multiple System Atrophy

Felix Geser and Gregor K. Wenning

INTRODUCTION

Multiple system atrophy (MSA) is a sporadic neurodegenerative disorder characterized clinically by various combinations of parkinsonian, autonomic, cerebellar, or pyramidal symptoms and signs and pathologically by cell loss, gliosis, and glial cytoplasmic inclusions in several brain and spinal cord structures. The term MSA was introduced in 1969, however cases of MSA were previously reported under the rubrics of striatonigral degeneration, olivopontocerebellar atrophy, Shy–Drager syndrome and idiopathic orthostatic hypotension. In the late 1990s, α-synuclein immunostaining was recognized as most sensitive marker of inclusion pathology in MSA: because of these advances in molecular pathogenesis, MSA has been firmly established as α-synucleinopathy along with Parkinson's disease (PD) and dementia with Lewy bodies. Recent epidemiological surveys have shown that MSA is not a rare disorder (~5 cases per 100,000 population), and that misdiagnosis, especially with PD, is still common due to variable clinical presentations of MSA. However, the clinical picture of MSA in its full-blown form is distinctive. The patient is hypomimic with orofacial and anterior neck dystonia resulting in a grinning smile akin to "risus sardonicus" and sometimes disproportionate antecollis. The voice is often markedly impaired with a characteristic quivering high-pitched dysarthria. The motor disorder of MSA is often mixed with parkinsonism, cerebellar ataxia, limb dystonia, myoclonus, and pyramidal features occurring at the same time. However, akinesia and rigidity are the predominating features in 80% of patients, and cerebellar ataxia within the remaining 20%. According to the predominant motor presentation, MSA patients may be labeled as parkinsonian or cerebellar variant (MSA-P, MSA-C). The diagnosis of MSA is largely based on clinical expertise, and this is well illustrated by the consensus diagnostic criteria, which comprise clinical features only (divided into four domains including autonomic dysfunction, parkinsonism, cerebellar dysfunction, and corticospinal tract dysfunction). Nevertheless, several autonomic function, imaging, neurophysiological, and biochemical studies have been proposed in the last decade to help in the differential diagnosis of MSA. No drug treatment consistently benefits patients with this disease. Indeed, parkinsonism often shows a poor or unsustained response to chronic levodopa therapy, however, one-third of the patients may show a moderate-to-good dopaminergic response initially. There is no effective drug treatment for cerebellar ataxia. On the other hand, features of autonomic failure such as orthostatic hypotension, urinary retention or incontinence, constipation, and impotence, may often be relieved if recognized by the treating physician. Novel symptomatic and neuroprotective therapies are urgently required.

From: *Current Clinical Neurology: Atypical Parkinsonian Disorders*
Edited by: I. Litvan © Humana Press Inc., Totowa, NJ

EPIDEMIOLOGY

Descriptive Epidemiology

There are only a few descriptive epidemiological studies on MSA. Bower and colleagues reported the incidence of MSA over a 14-yr period in Olmsted County, Minnesota. Nine incident cases of MSA were identified, none of which had an onset before the age of 50 yr. The reported crude incidence rate was 0.6 cases per 100,000 population per year; when the age band >50 yr was examined, the estimate rose to 3 cases per 100,000 population *(1)*.

Estimates of the prevalence of MSA (per 100,000 in the population) in five studies were 1.9 *(2)*, 4.4 *(3)*, 2.3 *(4)*, 4.9 *(5)* and—in individuals over 65 yr—310 *(6)*. The last three studies did not specifically address the prevalence of MSA, the primary aim of the work being to assess the prevalence of PD. In the Western Europe population, estimated on the basis of Bower's study *(1)*, 81.5% of the cases are concentrated in the 60- to 79-yr age band, whereas only 9.8% and 8.7% fall within the 50- to 59-yr and >80-yr age bands, respectively. These figures indicate a prevalence of MSA that is quite similar to that of other well-known neurological conditions such as Huntington's disease, myotonic dystrophy, and motor neuron disease.

Analytical Epidemiology

So far no single environmental factor has been clearly established as conferring increased or reduced risks to develop MSA. Only one case-control study, based on 60 MSA cases and 60 controls, has been published to date *(7)*. This study revealed a higher risk of disease onset associated with occupational exposure to organic solvents, plastic monomers and additives, pesticides, and metals. Moreover, a higher frequency of symptoms and neurological diseases has been observed in first relatives of MSA cases than in controls. This last finding points to a genetic predisposition to neurological diseases. A review of consecutive medical records of 100 patients who satisfied the diagnostic Consensus criteria for MSA *(8)* showed that 11 patients had a notable history of heavy exposure to environmental toxins including malathion, diazinon, formaldehyde, *n*-hexane, benzene, methyl isobutyl ketone, and pesticides *(9)*. Despite its methodical limits, this study implicates environmental factors in the pathogenesis of MSA. Smoking was less common among MSA patients compared to controls according to a cross-sectional study *(10)*. Prospective case-control studies are needed to clarify whether smoking is a protective factor against MSA.

CLINICAL DIAGNOSTIC CRITERIA

Clinical diagnostic criteria for MSA were first proposed by Quinn in 1989 *(11)* and later slightly modified in 1994 *(12)*. According to this schema, patients are classified as either striatonigral degeneration (SND) or olivopontocerebellar atrophy (OPCA) type MSA depending on the predominance of parkinsonism or cerebellar ataxia. There are three levels of diagnostic probability: possible, probable, and definite. Patients with sporadic adult-onset poorly levodopa-responsive parkinsonism fulfill criteria for *possible* SND. The presence of other atypical features such as severe autonomic failure, cerebellar or pyramidal signs, or a pathological sphincter electromyogram (EMG) is required for a diagnosis of *probable* SND. Patients with sporadic late-onset predominant cerebellar ataxia with additional mild parkinsonism or pyramidal signs are considered *possible* OPCA-type MSA. This may result in confusion since some patients with possible OPCA may also qualify for probable SND provided predominant cerebellar ataxia is accompanied by parkinsonian features. A diagnosis of *probable* OPCA-type MSA requires the additional presence of severe autonomic failure or a pathological sphincter EMG. A definite diagnosis rests on neuropathological confirmation. Predominant SND- or OPCA-type presentations may be distinguished from pure types on the basis of associated cerebellar (predominant SND) or parkinsonian features (predominant OPCA). Since some degree of autonomic failure is present in almost all SND- and OPCA-type MSA patients *(13,14)* a further "autonomic" subtype (Shy–Drager syndrome) was not considered useful *(15)*. A number of exclusion criteria were also proposed: onset should be age 30 yr or more, and in order to exclude inherited adult-onset ataxias there should be no family history of MSA.

The validity of Quinn's criteria was evaluated in a clinicopathologic study by Litvan and coworkers. This study revealed the criteria for the diagnosis of MSA proposed by Quinn present a suboptimal specificity (79% for possible MSA and 97% for probable MSA, at the first visit), a low sensitivity (53% for possible MSA and 44% for probable MSA, at the first visit), and a predictive value of 30% for possible MSA and 68% for probable MSA *(16)*. Because of the suboptimal diagnostic accuracy of Quinn's criteria, in 1998 an International Consensus Conference promoted by the American Academy of Neurology was convened to develop new and optimized criteria for a clinical diagnosis of MSA (Table 1) *(8)*. The Consensus criteria are now widely used for a clinical diagnosis of MSA. These criteria specify three diagnostic categories of increasing certainty: possible, probable, and definite. The diagnosis of possible and probable MSA are based on the presence of clinical features listed in Table 1. In addition, exclusion criteria have to be considered. A definite diagnosis requires a typical neuropathological lesion pattern as well as deposition of α-synuclein-positive glial cytoplasmic inclusions.

A subsequent study analyzed the agreement between Quinn's criteria and Consensus criteria in a clinical series of 45 MSA patients. Concordance was moderate for possible MSA and substantial for probable MSA *(17)*. Moreover, four cases with probable ($n = 2$) or possible ($n = 2$) MSA according to Quinn's criteria were unclassifiable according to the Consensus criteria.

A recent retrospective evaluation of the Consensus criteria on pathologically proven cases showed excellent positive predictive values (PPVs) for both possible (93%) and probable MSA (100%) at the first clinic visit; however, sensitivity for probable MSA was poor especially in early stages of the disease (16% at the first clinic visit) *(18)*. Interestingly, the Consensus criteria and Quinn's criteria had similar PPVs. Whether the Consensus criteria will improve recognition of MSA patients especially in early disease stages needs to be investigated by prospective surveys with neuropathological confirmation in as many cases as possible.

ONSET AND PROGRESSION

MSA usually manifests in middle age (the median age of onset is 53), affects both sexes, and progresses relentlessly with a mean survival of 6–9 yr *(13,19,20)*. MSA patients may present with akinetic-rigid parkinsonism that usually responds poorly to levodopa. This has been identified as the most important early clinical discriminator of MSA and PD *(11,21–23)*, although a subgroup of MSA patients may show a good or, rarely, excellent, but usually short-lived, response to levodopa *(24–26)*. Progressive ataxia, mainly involving gait, may also be the presenting feature of MSA *(27,28)*. A cerebellar presentation of MSA appears to be more common than the parkinsonian variant in Japan compared to Western countries *(29)*. Autonomic failure with symptomatic orthostatic hypotension and/or urogenital and gastrointestinal disturbance may accompany the motor disorder in up to 50% of patients at disease onset *(20)*. Besides the poor response to levodopa, and the additional presence of pyramidal or cerebellar signs or autonomic failure as major diagnostic clues, certain other features ("red flags") such as orofacial dystonia, stridor, or disproportionate antecollis (Fig. 1) may raise suspicion of MSA *(11)* (Table 2). Red flags often are early warning signs of MSA *(30)*.

MSA is a progressive disease characterized by the gradual accumulation of disability reflecting involvement of the systems initially unaffected. Thus, patients who present initially with extrapyramidal features commonly progress to develop autonomic disturbances, cerebellar disorders, or both (*see* video of an advanced MSA-P patient showing marked akinesia and rigidity as well as cerebellar incoordination, particularly of lower limbs). Conversely, patients who begin with symptoms of cerebellar dysfunction often progress to develop extrapyramidal or autonomic disorders, or both. Patients whose

Table 1
MSA Consensus Criteria

A. Nomenclature of clinical domains, features (disease characteristics) and criteria (defining features or composite of features) used in the diagnosis of MSA

Domain	Criterion	Feature
Autonomic and urinary dysfunction	Orthostatic fall in blood pressure (by 30 mmHg systolic or 15 mmHg diastolic) *or*	Orthostatic hypotension (by 20 mmHg systolic or 10 mmHg diastolic)
	persistent urinary incontinence with erectile dysfunction in men *or both*	Urinary incontinence or incomplete bladder emptying
Parkinsonism	Bradykinesia *plus* rigidity *or*	Bradykinesia (progressive reduction in speed and amplitude of voluntary movements during repetitive actions)
	postural instability *or*	Rigidity
	tremor	Postural instability (loss of primary postural reflexes) Tremor (postural, resting, or both)
Cerebellar dysfunction	Gait ataxia *plus* ataxic dysarthria *or*	Gait ataxia (wide-based stance with irregular steps)
	limb ataxia *or*	Ataxic dysarthria
	sustained gaze-evoked nystagmus	Limb ataxia Sustained gaze-evoked nystagmus
Corticospinal tract dysfunction	No defining features	Extensor plantar responses with hyperreflexia

B. Diagnostic categories of MSA

Possible MSA-P	Criterion for parkinsonism plus two features from separate other domains. A poor levodopa response qualifies already as one feature, hence only one additional feature is required.
Possible MSA-C	Criterion for cerebellar dysfunction plus two features from separate other domains.
Probable MSA-P	Criterion for autonomic failure/urinary dysfunction plus poorly levodopa-responsive parkinsonism.
Probable MSA-C	Criterion for autonomic failure/urinary dysfunction plus cerebellar dysfunction.
Definite MSA	Pathological confirmation: high density of α-synuclein-positive GCIs associated with degenerative changes in the nigrostriatal (SND) and olivopontocerebellar pathways (OPCA).

Modified from ref. 8.
Reproduced with kind permission from Whitehouse Publishing: Wenning and Geser, Diagnosis and treatment of multiple system atrophy: an update. ACNR 2004;3(6):5–10.

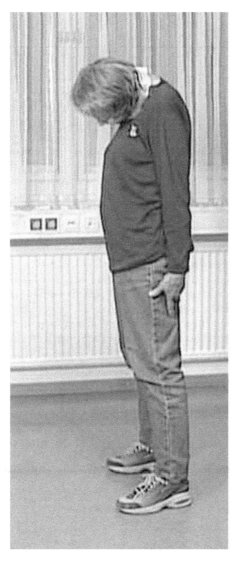

Fig. 1. Disproportionate antecollis of a patient with MSA-P.

symptoms initially are autonomic may later develop cerebellar, extrapyramidal, or both types of disorders. In a recent large study on 230 cases carried out in Japan, MSA-P patients had more rapid functional deterioration than MSA-C patients, but showed similar survival *(29)*.

INVESTIGATIONS

The diagnosis of MSA still rests on the clinical history and neurological examination. Attempts have been made, however, to improve diagnostic accuracy through analysis of cerebrospinal fluid (CSF) and serum biomarkers, autonomic function tests, structural and functional neuroimaging and neurophysiological techniques.

Table 2
"Red Flags": Warning Features of MSA[a]

Motor Red Flags	Definition
Orofacial dystonia	Atypical spontaneous or L-dopa-induced dystonia predominantly affecting orofacial muscles, occasionally resembling risus sardonicus of cephalic tetanus.
Pisa syndrome	Subacute axial dystonia with a severe tonic lateral flexion of the trunk, head, and neck (contracted and hypertrophic paravertebral muscles may be present).
Disproportionate antecollis	Chin-on-chest, neck can only with difficulty be passively and forcibly extended to its normal position. Despite severe chronic neck flexion, flexion elsewhere is minor.
Jerky tremor	Irregular (jerky) postural or action tremor of the hands and/or fingers.
Dysarthria	Atypical quivering, irregular, severely hypophonic or slurring high-pitched dysarthria, which tends to develop earlier, be more severe, and be associated with more marked dysphagia compared to PD.

Nonmotor Red Flags	
Abnormal respiration	Nocturnal (harsh or strained, high-pitched inspiratory sounds) or diurnal inspiratory stridor, involuntary deep inspiratory sighs/gasps, sleep apnea (arrest of breathing for ≥ 10 s), and excessive snoring (increase from premorbid level, or newly arising).
REM sleep behavior disorder	Intermittent loss of muscle atonia and appearance of elaborate motor activity (striking out with arms in sleep often with talking/shouting) associated with dream mentation.
Cold hands/feet	Coldness and color change (purple/blue) of extremities not resulting from drugs with blanching on pressure and poor circulatory return.
Raynaud's phenomenon	Painful "white finger," which may be provoked by ergot drugs.
Emotional incontinence	Crying inappropriately without sadness or laughing inappropriately without mirth.

[a]Excluding cardinal diagnostic features of MSA such as orthostatic hypotension, urinary incontinence/retention, levodopa-unresponsive parkinsonism, cerebellar (ataxia) and pyramidal signs. Also excluding nonspecific features suggesting atypical parkinsonism such as rapid progression or early instability and falls.

Reproduced with kind permission from John Wiley & Sons, Inc.: Wenning et al., Multiple system atrophy: an update. Mov Disord 2003;18(suppl 6):34–42.

CSF Analysis

Studies have attempted to identify biomarkers in the CSF to achieve early and accurate diagnosis, as well as to monitor response to treatment. Proteins in the CSF, including glial fibrillary acidic protein (GFAP) and neurofilament (NFL) protein have been studied. No difference was found in CSF concentrations of GFAP between patients with PD and MSA, but high concentrations of NFL seem to differentiate atypical parkinsonian disorders from PD *(31)*. Furthermore, CSF-NFL and levodopa tests combined with discriminant analysis may contribute even better to the differential diagnosis of parkinsonian syndromes *(32)*. Whereas the CSF-NFL and levodopa tests predicted 79 and 85% correct diagnoses (PD or non-PD [MSA and progressive supranuclear palsy—PSP]) respectively, the combined test predicted 90% correct diagnoses.

Hormonal Testing

In vivo studies in MSA, which involved testing of the endocrine component of the central autonomic nervous systems (the hypothalamopituitary axis) with a variety of challenge procedures, provided evidence of impaired humoral responses of the anterior and the posterior part of the pituitary gland with impaired secretion of adrenocorticotropic hormone (ACTH) *(33)*, growth hormone *(34)*, and vasopressin/ADH *(35)*. Although these observations can be made in virtually all advanced patients, their prevalence during the early course of MSA is unknown.

There is an ongoing debate about the diagnostic value of the growth hormone (GH) response to clonidine (CGH-test), a neuropharmacological assessment of central adrenoceptor function, in PD and MSA. Clonidine is a centrally active α2-adrenoceptor agonist that lowers blood pressure predominantly by reducing CNS (central nervous system) sympathetic outflow. In an early study, there was no increase in GH levels after clonidine in patients with MSA compared to those with PD or pure autonomic failure *(36)*. Kimber and colleagues confirmed a normal serum GH increase in response to clonidine in 14 PD patients (without autonomic failure) and in 19 patients with pure autonomic failure, whereas there was no GH rise in 31 patients with MSA *(34)*. However, these findings have been challenged subsequently *(37)*. More studies in well-defined patient cohorts are needed before the clonidine challenge test can be recommended as a helpful diagnostic test in patients with suspected MSA.

Autonomic Function Tests

Autonomic function tests are a mandatory part of the diagnostic process and clinical follow-up in patients with MSA. Findings of severe autonomic failure early in the course of the disease make the diagnosis of MSA more likely, although the specificity in comparison to other neurodegenerative disorders is unknown in a single patient. Pathological results of autonomic function tests may account for a considerable number of symptoms in MSA patients and should prompt specific therapeutic steps to improve quality of life and prevent secondary complications like injuries owing to hypotension-induced falls or ascending urinary infections.

Cardiovascular Function

A history of postural faintness or other evidence of orthostatic hypotension, e.g., neck ache on rising in the morning or posturally related changes of visual perception, should be sought in all patients in whom MSA is suspected. After taking a comprehensive history, testing of cardiovascular function should be performed. According the consensus statement of the American Autonomic Society and the American Academy of Neurology on the definition of orthostatic hypotension, pure autonomic failure, and MSA, a drop in systolic blood pressure (BP) of 20 mm Hg or more, or in diastolic BP of 10 mmHg or more, compared with baseline is defined as orthostatic hypotension (OH) and must lead to more specific assessment *(38)*. This is based on continuous noninvasive measurement of blood pressure and heart rate during tilt table testing *(39–41)*. Although abnormal cardiovascular test results may provide evidence of sympathetic and/or parasympathetic failure, they do not differentiate autonomic failure associated with PD vs MSA *(42)*.

In MSA, cardiovascular dysregulation appears to be caused by central rather than peripheral autonomic failure. During supine rest noradrenaline levels (representing postganglionic sympathethic efferent activity) are normal *(43)*, and there is no denervation hypersensitivity, which indicates a lack of increased expression of adrenergic receptors on peripheral neurons *(44)*. Uptake of the noradrenaline analog meta-iodobenzylguanidine is normal in postganglionic cardiac neurons *(45–48)* and the response to tilt is impaired with little increase in noradrenaline. In contrast, mainly postganglionic sympathetic dysfunction is thought to account for autonomic failure associated with PD. In keeping with this assumption, both basal and tilted noradrenaline levels are low.

Bladder Function

Assessment of bladder function is mandatory in MSA and usually provides evidence of involvement of the autonomic nervous system already at an early stage of the disease. Following a careful history regarding frequency of voiding, difficulties in initiating or suppressing voiding, and the presence and degree of urinary incontinence, a standard urine analysis should exclude an infection. Postvoid residual volume needs to be determined sonographically or via catheterization to initiate intermittent self-catheterization in due course. In some patients only cystometry can discriminate between hypocontractile detrusor function and a hyperreflexic sphincter-detrusor dyssynergy.

The nature of bladder dysfunction is different in MSA and PD. Although pollakiuria and urgency are common in both disorders, marked urge or stress incontinence with continuous leakage is not a feature of PD, apart from very advanced cases. Urodynamic studies show a characteristic pattern of abnormality in MSA patients (49). In the early stages there is often detrusor hyperreflexia, often with bladder neck incompetence resulting from abnormal urethral sphincter function, which result in early pollakiuria and urgency followed by urge incontinence. Later on, the ability to initiate a voluntary micturition reflex and the strength of the hyperreflexic detrusor contractions diminish, and the bladder may become atonic, accounting for increasing postmicturition residual urine volumes.

The detrusor hyperreflexia may result from a disturbance of the pontine micturition center (50,51). Alternatively, degeneration of substantia nigra and other regions of the basal ganglia that are important in the control of micturition, may contribute to urological symptoms. The atonic bladder in advanced MSA has been related to the progressive degeneration of the intermediolateral columns of the thoracolumbar spinal cord (50), however, this remains speculative.

IMAGING

Magnetic Resonance Imaging (MRI)

MRI scanning of patients with MSA often, but not always, reveals atrophy of cerebellar vermis and, less marked, of cerebellar hemispheres (52). There is also evidence of shrinkage of pons as well as middle cerebellar peduncles (27), differentiating MSA-C from cortical cerebellar atrophy (CCA). The pattern of infratentorial atrophy visible on MRI correlates with the pathological process of OPCA affecting the cerebellar vermis and hemispheres, middle cerebellar peduncles, pons, and lower brainstem (53). The MRI changes may be indistinguishable from those of patients with autosomal dominant cerebellar ataxias (54). MRI measures of basal ganglia pathology in MSA such as width of substantia nigra pars compacta, lentiform nucleus, and head of the caudate are less well established and naked-eye assessments are often unreliable. In advanced cases putaminal atrophy may be detectable and may correlate with severity of extrapyramidal symptoms (55). However, in one study MRI-based two-dimensional basal ganglia morphometry has proved unhelpful in the early differential diagnosis of patients with levodopa-unresponsive parkinsonism (56). A significant progression of atrophy to under the normal limit was observed in the cerebrum, frontal and temporal lobes, showing the involvement of the cerebral hemisphere, especially the frontal lobe (57). Abnormalities on MRI may include not only atrophy, but also signal abnormalities on T2-weighted images within the pontocerebellar system and putamen. Signal hyperintensities sometimes seen within the pons and middle cerebellar peduncles are thought to reflect degeneration of pontocerebellar fibers and therefore, together with marked atrophy in these areas, indicate a major site of pathology in OPCA type MSA (MSA-C) (27,58). The characteristic infratentorial signal change on T2-weighted 1.5 Tesla MRI ("hot cross bun" sign) may also corroborate the clinical diagnosis of MSA (52). Putaminal hypointensities in supposedly atypical parkinsonian disorders (APDs) were first reported in 1986 by two groups using a 1.5 Tesla magnet and T2-weighted images (59,60). This change has subsequently been observed by others in cases clinically thought to have MSA (27,55,61), and in some cases with pathological confirmation (62–64). A lateral to medial as well as posterior to anterior gradient is also well established with the most prominent changes in the posterolateral putamen (55,60,62). This putaminal hypointensity has been proposed as a sensitive and specific abnormality in patients with MSA, and to reflect increased iron deposition. However, similar abnormalities may occur in patients with classical PD (65,66) or may represent incidental findings in patients without basal ganglia disorders (Wenning G, unpublished observations). The notion of increased iron deposition has been challenged by Brooks and colleagues (67) and later by Schwarz and colleagues (64). Recently it was shown that hypointense putaminal signal changes were more often observed in MSA than in PD patients using T2*-weighted gradient echo (GE) but not T2-weighted fast-spin echo images, indicating that T2*-weighted GE sequences are of diagnostic value for patients with parkinsonism (68).

Increased putaminal relative to pallidal hypointensities may be seen as well as a slit-like hyperintense band lateral to the putamen *(64,69–71)*. These changes are consistent with a clinical diagnosis of MSA. However, they appear to be nonspecific and have also been noted in clinically diagnosed PD and PSP *(52,66)*. The pattern consisting of hypointense and hyperintense T2 changes within the putamen is a highly specific MRI sign of MSA, whereas hypointensity alone remains a sensitive, but nonspecific sign of MSA *(72)*. The hyperintense signal correlated with the most pronounced reactive microgliosis and astrogliosis or highest iron content in MRI-postmortem studies *(62,64)*. Konagaya et al. *(73)* reported that in a case of MSA, the slit hyperintensity at the putaminal margin represented widened intertissue space owing to a severe shrinkage and rarefaction of the putamen. However, in spite of these speculations the nature of this abnormal signal intensity remains uncertain.

Diffusion-weighted imaging (DWI) may represent a useful diagnostic tool that can provide additional support for a diagnosis of MSA-P. DWI, even if measured in the slice direction only, is able to discriminate MSA-P and both patients with PD and healthy volunteers on the basis of putaminal rADC (regional apparent diffusion coefficient) values *(74)*. The increased putaminal rADC values in MSA-P are likely to reflect ongoing striatal degeneration, whereas most neuropathologic studies reveal intact striatum in PD. But, since in PSP compared to PD patients' rADCs were also significantly increased in both putamen and globus pallidus *(75)*, increased putaminal rADC values do not discriminate MSA-P from PSP.

Whether magnetic resonance volumetry will contribute to the differential diagnosis of MSA from other parkinsonian disorders remains to be confirmed. Schulz et al. *(76)* found significant reductions in mean striatal and brainstem volumes in patients with MSA-P, MSA-C, and PSP, whereas patients with MSA-C and MSA-P also showed a reduction in cerebellar volume. Total intracranial volume-normalized MRI-based volumetric measurements provide a sensitive marker to discriminate typical and atypical parkinsonism. Voxel-based morphometry (VBM) confirmed previous region of interest (ROI)-based volumetric studies *(76)* showing basal ganglia and infratentorial volume loss in MSA-P patients *(77)*. These data revealed prominent cortical volume loss in MSA-P mainly comprising the cortical targets of striatal projections such as the primary sensorimotor, lateral premotor cortices, and the prefrontal cortex, but also the insula. These changes are consistent with the established frontal lobe impairment of MSA patients *(78)*.

Proton magnetic resonance spectroscopy (MRS) is a noninvasive method that provides information about the chemical pathology of disorders affecting the CNS. MRS has been used to identify striatal metabolic changes in MSA *(79–82)*. However, the available data are conflicting and further studies are clearly required to establish the role of MRS in the diagnosis of MSA.

Functional Imaging

Single-photon emission tomography (SPECT) or positron emission tomography (PET) studies of patients with MSA-P have demonstrated the combined nigral and striatal pathology using [(^{123})I]β-CIT [2β-carboxymethoxy-3β-(4-iodophenyl)tropane] (SPECT) or [^{10}F]fluorodopa (PET) and a variety of postsynaptic dopamine or opiate receptor ligands such as [^{123}I]iodobenzamide (IBZM) (SPECT), [^{11}C]raclopride or [^{11}C]diprenorphin (PET).

The Hammersmith Cyclotron Unit, using PET, found that putaminal uptake of the presynaptic dopaminergic markers [^{18}F]fluorodopa and S-[^{11}C]nomifensine *(83–85)* was similarly reduced in MSA and PD; in approximately half the MSA subjects, caudate uptake was also markedly reduced, as opposed to only moderate reduction in PD. However, discriminant function analysis of striatal [^{18}F]fluorodopa uptake separated MSA and PD patients poorly *(85)*. Patients with PD, PSP, and MSA share a marked loss of fluorodopa uptake in the putamen; however, uptake in the caudate nucleus differs among the three groups, with patients who have MSA showing uptake rates intermediate between those of patients with PD (normal uptake) and with PSP (markedly reduced uptake) *(83)*. Measurements of striatal dopamine D_2 receptor densities using raclopride and PET failed to differentiate between idiopathic and atypical parkinsonism, demonstrating a similar loss of densities in levodopa-treated patients with fluctuating PD, MSA, and PSP *(86)*. PET studies using other ligands such as [^{11}C]diprenorphine (nonselective opioid receptor antagonist) *(87)* and [^{18}F]fluoro-deoxyglucose *(88–90)* have proved more consistent in detecting striatal degeneration and in distinguishing patients with MSA-P from those with PD, particularly when combined with a dopamine D2 receptor scan *(91,92)*. Widespread functional abnormalities in MSA-C have been demonstrated using [^{18}F]fluorodeoxyglucose and PET *(93)*. Reduced metabolism was most marked in the brainstem and cerebellum, but other areas such as the putamen, caudate nucleus, thalamus, and cerebral cortex were also involved, differentiating MSA-C from spinocerebellar ataxias (SCAs). Subclinical evidence of striatal pathology in MSA-C, in the absence of extrapyramidal features, has been demonstrated using the nonselective opioid receptor ligand diprenorphine and PET *(94)*. In a PET study using [^{18}F]fluorodeoxyglucose, in comparison with normal controls putaminal hypometabolism was absent in sporadic OPCA patients without autonomic failure and extrapyramidal features, but present in those who were classified as OPCA-type MSA and therefore had autonomic dysfunction with or without parkinsonian features at the time of examination *(93)*. Striatal opiate receptors are reduced not only in MSA-P *(87)* but also in MSA-C with associated autonomic failure *(94)* supporting its nosological status as the cerebellar subtype of MSA. Differences in cerebellar benzodiazepine receptor binding densities have also been shown in MSA-C, CCA, and SCA using [^{11}C]flumazenil and PET *(95)*. Additionally, the poor levodopa response may be related to a deficiency in striatal D_1 receptor binding, as shown by PET studies in clinically diagnosed patients with MSA using the ligand [^{11}C]SCH 23390 *(96)*. This is a potentially helpful observation that may aid early differentiation of MSA and PD if corroborated by other groups.

SPECT imaging studies of patients with dopa naive parkinsonism have used [^{123}I]iodobenzamide (IBZM) as D2 receptor ligand *(21,22)*. A good response to apomorphine and subsequent benefit from chronic dopaminergic therapy was observed in subjects with normal IBZM binding whereas subjects with reduced binding failed to respond. Some of these patients developed other atypical clinical features suggestive of MSA during follow-up *(97)*. Other SPECT studies have also revealed significant reductions of striatal IBZM binding in clinically probable MSA subjects compared to PD patients *(27,98)*. Since [^{123}I]β-CIT SPECT reliably enables the visualization of the presynaptic dopaminergic lesion, this method was used as a label of dopamine transporter (DAT) to study the progression of presynaptic dopaminergic degeneration in PD and APD including MSA by Pirker and coworkers *(99)*. The results of the sequential [^{123}I]β-CIT SPECT imaging demonstrate a rapid decline of striatal β-CIT binding in patients with APD, exceeding the reduction in PD. Scintigraphic visualization of postganglionic sympathetic cardiac neurons was found to differentiate patients with MSA from patients with PD *(45–48)*, because patients in the latter group show a severely reduced cardiac uptake of the radioactive ligand [^{123}I]metaiodobenzylguanidine (MIBG). This method appears to be a highly sensitive and specific tool to discriminate between MSA and PD already within 2 year of onset of symptoms; however, the test cannot distinguish MSA from other APD such as PSP *(100)*.

NEUROPHYSIOLOGICAL TECHNIQUES

The external anal or urethral sphincter electromyogram (EMG) is a useful investigation in patients with suspected MSA. Because of degeneration of Onuf's nucleus, both anal and urethral external sphincter muscles undergo denervation and re-innervation. Abnormality of the striated urethral sphincter EMG in MSA was first shown by Martinelli and Coccagna in 1978 *(101)*. Subsequently, Kirby and colleagues *(49)* confirmed the presence of polyphasia and abnormal prolongation of individual motor units in MSA, and also examined the potential diagnostic role of sphincter EMG in patients with MSA and PD *(102)*. Sixteen (62%) of 26 patients with probable MSA, and only 1 (8%) of 13 with probable PD had a pathological EMG result (sensitivity 0.62, specificity 0.92). This test also helps to identify patients in whom incontinence may develop or worsen following surgery. Anal sphincter EMG is generally better tolerated, and yields identical results *(50)*. In at least 80% of patients with MSA, EMG of the external anal sphincter reveals signs of neuronal degeneration in Onuf's nucleus with spontaneous activity and increased polyphasia *(103–105)*. However, these findings do not reliably differentiate between MSA and other forms of APD. An abnormal anal sphincter examination was present in 5 of 12 (41.6%) PSP patients *(106)*. Furthermore, neurogenic changes of external anal sphincter muscle have also been demonstrated in advanced stages of PD by several investigators *(107,108)*. Also chronic constipation, previous pelvic surgery, or vaginal deliveries can be confounding factors to induce nonspecific abnormalities *(109)*. In summary, in patients with probable MSA, abnormal sphincter EMG, as compared to control subjects, has been found in the vast majority of patients, including those who, as yet, have no urological or anorectal problems. The prevalence of abnormalities in the early stages of MSA is as yet unclear. Patients with PD as a rule do not show severe sphincter EMG abnormalities in the early stage of the disease, unless other causes for sphincter denervation are present. However, sphincter EMG does not distinguish MSA from PSP *(110)*. For these reasons, this examination has not been included in the guidelines suggested by the Consensus Conference *(8)*.

In general, the value of evoked potential studies in the diagnosis of MSA is limited. Magnetic evoked potentials are often, but not always, normal in MSA *(111,112)*. Somatosensory, visual, and acoustic evoked potentials may show prolonged latencies in up to 40% of patients, but most patients show no abnormalities of central efferent and afferent neuronal pathways *(112–114)*.

Some investigators *(115,116)* have suggested that both somatic anterior horn cells and peripheral nerves are commonly affected in MSA, and their involvement has therefore been regarded as part of the clinical spectrum of MSA. Abnormalities of nerve conduction studies seem to be more frequent in MSA-P (43%) compared to MSA-C (14%), suggesting that the peripheral nervous system is differentially affected in the motor presentations of this disorder *(117)*.

Excessive auditory startle responses (ASRs) may also help differentiate MSA both from PD and other forms of APD *(118)*. Exaggerated ASRs may reflect disinhibition of lower brainstem nuclei owing to the degenerative disorder. ASRs appear to be more disinhibited in MSA-P than MSA-C, and there is a lack of ASR habituation in MSA-C unlike MSA-P, suggesting involvement of different neural structures in the two MSA-subtypes *(119)*.

PATHOLOGY

In MSA-P, the striatonigral system is the main site of pathology but less severe degeneration can be widespread and usually includes the olivopontocerebellar system *(51)*. The putamen is shrunken with gray-green discoloration. When putaminal pathology is severe there may be a cribriform appearance. In early stages the putaminal lesion shows a distinct topographical distribution with a predilection for the caudal and dorsolateral regions *(120)*. Later on during the course of disease, the entire putamen is usually affected with the result that bundles of striatopallidal fibres are narrowed and poorly stained for myelin. Degeneration of pigmented nerve cells occurs in the substantia nigra pars compacta (SNC), whereas nonpigmented cells of the pars reticulata are reported as normal. The topographical patterns of neurodegeneration involving the motor neostriatum, efferent pathways, and nigral neurons, reflect their anatomical relationship and suggest a common denominator or "linked" degeneration *(120)*.

In MSA-C, the brunt of pathology is in the olivopontocerebellar system whereas the involvement of striatum and substantia nigra is less severe. The basis pontis is atrophic, with loss of pontine neurons and transverse pontocerebellar fibers. In sections stained for myelin, the intact descending corticospinal tracts stand out against the degenerated transverse fibers and the atrophic middle cerebellar peduncles. There is a disproportionate depletion of fibers from the middle cerebellar peduncles compared with the loss of pontine neurons, an observation consistent with a "dying back" process.

A supraspinal contribution to the autonomic failure of MSA is now well established. Cell loss is reported in dorsal motor nucleus of the vagus *(121)* and involves catecholaminergic neurons of ventrolateral medulla *(122)*. It has also been described for the Edinger–Westphal nucleus and posterior hypothalamus *(123)* including the tuberomamillary nucleus *(124)*. Papp and Lantos *(125)* have shown marked involvement of brainstem pontomedullary reticular formation with glial cytoplasmic inclusions (GCIs), providing a supraspinal histological counterpart for impaired visceral function. Autonomic neuronal degeneration affects the locus ceruleus, too *(20)*. Disordered bladder, rectal, and sexual function in MSA-P and MSA-C have also been associated with cell loss in parasympathetic preganglionic nuclei of the spinal cord. These neurons are localized rostrally in the Onuf's nucleus between the sacral segments S2 and S3 and more caudally in the inferior intermediolateral nucleus chiefly in the S3 to S4 segments *(126)*. Degeneration of sympathetic preganglionic neurones in the intermediolateral column of the thoracolumbar spinal cord is considered contributory to orthostatic hypotension. If one considers only those reports in which formal cell counts have been made, with very few exceptions all cases of MSA with predominant pathology in either the striatonigral or olivopontocerebellar system show loss of intermediolateral cells *(127)*. However, it is noteworthy that there is not always a strong correlation between nerve cell depletion or gliosis and the clinical degree of autonomic failure. It is estimated that more than 50% of cells within the intermediolateral column need to decay before symptoms become evident *(128)*. In the peripheral component of the autonomic nervous system, Bannister and Oppenheimer have described atrophy of the glossopharyngeal and vagus nerves *(129)*.

A variety of other neuronal populations are noted to show cell depletion and gliosis with considerable differences in vulnerability from case to case. Only a few of the reported lesions are discussed here. Various degree of abnormalities in the cerebral hemisphere, including Betz cell loss, were detected in pathologically proven MSA cases *(57,130–132)*. Furthermore, anterior horn cells may show some depletion but rarely to the same extent as that occurring in motor neuron disease *(126,133)*. Depletion of large myelinated nerve fibres in the recurrent laryngeal nerve that innervates intrinsic laryngeal muscles has been demonstrated in MSA patients with vocal cord palsy *(134)*.

From a neuropathological viewpoint, there is little cause for confusion of MSA with other neurodegenerative conditions. The GCI is the hallmark that accompanies the signs of degeneration involving striatonigral and olivopontocerebellar systems. GCIs are distinctly different from filamentous oligodendroglial inclusions, called coiled bodies, found in other neurodegenerative diseases, including PSP, CBD, and argyrophilic grain disease *(135–138)*. Rarely MSA may be combined with additional pathologies. Lewy bodies (LBs) have been reported in 8–10% of MSA cases and show a distribution comparable with that of PD *(139)*. This frequency is similar to that of controls and suggests an incidental finding related to ageing and/or presymptomatic PD.

The discovery of GCIs in MSA brains in 1989 highlighted the unique glial pathology as biological hallmark of this disorder *(140)*. GCIs are argyrophilic and half-moon, oval, or conical in shape *(141)* and are composed of 20- to 30-nm tubular filaments *(142)*. Although inclusions have been described in five cellular sites, i.e., in oligodendroglial and neuronal cytoplasm and nuclei as well as in axons *(143)*, GCIs *(140)* are most ubiquitous and appear to represent the subcellular hallmark lesion of MSA *(141)*. Their distribution selectively involves basal ganglia, supplementary and primary motor cortex, the reticular formation, basis pontis, the middle cerebellar peduncles, and the cerebellar white matter *(125,141)*. GCIs contain classical cytoskeletal antigens, including ubiquitin and tau *(141,144)*. More recently, α-synuclein immunoreactivity has been recognized as the most sensitive marker of GCIs *(145)* (Fig. 2). In fact, α-synuclein, a presynaptic protein that is affected by point mutations in some families with autosomal dominant PD *(146)* and that is present in LBs *(147)*, has also been observed in both neuronal inclusions and GCIs *(148–152)* in brains of patients with MSA. GCI filaments are multilayered in structure, with α-synuclein oligomers forming the central core fibrils of the

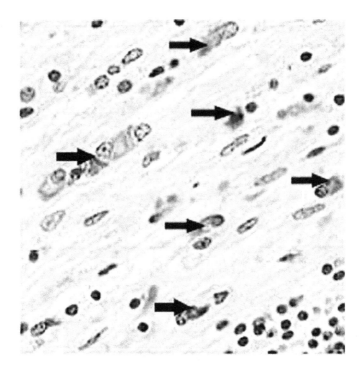

Fig. 2. α-Synuclein immunostaining reveals GCIs in subcortical white matter. Courtesy of Prof. K. Jellinger. Reproduced with kind permission of Whitehouse Publishing. Diagnosis and treatment of multiple system atrophy: an update. ACNR 2004;3(6):5–10.

filaments *(142)*. The accumulation of α-synuclein into filamentous inclusions appears to play a key role not only in MSA, but also in a growing number of α-synucleinopathies such as PD, dementia with Lbs (DLB), Down syndrome, familial Alzheimer's disease (AD), and sporadic AD *(153)*. The α-synuclein accumulation in GCIs as well as in neuronal inclusions associated with MSA precedes their ubiquitination *(154)*. Importantly, α-synuclein, but not ubiquitin, antibodies also reveal numerous degenerating neurites in the white matter of MSA cases *(154)*. This suggests that an as yet unrecognised degree of pathology may be present in the axons of MSA cases, although whether neuronal/axonal α-synuclein pathology precedes glial α-synuclein pathology has not been examined.

Recent findings support an important role for glial cells and inflammatory reactions in many neurodegenerative diseases including PD, DLB, and MSA *(155–157)*. Neuronal survival is critically dependent on glial function, which can exert both neuroprotective and neurotoxic influences. Glial cells are a primary target of cytokines and are activated in response to many cytokines, including tumor necrosis factor (TNF)-α *(158)*. This activation can trigger further release of cytokines that might enhance or suppress local inflammatory responses and neuronal survival. These cytokines may also participate in neurodegeneration either indirectly by activating other glial cells or directly by inducing apoptosis *(159–161)*. Several studies indicated that TNF-α is toxic for dopaminergic neurons in vitro *(162)* and in vivo *(163)*, thus supporting the potential involvement of this pro-inflammatory cytokine in the neurodegenerative processes in PD and other α-synucleinopathies. However, the relationship between intracellular α-synuclein-positive inclusions and the proinflammatory response in α-synucleinopathies remains obscure. The activation of microglial cells may be the final common pathway, contributing both to demyelination and neuronal removal, irrespective of the mode of cell death. PK 11195 selectively binds to benzodiazepine sites on activated microglia. [11]C PK 11195 PET has demonstrated activated microglia in vivo in the putamen, pallidum, substantia nigra, and pontine region in five patients with MSA *(164)*.

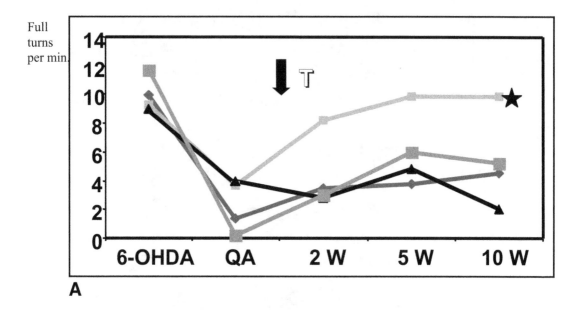

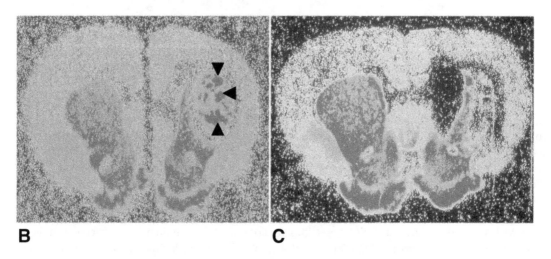

Fig. 3. Regeneration of apomorphine responsiveness following embryonic transplantation in the double lesion SND rat model as shown by behavioral studies and D-2 receptor autoradiography. (**A**) shows increased apomorphine-induced rotation rates following transplantation of embryonic striatal tissue (line marked with an asterisk) compared to nonsignificant changes in other transplant groups as well as sham controls (6-OHDA, 6-hydroxydopamine; QA, quinolinic acid; TP, transplantation; W, weeks). (**B**) shows surviving embroynic striatal graft tissue expressing foci of dompamine D-2 receptors (small arrows) within a severely lesioned host striatum, compared to a sham graft without evidence of regeneration (**C**). Modified from ref. *177.*

ANIMAL MODELS

A number of in vivo MSA models have become available as preclinical test bed for novel therapeutic interventions. Based on experiments in the early 1990s *(165)*, several attempts have been made to reproduce the core pathology of striatonigral degeneration (SND) that underlies L-Dopa-unresponsive parkinsonism in MSA-P *(166)*. The goal of these experimental studies was to replicate the unique lesion pattern present in human MSA-P/SND, i.e., the combined degeneration of dopaminergic nigrostriatal pathways as well as corresponding striatal projections. This work utilized well-established nigral and striatal lesion models that had been developed to mimic the core pathology of PD and Huntington's disease. These experiments produced several models mimicking various degrees of disease severity, each having its own advantages and pitfalls *(165,167–176)*. Embryonic striatal grafts have been shown to partially regenerate responsiveness to dopaminergic stimulation *(177)* *(see* Fig. 3) in the unilateral double lesion rat model. One principal problem encountered with the unilateral stereotaxic rat model was the interaction between the nigral and striatal lesion placement. Also the behavioral and motor impairments obtained were remote from those observed in the human disease. This was one of the reasons to move to a systemic primate model using the PD-like toxin, 1-methyl-4-phenyl-1,2,3,6-tetrahydropyridine (MPTP), and the HD-like toxin, 3-nitropropionic acid (3-NP). This strategy generated a reproducible symptomatology closer to human MSA-P/SND, i.e., levodopa-unresponsive parkinsonism/dystonia correlated with striatal outflow pathway lesions and severe nigral degeneration *(173,174)*. However, because of ethical considerations, time-consuming experiments, and the need for a great number of animals owing to a marked interindividual susceptibility to these mitochondrial toxins, the model strategy was switched to systemic MPTP + 3-NP mouse models *(171,172)*. These models allow screening of drugs in sufficient number of animals. The systemic double toxin paradigm may also be applied to transgenic mice with targeted expression of α-synuclein in oligodendrocytes *(175)*. However, more work is needed to confirm the stability of α-synuclein expression in these animals and particularly its deleterious effects upon oligodendroglial and neuronal function.

TREATMENT

Autonomic Failure

Unfortunately there is no causal therapy of autonomic dysfunction available. Therefore the therapeutic strategy is defined by clinical symptoms and impairment of quality of life in these patients. Because of the progressive course of MSA, a regular review of the treatment is mandatory to adjust measures according to clinical needs.

The concept to treat symptoms of orthostatic hypotension is based on the increase of intravascular volume and the reduction of volume shift to lower body parts when changing to upright position. The selection and combination of the following options depend on the severity of symptoms and their practicability in the single patient, but not on the extent of blood pressure drop during tilt test. Nonpharmacological options include sufficient fluid intake, high salt diet, more frequent, but smaller meals per day to reduce postprandial hypotension by spreading the total carbohydrate intake, and custom-made elastic body garments. During the night, head-up tilt increases intravascular volume up to 1 L within a week, which is particularly helpful to improve hypotension early in the morning. This approach is successful in particular in combination with fludrocortisone, which further supports sodium retention.

The next group of drugs to consider are the sympathomimetics. These include ephedrine (with both direct and indirect effects), which is often valuable in central autonomic disorders such as MSA. With higher doses, side effects include tremulousness, loss of appetite, and urinary retention in men.

Among the large number of vasoactive agents that have been evaluated in MSA, only one, the directly acting α-adrenergic agonist midodrine, meets the criteria of evidence-based medicine *(178–180)*. Side effects are usually mild and only rarely lead to discontinuation of treatment because of urinary retention or pruritus, predominantly on the scalp.

Another promising drug appears to be the norepinephrine precursor L-threo-dihydroxyphenylserine (L-threo-DOPS), which has been used in this indication in Japan for years and efficacy of which has now been shown by a recent open, dose-finding trial *(181)*.

In case the above-mentioned drugs do not produce the desired effects, selective targeting is needed. The somatostatin analog, octreotide, is often beneficial in postprandial hypotension *(182)*, presum-

Table 3
Practical Management of MSA

A. Pharmacotherapy
  I. For akinesia-rigidity
   • Levodopa up to 800–1000 mg/d, if tolerated (↔)
   • Dopamine agonists as second-line anti-parkinsonian drugs (dosing as for PD patients) (↔)
   • Amantadine as third-line drug, 100 mg up to three times daily (↔)
  II. For focal dystonia
   • Botulinum toxin A (↔)
  III. For orthostatic hypotension
   • Head-up tilt of bed at night (↔)
   • Elastic stockings or tights (↔)
   • Increased salt intake (↔)
   • Fludrocortisone 0,1-0, 3 mg/d (↔)
   • Ephedrine 15–45 mg t.i.d (↔)
   • L-threo-DOPS (300 mg b.i.d.) (↔)
   • Midodrine 2.5 µg–10 mg t.i.d. (↑↑)
  IV. For postprandial hypotension
   • Octreotide 25–50 µg s.c. 30 min before a meal (↔)
  V. For nocturnal polyuria
   • Desmopressin (spray: 10–40 mg/night or tablet: 100–400 mg/night) (↔)
  VI. For bladder symptoms
   • Oxybutynin for detrusor hyperreflexia (2.5–5 mg b.i.d-t.i.d.) (↔)
   • Intermittent self-catheterization for retention or residual volume >100 ml (↔)
B. Other therapies
   • Physiotherapy (↔)
   • Speech therapy (↔)
   • Occupational therapy (↔)
   • Percutaneous endoscopic gastrostomy (PEG) (rarely needed in late stage) (↔)
   • Provision of wheelchair (↔)
   • CPAP (↑) (rarely tracheostomy [↔]) for inspiratory stridor

Reproduced with kind permission from John Wiley & Sons, Inc.: Wenning et al., Multiple System atrophy: an update. Mov Disord 2003;18(suppl 6):34–42.

ably because it inhibits release of vasodilatory gastrointestinal peptides *(183)*; importantly it does not enhance nocturnal hypertension *(182)*.

The vasopressin analogue, desmopressin, which acts on renal tubular vasopressin-2 receptors, reduces nocturnal polyuria and improves morning postural hypotension *(184)*.

The peptide erythropoietin may be beneficial in some patients by raising red cell mass, secondarily improving cerebral oxygenation *(185,186)*.

A broad range of drugs (Table 3) have been used in the treatment of postural hypotension *(187)*. Unfortunately, the value and side effects of many of these drugs have not been adequately determined in MSA patients using appropriate endpoints.

In the management of neurogenic bladder including residual urine clean intermittent catheterization three to four times per day is a widely accepted approach to prevent secondary consequences of failure to micturate. It may be necessary to provide the patient with a permanent transcutaneous suprapubic catheter if mechanical obstruction in the urethra or motor symptoms of MSA prevent uncomplicated catheterization.

Pharmacological options with anti- or pro-cholinergic drugs or α-adrenergic substances are usually not successful to adequately reduce postvoid residual volume in MSA, but anticholinergic agents like oxybutynin can improve symptoms of detrusor hyperreflexia or sphincter-detrusor dyssynergy in the early course of the disease *(50)*. Recently, α-adrenergic receptor antagonists (prazosin and moxisylyte) have been shown to improve voiding with reduction of residual volumes in MSA patients *(188)*. Urological surgery must be avoided in these patients because postoperative worsening of bladder control is most likely *(50)*.

The necessity of a specific treatment for sexual dysfunction needs to be evaluated individually in each MSA patient. Male impotence can be partially circumvented by the use of intracavernosal papaverine, prostaglandin E1, or penile implants *(189)*. Preliminary evidence in PD patients *(190)* suggests that sildenafil may also be successful in treating erectile failure in MSA: a recent trial confirmed the efficacy of this compound in MSA, but also suggested caution because of the frequent cardiovascular side effects *(191)*. Erectile failure in MSA may also be improved by oral yohimbine *(50)*.

Constipation can be relieved by increasing the intraluminal volume, which may be achieved by using macrogol-water-solution *(192)*.

Inspiratory stridor develops in about 30% of patients. Continuous positive airway pressure (CPAP) may be helpful in some of these patients *(193)*. In only about 4% a tracheostomy is needed and performed.

Motor Disorder

General Approach

Because the results of drug treatment for the motor disorder of MSA are generally poor, other therapies are all the more important. Physiotherapy helps maintain mobility and prevent contractures, and speech therapy can improve speech and swallowing and provide communication aids. Dysphagia may require feeding via a nasogastric tube or even percutaneous endoscopic gastrostomy (PEG). Occupational therapy helps to limit the handicap resulting from the patient's disabilities and should include a home visit. Provision of a wheelchair is usually dictated by the liability to falls because of postural instability and gait ataxia but not by akinesia and rigidity *per se*. Psychological support for patients and partners needs to be stressed.

Parkinsonism

Parkinsonism is the predominant motor disorder in MSA and therefore represents a major target for therapeutic intervention. Although less effective than in PD and despite the lack of randomized-controlled trials, levodopa replacement represents the mainstay of anti-parkinsonian therapy in MSA. Open-label studies suggest that up to 30–40% of MSA patients may derive benefit from levodopa at least transiently *(13,26)*. Occasionally, a beneficial effect is evident only when seemingly unresponsive patients deteriorate after levodopa withdrawal *(25)*. Preexisting orthostatic hypotension is often unmasked or exacerbated in levodopa-treated MSA patients associated with autonomic failure. In contrast, psychiatric or toxic confusional states appear to be less common than in PD *(13)*. Results with dopamine agonists have been even more disappointing *(194)*. Severe psychiatric side effects occurred in a double-blind crossover trial of six patients on lisuride, with nightmares, visual hallucinations, and toxic confusional states *(195)*. Wenning et al. *(13)* reported a response to oral dopamine agonists only in 4 of 41 patients. None of 30 patients receiving bromocriptine improved, but 3 of 10 who received pergolide had some benefit. Twenty-two percent of the levodopa responders had good or excellent response to at least one orally active dopamine agonist in addition. Anti-parkinsonian effects were noted in 4 of 26 MSA patients treated with amantadine *(13)*, however, there was no significant improvement in an open study of 9 patients with atypical parkinsonism, including 5 subjects with MSA *(196)*.

Blepharospasm as well as limb dystonia, but not antecollis, may respond well to local injections of botulinum toxin A.

Ablative neurosurgical procedures such as medial pallidotomy fail to improve parkinsonian motor disturbance in MSA *(197)*. However, most recently a beneficial short-term and long-term effect of bilateral subthalamic nucleus high-frequency stimulation has been reported in four patients with MSA-P *(198)*. Further studies are needed to establish the scope of deep brain stimulation in MSA.

Cerebellar Ataxia

There is no effective therapy for the progressive ataxia of MSA-C. Occasional successes have been reported with cholinergic drugs, amantadine, 5-hydroxytryptophan, isoniazid, baclofen, and propanolol; for the large majority of patients these drugs proved to be ineffective.

One intriguing observation is the apparent temporary exacerbation of ataxia by cigarette smoking *(199,200)*. Nicotine is known to increase the release of acetylcholine in many areas of the brain and probably also releases noradrenaline, dopamine, 5-hydroxytryptophan, and other neurotransmitters. Nicotinic systems may therefore play a role in cerebellar function and trials of nicotinic antagonists such as dihydro-β-erythroidine might be worthwhile in MSA-C.

Practical Therapy

Because of the small number of randomized controlled trials, the practical management of MSA is largely based on empirical evidence (↔) or single randomized studies (↑), except for three randomized controlled trials of midodrine (↑↑) *(178–180)*. The present recommendations are summarized in Table 3.

Future Therapies

Two European research initiatives—European MSA-Study Group (EMSA-SG) and Neuroprotection and Natural History in Parkinson Plus Syndromes (NNIPPS)—are presently conducting multicentre intervention trials in MSA using candidate neuroprotective agents. For the first time, prospective progression data using novel rating tools such as the Unified MSA Rating Scale (UMSARS) *(201)* will become available. Furthermore, surrogate markers of disease progression will be evaluated using structural and functional neuroimaging. Even if the ongoing trials are negative, they will certainly stimulate further trial activity in MSA, which is desperately needed to tame this "beast."

LEGEND FOR THE VIDEO

60-yr-old patient with advanced MSA-P showing marked akinesia and rigidity as well as cerebellar incoordination, particularly of lower limbs.

MAJOR RESEARCH ISSUES IN MSA

1. Pathogenesis of neuronal degeneration
   - Interaction of glial and neuronal pathology
   - Genetic susceptibility toward inclusion pathology
2. Optimized diagnostic criteria
3. Biomarkers of disease progression
4. Screening of candidate neuroprotective agents
5. Transgenic animal models

REFERENCES

1. Bower J, Maraganore D, McDonnell S, Rocca W. Incidence of progressive supranuclear palsy and multiple system atrophy in Olmsted County, Minnesota, 1976 to 1990. Neurology 1997;49:1284–1288.
2. Tison F, Yekhlef F, Chrysostome V, Sourgen C. Prevalence of multiple system atrophy. Lancet 2000;355(9202):495–496.
3. Schrag A, Ben-Shlomo Y, Quinn NP. Prevalence of progressive supranuclear palsy and multiple system atrophy: a cross-sectional study. Lancet 1999;354:1771–1775.
4. Wermuth L, Joensen P, Bunger N, Jeune B. High prevalence of Parkinson's disease in the Faroe Islands. Neurology 1997;49(2):426–432.

5. Chio A, Magnani C, Schiffer D. Prevalence of Parkinson's disease in Northwestern Italy: comparison of tracer methodology and clinical ascertainment of cases. Mov Disord 1998;13(3):400–405.

6. Trenkwalder C, Schwarz J, Gebhard J, Ruland D, Trenkwalder P, Hense HW, et al. Starnberg trial on epidemiology of Parkinsonism and hypertension in the elderly. Prevalence of Parkinson's disease and related disorders assessed by a door-to-door survey of inhabitants older than 65 years. Arch Neurol 1995;52(10):1017–1022.

7. Nee LE, Gomez MR, Dambrosia J, Bale S, Eldridge R, Polinsky RJ. Environmental-occupational risk factors and familial associations in multiple system atrophy: a preliminary investigation. Clin Auton Res 1991;1:9–13.

8. Gilman S, Low P, Quinn N, Albanese A, Ben-Shlomo Y, Fowler CJ, et al. Consensus statement on the diagnosis of multiple system atrophy. Clin Auton Res 1998;8:359–362.

9. Hanna P, Jankovic J, Kirkpatrick JB. Multiple system atrophy: the putative causative role of environmental toxins. Arch Neurol 1999;56:90–94.

10. Vanacore N, Bonifati V, Fabbrini G, Colosimo C, Marconi R, Nicholl D, et al. Smoking habits in multiple system atrophy and progressive supranuclear palsy. Neurology 2000;54:114–119.

11. Quinn N. Multiple system atrophy—the nature of the beast. J Neurol Neurosurg Psychiatry 1989;52(Suppl):78–89.

12. Quinn N. Multiple system atrophy. In: Marsden CD, Fahn S, eds. Movement Disorders 3. London: Butterworth-Heinemann, 1994:262–281.

13. Wenning GK, Ben Shlomo Y, Magalhaes M, Daniel SE, Quinn NP. Clinical features and natural history of multiple system atrophy. An analysis of 100 cases. Brain 1994;117(Pt 4):835–845.

14. Magalhaes M, Wenning GK, Daniel SE, Quinn NP. Autonomic dysfunction in pathologically confirmed multiple system atrophy and idiopathic Parkinson's disease—a retrospective comparison. Acta Neurol Scand 1995;91(2):98-102.

15. Quinn NP, Wenning G, Marsden CD. The Shy Drager syndrome. What did Shy and Drager really describe? Arch Neurol 1995;52(7):656–657.

16. Litvan I, Booth V, Wenning GK, Bartko JJ, Goetz CG, McKee A, et al. Retrospective application of a set of clinical diagnostic criteria for the diagnosis of multiple system atrophy. J Neural Transm 1998;105(2–3):217–227.

17. Colosimo C, Vanacore N, Bonifati V, Fabbrini G, Rum A, De Michele G, et al. Clinical diagnosis of multiple system atrophy: level of agreement between Quinn's criteria and the consensus conference guidelines. Acta Neurol Scand 2001;103:261–264.

18. Osaki Y, Wenning GK, Daniel SE, Hughes A, Lees AJ, Mathias CJ, et al. Do published criteria improve clinical diagnostic accuracy in multiple system atrophy? Neurology 2002;59(10):1486–1491.

19. Ben Shlomo Y, Wenning GK, Tison F, Quinn NP. Survival of patients with pathologically proven multiple system atrophy: a meta-analysis. Neurology 1997;48(2):384–393.

20. Wenning G, Tison F, Ben-Shlomo Y, Daniel SE, Quinn NP. Multiple system atrophy: a review of 203 pathologically proven cases. Mov Disord 1997;12(2):133–147.

21. Schwarz J, Tatsch K, Arnold G, Gasser T, Trenkwalder C, Kirsch C. 123I-iodobenzamide-SPECT predicts dopaminergic responsiveness in patients with de novo parkinsonism. Neurology 1992;42:556–561.

22. Schelosky L, Hierholzer J, Wissel J, Cordes M, Poewe W. Correlation of clinical response in apomorphine test with D2-receptor status as demonstrated by 123I IBZM-SPECT. Mov Disord 1993;8(4):453–458.

23. Wenning GK, Ben Shlomo Y, Hughes A, Daniel SE, Lees A, Quinn NP. What clinical features are most useful to distinguish definite multiple system atrophy from Parkinson's disease? J Neurol Neurosurg Psychiatry 2000;68(4):434–440.

24. Boesch SM, Wenning GK, Ransmayr G, Poewe W. Dystonia in multiple system atrophy. J Neurol Neurosurg Psychiatry 2002;72(3):300–303.

25. Hughes A, Colosimo C, Kleedorfer B, Daniel SE, Lees AJ. The dopaminergic response in multiple system atrophy. J Neurol Neurosurg Psychiatry 1992;55:1009–1013.

26. Parati E, Fetoni V, Geminiani C, Soliveri P, Giovannini P, Testa D, et al. Response to L-Dopa in multiple system atrophy. Clin Neuropharmacol 1993;16(2):139–144.

27. Schulz J, Klockgether T, Petersen D, Jauch M, Müller-Schauenburg W, Spieker S, et al. Multiple system atrophy: natural history, MRI morphology, and dopamine receptor imaging with 123IBZM-SPECT. J Neurol Neurosurg Psychiatry 1994;57:1047–1056.

28. Wenning GK, Kraft E, Beck R, Fowler CJ, Mathias CJ, Quinn NP, et al. Cerebellar presentation of multiple system atrophy. Mov Disord 1997;12(1):115–117.

29. Watanabe H, Saito Y, Terao S, Ando T, Kachi T, Mukai E. Progression and prognosis in multiple system atrophy: an analysis of 230 Japanese patients. Brain 2002;125:1070–1083.

30. Gouider-Khouja N, Vidailhet M, Bonnet AM, Pichon J, Agid Y. "Pure" striatonigral degeneration and Parkinson's disease: a comparative clinical study. Mov Disord 1995;10(3):288–294.

31. Holmberg B, Rosengren L, Karlsson JE, Johnels B. Increased cerebrospinal fluid levels of neurofilament protein in progressive supranuclear palsy and multiple-system atrophy compared with Parkinson's disease. Mov Disord 1998;13(1):70–77.

32. Holmberg B, Johnels B, Ingvarsson P, Eriksson B, Rosengren L. CSF-neurofilament and levodopa tests combined with discriminant analysis may contribute to the differential diagnosis of Parkinsonian syndromes. Parkinsonism Relat Disord 2001;8(1):23–31.

33. Polinsky RJ, Brown RT, Lee GK, Timmers K, Culman J, Foldes O, et al. Beta-endorphin, ACTH, and catecholamine responses in chronic autonomic failure. Ann Neurol 1987;21(6):573–577.

34. Kimber JR, Watson L, Mathias CJ. Distinction of idiopathic Parkinson's disease from multiple-system atrophy by stimulation of growth-hormone release with clonidine. Lancet 1997;349(9069):1877–1881.

35. Kaufmann H, Oribe E, Miller M, Knott P, Wiltshire-Clement M, Yahr MD. Hypotension-induced vasopressin release distinguishes between pure autonomic failure and multiple system atrophy with autonomic failure. Neurology 1992;42(3 Pt 1):590–593.

36. Zoukos Y, Thomaides T, Pavitt DV, Cuzner ML, Mathias CJ. Beta-adrenoceptor expression on circulating mononuclear cells of idiopathic Parkinson's disease and autonomic failure patients before and after reduction of central sympathetic outflow by clonidine. Neurology 1993;43(6):1181–1187.

37. Clarke CE, Ray PS, Speller JM. Failure of the clonidine growth hormone stimulation test to differentiate multiple system atrophy from early or advanced idiopathic Parkinson's disease. Lancet 1999;353(9161):1329–1330.

38. Consensus statement on the definition of orthostatic hypotension, pure autonomic failure, and multiple system atrophy. J Neurol Sci 1996;144(1–2):218–219.

39. Bannister R, Mathias C. Investigation of autonomic disorders. In: Mathias C, Bannister R, eds. Autonomic Failure: A Textbook of Clinical Disorders of the Autonomic Nervous System. Oxford: Oxford University Press, 1999:169–195.

40. Braune S, Auer A, Schulte-Mönting J, Schwerbrock S, Lücking C. Cardiovascular parameters: sensitivity to detect autonomic dysfunction and influence of age and sex in normal subjects. Clin Auton Res 1996;6:3–15.

41. Braune S, Schulte-Mönting J, Schwerbrock S, Lücking CH. Retest variation of cardiovascular parameters in autonomic testing. J Auton Nerv Syst 1996;60(3):103–107.

42. Riley D, Chemlinsky T. Autonomic nervous system testing may not distinguish multiple system atrophy from Parkinson's disease. J Neurol Neurosurg Psychiatry 2003;74(1):56–60.

43. Ziegler M, Lake C, Kopin I. The sympathetic-nervous-system defect in primary orthostatic hypotension. N Engl J Med 1977;296:293–297.

44. Polinsky R, Kopin I, Ebert M, Weise V. Pharmacologic distinction of different orthostatic hypotension syndromes. Neurology 1981;31:1–7.

45. Braune S, Reinhardt M, Schnitzer R, Riedel A, Lücking CH. Cardiac uptake of (123I)MIBG separates Parkinson's disease from multiple system atrophy. Neurology 1999;53(5):1020–1025.

46. Orimo S, Ozawa E, Nakade S, Sugimoto T, Mizusawa H. (123)I-metaiodobenzylguanidine myocardial scintigraphy in Parkinson's disease. J Neurol Neurosurg Psychiatry 1999;67(2):189–194.

47. Takatsu H, Nagashima K, Murase M, Fujiwara H, Nishida H, Matsuo H, et al. Differentiating Parkinson disease from multiple-system atrophy by measuring cardiac iodine-123 metaiodobenzylguanidine accumulation. JAMA 2000;284(1):44–45.

48. Taki J, Nakajima K, Hwang EH, Matsunari I, Komai K, Yoshita M, et al. Peripheral sympathetic dysfunction in patients with Parkinson's disease without autonomic failure is heart selective and disease specific. Eur J Nucl Med 2000;27(5):566-573.

49. Kirby R, Fowler CJ, Gosling J, Bannister R. Urethro-vesical dysfunction in progressive autonomic failure with multiple system atrophy. J Neurol Neurosurg Psychiatry 1986;49:554–562.

50. Beck R, Betts C, Fowler C. Genitourinary dysfunction in multiple system atrophy: clinical features and treatment in 62 cases. J Urol 1994;151(5):1336–1341.

51. Wenning GK, Tison F, Elliott L, Quinn NP, Daniel SE. Olivopontocerebellar pathology in multiple system atrophy. Mov Disord 1996;11(2):157–162.

52. Schrag A, Good CD, Miszkiel K, Morris HR, Mathias CJ, Lees AJ, et al. Differentiation of atypical parkinsonian syndromes with routine MRI. Neurology 2000;54(3):697–702.

53. Klockgether T, Schroth G, Diener HC, Dichgans J. Idiopathic cerebellar ataxia of late onset: natural history and MRI morphology. J Neurol Neurosurg Psychiatry 1990;53:297–305.

54. Wüllner U, Klockgether T, Petersen D, Naegele T, Dichgans J. Magnetic resonance imaging in hereditary and idiopathic ataxia. Neurology 1993;43:318–325.

55. Wakai M, Kume A, Takahashi A, Ando T, Hashizume Y. A study of parkinsonism in multiple system atrophy: clinical and MRI correlation. Acta Neurol Scand 1994;90(4):225–231.

56. Albanese A, Colosimo C, Bentivoglio A, Fenici R, Melillo G, Colosimo C, et al. Multiple system atrophy presenting as parkinsonism: clinical features and diagnostic criteria. J Neurol Neurosurg Psychiatry 1995;59:144–151.

57. Konagaya M, Konagaya Y, Sakai M, Matsuoka Y, Hashizume Y. Progressive cerebral atrophy in multiple system atrophy. J Neurol Sci 2002;195(2):123–127.

58. Savoiardo M, Strada L Girotti F. Olivopontocerebellar atrophy: MR diagnosis and relationship to multisystem atrophy. Radiology 1990;174:693–696.

59. Drayer B, Olanow W, Burger P, Johnson GA, Herfkens R, Riederer S. Parkinson Plus syndrome: diagnosis using high field MR imaging of brain iron. Radiology 1986;159:493-498.

60. Pastakia B, Polinsky R, Di Chiro G, Simmon JT, Brown R, Wener L. Multiple system atrophy (Shy–Drager syndrome): MR imaging. Radiology 1986;159:499–502.

61. Olanow C. Magnetic resonance imaging in parkinsonism. Neurol Clin 1992;10:405–420.

62. Lang A, Curran T, Provias J, Bergeron C. Striatonigral degeneration: iron deposition in putamen correlated with the slit-like void signal of magnetic resonance imaging. Can J Neurol Sci 1994;21:311–318.

63. O'Brien C, Sung JH, McGeachie RE, Lee MC. Striatonigral degeneration: Clinical, MRI, and pathologic correlation. Neurology 1990;40:710–711.

64. Schwarz J, Weis S, Kraft E. Signal changes on MRI and increases in reactive microgliosis, astrogliosis, and iron in the putamen of two patients with multiple system atrophy. J Neurol Neurosurg Psychiatry 1996;60:98–101.

65. Stern M, Braffman BH, Skolnick BE, Hurtig HI, Grossman RI. Magnetic resonance imaging in Parkinson's disease and parkinsonian syndromes. Neurology 1989;39:1524–1526.

66. Schrag A, Kingsley D, Phatouros C, Mathias CJ, Lees AJ, Daniel SE, et al. Clinical usefulness of magnetic resonance imaging in multiple system atrophy. J Neurol Neurosurg Psychiatry 1998;65(1):65–71.

67. Brooks D, Luthert P, Gadian D, Marsden C. Does signal-attentuation on high-field T2-weighted MRI of the brain reflect regional cerebral iron deposition? Observations on the relationship between regional cerebral water proton T2-values and iron levels. J Neurol Neurosurg Psychiatry 1989;52:108–111.

68. Kraft E, Trenkwalder C, Auer DP. T2*-weighted MRI differentiates multiple system atrophy from Parkinson's disease. Neurology 2002;59(8):1265–1267.

69. Konagaya M, Konagaya Y, Iida M. Clinical and magnetic resonance imaging study of extrapyramidal symptoms in multiple system atrophy. J Neurol Neurosurg Psychiatry 1994;57:1528–1531.

70. Konagaya M, Konagaya Y, Honda H, Iida M. A clinico-MRI study of extrapyramidal symptoms in multiple system atrophy—linear hyperintensity in the outer margin of the putamen. No To Shinkei 1993;45(6):509–513.

71. Yekhlef F, Ballan G, Macia F, Delmer O, Sourgen C, Tison F. Routine MRI for the differential diagnosis of Parkinson's disease, MSA, PSP, and CBD. J Neural Transm 2003;110(2):151–169.

72. Kraft E, Schwarz J, Trenkwalder C, Vogl T, Pfluger T, Oertel WH. The combination of hypointense and hyperintense signal changes on T2-weighted magnetic resonance imaging sequences: a specific marker of multiple system atrophy? Arch Neurol 1999;56(2):225–228.

73. Konagaya M, Sakai M, Matsuoka Y, Goto Y, Yoshida M, Hashizume Y. Patho-MR imaging study in the putaminal margin in multiple system atrophy. No To Shinkei 1998;50(4):383–385.

74. Schocke M, Seppi K, Esterhammer R, Kremser C, Jaschke W, Poewe W. Diffusion-weighted MRI differentiates the Parinson variant of multiple system atrophy from PD. Neurology 2002;58:575–580.

75. Seppi K, Schocke MF, Esterhammer R, Kremser C, Brenneis C, Mueller J, et al. Diffusion-weighted imaging discriminates progressive supranuclear palsy from PD, but not from the parkinson variant of multiple system atrophy. Neurology 2003;60(6):922–927.

76. Schulz J, Skalej M, Wedekind D, Luft AR, Abele M, Voigt K, et al. Magnetic resonance imaging-based volumetry differentiates idiopathic Parkinson's syndrome from multiple system atrophy and progressive supranuclear palsy. Ann Neurol 1999;45:65–74.

77. Brenneis C, Seppi K, Schocke M, Müller J, Luginger E, Bösch S, et al. Voxel-based morphometry detects cortical atrophy in the parkinson variant of multiple system atrophy. Mov Disord 2003;18(10):1132–1138.

78. Robbins TW, James M, Lange KW, Owen AM, Quinn NP, Marsden CD. Cognitive performance in multiple system atrophy. Brain 1992;115(Pt 1):271–291.

79. Davie CA, Wenning GK, Barker GJ, Tofts PS, Kendall BE, Quinn N, et al. Differentiation of multiple system atrophy from idiopathic Parkinson's disease using proton magnetic resonance spectroscopy. Ann Neurol 1995;37(2):204–210.

80. Federico F, Simone IL, Lucivero V, Mezzapesa DM, de Mari M, Lamberti P, et al. Usefulness of proton magnetic resonance spectroscopy in differentiating parkinsonian syndromes. Ital J Neurol Sci 1999;20(4):223–229.

81. Ellis C, Lemmens G, Williams S, Simmons A, Leigh PN, Chaudhuri K. Striatal changes in striatonigral degeneration and Parkinson's disease: a proton magnetic resonance spectroscopy study. Mov Disord 1996;11:104.

82. Hu M, Simmons A, Glover A. Proton magnetic resonance spectroscopy of the putamen in Parkinson's disease and multiple system atrophy. Mov Disord 1998;13:182.

83. Brooks D, Ibanez V, Sawle GV, Quinn N, Lees AJ, Mathias CJ, et al. Differing patterns of striatal 18F-dopa uptake in Parkinson's disease, multiple system atrophy, and progressive supranuclear palsy. Ann Neurol 1990;28:547–555.

84. Brooks D, Salmon E, Mathias C, Quinn N, Leenders K, Bannister R, et al. The relationship between locomotor disability, autonomic dysfunction, and the integrity of the striatal dopaminergic system in patients with multiple system atrophy, pure autonomic failure, and Parkinson's disease, studied with PET. Brain 1990;113:1539–1552.

85. Burn D, Sawle G, Brooks D. Differential diagnosis of Parkinson's disease, multiple system atrophy, and Steele–Richardson–Olszewski syndrome: discriminant analysis of striatal 18F-dopa PET data. J Neurol Neurosurg Psychiatry 1994;57(3):278–284.

86. Brooks D, Ibanez V, Sawle G, Playford E, Quinn N, Mathias C, et al. Striatal D2 receptor status in patients with Parkinson's disease, striatonigral degeneration, and progressive supranuclear palsy, measured with 11C-raclopride and positron emission tomography. Ann Neurol 1992;31(2):184–192.

87. Burn D, Rinne J, Quinn N, Lees A, Marsden C, Brooks D. Striatal opioid receptor binding in Parkinson's disease, striatonigral degeneration and Steele–Richardson–Olsewski syndrome. A (11C)diprenorphine PET study. Brain 1995;118:951–958.

88. De Volder A, Francart J, Laterre C, Dooms G, Bol A, Michel C, et al. Decreased glucose utilization in the striatum and frontal lobe in probable striatonigral degeneration. Ann Neurol 1989;26:239–247.

89. Eidelberg D, Takikawa S, Moeller JR, Dhawan V, Redington K, Chaly T, et al. Striatal hypometabolism distinguishes striatonigral degeneration from Parkinson's disease. Ann Neurol 1993;33:518–527.

90. Perani D, Bressi S, Testa D, Grassi F, Cortelli P, Gentrini S, et al. Clinical/metabolic correlations in multiple system atrophy. A fludeoxyglucose F18 positron emission tomography study. Arch Neurol 1995;52:179-185.

91. Antonini A, Kazamuta k, Feigin A, Mandel F, Dhawan V, Margouleff C, et al. Differential diagnosis of parkinsonism with 18F-fluorodeoxyglucose and PET. Mov Disord 1998;13(2):268–274.

92. Ghaemi M, Hilker R, Rudolf J, Sobesky J, Heiss WD. Differentiating multiple system atrophy from Parkinson's disease: contribution of striatal and midbrain MRI volumetry and multi-tracer PET imaging. J Neurol Neurosurg Psychiatry 2002;73(5):517–523.

93. Gilman S, Koeppe RA, Junck L, Kluin KJ, Lohman M, St. Laurent RT. Patterns of cerebral glucose metabolism detected with positron emission tomography differ in multiple system atrophy and olivopontocerebellar atrophy. Ann Neurol 1994;36:166–175.

94. Rinne J, Burn DJ, Mathias CJ, Quinn NP, Marsden CD, Brooks DJ. Positron emission tomography studies on the dopaminergic system and striatal opioid binding in the olivopontocerebellar atrophy variant of multiple system atrophy. Ann Neurol 1995;37:568–573.

95. Gilman S, Koeppe RA, Junck L, Kluin KJ, Lohman M, St. Laurent RT. Benzodiazepine receptor binding in cerebellar degenerations studied with positron emission tomography. Ann Neurol 1995;38:176–185.

96. Shinotoh H, Inoue O, Hirayama K. Dopamine D1 receptors in Parkinson's disease and striatonigral degeneration: a positron emission tomography study. J Neurol Neurosurg Psychiatry 1993;56:467–472.

97. Schwarz J, Tatsch K, Arnold G, Ott M, Trenkwalder C, Kirsch CM, et al. 123I-iodobenzamide-SPECT in 83 patients with *de novo* parkinsonism. Neurology 1993;43(6):17–20.

98. Brücke T, Wenger S, Asenbaum S. Dopamine D2 receptor imaging and measurement with SPECT. Adv Neurol 1993;60:494–500.

99. Pirker W, Djamshidian S, Asenbaum S, Gerschlager W, Tribl G, Hoffmann M, et al. Progression of dopaminergic degeneration in Parkinson's disease and atypical parkinsonism: a longitudinal beta-CIT SPECT study. Mov Disord 2002;17:45–53.

100. Yoshita M. Differentiation of idiopathic Parkinson's disease from striatonigral degeneration and progressive supranuclear palsy using iodine-123 meta-iodobenzylguanidine myocardial scintigraphy. J Neurol Sci 1998;155:60–67.

101. Martinelli P, Coccagna G. Etude electromyographique du sphincter strie de l'anus dans trois cas de syndrome de Shy–Drager. In: Arbus L, Cadilhac J, eds. Electromyographie. Toulouse: Premieres Journees Languedociennes d'Electro-myographie, 1978:321-326.

102. Eardley I, Quinn NP, Fowler CJ, Kirby RS, Parkhouse HF, Marsden CD, et al. The value of urethral sphincter electromyography in the differential diagnosis of parkinsonism. Br J Urol 1989;64:360–362.

103. Pramstaller PP, Wenning GK, Smith SJ, Beck RO, Quinn NP, Fowler CJ. Nerve conduction studies, skeletal muscle EMG, and sphincter EMG in multiple system atrophy. J Neurol Neurosurg Psychiatry 1995;58(5):618–621.

104. Palace J, Chandiramani VA, Fowler CJ. Value of sphincter electromyography in the diagnosis of multiple system atrophy. Muscle Nerve 1997;20(11):1396–1403.

105. Tison F, Arne P, Sourgen C, Chrysostome V, Yeklef F. The value of external anal sphincter electromyography for the diagnosis of multiple system atrophy. Mov Disord 2000;15(6):1148–1157.

106. Valldeoriola F, Valls-Sole J, Tolosa ES, Marti MJ. Striated anal sphincter denervation in patients with progressive supranuclear palsy. Mov Disord 1995;10(5):550–555.

107. Giladi N, Simon ES, Korczyn AD, Groozman GB, Orlov Y, Shabtai H, et al. Anal sphincter EMG does not distinguish between multiple system atrophy and Parkinson's disease. Muscle Nerve 2000;23:731–734.

108. Libelius R, Johannson F. Quantitative electromyography of the external anal sphincter in Parkinson's disease and multiple system atrophy. Muscle Nerve 2000;23:1250–1256.

109. Colosimo C, Inghilleri M, Chaudhuri KR. Parkinson's disease misdiagnosed as multiple system atrophy by sphincter electromyography. J Neurol 2000;247:559–561.

110. Vodusek B. Sphincter EMG and differential diagnosis of multiple system atrophy. Mov Disord 2001;16(4):600–607.

111. Wenning G, Smith SJM. Magnetic brain stimulation in multiple system atrophy. Mov Disord 1997;12(3):452–453.

112. Abbruzzese G, Marchese R, Trompetto C. Sensory and motor evoked potentials in multiple system atrophy: comparative study with Parkinson's disease. Mov Disord 1997;12(3):315–321.

113. Abele M, Schulz JB, Burk K, Topka H, Dichgans J, Klockgether T. Evoked potentials in multiple system atrophy (MSA). Acta Neurol Scand 2000;101(2):111–115.

114. Delalande I, Hache JC, Forzy G, Bughin M, Benhadjali J, Destee A. Do visual-evoked potentials and spatiotemporal contrast sensitivity help to distinguish idiopathic Parkinson's disease and multiple system atrophy? Mov Disord 1998;13(3):446–452.

115. Montagna P, Martinelli P, Rizzuto N, Salviati A, Rasi F, Lugaresi E. Amyotrophy in Shy–Drager syndrome. Acta Neurol Belg 1983;83:142–157.

116. Cohen J, Low P, Fealey R, Sheps S, Jiang NS. Somatic and autonomic function in progressive autonomic failure and multiple system atrophy. Ann Neurol 1987;22:692–699.

117. Abele M, Schulz J, Burk K, Topka H, Dichgans J, Klockgether T. Nerve conduction studies in multiple system atrophy. Eur Neurol 2000;43(4):221–223.

118. Kofler M, Muller J, Wenning GK, Reggiani L, Hollosi P, Bosch S, et al. The auditory startle reaction in parkinsonian disorders. Mov Disord 2001;16(1):62–71.

119. Kofler M, Muller J, Seppi K, Wenning GK. Exaggerated auditory startle responses in multiple system atrophy: a comparative study of parkinson and cerebellar subtypes. Clin Neurophysiol 2003;114(3):541–547.

120. Kume A, Takahashi A, Hashizume Y. Neuronal cell loss of the striatonigral system in multiple system atrophy. J Neurol Sci 1993;117:33–40.

121. Sung J, Mastri A, Segal E. Pathology of Shy–Drager syndrome. J Neuropathol Exp Neurol 1979;38:353–368.

122. Benarroch EE, Smithson IL, Low PA, Parisi JE. Depletion of catecholaminergic neurons of the rostral ventrolateral medulla in multiple systems atrophy with autonomic failure. Ann Neurol 1998;43(2):156–163.

123. Shy G, Drager GA. A neurological syndrome associated with orthostatic hypotension. A clinicopathological study. Arch Neurol 1960;2:511–527.

124. Nakamura S, Ohnishi K, Nishimura M, Suenaga T, Akiguchi I, Kimura J, et al. Large neurons in the tuberomammillary nucleus in patients with Parkinson's disease and multiple system atrophy. Neurology 1996;46(6):1693–1696.

125. Papp M, Lantos PL. The distribution of oligodendroglial inclusions in multiple system atrophy and its relevance to clinical symptomatology. Brain 1994;117:235–243.

126. Konno H, Yamamoto T, Iwasaki Y, Iizuka H. Shy–Drager syndrome and amyotrophic lateral sclerosis. Cytoarchitectonic and morphometric studies of sacral autonomic neurons. J Neurol Sci 1986;73(2):193–204.

127. Daniel S. The neuropathology and neurochemistry of multiple system atrophy. In: Mathias C, Bannister R, eds. Autonomic Failure: A Textbook of Clinical Disorders of the Autonomic Nervous System. Oxford: Oxford University Press, 1999:321–328.

128. Oppenheimer DR. Lateral horn cells in progressive autonomic failure. J Neurol Sci 1980;46(3):393–404.

129. Bannister R, Oppenheimer D. Degenerative diseases of the nervous system associated with autonomic failure. Brain 1972;95:457–474.

130. Tsuchiya K, Ozawa E, Haga C, Watabiki S, Ikeda M, Sano M, et al. Constant involvement of the Betz cells and pyramidal tract in multiple system atrophy: a clinicopathological study of seven autopsy cases. Acta Neuropathol (Berl) 2000;99:628–636.

131. Wakabayashi K, Ikeuchi T, Ishikawa A, Takahashi H. Multiple system atrophy with severe involvement of the motor cortical areas and cerebral white matter. J Neurol Sci 1998;156(1):114–117.

132. Konagaya M, Sakai M, Matsuoka Y, Konagaya Y, Hashizume Y. Multiple system atrophy with remarkable frontal lobe atrophy. Acta Neuropathol (Berl) 1999;97(4):423–428.

133. Sima A, Caplan M, D'Amato CJ, Pevzner M, Furlong JW. Fulminant multiple system atrophy in a young adult presenting as motor neuron disease. Neurology 1993;43:2031–2035.

134. Hayashi M, Isozaki E, Oda M, Tanabe H, Kimura J. Loss of large myelinated nerve fibres of the recurrent laryngeal nerve in patients with multiple system atrophy and vocal cord palsy. J Neurol Neurosurg Psychiatry 1997;62:234–238.

135. Braak H, Braak E. Cortical and subcortical argyrophilic grains characterize a disease associated with adult onset dementia. Neuropathol Appl Neurobiol 1989;15(1):13-26.

136. Yamada T, McGeer PL. Oligodendroglial microtubular masses: an abnormality observed in some human neurodegenerative diseases. Neurosci Lett 1990;120:163–166.

137. Arima K, Nakamura M, Sunohara N, Ogawa M, Anno M, Izumiyama Y, et al. Ultrastructural characterization of the tau-immunoreactive tubules in the oligodendroglial perikarya and their inner loop processes in progressive supranuclear palsy. Acta Neuropathol (Berl) 1997;93(6):558–566.

138. Chin SS, Goldman JE. Glial inclusions in CNS degenerative diseases. J Neuropathol Exp Neurol 1996;55(5):499–508.

139. Wenning G, Quinn N. Are Lewy bodies non-specific epiphenomena of nigral damage? Mov Disord 1994;9(3):378–379.

140. Papp M, Kahn JE, Lantos PL. Glial cytoplasmic inclusions in the CNS of patients with multiple system atrophy (striatonigral degeneration, olivopontocerebellar atrophy and Shy–Drager syndrome). J Neurol Sci 1989;94:79–100.

141. Lantos PL. The definition of multiple system atrophy: a review of recent developments. J Neuropathol Exp Neurol 1998;57(12):1099-1111.

142. Gai WP, Pountney DL, Power JH, Li QX, Culvenor JG, McLean CA, et al. alpha-Synuclein fibrils constitute the central core of oligodendroglial inclusion filaments in multiple system atrophy. Exp Neurol 2003;181(1):68–78.

143. Papp M, Lantos PI. Accumulation of tubular structures in oligodendroglial and neuronal cells as the basic alteration in multiple system atrophy. J Neurol Sci 1992;107:172–182.

144. Cairns NJ, Atkinson PF, Hanger DP, Anderton BH, Daniel SE, Lantos PL. Tau protein in the glial cytoplasmic inclusions of multiple system atrophy can be distinguished from abnormal tau in Alzheimer's disease. Neurosci Lett 1997;230(1):49–52.

145. Dickson DW, Lin W, Liu WK, Yen SH. Multiple system atrophy: a sporadic synucleinopathy. Brain Pathol 1999;9(4):721–732.

146. Goedert M, Spillantini MG. Lewy body diseases and multiple system atrophy as alpha-synucleinopathies. Mol Psychiatry 1998;3(6):462–465.

147. Spillantini MG, Schmidt ML, Lee VM, Trojanowski JQ, Jakes R, Goedert M. Alpha-synuclein in Lewy bodies. Nature 1997;388(6645):839–840.

148. Wakabayashi K, Yoshimoto M, Tsuji S, Takahashi H. Alpha-synuclein immunoreactivity in glial cytoplasmic inclusions in multiple system atrophy. Neurosci Lett 1998;249(2–3):180–182.

149. Wakabayashi K, Hayashi S, Kakita A, Yamada M, Toyoshima Y, Yoshimoto M, et al. Accumulation of alpha-synuclein/NACP is a cytopathological feature common to Lewy body disease and multiple system atrophy. Acta Neuropathol (Berl) 1998;96:445–452.

150. Arima K, Ueda K, Sunohara N, Arakawa K, Hirai S, Nakamura M, et al. NACP/alpha-synuclein immunoreactivity in fibrillary components of neuronal and oligodendroglial cytoplasmic inclusions in the pontine nuclei in multiple system atrophy. Acta Neuropathol (Berl) 1998;96:439–444.

151. Tu P, Galvin JE, Baba M, Giasson B, Tomita T, Leight S, et al. Glial cytoplasmic inclusions in white matter oligodendrocytes of multiple system atrophy brains contain insoluble alpha-synuclein. Ann Neurol 1998;44(3):415–422.

152. Spillantini MG, Crowther RA, Jakes R, Cairns NJ, Lantos PL, Goedert M. Filamentous alpha-synuclein inclusions link multiple system atrophy with Parkinson's disease and dementia with Lewy bodies. Neurosci Lett 1998;251(3):205–208.

153. Trojanowski JQ. Tauists, Baptists, Syners, Apostates, and new data. Ann Neurol 2002;52(3):263–265.

154. Gai WP, Power JH, Blumbergs PC, Blessing WW. Multiple-system atrophy: a new alpha-synuclein disease? Lancet 1998;352(9127):547–548.

155. Hirsch EC, Hunot S, Damier P, Faucheux B. Glial cells and inflammation in Parkinson's disease: a role in neurodegeneration? Ann Neurol 1998;44(3 Suppl 1):S115–S120.

156. Togo T, Iseki E, Marui W, Akiyama H, Ueda K, Kosaka K. Glial involvement in the degeneration process of Lewy body-bearing neurons and the degradation process of Lewy bodies in brains of dementia with Lewy bodies. J Neurol Sci 2001;184(1):71–75.

157. Vila M, Jackson-Lewis V, Guegan C, Wu DC, Teismann P, Choi DK, et al. The role of glial cells in Parkinson's disease. Curr Opin Neurol 2001;14(4):483–489.

158. Allan SM, Rothwell NJ. Cytokines and acute neurodegeneration. Nat Rev Neurosci 2001;2(10):734–744.

159. Boka G, Anglade P, Wallach D, Javoy-Agid F, Agid Y, Hirsch EC. Immunocytochemical analysis of tumor necrosis factor and its receptors in Parkinson's disease. Neurosci Lett 1994;172(1–2):151–154.

160. Hunot S, Dugas N, Faucheux B, Hartmann A, Tardieu M, Debre P, et al. FcepsilonRII/CD23 is expressed in Parkinson's disease and induces, in vitro, production of nitric oxide and tumor necrosis factor-alpha in glial cells. J Neurosci 1999;19(9):3440–3447.

161. Mogi M, Harada M, Riederer P, Narabayashi H, Fujita K, Nagatsu T. Tumor necrosis factor-alpha (TNF-alpha) increases both in the brain and in the cerebrospinal fluid from parkinsonian patients. Neurosci Lett 1994;165(1–2):208–210.

162. McGuire SO, Ling ZD, Lipton JW, Sortwell CE, Collier TJ, Carvey PM. Tumor necrosis factor alpha is toxic to embryonic mesencephalic dopamine neurons. Exp Neurol 2001;169(2):219–230.

163. Aloe L, Fiore M. TNF-alpha expressed in the brain of transgenic mice lowers central tyroxine hydroxylase immunoreactivity and alters grooming behavior. Neurosci Lett 1997;238(1–2):65–68.

164. Gerhard A, Banati RB, Goerres GB, Cagnin A, Myers R, Gunn RN, et al. [(11)C](R)-PK11195 PET imaging of microglial activation in multiple system atrophy. Neurology 2003;61(5):686–689.

165. Wenning G, Granata R, Laboyrie PM, Quinn NP, Jenner P, Marsden CD. Reversal of behavioural abnormalities by fetal allografts in a novel rat model of striatonigral degeneration. Mov Disord 1996;11(5):522–532.

166. Wenning G, Granata R, Puschban Z, Scherfler C, Poewe W. Neural transplantation in animal models of multiple system atrophy: a review. J Neural Transm 1999;55:103–113.

167. Scherfler C, Puschban Z, Ghorayeb I, Goebel GP, Tison F, Jellinger K, et al. Complex motor disturbances in a sequential double lesion rat model of striatonigral degeneration (multiple system atrophy). Neuroscience 2000;99(1):43–54.

168. Ghorayeb I, Puschban Z, Fernagut PO, Scherfler C, Rouland R, Wenning GK, et al. Simultaneous intrastriatal 6-hydroxydopamine and quinolinic acid injection: a model of early-stage striatonigral degeneration. Exp Neurol 2001;167(1):133–147.

169. Waldner R, Puschban Z, Scherfler C, Seppi K, Jellinger K, Poewe W, et al. No functional effects of embryonic neuronal grafts on motor deficits in a 3-nitropropionic acid rat model of advanced striatonigral degeneration (multiple system atrophy). Neuroscience 2001;102(3):581–592.

170. Ghorayeb I, Fernagut PO, Hervier L, Labattu B, Bioulac B, Tison F. A "single toxin-double lesion" rat model of striatonigral degeneration by intrastriatal 1-methyl-4-phenylpyridinium ion injection: a motor behavioural analysis. Neuroscience 2002;115(2):533–546.

171. Stefanova N, Puschban Z, Fernagut PO, Brouillet E, Tison F, Reindl M, et al. Neuropathological and behavioral changes induced by various treatment paradigms with MPTP and 3-nitropropionic acid in mice: towards a model of striatonigral degeneration (multiple system atrophy). Acta Neuropathol (Berl) 2003;106(2):157–166.

172. Fernagut PO, Diguet E, Bioulac B, Tison F. MPTP potentiates 3-nitropronionic acid-induced striatal damage in mice: reference to striatonigral degeneration. Exp Neurol. 2004;185(1):47–62.

173. Ghorayeb I, Fernagut PO, Aubert I, Bezard E, Poewe W, Wenning GK, et al. Toward a primate model of L-dopa-unresponsive parkinsonism mimicking striatonigral degeneration. Mov Disord 2000;15(3):531–536.

174. Ghorayeb I, Fernagut PO, Stefanova N, Wenning GK, Bioulac B, Tison F. Dystonia is predictive of subsequent altered dopaminergic responsiveness in a chronic 1-methyl-4-phenyl-1,2,3,6-tetrahydropyridine+3-nitropropionic acid model of striatonigral degeneration in monkeys. Neurosci Lett 2002;335(1):34–38.

175. Kahle PJ, Neumann M, Ozmen L, Muller V, Jacobsen H, Spooren W, et al. Hyperphosphorylation and insolubility of alpha-synuclein in transgenic mouse oligodendrocytes. EMBO Rep 2002;3(6):583–588.

176. Zuscik M, Sands S, Ross SA, Waugh DJJ, Gaivin RJ, Morilak D, et al. Overexpression of the alpha1B-adrenergic receptor causes apoptotic neurodegeneration: multiple system atrophy. Nat Med 2000;6(12):1388–1394.

177. Puschban Z, Scherfler C, Granata R, Laboyrie P, Quinn NP, Jenner P, et al. Autoradiographic study of striatal dopamine re-uptake sites and dopamine D1 and D2 receptors in a 6-hydroxydopamine and quinolinic acid double-lesion rat model of striatonigral degeneration (multiple system atrophy) and effects of embryonic ventral mesencephalic, striatal or co-grafts. Neuroscience 2000;95(2):377–388.

178. Jankovic J, Gilden JL, Hiner BC, Kaufmann H, Brown DC, Coghlan CH, et al. Neurogenic orthostatic hypotension: a double-blind, placebo-controlled study with midodrine. Am J Med 1993;95(1):38–48.

179. Low PA, Gilden JL, Freeman R, Sheng KN, McElligott MA. Efficacy of midodrine vs placebo in neurogenic orthostatic hypotension. A randomized, double-blind multicenter study. Midodrine Study Group. JAMA 1997;277(13):1046–1051.

180. Wright RA, Kaufmann HC, Perera R, Opfer-Gehrking TL, McElligott MA, Sheng KN et al. A double-blind, dose-response study of midodrine in neurogenic orthostatic hypotension. Neurology 1998;51(1):120–124.

181. Mathias CJ, Senard JM, Braune S, Watson L, Aragishi A, Keeling JE, et al. L-threo-dihydroxyphenylserine (L-threo-DOPS; droxidopa) in the management of neurogenic orthostatic hypotension: a multi-national, multi-center, dose-ranging study in multiple system atrophy and pure autonomic failure. Clin Auton Res 2001;11(4):235–242.

182. Alam M, Smith G, Bleasdale-Barr K, Pavitt DV, Mathias CJ. Effects of the peptide release inhibitor, octreotide, on day-time hypotension and on nocturnal hypertension in primary autonomic failure. J Hypertens 1995;13(12 Pt 2):1664–1669.

183. Raimbach SJ, Cortelli P, Kooner JS, Bannister R, Bloom SR, Mathias CJ. Prevention of glucose-induced hypotension by the somatostatin analogue octreotide (SMS 201-995) in chronic autonomic failure: haemodynamic and hormonal changes. Clin Sci (Lond) 1989;77(6):623–628.

184. Mathias CJ, Fosbraey P, da Costa DF, Thornley A, Bannister R. The effect of desmopressin on nocturnal polyuria, overnight weight loss, and morning postural hypotension in patients with autonomic failure. Br Med J (Clin Res Ed) 1986;293(6543):353–354.

185. Perera R, Isola L, Kaufmann H. Effect of recombinant erythropoietin on anemia and orthostatic hypotension in primary autonomic failure. Clin Auton Res 1995;5(4):211–213.

186. Winkler A, Marsden J, Parton M, Watkins P, Chaudhuri K. Erythropoietin deficiency and anaemia in multiple system atrophy. Mov Disord 2001;16:233–239.

187. Mathias C, Kimber JR. Postural hypotension: causes, clinical features, investigation, and management. Annu Rev Med 1999;50:317–326.

188. Sakakibara R, Hattori T, Uchiyama T, Suenaga T, Takahashi H, Yamanishi T, et al. Are alpha-blockers involved in lower urinary tract dysfunction in multiple system atrophy? A comparison of prazosin and moxisylyte. J Auton Nerv Syst 2000;79:191–195.

189. Colosimo C, Pezzella FR. The symptomatic treatment of multiple system atrophy. Eur J Neurol 2002;9(3):195–199.

190. Zesiewicz T, Helal M, Hauser RA. Sildenafil Citrate (Viagra) for the treatment of erectile dysfunction in men with Parkinson's disease. Mov Disord 2000;15(2):305–308.

191. Hussain IF, Brady CM, Swinn MJ, Mathias CJ, Fowler CJ. Treatment of erectile dysfunction with sildenafil citrate (Viagra) in parkinsonism due to Parkinson's disease or multiple system atrophy with observations on orthostatic hypotension. J Neurol Neurosurg Psychiatry 2001;71(3):371–374.

192. Eichhorn TE, Oertel WH. Macrogol 3350/electrolyte improves constipation in Parkinson's disease and multiple system atrophy. Mov Disord 2001;16(6):1176–1177.

193. Iranzo A, Santamaria J, Tolosa E, Barcelona Multiple System Atrophy Study Group. Continuous positive air pressure eliminates nocturnal stridor in multiple system atrophy. Lancet 2000;356:1329–1330.

194. Lees A. The treatment of the motor disorder of multiple system atrophy. In: Mathias C, Bannister R, eds. Autonomic Failure. Oxford: Oxford University Press, 1999:357–363.

195. Lees A, Bannister R. The use of lisuride in the treatment of multiple system atrophy with autonomic failure (Shy–Drager syndrome). J Neurol Neurosurg Psychiatry 1981;44:347–351.

196. Colosimo C, Merello M, Pontieri FE. Amantadine in parkinsonian patients unresponsive to levodopa: a pilot study. J Neurol 1996;243(5):422–425.

197. Lang AE, Lozano A, Duff J, Tasker R, Miyasaki J, Galvez-Jimenez N, et al. Medial pallidotomy in late-stage Parkinson's disease and striatonigral degeneration. Adv Neurol 1997;74:199–211.

198. Visser-Vandewalle V, Temel Y, Colle H, van der LC. Bilateral high-frequency stimulation of the subthalamic nucleus in patients with multiple system atrophy—parkinsonism. Report of four cases. J Neurosurg 2003;98(4):882–887.

199. Graham J, Oppenheimer DR. Orthostatic-hypotension and nicotine sensitivity in a case of multiple system atrophy. J Neurol Neurosurg Psychiatry 1969;32:28–34.

200. Johnsen J, Miller VT. Tobacco intolerance in multiple system atrophy. Neurology 1986;36:986–988.

201. Wenning GK, Seppi K, Sampaio C, Quinn NP, Poewe W, Tison F. European Multiple System Atrophy Study Group (EMSA-SG): Validation of the Unified MSA Rating Scale (UMSARS). Mov Disord 2002;17(Suppl 5):252.

21

Clinical Diagnosis of Dementia With Lewy Bodies

David J. Burn, Urs P. Mosimann, and Ian G. McKeith

INTRODUCTION

Dementia with Lewy bodies (DLB) is a dementia syndrome associated with visual hallucinations, parkinsonism, and fluctuating levels of attention. "Necroepidemiological" studies place DLB second to Alzheimer's disease (AD) in prevalence, accounting for 15–20% of all autopsy-confirmed dementias. The prevalence of clinically diagnosed DLB in a Finnish population aged 75 yr or older was found to be 5%, comprising 22% of all demented subjects (1).

The association of Lewy bodies with Parkinson's disease (PD) was made in 1912, but it was not until nearly 50 yr later, in 1961, that Okazaki and colleagues reported the association of the same inclusion body with severe dementia in two elderly male patients (2). In contrast to their brainstem counterparts, cortical Lewy bodies are less eosinophilic and lack a clear halo, making them more difficult to recognize using older haematoxylin and eosin staining methods. With the advent of more sensitive immunohistochemical techniques, notably ubiquitin and α-synuclein antibodies, a significantly greater burden of cortical Lewy body and neuritic pathology may be identified.

Cortical Lewy bodies may also be found in the majority of PD cases, with or without dementia, as well as in DLB. Alzheimer's-type pathological features, notably senile plaques, frequently coexist in both DLB and PD with dementia (PDD). This "dual pathology" and clinicopathological overlap between PDD and DLB on the one hand and AD and DLB on the other, encapsulates the nosological debate currently surrounding DLB. Indeed, some authorities refer to DLB as the "Lewy body variant of Alzheimer's disease," although "dementia with Lewy bodies" is the preferred term, following a Consensus meeting in 1996 (3).

This chapter will discuss the various components of the DLB clinical syndrome and explore the diagnostic issues that arise in differentiating DLB from PDD and AD. For details on the pathology the reader should see Chapters 4 and 8, and for the genetic aspects, Chapter 6.

CLINICAL FEATURES OF DEMENTIA WITH LEWY BODIES

The central feature of DLB is a progressive cognitive decline of sufficient magnitude to interfere with normal social or occupational function, whereas core clinical components comprise fluctuating cognition, recurrent and persistent visual hallucinations, and extrapyramidal signs (EPS). Supportive features may increase diagnostic sensitivity, though exclusion criteria also need to be considered (Table 1). Depression and REM sleep behavior disorder (RBD) have been suggested as additions to the list of supportive features (4).

From: *Current Clinical Neurology: Atypical Parkinsonian Disorders*
Edited by: I. Litvan © Humana Press Inc., Totowa, NJ

Table 1
Consensus Criteria for Clinical Diagnosis of Probable and Possible DLB

1. The central feature required for a diagnosis of DLB is progressive cognitive decline of sufficient magnitude to interfere with normal social and occupational function. Prominent or persistent memory impairment may not necessarily occur in the early stages but is usually evident with progression. Deficits on tests of attention and of frontal-subcortical skills and visuospatial ability may be especially prominent.

2. *Two* of the following core features are essential for a diagnosis of *probable DLB* and *one* is essential for *possible DLB*:

   a. fluctuation of cognition with pronounced variations in attention and alertness
   b. recurrent visual hallucinations that are typically well formed and detailed
   c. spontaneous motor features of parkinsonism

3. Features supportive of the diagnosis are:

   a. repeated falls
   b. syncope
   c. transient loss of consciousness
   d. neuroleptic sensitivity
   e. systematized delusions
   f. hallucinations in other modalities
   g. REM sleep behavior disorder *(4)*
   h. depression *(4)*

4. A diagnosis of DLB is less likely in the presence of:

   a. stroke disease, evident as focal neurological signs or on brain imaging
   b. evidence on physical examination and investigation of any physical illness or other brain disorder sufficient to account for the clinical picture

Adapted from ref. *3*.

Cognitive and Neuropsychological Profile

A meta-analysis of 21 controlled comparisons has shown a clear and profound pattern of visual-perceptual and attentional-executive impairments in DLB *(5)*. In terms of group differences, patients with DLB always do worse than age-matched controls on neuropsychological tasks, with particularly poor performance on visual perceptual and learning tasks, visual semantic tasks, and praxis tasks. Simple global measures of performance (e.g., the Mini Mental State Examination [MMSE]) are usually equivalent to those of patients with AD of comparable severity, highlighting the insensitivity of these tests to executive dysfunction. There are trends for better performance in DLB than AD patients on verbal memory and orientation tasks, for example, logical memory from the Wechsler Memory Scale. Patients with DLB lack the poor retention over delay intervals and increased propensity to produce intrusion errors in the cued recall condition, typical of AD. Performance on visual tasks, particularly praxis tasks, for example, Block Design from the Wechsler Adult Intelligence Scale, is consistently more impaired in DLB than in AD. A DLB patient will perform more poorly on simple bedside constructional tasks, for example copying a clock face, than an AD patient of comparable MMSE *(6)*.

The neuropsychological changes with progression of DLB are not well characterized, though the clinical impression is that differences with AD are particularly pronounced in the early stages and, as the disease evolves, these lessen. Rate of progression, as evidenced by change in mental test scores, is equivalent to that seen in AD and vascular dementia *(7)*.

Fluctuating Cognition

Variation in cognitive performance is commonly observed in all the major late-onset dementias. It is frustrating to carers and has a major impact upon the patient's ability to reliably perform everyday activities. Fluctuating cognition (FC) may present in several ways, previously described as "sundowning" or "intermittent delirium," depending upon the severity and diurnal pattern. FC occurs in 80% or more of DLB patients. The profile of attentional impairment and fluctuating attention in DLB is indistinguishable from that recorded in PDD *(8)*.

The severity of FC can be judged by experienced clinicians and is highly correlated with variability in performance on computer-based attentional tasks. The variation can be detected over very short periods of time (on a second-to-second basis), suggesting that FC derives from dysfunction of continuously active arousal systems *(9)*. Questions posed to the carer such as "are there times when his or her thinking seems quite clear and then becomes muddled" may be useful probes for this symptom. Substantial variability in attentiveness may also be observed throughout the consultation, or between one appointment and the next. The Clinician Assessment of Fluctuation and the One Day Fluctuation Assessment Scale are validated instruments to record FC, correlating with both neuropsychological and electrophysiological measures of fluctuation *(10)*.

Neuropsychiatric Features

A majority of DLB patients (80%) experience neuropsychiatric symptoms, particularly hallucinations, delusions, apathy, anxiety, and depression, at some stage of their illness *(11)*. These symptoms may be quantified using the Neuropsychiatric Inventory (NPI), a 12-item interview with the caregiver rating frequency, severity, and associated carer distress of delusions, hallucinations, agitation, depression, anxiety, elation, apathy, disinhibition, irritability, aberrant motor behavior, sleep, and appetite disturbances *(12)*. The NPI-4, comprising delusions, hallucinations, depression, and apathy, may represent a sufficiently sensitive abbreviated form of the NPI for practical use in the busy clinic setting for patient assessment *(13)*.

Visual hallucinations (VHs) are a core feature in the Consensus Criteria for the clinical diagnosis of DLB. They are present in 33% of patients at the time of presentation (range 11–64%) and occur at some point in the course of the illness in 46% (13–80%) *(14)*.

VHs are the most common form of hallucination in DLB, although tactile, olfactory, and auditory hallucinations may also occur. The VHs are complex in type, often containing detailed scenes featuring mute people and animals *(15)*. Affective responses to the hallucinations vary from indifference, to amusement, or fear and combativeness. VHs and delusions often coexist, common delusions being phantom border delusions (i.e., the belief that strangers live in the home), or paranoid delusions of persecution, theft, and spousal infidelity. Delusions and hallucinations often trigger other behavioral problems, such as aggression and agitation, leading to profound caregiver distress and precipitating early nursing home admission.

VHs in DLB correlate strongly with Lewy body density in parahippocampal and inferior temporal lobe cortices *(16)*. *See also* Chapter 11.

Extrapyramidal Signs

The frequency of parkinsonian features at presentation in DLB ranges between 10% and 78%, with 40–100% of DLB cases displaying EPS at some stage of the illness *(17–19)*, with differences likely to represent ascertainment bias, use of neuroleptic agents, and variable definition of clinical phenomenology.

The Phenomenology of the Extrapyramidal Syndrome in DLB

Louis and coworkers compared EPS in 31 DLB and 34 PD pathologically confirmed cases *(17)*. Clinical information was obtained prospectively in some patients. DLB patients presenting with parkinsonism were, on average, 10 yr younger than the DLB patients presenting with neuropsychiatric features (60.0 vs 70.9 yr). Of the DLB patients, 92% had at least one sign of parkinsonism, with 92% having either rigidity or bradykinesia. A tremor of any type or a specific rest tremor was recorded in 76% and 55%, respectively, of the DLB patients. This compared with 88% and 85%, respectively, of the PD group. Myoclonus was documented in 18.5% of the DLB patients but none of the PD group.

A trial of levodopa was used in 42% of the DLB group, with a clinical response recorded in 7 of the 10 patients (70%). The dose of levodopa required and the precise nature of the response were not stated. In attempting to differentiate DLB from PD on the basis of the Parkinsonian syndrome, the authors concluded that patients with DLB were 10 times more likely to have one of four clinical features (myoclonus, absence of rest tremor, no perceived need to treat with levodopa, and no response to levodopa). The positive predictive value for having DLB, given any one of these features was 85.7% (sensitivity 66.7%, specificity 85.7%).

Gnanalingham and colleagues reported a comparison of clinical features, including EPS, in 16 DLB, 15 PD, and 25 AD patients, diagnosed according to published clinical criteria *(20)*. Nine of 16 DLB patients (56%) presented with EPS and 15 (94%) qualified for a "second diagnosis" of PD. A greater rigidity score, assessed using the Unified Parkinson's Disease Rating Scale (UPDRS), and lower scores on a finger-tapping test were more frequently noted in the DLB patients compared with the PD group, whereas resting tremor and left/right asymmetry were less common. Twelve of 16 (75%) DLB patients had received levodopa at some stage of their disease, and 10 were taking anti-parkinsonian drugs at the time of the study. All cases were noted to have treatment "responsiveness," although the degree of motor improvement and the doses required were not stated.

An international, multicenter study reported parkinsonism in 92.4% of 120 DLB patients *(19)*. There was a small but statistically significant difference between male and female patients on a five-item UPDRS subscale (the UPDRS-5), with male DLB patients more severely affected. This modified subscale comprising rest tremor, action tremor, bradykinesia, facial expression, and rigidity, is independent of the severity of cognitive impairment *(21)*. Older DLB patients tended to have higher UPDRS scores, but the difference was not statistically significant. Cases with severe cognitive impairment (MMSE < 18) had significantly more severe EPS than those with less cognitive decline using the full UPDRS part III, but when this relationship was reexamined using the UPDRS-5 there was no difference between the groups. Patients with more severe dementia may thus have difficulty understanding and executing some of the instructions. It is thus likely that severity of parkinsonism is independent of cognitive decline.

Aarsland and colleagues compared EPS in 98 DLB and 130 PD patients *(18)*. The DLB group was older at time of assessment and had a shorter duration of disease compared with the PD patients. Sixty-seven of the DLB patients (68%) had EPS. More severe action tremor, rigidity, bradykinesia, difficulty arising from a chair, greater facial impassivity, and gait disturbance were described in the DLB group.

The Spectrum of Parkinsonism in PD With and Without Dementia and DLB

Does the parkinsonian syndrome associated with DLB differ fundamentally from that seen in PD? This seems highly improbable, and though clinical series may describe higher or lower frequencies of certain EPS in DLB compared with PD, there are no *absolute* discriminating features. The pattern of EPS in DLB does, however, seem to show an axial bias (e.g., greater postural instability and facial impassivity), with a tendency toward less tremor, consistent with greater "non-dopaminergic" motor involvement. According to the classification proposed by Jankovic based upon the UPDRS II and III *(22)*, the postural instability-gait difficulty (PIGD) phenotype of parkinsonism is overrepresented in DLB, as indeed it may be in PDD *(23)*. EPS in PD, PDD, and DLB may thus be a spectrum, with a shift toward greater non-dopaminergic motor system involvement through PD to DLB. This is consistent with previous studies reporting motor features mediated by non-dopaminergic pathways (speech, posture, and balance) correlating with incident dementia in PD *(24)*.

Progression of Parkinsonism in DLB

DLB patients with established parkinsonism have an annual increase in severity, assessed using the UPDRS, of 9%, a figure comparable with PD *(25)*. In contrast, and again in common with PD, progression is more rapid in DLB patients with early parkinsonism (49% increase in motor UPDRS score in 1 yr).

Falls, Syncope, Sleep Disorders, and Other Neurological Features

A retrospective clinical analysis of pathologically confirmed cases of PD and DLB revealed that falls occurred at some point in the disease duration in 91% of 11 and 79% of 14 cases, respectively *(26)*. The mean latency to onset of recurrent falls was, however, much shorter in the DLB group at 48 months, compared with 118 mo in the PD group. In a prospective study, multiple falls (defined as more than five falls) occurred in 37% of 30 DLB patients and only 6% of 35 AD patients *(27)*. The falls often resulted in injury. Other than having DLB, multiple falls were associated with parkinsonism, previous falls, greater impairment of activities of daily living, and older age.

Several pathophysiological mechanisms could underlie the falls in DLB, including degeneration of brainstem nuclei, for example, the pedunculopontine nucleus, and impaired visuospatial processing. Orthostatic hypotension, vasovagal syncope, and carotid sinus hypersensitivity, collectively referred to as neurovascular instability, are common in patients with neurodegenerative dementia, and also contribute to falls. Cardioinhibitory carotid sinus hypersensitivity occurs in over 40% of DLB patients, compared with 28% AD cases and may reflect monoaminergic neuronal loss within cardioregulatory brainstem centers *(28)*.

A supranuclear gaze paresis has been described in DLB *(29–31)*. In combination with cognitive impairment and falls, this may cause diagnostic confusion with Steele–Richardson–Olszewski syndrome (progressive supranuclear palsy [PSP]). Other neurological features rarely described in DLB include an alien limb *(32)*, chorea and dystonia *(33)*.

Sleep disturbance is more common in DLB than in AD, as are daytime drowsiness and confusion on waking *(34)*. RBD is characteristic of synucleinopathic disorders and frequently commences before the onset of dementia in DLB, sometimes by up to 20 yr *(35)*. Over 90% of patients with RBD and degenerative dementia meet criteria for possible or probable DLB *(36)*.

DIAGNOSTIC ACCURACY AND DIFFERENTIAL DIAGNOSIS

Five sets of diagnostic criteria have been proposed to date to assist in the accurate diagnosis of DLB *(37)*. The most rigorous approach led to the formulation of the Consensus criteria (Table 1) *(3)*. Considering all the published studies together that have reported the diagnostic accuracy of the Consensus criteria yields a mean sensitivity of 49% (range 0–83%) and specificity of 92% (79–100%) *(37)*. All these studies compared DLB to other dementia syndromes, including AD or vascular dementia, and the majority was retrospective. Discriminating value for the Consensus criteria is greatest at an early stage, suggesting that DLB should be considered in any new dementia presentation *(38)*.

Interrater reliability for the core clinical features of parkinsonism and hallucinations in DLB is generally good, but only poor or moderate for fluctuating cognition. The application of validated methods to recognize the latter may thus increase diagnostic accuracy.

Perhaps unsurprisingly, AD is the most frequent misdiagnosis in autopsy-confirmed DLB cases *(39,40)*. Pathologically, of course, the situation is frequently not clear-cut, with a variable admixture of plaques and tangles, in addition to synuclein-positive inclusions. The degree of concomitant AD tangle pathology has an important influence upon both the clinical diagnostic accuracy of DLB and the clinical phenotype. In one study, the clinical diagnostic accuracy for DLB cases with low Braak staging was 75% compared to only 39% in those cases with high Braak stages *(41)*. High–Braak stage DLB cases are also less likely to experience VHs during the disease course.

Despite a significant overlap in neuropathological and clinical features with DLB, Consensus guidelines suggest that PD patients developing dementia more than 12 mo after the initial motor symptoms should be diagnosed as PDD rather than DLB. At least 25–30% of PD patients are demented in cross-sectional studies *(18)* although the cumulative incidence of dementia is nearer 80% *(42)*. Future research needs to clarify whether PDD and DLB are different representations of the same neuropathological process, with different early clinical manifestations, or whether they are independent disease processes ending in a similar common pathway.

When DLB presents as a primary dementia syndrome the key differential diagnoses are AD, vascular dementia, delirium secondary to systemic or pharmacological toxicity, Creutzfeldt–Jakob disease, or other neurodegenerative syndromes characterized by EPS and dementia. The latter include PSP and corticobasal degeneration (CBD). These conditions need to be excluded as far as possible by taking a careful history (including the carer whenever possible) and performing a thorough neurological examination, supplemented where necessary by ancillary investigations (*see* next section, Investigation). Table 2 summarizes the key clinical features in several neurodegenerative syndromes featuring parkinsonism and cognitive impairment.

The value of simple bedside tests of cognitive function should not be overlooked. For example, the inability of moderately impaired DLB patients to accurately copy pentagons has been reported with a sensitivity of 88% and specificity of 59% compared with AD *(6)*.

INVESTIGATION

No specific serum or cerebrospinal fluid biomarkers are yet available to increase diagnostic accuracy for DLB. Genetic testing cannot be recommended at present as part of the routine diagnostic process. Most DLB cases are sporadic, although there are a few reports of autosomal dominant Lewy body disease families *(43,44)*. The APOE4 allele is overrepresented in DLB as in AD but not in PD without dementia *(45)*. No robust associations have been found between polymorphisms linked with familial AD and DLB. The APP717 mutation, however, may be associated with familial AD and extensive cortical Lewy bodies *(46)*.

The additional value of ancillary investigations in the diagnostic process for DLB is also uncertain, although the development and validation of functional neuroimaging techniques, in particular, will almost certainly improve upon current clinical diagnostic sensitivity.

Neuroimaging

Structural Imaging Changes in DLB

Relative preservation of the hippocampal and medial temporal lobe compared to AD is characteristic of DLB *(47)*, possibly helping to explain the preservation of mnemonic function. Although hippocampal volume is reduced, by around 15% compared to controls, the reduction is considerably less than that seen in AD, with some 40% of DLB cases having no evidence of any atrophy. Rate of volume loss over time using serial magnetic resonance imaging (MRI) is comparable with AD (2% per year in AD and DLB compared with 0.5% in controls) *(48)*. There are increased white matter lesions in AD and these may contribute to the cognitive impairment. A similar increase has been described in DLB cases *(49)*, though effects on cognitive function have not yet been determined.

Functional Imaging Changes in DLB

Fluorodeoxyglucose positron emission tomography (PET) and single photon computed tomography (SPECT) studies using blood flow markers such as ^{99m}Tc-HMPAO demonstrate many similarities between DLB and AD subjects *(50,51)*, with pronounced biparietal hypoperfusion and variable, usually symmetric, deficits in frontal and temporal lobes. The biparietal hypoperfusion in DLB is, however, more extensive than in AD cases matched for age and dementia severity, particularly in Brodmann area 7, an area subserving visuospatial function *(52)*.

Occipital hypometabolism on PET and SPECT is characteristic of DLB and affects both primary visual cortex as well as visual association areas (Brodmann areas 17–19). Occipital hypoperfusion has reasonable specificity (86%) for distinguishing DLB from AD and controls, although the sensitivity for this finding is relatively low (64%) *(51)*. Consistent with findings from structural imaging studies, temporal lobe perfusion is relatively preserved in DLB.

Significant reductions in striatal binding of β-carbomethoxy-iodophenyl-tropane (a ligand for the dopamine transporter) using PET have been demonstrated in DLB but not AD, a difference that

Table 2
Comparison of Neurodegenerative Diseases Featuring Parkinsonism and Cognitive Impairment

	DLB	PD	AD	PSP	CBD	MSA
Parkinsonism phenotype	symmetric, PIGD	asymmetric, TD, and late PIGD	variable, usually mild, late	symmetric bradykinesia ++, PIGD	marked asymmetry, rigidity dominant	symmetric bradykinesia, PIGD
*L-dopa response	++	+++	–	–	–	–/++ (waning)
Other motor features	myoclonus		Gegenhalten (paratonia)		alien limb, stimulus-sensitive myoclonus, dystonia, ideomotor apraxia	cerebellar ataxia, myoclonus
Eye movements	impaired saccade triggering	normal	normal	SNGP/slow vertical saccades	increased saccadic latency (speed N)	mild saccadic slowing
Autonomic failure	++ (may be early)	++ (often late)	–	–	–	+++ (often early)
Dementia	early, executive, and visuospatial	often late, executive, and visuospatial	early, severe memory deficit	fronto-subcortical and apathy	frontal dementia may be early feature	mild (dementia an exclusion feature)
Neuropsychiatric features						
*VH	+++	++ (usually late)	+	–	–	–
*depression	++	+++	+	+ (<apathy)	++	++

–, absent; + to +++ frequency of feature; N, normal; SNGP, supranuclear gaze palsy; PIGD, postural instability-gait difficulty; TD, tremor dominant; VH, visual hallucination.

would be predicted from the nigrostriatal dopaminergic pathology associated with DLB *(53)*. FP-CIT SPECT can also differentiate DLB from AD *(54)*.

Scintigraphy with [^{123}I]metaiodobenzyl guanidine (MIBG) enables quantification of postganglionic sympathetic cardiac innervation. Cardiac MIBG scanning can differentiate DLB (where the signal is reduced) from AD (where the signal is similar to control values) *(55,56)*.

Neurophysiological Studies

The electroencephalogram (EEG) is diffusely abnormal in over 90% of DLB patients. Early slowing of the dominant rhythm, with 4- to 7-Hz transient activity over the temporal lobe area, is characteristic and correlates with a clinical history of loss of consciousness *(57)*. It is not possible to reliably differentiate DLB and AD subjects on the basis of the EEG, however *(58)*. The diagnostic significance of bursts of bilateral frontal rhythmic delta activity, reported to be more common in DLB than AD, has yet to be established *(59)*.

Multifocal action myoclonus, which occurs in approx 15% of DLB patients, is clinically more severe than that associated with PD, although it has the same electrophysiologcal characteristics. The balance of evidence favors a cortical source for the myoclonus *(60)*. Since myoclonus also occurs in AD, it will be interesting to determine whether concomitant cortical Alzheimer's-type pathology influences the presence and severity of the myoclonus in Lewy body disorders.

DLB patients have fewer and abnormally delayed auditory startle responses (ASRs) of low amplitude and short duration in extremity muscles compared with healthy controls *(61)*. Virtually no responses may be elicited in the lower limbs. Interestingly, the reduced ASR probability in advanced DLB is similar to that found in PD patients with postural instability and recurrent falls, suggesting a common brainstem pathophysiological mechanism for both disorders.

MANAGEMENT

General Considerations

Nonpharmacologic strategies for cognitive symptoms in DLB include orientation and memory prompts and attentional cues, although such approaches are of limited benefit. For psychiatric symptoms, explanation, education, reassurance, and targeted behavioral interventions may alleviate patient and carer distress.

In the acutely confused and psychotic patient, intercurrent infection and subdural haematoma should be excluded. Other nonessential medication capable of causing confusion should be discontinued. Potential therapeutic conflict may arise in the management of DLB over the so-called "motion-emotion" conundrum, whereby measures to alleviate psychosis and cognitive deficits may lead to deterioration in motor function and vica versa. Anti-parkinsonian drug treatment, if necessary, should be restricted to levodopa. Anticholinergics, amantadine, selegiline, and dopamine agonists should generally be avoided *(14)* (Fig. 1).

Nearly 50% of DLB patients receiving conventional high-affinity dopamine D_2 receptor antipsychotic agents experience life-threatening adverse effects, termed neuroleptic sensitivity reactions, characterized by sedation, rigidity, postural instability, falls, and increased confusion, and associated with a two- to threefold increased mortality *(62)*. Even the use of so-called "atypical" antipsychotic drugs may be associated with neuroleptic sensitivity reactions and low dosing may be more important than the use of any specific drug *(63–65)*.

Cholinesterase Inhibitors in DLB

There is converging and consistent evidence that cholinesterase inhibitors (ChEIs) are effective and relatively safe in the treatment of neuropsychiatric and cognitive symptoms in DLB. Open studies of donepezil and rivastigmine have reported improvement in cognitive and noncognitive symptoms, without significant deterioration in motor function *(66,67)*. A placebo-controlled, double-blind

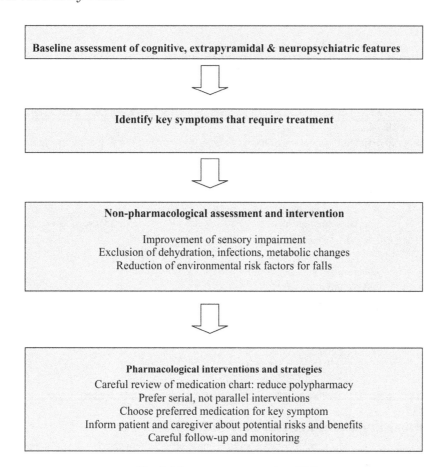

Fig. 1. Management approach to DLB.

study assessed the effect of rivastigmine (mean dose 7mg/d) in 120 DLB patients over 20 wk, followed by a 3-wk withdrawal period *(68)*. Patients taking rivastigmine were less apathetic, less anxious, and had fewer delusions and hallucinations compared to placebo controls. Treatment effects disappeared on drug withdrawal.

The long-term efficacy of rivastigmine was further assessed in an open-label study over 96 wk *(69)*. Improvements in cognitive and neuropsychiatric symptoms were noted after 24 wk, returning to pretreatment levels after 36 wk. The presence, rather than absence, of VHs in DLB may predict a good response to ChEIs, as evidenced by improved attention measures *(70)*. In autopsy studies, DLB cases with VHs have lower levels of cortical choline acetyltransferase, particularly in temporoparietal regions, compared with DLB patients without VHs *(71)*. This may allow greater clinical improvements to occur, with cholinergic replacement therapy having a more marked effect upon a lower neurochemical baseline.

ChEIs are well tolerated in DLB subjects, with dropout rates (10–31%) and gastrointestinal side effects similar to those found in AD. Hypersalivation, rhinorrhea, and lacrimation may also occur in approx 15% of DLB and PDD patients treated with donepezil *(72)*. An early report of worsening of parkinsonism in two of nine patients treated with donepezil has not been replicated in other studies, which have consistently demonstrated either no change or improvement in EPS during ChEI therapy *(73)*.

Table 3
Future Research Directions for DLB

1. to improve the understanding of molecular mechanisms underpinning α-synuclein processing and aggregation "upstream" to Lewy neurite and body formation
2. to better define the clinicopathological boundaries between DLB and PD with dementia
3. to define the role of ancillary investigations in increasing diagnostic accuracy
   - diagnostic algorithm
   - serum and cerebrospinal fluid biomarkers
4. to establish the extent of a genetic predisposition toward DLB
5. to define L-dopa responsiveness and tolerability
6. to determine the pharmacogenetic basis for variable treatment responsiveness with ChEI
7. the development of disease modifying therapies, for example:
   - α-synuclein anti-aggregation agents
   - anti-β-amyloid agents
   - tau de-phosphorylating agents

Other Pharmacological Management of DLB

No placebo-controlled study has assessed the effects of antidepressant drugs in DLB. Tricyclic antidepressants (e.g., amitriptyline, clomipramine, nortriptyline) should be avoided because of their anticholinergic side effects and potential to exacerbate orthostatic hypotension. Selective serotonin reuptake inhibitors (e.g., citalopram, sertraline, paroxetine) and the multireceptor antidepressants (e.g., nefazodone, mirtazapine, and venlafaxine) may therefore be better options for the treatment of depressed DLB patients *(74)*.

Sleep disturbances, particularly RBD, may be cautiously treated with low-dose clonazepam (0.25–1.0 mg) at bedtime *(36)*. Anticonvulsant drugs (e.g., carbamazepine, sodium valproate) may be occasionally necessary to treat significant behavioral disturbances, although randomized controlled trial data are lacking *(75)*.

CONCLUSION AND FUTURE DIRECTIONS

DLB is a relatively "young" disease, in which the clinicopathological overlap between PD and AD needs to be better defined. An accurate diagnosis of DLB has significant management and prognostic implications for the patient; an improved diagnostic awareness is therefore important. Information derived through the study of DLB may ultimately benefit patients with other synucleinopathies. For example, the successful use of ChEI drugs in DLB has encouraged the design of trials and use of these agents in PDD, strengthened by our knowledge of similar underlying pathophysiological mechanisms.

Table 3 lists a number of future research directions for DLB. These include a better understanding of underlying molecular biological mechanisms underpinning the disease, defining the role of additional investigations in refining diagnostic accuracy, and improved therapeutic approaches. Although clearly something of a "wish list," studies are already under way to address several of these issues.

LEGEND TO VIDEOTAPE

This video shows a 67-yr-old patient with a two-year history of probable DLB (MMSE 21), with no previous neurological, psychiatric or medical history. Parkinsonian features appeared within the first year of cognitive impairment. Medication comprised a cholinesterase inhibitor and low dose co-careldopa.

Sequence 1: The caregiver's view of early symptoms (including visuospatial problems and REM-sleep behaviour disorder)

Sequence 2: The patient's description of his visual hallucinations, occurring usually at night, but not when falling asleep or waking up.

Sequence 3: Assessment of parkinsonian features, including reduced blink rate, significant hypomimia, monotonous speech, bradyphrenia, limb bradykinesia and reduced arm swing when walking.

Sequence 4: Illustrative components of the bed-side cognitive assessment. Memory function is relatively preserved (learning of three words and recall), but there are difficulties in visuo-constructional function (slowing and errors on the clock face including clock hands having the same length, and use of a "0" instead of "9").

REFERENCES

1. Rahkonen T, Eloniemi-Sulkava U, Rissanen S, Vatanen A, Viramo P, Sulkava R. Dementia with Lewy bodies according to the consensus criteria in a general population aged 75 years or older. J Neurol Neurosurg Psychiatry 2003;74:720–724.
2. Okazaki H, Lipton LS, Aronson SM. Diffuse intracytoplasmic ganglionic inclusions (Lewy type) associated with progressive dementia and quadraparesis in flexion. J Neuropathol Exp Neurol 1961;20:237–244.
3. McKeith IG, Galasko D, Kosaka K, et al. Consensus guidelines for the clinical and pathological diagnosis of dementia with Lewy bodies (DLB): report of the consortium on DLB international workshop. Neurology 1996;47:1113–1124.
4. McKeith IG, Perry EK, Perry RH. Report of the second dementia with Lewy body international workshop. Neurology 1999;53:902–905.
5. Collerton D, Burn D, McKeith I, O' Brien J. Systematic review and meta-analysis show dementia with Lewy bodies is a visual perceptual and attentional-executive dementia. Dement Geriat Cog Disord, 2003;16:229–237.
6. Ala TA, Hughes LF, Kyrouac GA, Ghobrial MW, Elble RJ. Pentagon copying is more impaired in dementia with Lewy bodies than in Alzheimer's disease. J Neurol Neurosurg Psychiatry 2001;70:483–488.
7. Ballard CG, O'Brien J, Morris CM, et al. The progression of cognitive impairment in dementia with Lewy bodies, vascular dementia and Alzheimer's disease. Int J Geriatr Psychiatry 2001;16:499–503.
8. Ballard CG, Aarsland D, McKeith I, et al. Fluctuations in attention: PD dementia vs DLB with parkinsonism. Neurology 2002;59:1714–1720.
9. Walker MP, Ayre GA, Cummings JL, et al. Quantifying fluctuation in dementia with Lewy bodies, Alzheimer's disease, and vascular dementia. Neurology 2000;54:1616–1625.
10. Walker MP, Ayre GA, Cummings JL, et al. The Clinician Assessment of Fluctuation and the One Day Fluctuation Assessment Scale. Two methods to assess fluctuating confusion in dementia. Brit J Psychiatry 2000;177:252–256.
11. Ballard CG, Holmes C, McKeith IG, et al. Psychiatric morbidity in dementia with Lewy bodies: a prospective clinical and neuropathological comparative study with Alzheimer's disease. Am J Psychiatry 1999;156:1039–1045.
12. Cummings JL, Mega M, Gray K, Rosenberg-Thompson S, Carusi DA, Gornbein J. The neuropsychiatric inventory: comprehensive assessment of psychopathology in dementia. Neurology 1994;44:2308–2314.
13. McKeith IG, Del Ser T, Spano P, et al. Efficacy of rivastigmine in dementia with Lewy bodies: a randomised, double-blind, placebo-controlled international study. Lancet 2000;356:2031–2036.
14. McKeith IG, Burn DJ. Spectrum of Parkinson's disease, Parkinson's dementia, and Lewy body dementia. In: DeKosky ST, ed. Neurologic Clinics: Dementia, vol. 18. Philadelphia: Saunders, 2000:865–883.
15. Ballard C, McKeith I, Harrison R, et al. A detailed phenomenological comparison of complex visual hallucinations in dementia with Lewy bodies and Alzheimer's disease. Int Psychogeriatr 1997;9:381–388.
16. Harding AJ, Broe GA, Halliday GM. Visual hallucinations in Lewy body disease relate to Lewy bodies in the temporal lobe. Brain 2002;125:391–403.
17. Louis ED, Klatka LA, Liu Y, Fahn S. Comparison of extrapyramidal features in 31 pathologically confirmed cases of diffuse Lewy body disease and 34 pathologically confirmed cases of Parkinson's disease. Neurology 1997;48:376–380.

18. Aarsland D, Ballard C, McKeith I, Perry RH, Larsen JP. Comparison of extrapyramidal signs in dementia with Lewy bodies and Parkinson's disease. J Neuropsychiatry Clin Neurosci 2001;13:374–379.

19. Del Ser T, McKeith I, Anand R, Cicin-Sain A, Ferrara R, Spiegel R. Dementia with Lewy bodies: findings from an international multicentre study. Int J Geriatr Psychiatry 2000;15:1034–1045.

20. Gnanalingham KK, Byrne EJ, Thornton A, Sambrook MA, Bannister P. Motor and cognitive function in Lewy body dementia: comparison with Alzheimer's and Parkinson's disease. J Neurol Neurosurg Psychiatry 1997;62:243–252.

21. Ballard C, McKeith I, Burn D, et al. The UPDRS scale as a means of identifying extrapyramidal signs in patients suffering from dementia with Lewy bodies. Acta Neurol Scand 1997;96:366–371.

22. Jankovic J, McDermott M, Carter J, et al. Variable expression of Parkinson's disease: a baseline analysis of the DATATOP cohort. Neurology 1990;40:1529–1534.

23. Burn DJ, Rowan EN, Minnett T, et al. Extrapyramidal features in Parkinson's disease with and without dementia and dementia with Lewy bodies: a cross-sectional comparative study. Mov Disord 2003;18:884–889.

24. Foltynie T, Brayne C, Barker RA. The heterogeneity of idiopathic Parkinson's disease. J Neurol 2002;249:138–145.

25. Ballard CG, O'Brien J, Swann A, et al. One year follow-up of parkinsonism in dementia with Lewy bodies. Dement Geriatr Cogn Disord 2000;11:219–222.

26. Wenning GK, Ebersbach G, Verny M, et al. Progression of falls in postmortem-confirmed parkinsonian disorders. Mov Disord 1999;14:947–950.

27. Ballard CG, Shaw F, Lowery K, McKeith I, Kenny R. The prevalence, assessment and associations of falls in dementia with Lewy bodies and Alzheimer's disease. Dement Geriatr Cogn Disord 1999;10:97–103.

28. Ballard C, Shaw F, McKeith I, Kenny R. High prevalence of neurovascular instability in neurodegenerative dementias. Neurology 1998;51:1760–1762.

29. Fearnley JM, Revesz T, Brooks DJ, Frackowiak RS, Lees AJ. Diffuse Lewy body disease presenting with a supra-nuclear gaze palsy. J Neurol Neurosurg Psychiatry 1991;54:159–161.

30. de Bruin VM, Lees AJ, Daniel SE. Diffuse Lewy body disease presenting with supranuclear gaze palsy, parkinsonism, and dementia: a case report. Mov Disord 1992;7:355–358.

31. Brett FM, Henson C, Staunton H. Familial diffuse Lewy body disease, eye movement abnormalities, and distribution of pathology. Arch Neurol 2002;59:464–467.

32. Santacruz P, Torner L, Cruz-Sánchez F, Lomena F, Catafau A, Blesa R. Corticobasal degeneration syndrome: a case of Lewy body variant of Alzheimer's disease. Int J Geriatr Psychiatry 1996;11:559–564.

33. Lennox GG, Lowe JS. Dementia with Lewy bodies. Baillieres Clinical Neurology 1997;6:147–166.

34. Grace JB, Walker MP, McKeith IG. A comparison of sleep profiles in patients with dementia with lewy bodies and Alzheimer's disease. Int J Geriatr Psychiatry 2000;15:1028–1033.

35. Boeve BF, Silber MH, Parisi JE, et al. Synucleiopathy pathology and REM sleep behavior disorder plus dementia or parkinsonism. Neurology 2003;61:40–45.

36. Boeve BF, Silber MH, Ferman TJ, et al. REM sleep behavior disorder and degenerative dementia: an association likely reflecting Lewy body disease. Neurology 1998;51:363–370.

37. Litvan I, Bhatia KP, Burn DJ, et al. SIC task force appraisal of clinical diagnostic criteria for parkinsonian disorders. Mov Disord 2003;18:467–486.

38. McKeith IG, Ballard CG, Perry RH, et al. Prospective validation of consensus criteria for the diagnosis of dementia with Lewy bodies. Neurology 2000;54:1050–1058.

39. McKeith IG, Galasko D, Wilcock GK, Byrne EJ. Lewy body dementia: diagnosis and treatment. Brit J Psychiatry 1995;167:709–717.

40. Lopez OL, Becker JT, Kaufer DI, et al. Research evaluation and prospective diagnosis of dementia with Lewy bodies. Arch Neurol 2002;59:43–46.

41. Merdes AR, Hansen LA, Jeste DV, et al. Influence of Alzheimer pathology on clinical diagnostic accuracy in dementia with Lewy bodies. Neurology 2003;60:1586–1590.

42. Aarsland D, Andersen K, Larsen JP, Lolk A, Kragh-Sørensen P. Prevalence and characteristics of dementia in Parkinson disease. Arch Neurol 2003;60:387–392.

43. Wakabayashi K, Hayashi S, Ishikawa A, et al. Autosomal dominant diffuse Lewy body disease. Acta Neuropathol (Berl) 1998;96:207–210.

44. Gwinn-Hardy K. Genetics of parkinsonism. Mov Disord 2002;17:645–656.

45. Galasko D, Saitoh T, Xia Y, et al. The apolipoprotein E allele epsilon 4 is overrepresented in patients with the Lewy body variant of Alzheimer's disease. Neurology 1994;44:1950–1951.

46. Revesz T, McLaughlin JL, Rossor MN, Lantos PL. Pathology of familial Alzheimer's disease with Lewy bodies. J Neural Transm 1997;51:121–135.

47. Barber R, Ballard C, McKeith IG, Gholkar A, O'Brien JT. MRI volumetric study of dementia with Lewy bodies: a comparison with AD and vascular dementia. Neurology 2000;54:1304–1309.

48. O'Brien JT, Paling S, Barber R, et al. Progressive brain atrophy on serial MRI in dementia with Lewy bodies, AD and vascular dementia. Neurology 2001;56:1386–1388.

49. Barber R, Scheltens P, Gholkar A, et al. White matter lesions on magnetic resonance imaging in dementia with Lewy bodies, Alzheimer's disease, vascular dementia, and normal aging. J Neurol Neurosurg Psychiatry 1999;67:66–72.

50. Minoshima S, Foster NL, Sima AA, Frey KA, Albin RL, Kuhl DE. Alzheimer's disease versus dementia with Lewy bodies: cerebral metabolism distinction with autopsy confirmation. Ann Neurol 2001;50:358–365.

51. Lobotesis K, Fenwick J, Phipps A, et al. Occipital hypoperfusion on SPECT in dementia with Lewy bodies but not AD. Neurology 2001;56:643–649.

52. Colloby SJ, Fenwick JD, Williams ED, et al. A comparison of (99m)Tc-HMPAO SPET changes in dementia with Lewy bodies and Alzheimer's disease using statistical parametric mapping. Eur J Nucl Med Mol Imaging 2002;29:615–622.

53. Donnemiller E, Heilmann J, Wenning GK, et al. Brain perfusion scintigraphy with ^{99m}Tc-HMPAO or ^{99m}Tc-ECD and ^{123}I-beta-CIT single-photon emission tomography in dementia of the Alzheimer-type and diffuse Lewy body disease. Eur J Nucl Med 1997;24:320–325.

54. Walker Z, Costa DC, Walker RWH, et al. Differentiation of dementia with Lewy bodies from Alzheimer's disease using a dopaminergic presynaptic ligand. J Neurol Neurosurg Psychiatry 2002;73:134–140.

55. Yoshita M, Taki J, Yamada M. A clinical role for [^{123}I]MIBG myocardial scintigraphy in the distinction between dementia of the Alzheimer's-type and dementia with Lewy bodies. J Neurol Neurosurg Psychiatry 2001;71:583–588.

56. Watanabe H, Ieda T, Katayama T, et al. Cardiac ^{123}I-meta-iodobenzylguanidine (MIBG) uptake in dementia with Lewy bodies: comparison with Alzheimer's disease. J Neurol Neurosurg Psychiatry 2001;70:781–783.

57. Briel RC, McKeith IG, Barker WA, et al. EEG findings in dementia with Lewy bodies and Alzheimer's disease. J Neurol Neurosurg Psychiatry 1999;66:401–403.

58. Barber PA, Varma AR, Lloyd JJ, Haworth B, Snowden JS, Neary D. The electroencephalogram in dementia with Lewy bodies. Acta Neurol Scand 2000;101:53–56.

59. Calzetti S, Bortone E, Negrotti A, Zinno L, Mancia D. Frontal intermittent rhythmic delta activity (FIRDA) in patients with dementia with Lewy bodies: a diagnostic tool? Neurol Sci 2002;23:S65–S66.

60. Caviness JN, Adler CH, Caselli RJ, Hernandez JL. Electrophysiology of the myoclonus in dementia with Lewy bodies. Neurology 2003;60:523–524.

61. Kofler M, Muller J, Wenning GK, et al. The auditory startle reaction in parkinsonian disorders. Mov Disord 2001;16:62–71.

62. McKeith IG, Fairbairn A, Perry RH, Thompson P, Perry EK. Neuroleptic sensitivity in patients with senile dementia of Lewy body type. Brit Med J 1992;305:673–678.

63. McKeith IG, Ballard CG, Harrison RW. Neuroleptic sensitivity to risperidone in Lewy body dementia. Lancet 1995;346:699.

64. Burke WJ, Pfeiffer RF, McComb RD. Neuroleptic sensitivity to clozapine in dementia with Lewy bodies. J Neuropsychiatry Clin Neurosci 1998;10:227–229.

65. Walker Z, Grace J, Overshot R, et al. Olanzapine in dementia with Lewy bodies: a clinical study. Int J Geriatr Psychiatry 1999;14:459–466.

66. Samuel W, Caligiuri M, Galakso D, et al. Better cognitive and psychopathologic response to donepezil in patients prospectively diagnosed as dementia with Lewy bodies: a preliminary study. Int J Geriatr Psychiatry 2000;15:794–802.

67. McKeith IG, Grace JB, Walker Z, et al. Rivastigmine in the treatment of dementia with Lewy bodies: preliminary findings from an open trial. Int J Geriatr Psychiatry 2000;15:387–392.

68. McKeith IG, Spano PF, Del Ser T, et al. Efficacy of rivastigmine in dementia with Lewy bodies: a randomised, double-blind, placebo-controlled international study. Lancet 2000;356:2031–2036.

69. Grace J, Daniel S, Stevens T, et al. Long-term use of rivastigmine in patients with dementia with Lewy bodies: an open label trial. Int Psychogeriatr 2001;13:199–205.

70. Wesnes KA, McKeith IG, Ferrara R, et al. Effects of rivastigmine on cognitive function in dementia with Lewy bodies: a randomised placebo-controlled international study using the cognitive drug research computerised assessment system. Dement Geriatr Cogn Disord 2002;13:183–192.

71. Perry EK, Marshall E, Kerwin J, et al. Evidence of a monoaminergic-cholinergic imbalance related to visual hallucinations in Lewy body dementia. J Neurochem 1990;55:1454–1456.

72. Thomas AJ, Burn DJ, Rowan EN, et al. Efficacy of donepezil in Parkinson's disease with dementia and dementia with Lewy bodies. submitted 2003.

73. Shea C, MacKnight C, Rockwood K. Donepezil for treatment of dementia with Lewy bodies: a case series of nine patients. Int Psychogeriatr 1998;10:229–238.

74. Nyth Al, Gottfries CG. The clinical efficacy of citalopram in treatment of emotional disturbances in dementia disorders. A Nordic multicentre study. Brit J Psychiatry 1990;157:894–901.

75. Sival RC, Haffmans PM, Jansen PA, Duursma SA, Eikelenboom P. Sodium valproate in the treatment of aggressive behaviour in patients with dementia: a randomised placebo controlled clinical trial. Int J Geriatr Psychiatry 2002;17:579–585.

22

Clinical Diagnosis of Familial Atypical Parkinsonian Disorders

Yoshio Tsuboi, Virgilio H. Evidente, and Zbigniew K. Wszolek

INTRODUCTION

Parkinson's disease (PD) is defined clinically as a disorder characterized by the presence of at least two of four cardinal signs, i.e., resting tremor, bradykinesia, rigidity, and postural instability, along with a good response to levodopa *(1)*. Patients with typical PD do not manifest ataxia, chorea, orthostatic hypotension unrelated to medications, vertical downward-gaze deficits, amyotrophy, early dementia, or early hallucinations. When present, these signs suggest a diagnosis of atypical parkinsonism or parkinsonism-plus syndrome *(2)*.

Both typical and atypical parkinsonism can be either sporadic or familial. The etiology of sporadic forms remains unknown. However, recent advances in molecular genetics have allowed us to classify familial forms into several separate categories. Typical forms of familial parkinsonism are found in patients carrying PARK1-10 chromosomal abnormalities (Table 1). Although even these patients may exhibit some atypical clinical features, the detailed discussion of kindreds with PARK1-10 is beyond the scope of this chapter.

Atypical forms of familial parkinsonism with known chromosomal loci or mutations discussed in this chapter are found in kindreds with frontotemporal dementia, ataxia, dystonia, abnormal copper and iron accumulation, and mitochondrial dysfunction (Table 2). We have also included a brief discussion of Perry syndrome, a rare atypical familial parkinsonian disorder with an unknown genetic abnormality but with worldwide occurrence.

CLINICAL DIAGNOSIS OF FAMILIAL ATYPICAL PARKINSONIAN DISORDERS

Frontotemporal Dementia and Parkinsonism Linked to Chromosome 17

The term *frontotemporal dementia and parkinsonism linked to chromosome 17* (FTDP-17) was defined in 1996 during the International Consensus Conference in Ann Arbor, Michigan *(3)*. At the time of this meeting, only 13 families with syndromes linked to the chromosome 17q21-22 locus were known *(4–12)*. Currently, over 80 families with FTDP-17 are known *(13)*. Data indicate that some of these kindreds may share a common founder *(14,15)*. However, distribution is worldwide, with families described in North America, Europe, Asia, and Australia *(4–14,16)*.

Molecular genetic studies have identified 31 unique tau gene mutations associated with FTDP-17 *(8,10–12,14,16)*. The three most prevalent are P301L, exon 10 5' +16, and N279K. These mutations account for about 60% of known cases of FTDP-17 *(16)*. Thus, the concept of FTDP-17 has evolved

From: *Current Clinical Neurology: Atypical Parkinsonian Disorders*
Edited by: I. Litvan © Humana Press Inc., Totowa, NJ

Table 1
Familial Parkinsonism Associated With Known Gene Mutations or Loci

Nomenclature	Chromosome/loci	Gene	Range of Age at Onset, yr (mean)	Phenotype	Response to Levodopa	Pathology
Autosomal dominant						
PARK1	4q21	α-Synuclein (2 mutations)	20–85 (46)	PD, some cases with dementia	Good	Lewy body
PARK3	2p13	Unknown	36–89 (58)	PD, some cases with dementia	Good	Lewy body
PARK4	4p15	Unknown	24–48 (30s)	PD, some cases with dementia	Good	Lewy body
PARK5	4p14-15	UCH-L1	49–51 (50)	PD	Good	Unknown
PARK8	12p11.2-q13.11	Unknown	38–68 (51)	PD	Good	Pure nigral degeneration
PARK10	1p32	Unknown	(65.8)	PD	Good	Unknown
Autosomal recessive						
PARK2	6q25.2-27	Parkin (multiple mutations)	6–58 (26)	PD	Good	Nigral degeneration sometimes with tau inclusions or Lewy bodies
PARK6	1p35-36	Unknown	32–48 (41)	PD	Good	Unknown
PARK7	1p36	DJ-1 (2 mutations)	27–40 (33)	PD	Good	Unknown
PARK9 (Kufor-Rakeb syndrome)	1p36	Unknown	11-16	PD, spasticity, dementia, gaze palsy	Good	Unknown

PD, Parkinson's disease; UCH-L1, ubiquitin carboxyterminal hydrase L1.

Table 2
Familial Atypical Parkinsonism Associated With Known Gene Mutations or Loci

Nomenclature	Chromosome/loci	Gene	Range of Age at Onset, yr (mean)	Parkinsonism	Other Features	Response to Levodopa
Autosomal dominant						
FTDP-17	17q21-22	Tau	25–76 (49)	PD	FTD, CBD, PSP, ALS	Poor
SCA2	12q23-24.1	SCA2 (Ataxin-2)	19–61 (39)	PD	Ataxia	Good
SCA3	14q32.1	SCA3 (Ataxin-3)	31–57 (42)	PD	Ataxia	Good
DYT5	14q22.1	GCH	<16	PD	Diurnal fluctuation, dystonia	Good
DYT12	19q13	Unknown	12–45 (22)	Bradykinesia, PI	Rapid-onset dystonia	Poor
DYT14	14q13	Unknown	3	Rigidity, akinesia	Dystonia	Good
Huntington's disease	4p16.3	Huntingtin	35–50	Rigidity, akinesia	Chorea	Poor, occasionally good
Perry syndrome	Unknown	Unknown	35–61 (48)	PD	Depression, weight loss, hypoventilation	Fair
Autosomal recessive						
Wilson's disease	13q14-q21	ATP7B	7–58	Tremor, rigidity	Intention tremor, K–F ring, behavioral disturbances	Poor
NBIA	20p12.3-13	PANK2	<20	Rigidity	Chorea, dystonia, pyramidal signs, dementia	Occasionally fair
X-linked recessive						
DYT3 (Lubag)	Xq13.1	Unknown	12–60 (35)	PD	Dystonia, focal tremor, chorea, myoclonus, myorhythmia	Poor, occasionally good
Mitochondrial						
	Complex 1	Unknown	41–79 (42)	PD	None	Good
	Complex 1	ND4	(31)	PD	Dementia, dystonia, ophthalmoplegia	Good

ALS, amyotrophic lateral sclerosis; ATP7B, P-type adenosine triphosphatase; CBD, corticobasal degeneration; FTD, frontotemporal dementia; FTDP-17, frontotemporal dementia and parkinsonism linked on chromosome 17; GCH, guanosine triphosphate cyclohydrolase I; K–F, Kayser-Fleischer; NBIA, neurodegeneration with brain iron accumulation; PANK2, pantothenate kinase 2; PD, Parkinson's disease; PI, postural instability; PSP, progressive supranuclear palsy; SCA, spinocerebellar ataxia.

over the past several years to include the association with tau mutations. Some investigators now refer to FTDP-17 as familial tauopathies or frontotemporal dementia and parkinsonism linked to chromosome 17 associated with tau gene mutations (FTDP-17T). Of note, there are five kindreds linked to the *wld* locus on chromosome 17 but no mutations have so far been identified in this critical region, suggesting the presence of another gene *(17–21)*. The molecular genetic aspects of FTDP-17 are discussed separately in Chapter 5. Neuropathologic studies demonstrate tau deposition in neurons alone or in both neurons and glial cells in multiple areas of the central nervous system, particularly in the cerebral cortex and some subcortical nuclei (e.g., substantia nigra).

Clinical Description

FTDP-17 is characterized clinically by a combination of personality and behavioral dysfunction, cognitive impairment, and motor signs. The average age at symptomatic onset is 49 yr (range, 25–76 yr). The average duration of survival after onset is 9 yr (range, 2–26 yr). Personality and behavioral changes are the most common symptoms and are described in almost all known kindreds. Cognitive impairment is also common and can occur in the initial or later stages of the illness. The motor manifestations usually include atypical parkinsonism and can in fact be the presenting and dominating clinical feature, often leading to disability within 2–3 yr.

The personality and behavioral manifestations of FTDP-17 include disinhibition, apathy, impaired judgment, compulsive behavior, hyperreligiosity, neglect of personal hygiene, alcoholism, illicit drug addiction, verbal and physical aggressiveness, and family abuse. Early in the disease, cognition is characterized by relative preservation of memory, orientation, and visuospatial functions. Progressive speech impairment with nonfluent aphasia, as well as executive dysfunction, may be seen in the initial stages. Later in the course of the disease, progressive deterioration of memory, orientation, and visuospatial functions occurs. Echolalia, palilalia, and verbal and vocal perseverations are frequently observed. Finally, progressive dementia and mutism develop.

The motor signs consist mainly of parkinsonism and can be the initial manifestation of the disease. In fact, some FTDP-17 patients are misdiagnosed as having PD or progressive supranuclear palsy (PSP). However, in some families, parkinsonism is absent or occurs late in the course of the disease. The parkinsonism in FTDP-17 is characterized by symmetrical bradykinesia, rigidity equally affecting the axial and appendicular musculature, absence of resting tremor *(13)*, postural instability, and poor or no response to levodopa *(22)*. Other motor disturbances seen in FTDP-17 include dystonia unrelated to medications, supranuclear gaze palsy, upper and lower motor neuron dysfunction, myoclonus, postural and action tremors, apraxia of eyelid opening and closing, dysphagia, and dysarthria.

Notably, considerable phenotypic heterogeneity exists in individuals with different mutations *(13,14,16)*. In addition, phenotypic variability is often seen in individuals carrying the same mutation. The correlation between clinical signs and different tau mutations is presented in Table 3.

Determining the precise relationship between phenotype and genotype in FTDP-17 remains challenging because clinical information is often unavailable or insufficient. Nevertheless, some patterns have emerged. Two major phenotypes are associated with FTDP-17: one in which dementia is predominant and one in which parkinsonism-plus is predominant *(13,14,16)*. The dementia-predominant phenotype is more common and is usually associated with exonic mutations sparing the splicing of exon 10. The parkinsonism-plus–predominant phenotype is often associated with intronic and exonic mutations that affect exon 10 splicing, leading to an overproduction of four-repeat tau isoforms.

Case 1: (Video 1) Pallido-Ponto-Nigral Degeneration (PPND) With the N279K Tau Mutation (23)

This right-handed man first noted a tremor in his right leg at age 40. When he drove an automobile, his left leg sometimes felt stiff and occasionally shook. His wife also noted that he turned his body en bloc (*see* accompanying DVD video 1, segments A and B). At age 41, he was noted to have

Table 3
Clinical Features of Specific Mutations in the Tau Gene

	Not in Exon 10					Exon 10	Exon 10 5' splice site
	Exon 1	Exon 9	Exon 11	Exon 12	Exon 13		
Average age at onset, yr							
≤30						P301S	
31–40		L266V, G272V	S320F	E342V, V337M, K369I	G389R	delN296	−2
41–50	R5H, R5L				R406W	N279K, P301L	+3, +11, +14, +16
>50						del280K, L284L, N296H, S305S	+12, +13
Average survival, yr							
≤5	R5H, R5L	L266V, G272V		E342V, K369I	G389R	del280, delN296, N296H	−2
6–10			S320F			N279K, L284L, P301L, P301S, S305S	−1, +11, +12
11–15				V337M	R406W		+3, +14, +16
>15					R406W		
First sign							
Parkinsonism	R5L					N279K, P301L, delN296	−1, +3, +11
Dementia	R5H		S320F		R406W	L284L, delN296	+3, +12
Personality change		L266V, G272V		V337M, E342V, K369I		P301L, N296H	−2, −1, +12, +14, +16
Parkinsonism							
Early-prominent						N279K, delN296	−1, +11
Late-prominent						P301S, N296H	+3, +12, +14, +16
Rare-minimal	R5L	G272V				P301L	−2
Dementia							
Early-prominent		L266V, G272V	S320F	V337M, K369I	R406W	delN296	−1, +12
Late-prominent						del280K, L284L, P301L, P301S, N279K	−2, +3, +11, +13
Rare-minimal							
Personality change							
Early-prominent		L266V, G272V			R406W	del280K, L284L, P301L, P301S	−2, −1, +12, +14, +16
Language difficulties		G272V	S320F	V337M	G389R	N279K, L284L, N296H, P301L	−1, +14, +16
Late mutism					R406W	N279K, del280K, N296H, P301S	−2
Eye movement abnormalities						N279K, N296H, P301S, delN296, S305S	−1, +3
Epilepsy						P301S	
Myoclonus				V337M		N279K, P301S	+11
Pyramidal signs						N279K, P301S	−1, +3, +12
Amyotrophy						P301L	+14

Modified from Wszolek et al. (*13*) and Ghetti et al. (*16*). By permission of Lippincott Williams & Wilkins and ISN Neuropath Press.

a shuffling gait and reduced arm swing. His facial expression also had changed considerably, and drooling became a problem. Subsequently, a resting tremor developed in both legs (in the left more than the right) and occasionally in both hands. His balance deteriorated steadily over the next 2 yr. He experienced many falls throughout the day and had difficulty standing up (*see* video 1, segments C and D). His balance was better in the morning than in the evening. Treatment with carbidopa-levodopa was of limited benefit.

At age 44, the patient reported generalized stiffness in the muscles of his neck, tongue, and extremities. The stiffness was more pronounced in the afternoon and after the carbidopa-levodopa effect had worn off (i.e., after 3 h). The tremor in his legs (particularly the left) was also worse several hours after carbidopa-levodopa administration. He complained of frequent and uncontrollable yawning. He chewed gum almost constantly to avoid yawning and excessive drooling. He remained independent in most activities of daily living but needed occasional assistance with cutting food.

When examined at age 44, his Mini-Mental State Examination score was 30/30. His neck was anteroflexed, and he had obvious parkinsonism in the form of facial hypomimia, markedly reduced blinking, prominent drooling, and generalized body bradykinesia. He had severe postural instability, and while walking he needed assistance from at least one person to prevent falls (video 1, segments E–G). Muscle tone was increased and was a mixture of rigidity and spasticity; the tone was more pronounced in axial than in appendicular muscles. Muscle strength was normal. Deep tendon reflexes were exaggerated, with bilateral ankle clonus (right more than left). Bilateral extensor plantar responses were also noted.

At the time of this writing, he was 46 yr old, lived in a skilled nursing facility, and required assistance in all activities of daily living.

Familial Parkinsonism With Ataxia

The inherited spinocerebellar ataxias (SCAs) are a heterogeneous group of disorders characterized by dysfunction and degeneration of systems involved in motor coordination (24). The clinical phenotypes vary. Additional clinical features include pyramidal signs, eye movement abnormalities, dementia, chorea, and peripheral neuropathy. Currently, 19 SCA loci and mutations have been identified.

Parkinsonism has been recognized as a clinical phenotype in the SCA3 mutation (25,26). The autopsies performed on individuals with the SCA3 mutation demonstrated Purkinje cell loss and torpedo-like structures in the axons of Purkinje cells. Cell loss is also frequently seen in brainstem nuclei, including the substantia nigra, inferior olive, and pontine nuclei.

Recently, several families with the SCA2 mutation were described whose members manifested with either ataxia and parkinsonism or with parkinsonism alone (27–30). However, no autopsies have been reported from these kindreds.

Clinical Description

Table 4 outlines clinical data on all known SCA2 families with parkinsonism. Although parkinsonism is rare with the SCA2 mutation, it can be the only manifestation of the disease in some SCA2 families. For example, before the SCA2 mutation was identified in the Canadian (Alberta) kindred (29), affected individuals in this family were thought to have PD. The parkinsonism in SCA2 is characterized by asymmetrical rigidity, bradykinesia, resting tremor, and responsiveness to levodopa. In a Taiwanese family, two affected individuals had supranuclear gaze palsy (27). The average age at onset of parkinsonian symptoms in SCA2 kindreds is 47 yr (range, 19–86 yr). Because many of the affected individuals in these kindreds are still living, the average disease duration remains unclear.

Table 5 summarizes the clinical signs observed in SCA3 kindreds. In these families, parkinsonism is usually associated not only with ataxia but also with oculomotor dysfunction and upper and lower motor signs. However, in the African-American population, some affected members of families with the SCA3 mutation exhibit a phenotype indistinguishable from that of idiopathic PD (31,32). The

Table 4
Clinical Features of SCA2 Families With Parkinsonism

| Feature | Published Report | | | |
	Gwinn-Hardy et al., 2000 (27)	Shan et al., 2001 (28)	Furtado et al., 2002 (29)	Lu et al., 2002 (30)
Origin	Taiwanese-American	Taiwan (2 families)	Canada	Taiwan
Number of affected individuals	9	5	10	2
Age at disease onset, yr	19–61	50	31–86	40–43
Initial symptoms	B	T	B, T, dystonia	T
Parkinsonism				
Bradykinesia	+	+	+	+
Rigidity	+	+	+	+
Resting tremor	–	+	+	+
Postural instability	+	+	+	+
Response to levodopa	+	+	+	+
Ataxic gait	+	–	–	–
Dementia	–	–	–	–
Peripheral neuropathy	–	–	–	Mild
Dystonia	+	–	+	–
Gaze palsy	+	–	–	–
Length of CAG repeats	33–43	36–37	39	36

B, bradykinesia; T, tremor; +, present; –, not present.

Table 5
Cerebellar and Extrapyramidal Signs in SCA3 Families

Signs	Frequency (%)
Cerebellar	
Gait ataxia	100
Limb ataxia	93.5
Nystagmus	92
Dysarthria	85.5
Extrapyramidal	
Dystonia	23
Rigidity/bradykinesia	23

Modified from Jardim et al. (26). By permission of the American Medical Association.

average age at onset of parkinsonian symptoms in SCA3 kindreds is 42 yr (range, 31-57 yr) (31). In general, the average disease duration spans decades. However, as in SCA2 families, the length of survival is unknown because many affected individuals are still living (31).

Familial Parkinsonism With Dystonia

Clinically, dystonia is defined as a syndrome of sustained muscle contractions causing twisting and repetitive movement or abnormal postures (33). Familial dystonia syndromes are termed "DYT" and numbered from 1 to 14 according to the associated chromosomal loci. Familial dystonias can be focal or generalized, with onset in childhood or adulthood. Dystonia can respond to levodopa (DYT5),

Table 6
Clinical Features Seen in Dystonia Kindreds Associated With Parkinsonism

Feature	Lubag Disease (DYT3)	Dopa-Responsive Dystonia (DYT5)	Rapid-Onset Dystonia and Parkinsonism (DYT12)	Dopa-Responsive Dystonia (DYT14)
Inheritance	X-linked recessive	AD	AD	AD
Average age at disease onset, yr	35	<10	24	3
Initial symptoms	Parkinsonism or Dy	Dy	Dy	Dy
Parkinsonism				
Bradykinesia	+	+	+	+
Rigidity	+	+	–	+
Resting tremor	+	+	–	–
Postural instability	+	+	+	+
Response to levodopa	+/–	+	–	+
Dystonia	Focal-generalized	Focal-generalized	Focal-segmental	Focal-generalized

AD, autosomal dominant; Dy, dystonia; +, present; –, not present.

alcohol (DYT8 and DYT9), or anticonvulsant medications (DYT10). Parkinsonian features have been recognized in DYT3, DYT5, and DYT12. Clinical features of dystonia kindreds associated with parkinsonism are summarized in Table 6.

Clinical Description

DYT3, also known as X-linked dystonia-parkinsonism (XDP) or Lubag disease, was first identified in families residing on the Philippine island of Panay. The disease is inherited as an X-linked recessive trait with high penetrance and is thus transmitted to men by their mothers. Female carriers can manifest symptoms, although these are rare and much less severe than those in men. Onset is at a mean age of 35 yr but can range from age 12–60 yr.

The earliest feature in most DYT3 patients is mild parkinsonism. In particular, breakdown of rapid alternating movements and subtle body bradykinesia are often seen early. In some patients, an asymmetrical resting limb tremor similar to that in PD may in fact be misdiagnosed as PD. Other patients may have a coarse type of action and postural appendicular or axial tremor similar to essential tremor. With time, dystonia develops in the majority of patients. Those who develop segmental or multifocal dystonia within the first year of the disease, especially in combination with parkinsonism, usually have a more rapid progression. Patients with pure or predominant parkinsonism and either negative or late-onset dystonia have a more benign course. These parkinsonian patients may be levodopa-responsive. However, the dystonia can sometimes be exacerbated by levodopa.

When the family history cannot be adequately determined or when the maternal roots cannot be traced back to the Philippine island of Panay, some patients with XDP can be misdiagnosed as suffering from idiopathic torsion dystonia, essential tremor, PD, or other forms of parkinsonism-plus syndrome *(34,35)*. Neuropathologic studies demonstrate a patchy or mosaic pattern of neuronal loss and gliosis in the striatum, with dorsal-to-ventral, rostral-to-caudal, and medial-to-lateral gradients *(36)*. Furthermore, gliotic changes occur in the globus pallidus and substantia nigra pars reticularis.

DYT5 is a dopa-responsive dystonia also known as autosomal dominant progressive dystonia with marked diurnal fluctuation. This form of dystonia is caused by mutations in the guanosine triphosphate cyclohydrolase I gene (GTPCHI) on chromosome 14q22.1-q22.2 *(37)*. More than 70 mutations have been found in patients with DYT5. The age at onset is usually in the first decade and only occasionally in adulthood. Dystonia in DYT5 can be focal (frequently affecting a foot) or it can be generalized. Parkinsonian features include resting tremor, bradykinesia, rigidity, and postural instability. Parkinsonism usually occurs in adult-onset cases and at times can develop early in the course of the disease. The most characteristic features of DYT5 include marked diurnal fluctuation and excellent response to levodopa therapy. Some families with DYT5 can be difficult to distinguish from kindreds with autosomal recessive juvenile parkinsonism carrying the parkin mutation PARK2. There is considerable overlapping of clinical features between these two genetic conditions regarding age at onset, clinical signs and symptoms, and response to dopaminergic therapy. However, the pattern of inheritance is different: autosomal dominant in DYT5 and autosomal recessive in PARK2 families *(38)*. Neuropathologic studies of DYT5 brains revealed no degenerative changes.

DYT12 has been described in only three families: two from the United States and one from Ireland *(39,40)*. Linkage analyses of the three families revealed a disease locus on chromosome 19q13. The syndrome was termed "rapid-onset dystonia and parkinsonism" because of the acute development of symptoms within hours (or at most a few days). The dystonia usually affects bulbar and upper limb muscles, and the parkinsonian features include bradykinesia and postural instability. Resting tremor and rigidity are not seen. Response to levodopa and dopamine agonists is poor. Despite the initial rapid progression, the clinical course eventually levels off with no further deterioration. No brain pathologic changes were seen in one autopsied case of DYT12.

A family from Switzerland with levodopa-responsive dystonia (DYT14) has also been described *(41)*. Linkage analysis showed a locus on chromosome 14q13 in close proximity to the GCH-1 gene. The patients from this family developed dystonia in both legs at a mean age of 3 yr. Later in the course of the disease, postural instability, frequent falls, and dystonia affecting the upper limbs were also observed. In one family member, a severe akinetic rigid syndrome developed at age 73 yr. Treatment with low-dose levodopa dramatically improved his symptoms. Neuropathologic studies revealed neuronal loss in the substantia nigra without Lewy bodies.

Case 2: (Video 2, see accompanying DVD) DYT3 (XDP/Lubag Disease)

The patient was a 39-yr-old right-handed Filipino man who was born and raised in the province of Iloilo on the Philippine island of Panay. At age 34, he noted a resting tremor of the right foot, difficulty in handwriting, and intermittent hyperextension of the neck. One year later, he experienced spontaneous jaw opening, slurring of speech, drooling, difficulty swallowing, and involuntary turning of the head to the left. By this time, he was forced to quit his profession as a dentist. By the third year of his disorder, the patient was already severely disabled and had lost 30 pounds because of difficulty in swallowing.

His medical history revealed no notable illness in the past. A review of the family history showed similar symptoms in an uncle (brother of his mother), whose symptoms started during his late 30s.

On examination 3 yr after onset (at age 37), the patient's dystonia was generalized in distribution and included inversion of the right foot at rest, dorsiflexion of the toes on raising the left foot (video 2, segment A), spontaneous jaw-opening, retrocollis and torticollis (with abundant phasic movements), hyperextension or arching of the back (video 2, segment B), and hyperextension and adduction of both arms on walking. As a sensory trick, the patient puts both hands in the occipital region in order to partially alleviate the retrocollis (video 2, segment C). He also had moderate parkinsonism in the form of hypophonic speech, reduced blinking, resting tremor of the right foot, diffuse rigidity, bradykinesia, breakdown of rapid alternating movements on finger/hand/foot tapping and hand opening/closing bilaterally, reduced arm swing, slowness in arising from a seated position, and retropulsion (video 2, segment D).

He received bromocriptine, diphenhydramine, tetrabenazine, reserpine, baclofen, tizanidine, trihexyphenidyl, clonazepam, and haloperidol as monotherapy and in different combinations at maximally tolerated doses, with no change in his dystonia. Some improvement of the dystonia was achieved with trihexyphenidyl (10 mg/d) and clonazepam (2 mg/d). Levodopa (375 mg/d) slightly improved the resting tremor of the right foot but did not affect the bradykinesia. Levodopa was stopped after 3 mo because of subjective worsening of his cervical dystonia. Botulinum toxin type A injections to the neck muscles gave the best, albeit temporary, relief of his cervical dystonia but caused considerable worsening of his dysphagia.

Familial Parkinsonism With Chorea (Huntington's Disease)

Huntington's disease (HD) is an adult-onset, progressive autosomal dominant neurodegenerative disorder caused by an abnormal expansion of CAG trinucleotide repeats in a gene on chromosome 4 coding for the huntingtin protein *(42)*. In most cases of HD, the phenotype is characterized by hyperkinetic movements (chorea), dementia, and personality disorder. However, phenotypic presentation and age at onset of symptoms in HD are variable and depend on the length of the CAG repeat expansion, with an inverse correlation between age at onset and the CAG repeat length *(43)*. In addition, patients with early onset and larger CAG repeat sizes present more often with parkinsonism, dystonia, or eye movement abnormalities rather than chorea *(44,45)*. Neuropathology in HD is characterized by a striking neuronal loss in the caudate and putamen, as well as a moderate neuronal loss in the thalamus and cerebral cortex *(46)*.

Clinical Description

The clinical features seen in HD patients with parkinsonism, which include rigidity and bradykinesia, are summarized in Table 7 *(47,48)*. In patients with classic HD, age at onset is between 35 and 44 yr, but in those with prominent parkinsonism, onset occurs at a substantially younger age *(49,50)*. The parkinsonism in HD responds poorly to dopaminergic therapy. The akinetic rigid state is not associated with chorea, but rather with dementia and seizures. This form of HD is more rapidly progressive and is fatal within 10 yr.

A few cases of the akinetic rigid form of HD with later onset (age over 40 yr) have been reported. Levodopa therapy can be beneficial in these late-onset akinetic rigid forms of HD *(51,52)*. In the terminal stages of the classic form of HD, rigidity and dystonia tend to replace chorea *(53,54)*.

Familial Parkinsonism With Depression, Weight Loss, and Central Hypoventilation (Perry Syndrome)

In 1975, Perry et al. *(55,56)* described a family presenting with parkinsonism, depression, weight loss, and central hypoventilation. Subsequently, six other families with a similar phenotype were identified in North America, Europe, and Asia *(57–62)*. The phenotype differs from other familial autosomal dominant or recessive parkinsonian syndromes linked to known mutations or loci. Molecular genetic study in these families is in progress, but the gene locus has not yet been identified. Neuropathologic findings include severe neuronal loss and gliosis in the substantia nigra with few or no Lewy bodies *(57–61)*.

Clinical Presentation

The pattern of inheritance is autosomal dominant with high penetrance. Table 8 summarizes the clinical and pathologic features of seven kindreds described with this syndrome. The mean age at onset is 46 yr (range, 35–57). The phenotype consists of parkinsonism, weight loss, respiratory dysfunction, and depression. The parkinsonian features include a resting tremor, bradykinesia, and rigidity. Depression and severe weight loss are usually seen in the early stages of the disease. Affected individuals may die suddenly or die of respiratory failure *(57,58,61)*. Suicide attempts also occur. The most consistent clinical signs include parkinsonism and hypoventilation. A good response to levodopa is seen in some but not all kindreds. The disease progression is relentless, leading to death in 2–8 yr.

Case 3: (Video 3, see accompanying DVD) Perry Syndrome (Fukuoka Family, Unknown Genetic Locus)

This 43-yr-old right-handed man *(61)* was referred by his employer to the company physician because of inability to perform his regular job duties. The examination performed at that time demon-

Table 7
Clinical Features Seen in Juvenile HD vs Adult-Onset HD Associated With Parkinsonism

Feature	Juvenile HD	Adult Form of HD Associated with Parkinsonism
Average age at disease onset, yr	<20	45–64
Initial symptoms	Parkinsonism	Parkinsonism
Parkinsonism		
Bradykinesia	+	+
Rigidity	+	+
Resting tremor	–	–
Postural instability	+	+
Response to levodopa	–	+
Dystonia	+	+
Chorea	+/–	+/–

HD, Huntington's disease; +, present; –, not present.

strated bradykinesia and depressed mood, which the patient was not aware of. When the patient was examined in a tertiary care facility 6 mo later, the parkinsonian features noted included a masklike facial expression, hypophonic speech, rigidity, and bradykinesia. His cognition was intact. The rigidity was moderately severe and symmetrical in all four extremities, with no axial involvement noted. His muscle strength was preserved. A mild bilateral postural hand tremor was present. Deep tendon reflexes were symmetrical and hyperactive, especially in the lower extremities. Bilateral ankle clonus was observed. Posture was stooped, gait was slow, and arm swing was reduced bilaterally. Postural stability was preserved. No sensory, cerebellar, or lower motor deficits were present. Therapy with carbidopa-levodopa was initiated, with mild improvement initially. However, his health deteriorated. He lost 10 kg over the next 2 mo and began to require assistance in all activities of daily living. Six months later, he was admitted to a psychiatric hospital for treatment of anxiety, nighttime dyspnea, and progressive weight loss. Discontinuation of the carbidopa-levodopa resulted the next day in confusion and exacerbation of his tremor, akinesia, and rigidity. Prompt reinstatement of carbidopa-levodopa therapy led to resolution of the confusion and improvement of the parkinsonism.

Clinical examination of the patient revealed a weight of 37 kg and notable tachypnea (30 breaths/min). Orientation was intact, but calculation skills and immediate recall were impaired. Extraocular movements were preserved. The parkinsonism was considerably more pronounced than it had been 14 mo earlier (video 3, segment A). The rigidity was present in both axial and appendicular muscles. The patient was also more bradykinetic, and striking postural instability was noted (video 3, segment B). A severe postural and resting tremor affecting all four extremities was seen. Bilateral ankle clonus and a right Babinski sign were present.

Chest radiography, chest computed tomography, and pulmonary function tests were normal. Polysomnography showed an apnea index of 6.96. The arterial blood gases measured on room air showed a PCO_2 of 47 mmHg and PO_2 of 85.2 mmHg. A repeat arterial blood gas measurement made 1 mo later showed further deterioration, with a PCO_2 of 51 mmHg. Two days later, PCO_2 increased to 61 mmHg, necessitating ventilator support. Repeat polysomnography demonstrated irregular breathing and central hypoventilation with hypoxia. At the time of writing, the patient was 47 yr old, severely disabled, and in need of assisted breathing support and total nursing care. He was also depressed and receiving antidepressant therapy. His parkinsonism was severe and not responsive to carbidopa-levodopa.

Table 8

Characteristic Clinical and Pathologic Features of Families With Parkinsonism, Depression, Weight Loss, and Central Hypoventilation (Perry Syndrome)

Feature	Published Reports						
	Perry et al., 1975 (55); Perry et al., 1990 (56)	Purdy et al., 1979 (57)	Roy et al., 1988 (58)	Lechevalier et al., 1992 (59)	Bhatia et al., 1993 (60)	Tsuboi et al., 2002 (61)	Elibol et al., 2002 (62)
Residence	Canada	Canada	USA	France	UK	Japan	Turkey
No. of affected individuals	8	5	6	5	8	6	3
Mean age at onset, y (range)	48 (42–52)	46	51 (45–57)	52 (45–57)	35, 43	41 (38–43)	Proband 46/M Sister 49/F
Disease duration, y (range)	5 (4–6)	2, 3	3 (3–4)	7 (6–8)	3, 4	6	3, 5
Initial signs	D, WL	D, WL	P, D	P, D	P	P, D	Apathy, P
Clinical features							
P	+	+	+	+	+	+	+
D	+	+	+	+	+	+	–
WL	+	+	+	+	–	+	+
HV	+	+	+	+	–	+	+
Resp. to L-dopa	–	–	+	+	+	+	+
Outcome	1 suicide	1 sudden death	3 sudden deaths	2 deaths owing to respiratory failure	1 sudden death	1 suicide	1 sudden death
Pathologic features							
Cell loss	SN	SN, caudate, globus pallidus, pons, medulla	SN, locus ceruleus	SN, dorsal medullary nuclei	SN, locus ceruleus	SN, locus ceruleus	NA
Lewy bodies	Few	Few	No	No	2 in SN, 1 in bnM	No	NA

bnM, basal nucleus of Meynert; D, depression; HV, hypoventilation; LB, Lewy body; NA, not available; P, parkinsonism; Resp., response; SN, substantia nigra; WL, weight loss; +, present; –, not present.

Familial Parkinsonism Owing to a Defect in Copper Metabolism (Wilson's Disease)

Wilson's disease (WD) is an autosomal recessive disorder in which copper metabolism is impaired. The causative "WD gene," known as ATP7B, is located on chromosome 13q14-q21 and is involved in the copper-transporting P-type adenosine triphosphatase interaction between copper and ceruloplasmin *(63–65)*. More than 200 mutations have been found in this gene, and WD occurs worldwide. It is a progressive disorder with a variable age at onset, ranging from 7 to 58 yr. The initial symptoms can be hepatic, behavioral, or neurological *(66)*. Most patients exhibit intracorneal pigmentation (Kayser–Fleischer ring) at the initial presentation *(67)*. Neurological symptoms include various combinations of resting tremor, intention tremor, dysarthria, unsteady gait, dystonia, bradykinesia, and rigidity *(68)*. On neuropathologic examination, the most striking changes, consisting of pigmentation and spongy degeneration, are seen in the basal ganglia. Microscopically, the basal ganglia exhibit neuronal loss as well as abundant protoplasmic astrocytes, including giant cells called "Alzheimer cells" *(69)*.

Clinical Presentation

Tremor and rigidity are the most common parkinsonian manifestations of WD *(70)*. Throughout the course of the illness, the tremor may be unilateral and present only at rest, and it may be indistinguishable from PD tremor. In the advanced stages of WD, some patients develop a "wing-beating" type of tremor. Rigidity is frequently present, together with dystonia. A fixed open mouth and drooling are common. If no treatment is administered, the disease is relentlessly progressive *(68)*.

Familial Parkinsonism With Iron Metabolism Deficiency (Neurodegeneration With Brain Iron Accumulation, Hallervorden–Spatz Syndrome)

Neurodegeneration with brain iron accumulation (NBIA) is a heterogeneous group of disorders with sporadic and familial forms. This syndrome was previously known as Hallervorden–Spatz disease. It typically begins in childhood with extrapyramidal features, including chorea, rigidity, and dystonia. In addition, pyramidal signs, progressive dementia, and, less commonly, retinitis pigmentosa and seizures are also seen *(71,72)*. Some familial cases present with late-onset parkinsonism that can occasionally be responsive to levodopa *(73,74)*.

The molecular genetic study of an Amish family with NBIA demonstrated linkage to a locus on chromosome 20p12.3-p13 *(75)*. More recently, a mutation in the coding sequence of a pantothenate kinase gene called PANK2 was found in this family *(76)*. Additional missense and null mutations have been identified in other familial forms of NBIA *(77)*. The term "PKAN" (pantothenate kinase–associated neurodegeneration) means a defect of the gene PANK2 leading to a deficiency of the enzyme pantothenate kinase. Interestingly, missense mutations in PANK2 were identified in individuals with atypical PKAN. There are also families with NBIA with no linkage to the PANK2 locus *(77–79)*, suggesting the existence of another chromosomal locus for this disorder. Clinical features similar to NBIA were seen in families with neuroferritinopathy who had mutations in the ferritin light chain *(78)* and in families with aceruloplasminemia who had mutations in the gene encoding for ceruloplasmin *(79)*. A striking rust-brown pigmentation is seen in the globus pallidus and substantia nigra pars reticulata (80). In these structures, many axonal spheroids are seen. The presence of Lewy bodies and neurofibrillary tangles was also reported in NBIA *(81,82)*.

Clinical Presentation

NBIA is characterized by extrapyramidal features, including rigidity and dystonia. Age at onset in familial forms is usually in the first or second decade. However, a later onset has also been reported *(73,74)*. Rigidity usually starts first in the lower extremities but later affects the upper extremities as well. Involuntary choreoathetoid movements sometimes precede or accompany rigidity. Orobuccolingual rigidity may be a presenting feature and can lead to difficulties in articulation and swallowing. Pyramidal tract involvement is common. Cognitive dysfunction and epilepsy occur rarely *(71)*.

Familial Parkinsonism With Mitochondrial Abnormality

Increasingly, mitochondrial dysfunction (particularly of complex I) has been recognized to play an important role in the pathogenesis of PD. Complex I activity is decreased in the substantia nigra of PD patients compared to normal controls *(83)*. Similarly, cytoplasmic hybrid (cybrid) cell lines expressing mitochondrial DNA (mtDNA) from the platelets of PD patients have impaired complex I activity compared to platelets of normal controls *(84,85)*. 1-Methyl-4-phenyl-1,2,3,6-tetrahydropyridine (MPTP) or rotenone may produce PD in animal models by inhibiting complex I mitochondrial activity. These data suggest that mitochondrial dysfunction plays an important role in the pathogenesis of PD. In addition, mtDNA dysfunction has been identified in two large PD families with a maternal mode of inheritance *(86,87)*.

Clinical Description

In the first family with maternally inherited PD, in which three generations were studied, cybrid cell line cultures demonstrated decreased complex I activity *(86)*. The average age at onset was 42 yr (range, 41–79 yr). The phenotype resembled "classic" PD, with a resting tremor, bradykinesia, and rigidity. A good response to levodopa was observed. So far, no specific mutation has been identified in this family. The second family had a mixed phenotype resembling adult-onset multisystem degeneration. The clinical features included levodopa-responsive parkinsonism, dementia, dystonia, extraocular movement abnormalities, and pyramidal signs. A missense mtDNA mutation in the gene for the nicotinamide dehydrogenase 4 (ND4) subunit of complex I was identified in this family *(87)*. One case was autopsied, showing loss of pigmented neurons in the substantia nigra and absence of Lewy bodies.

GENETIC TESTING FOR ATYPICAL PARKINSONIAN DISORDERS

Recent discoveries on chromosomal loci and mutations in familial neurodegenerative conditions have expanded our knowledge about the basic cellular mechanisms involved in neurodegeneration. These have provided us with the option of genetic testing to establish a more precise diagnosis in symptomatic individuals with or without an obvious family history. Presymptomatic (predictive) and prenatal diagnosis are possible for several movement disorders, including some of those discussed here, although a detailed discussion of molecular genetic testing is beyond the scope of this chapter. A recent review on this subject was published by the Movement Disorders Society Task Force on Molecular Diagnosis *(88)*. Molecular genetic testing can be readily performed in affected individuals presenting with parkinsonism with ataxia (SCA2 and SCA3), dystonia (DYT1), and chorea (HD). The genetic tests for these conditions are commercially available. Appropriate genetic counseling can be provided by a neurologist requesting such tests. However, presymptomatic and prenatal molecular testing, if requested by family members, should be performed by experienced personnel in specialized genetic centers. Clinical geneticists can also help locate laboratories where molecular genetic testing can be performed for parkinsonian patients in whom known mutations are suspected. Testing for such mutations is currently performed only on an experimental basis.

SUMMARY

Our knowledge of familial atypical parkinsonian disorders has increased greatly over the past decade. Families with unique phenotypes have been newly discovered, and the molecular basis for some of these phenotypes has been established. These molecular genetic discoveries allow us to make more precise clinical diagnoses of several neurodegenerative conditions, including HD, SCA, and dystonia. Future discoveries using transgenic animal models can be expected to lead to a better classification of these disorders and to the development of improved treatments (and cures).

The refinement of molecular genetic techniques and a growing interest in the genetics of parkinsonism will undoubtedly lead to improved characterization and classification of familial atypical parkinsonian syndromes. It is hoped that a classification based on genotype (rather than phenotype alone) will lead to earlier and more accurate diagnoses and more timely and appropriate genetic counseling. Differentiating atypical parkinsonism from idiopathic PD is important because prognosis for each of these conditions varies. There is also a need to develop clinical and pathological criteria for atypical parkinsonian conditions. If specific disease biomarkers are identified, they can further improve accuracy of diagnosis, even in the early or presymptomatic stages.

Probands and families may be interested in genetic counseling; thus, appropriate referral needs to be arranged by the treating neurologist. Genetic testing is already commercially available for some of the atypical parkinsonian disorders and undoubtedly more diagnostic tests will become available in the near future. Treatment for these rare conditions is still supportive in nature. It is hoped that better symptomatic and curative therapies will eventually be developed. This will require a multifaceted approach involving molecular genetics, transgenic animal models, cell biology, and a deeper understanding of the underlying pathologic features in each of these disorders.

DIRECTIONS FOR FUTURE RESEARCH

- Better clinical and pathological characterization
- Establishment of clinical and pathological diagnostic criteria
- Search for biomarkers that will facilitate earlier diagnosis
- Development of commercially available genetic testing
- Development of better symptomatic and curative therapies

REFERENCES

1. Calne DB, Snow BJ, Lee C. Criteria for diagnosing Parkinson's disease. Ann Neurol 1992;32(Suppl):S125–127.
2. Jankovic J. Parkinsonism-plus syndromes. Mov Disord 1989;4(Suppl 1): S95–S119.
3. Foster NL, Wilhelmsen K, Sima AA, Jones MZ, D'Amato CJ, Gilman S. Frontotemporal dementia and parkinsonism linked to chromosome 17: a consensus conference. Conference Participants. Ann Neurol 1997;41:706–715.
4. Pickering-Brown S, Baker M, Yen SH, et al. Pick's disease is associated with mutations in the tau gene. Ann Neurol 2000;48:859–867.
5. Lanska DJ, Currier RD, Cohen M, et al. Familial progressive subcortical gliosis. Neurology 1994;44:1633–1643.
6. Sumi SM, Bird TD, Nochlin D, Raskind MA. Familial presenile dementia with psychosis associated with cortical neurofibrillary tangles and degeneration of the amygdala. Neurology 1992;42:120–127.
7. Wszolek ZK, Pfeiffer RF, Bhatt MH, et al. Rapidly progressive autosomal dominant parkinsonism and dementia with pallido-ponto-nigral degeneration. Ann Neurol 1992;32:312–320.
8. Spillantini MG, Goedert M, Crowther RA, Murrell JR, Farlow MR, Ghetti B. Familial multiple system tauopathy with presenile dementia: a disease with abundant neuronal and glial tau filaments. Proc Natl Acad Sci USA 1997;94:4113–4118.
9. Lynch T, Sano M, Marder KS, et al. Clinical characteristics of a family with chromosome 17-linked disinhibition-dementia-parkinsonism-amyotrophy complex. Neurology 1994;44:1878–1884.
10. Hutton M, Lendon CL, Rizzu P, et al. Association of missense and 5'-splice-site mutations in tau with the inherited dementia FTDP-17. Nature 1998;393:702–705.
11. Poorkaj P, Bird TD, Wijsman E, et al. Tau is a candidate gene for chromosome 17 frontotemporal dementia. Ann Neurol 1998;43:815–825.
12. Spillantini MG, Murrell JR, Goedert M, Farlow MR, Klug A, Ghetti B. Mutation in the tau gene in familial multiple system tauopathy with presenile dementia. Proc Natl Acad Sci USA 1998;95:7737–7741.
13. Wszolek ZK, Tsuboi Y, Farrer M, Uitti RJ, Hutton ML. Hereditary tauopathies and parkinsonism. Adv Neurol 2003;91:153–163.
14. Reed LA, Wszolek ZK, Hutton M. Phenotypic correlations in FTDP-17. Neurobiol Aging 2001;22:89–107.
15. Tsuboi Y, Baker M, Hutton ML, et al. Clinical and genetic studies of families with the tau N279K mutation (FTDP-17). Neurology 2002;59:1791–1793.
16. Ghetti B, Hutton M, Wszolek ZK. Frontotemporal dementia and parkinsonism linked to chromosome 17 associated with tau gene mutations (FTDP-17T). In: Dickson D, ed. Neurodegeneration: The Molecular Pathology of Dementia and Movement Disorders. Basel: International Society of Neuropathology Press, 2003:86–102.
17. Basun H, Almkvist O, Axelman K, et al. Clinical characteristics of a chromosome 17-linked rapidly progressive familial frontotemporal dementia. Arch Neurol 1997;54:539–544.

18. Lendon CL, Lynch T, Norton J, et al. Hereditary dysphasic disinhibition dementia: a frontotemporal dementia linked to 17q21-22. Neurology 1998;50:1546–1555.

19. Heutink P, Stevens M, Rizzu P, et al. Hereditary frontotemporal dementia is linked to chromosome 17q21-q22: a genetic and clinicopathological study of three Dutch families. Ann Neurol 1997;41:150–159.

20. Rademakers R, Cruts M, Dermaut B, et al. Tau negative frontal lobe dementia at 17q21: significant finemapping of the candidate region to a 4.8 cM interval. Mol Psychiatry 2002;7:1064–1074.

21. Froelich S, Basun H, Forsell C, et al. Mapping of a disease locus for familial rapidly progressive frontotemporal dementia to chromosome 17q12-21. Am J Med Genet 1997;74:380–385.

22. Wszolek ZK, Tsuboi Y, Uitti RJ, Reed L. Two brothers with frontotemporal dementia and parkinsonism with an N279K mutation of the tau gene. Neurology 2000;55:1939.

23. Tsuboi Y, Uitti RJ, Delisle MB, et al. Clinical features and disease haplotypes of individuals with the N279K tau gene mutation: a comparison of the pallidopontonigral degeneration kindred and a French family. Arch Neurol 2002;59:943–950.

24. Harding AE. The clinical features and classification of the late onset autosomal dominant cerebellar ataxias: a study of 11 families, including descendants of "the Drew family of Walworth." Brain 1982;105:1–28.

25. Schols L, Peters S, Szymanski S, et al. Extrapyramidal motor signs in degenerative ataxias. Arch Neurol 2000;57:1495–1500.

26. Jardim LB, Pereira ML, Silveira I, Ferro A, Sequeiros J, Giugliani R. Neurologic findings in Machado–Joseph disease: relation with disease duration, subtypes, and (CAG)n. Arch Neurol 2001;58:899–904.

27. Gwinn-Hardy K, Chen JY, Liu HC, et al. Spinocerebellar ataxia type 2 with parkinsonism in ethnic Chinese. Neurology 2000;55:800–805.

28. Shan DE, Soong BW, Sun CM, Lee SJ, Liao KK, Liu RS. Spinocerebellar ataxia type 2 presenting as familial levodopa-responsive parkinsonism. Ann Neurol 2001;50:812–815.

29. Furtado S, Farrer M, Tsuboi Y, et al. SCA-2 presenting as parkinsonism in an Alberta family: clinical, genetic, and PET findings. Neurology 2002;59:1625–1627.

30. Lu CS, Wu Chou YH, Yen TC, Tsai CH, Chen RS, Chang HC. Dopa-responsive parkinsonism phenotype of spinocerebellar ataxia type 2. Mov Disord 2002;17:1046–1051.

31. Gwinn-Hardy K, Singleton A, O'Suilleabhain P, et al. Spinocerebellar ataxia type 3 phenotypically resembling Parkinson disease in a black family. Arch Neurol 2001;58:296–299.

32. Subramony SH, Hernandez D, Adam A, et al. Ethnic differences in the expression of neurodegenerative disease: Machado–Joseph disease in Africans and Caucasians. Mov Disord 2002;17:1068–1071.

33. Fahn S, Marsden CD, Calne DB. Classification and investigation of dystonia. In: Marsden CD, Fahn S, eds. Movement Disorders 2. London: Butterworths, 1987:332–358.

34. Evidente VG, Advincula J, Esteban R, et al. Phenomenology of "Lubag" or X-linked dystonia-parkinsonism. Mov Disord 2002;17:1271–1277.

35. Evidente VG, Gwinn-Hardy K, Hardy J, Hernandez D, Singleton A. X-linked dystonia ("Lubag") presenting predominantly with parkinsonism: a more benign phenotype? Mov Disord 2002;17:200–202.

36. Evidente VGH, Dickson D, Singleton A, Natividad F, Hardy D. Novel neuropathological findings in Lubag or X-linked dystonia-parkinsonism (abstract). Mov Disord 2002;17(Suppl 5):S294.

37. Ichinose H, Ohye T, Takahashi E, et al. Hereditary progressive dystonia with marked diurnal fluctuation caused by mutations in the GTP cyclohydrolase I gene. Nat Genet 1994;8:236–242.

38. Tassin J, Durr A, Bonnet AM, et al. Levodopa-responsive dystonia: GTP cyclohydrolase I or parkin mutations? Brain 2000;123:1112–1121.

39. Kramer PL, Mineta M, Klein C, et al. Rapid-onset dystonia-parkinsonism: linkage to chromosome 19q13. Ann Neurol 1999;46:176–182.

40. Pittock SJ, Joyce C, O'Keane V, et al. Rapid-onset dystonia-parkinsonism: a clinical and genetic analysis of a new kindred. Neurology 2000;55:991–995.

41. Grotzsch H, Pizzolato GP, Ghika J, et al. Neuropathology of a case of dopa-responsive dystonia associated with a new genetic locus, DYT14. Neurology 2002;58:1839–1842.

42. The Huntington's Disease Collaborative Research Group. A novel gene containing a trinucleotide repeat that is expanded and unstable on Huntington's disease chromosomes. Cell 1993;72:971–983.

43. Rubinsztein DC, Leggo J, Chiano M, et al. Genotypes at the GluR6 kainate receptor locus are associated with variation in the age of onset of Huntington disease. Proc Natl Acad Sci USA 1997;94:3872–3876.

44. Squitieri F, Berardelli A, Nargi E, et al. Atypical movement disorders in the early stages of Huntington's disease: clinical and genetic analysis. Clin Genet 2000;58:50–56.

45. Louis ED, Anderson KE, Moskowitz C, Thorne DZ, Marder K. Dystonia-predominant adult-onset Huntington disease: association between motor phenotype and age of onset in adults. Arch Neurol 2000;57:1326–1330.

46. de la Monte SM, Vonsattel JP, Richardson EP Jr. Morphometric demonstration of atrophic changes in the cerebral cortex, white matter, and neostriatum in Huntington's disease. J Neuropathol Exp Neurol 1988;47:516–525.

47. Campbell AMG, Corner BD, Norman RM, Urich H. The rigid form of Huntington's disease. J Neurol Neurosurg Psychiatry 1961;24:71–77.
48. van Dijk JG, van der Velde EA, Roos RA, Bruyn GW. Juvenile Huntington disease. Hum Genet 1986;73:235–239.
49. Bittenbender JB, Quadfasel FA. Rigid and akinetic forms of Huntington's chorea. Arch Neurol 1962;7:37–50.
50. Roos RA, Vegter-van der Vlis M, Hermans J, et al. Age at onset in Huntington's disease: effect of line of inheritance and patient's sex. J Med Genet 1991;28:515–519.
51. Racette BA, Perlmutter JS. Levodopa responsive parkinsonism in an adult with Huntington's disease. J Neurol Neurosurg Psychiatry 1998;65:577–579.
52. Reuter I, Hu MT, Andrews TC, Brooks DJ, Clough C, Chandhuri KR. Late onset levodopa responsive Huntington's disease with minimal chorea masquerading as Parkinson plus syndrome. J Neurol Neurosurg Psychiatry 2000;68: 238–241.
53. Thompson PD, Berardelli A, Rothwell JC, et al. The coexistence of bradykinesia and chorea in Huntington's disease and its implications for theories of basal ganglia control of movement. Brain 1988;111:223–244.
54. Garcia Ruiz PJ, Gomez Tortosa E, Sanchez Bernados V, Rojo A, Fontan A, Garcia de Yebenes J. Bradykinesia in Huntington's disease. Clin Neuropharmacol 2000;23:50–52.
55. Perry TL, Bratty PJ, Hansen S, Kennedy J, Urquhart N, Dolman CL. Hereditary mental depression and Parkinsonism with taurine deficiency. Arch Neurol 1975;32:108–113.
56. Perry TL, Wright JM, Berry K, Hansen S, Perry TL Jr. Dominantly inherited apathy, central hypoventilation, and Parkinson's syndrome: clinical, biochemical, and neuropathologic studies of 2 new cases. Neurology 1990;40:1882–1887.
57. Purdy A, Hahn A, Barnett HJ, et al. Familial fatal Parkinsonism with alveolar hypoventilation and mental depression. Ann Neurol 1979;6:523–531.
58. Roy EP III, Riggs JE, Martin JD, Ringel RA, Gutmann L. Familial parkinsonism, apathy, weight loss, and central hypoventilation: successful long-term management. Neurology 1988;38:637–639.
59. Lechevalier B, Schupp C, Fallet-Bianco C, et al. Familial parkinsonian syndrome with athymhormia and hypoventilation [French]. Rev Neurol (Paris) 1992;148:39–46.
60. Bhatia KP, Daniel SE, Marsden CD. Familial parkinsonism with depression: a clinicopathological study. Ann Neurol 1993;34:842–847.
61. Tsuboi Y, Wszolek ZK, Kusuhara T, Doh-ura K, Yamada T. Japanese family with parkinsonism, depression, weight loss, and central hypoventilation. Neurology 2002;58:1025–1030.
62. Elibol B, Kobayashi T, Atac FB, et al. Familial parkinsonism with apathy, depression and central hypoventilation (Perry's syndrome). In: Mizuno Y, Fisher A, Hanin I, eds. Mapping the progress of Alzheimer's and Parkinson's disease. New York: Kluwer Academic/Plenum Publishers, 2002:285–290.
63. Bowcock AM, Farrer LA, Hebert JM, et al. Eight closely linked loci place the Wilson disease locus within 13q14-q21. Am J Hum Genet 1988;43:664–674.
64. Bull PC, Thomas GR, Rommens JM, Forbes JR, Cox DW. The Wilson disease gene is a putative copper transporting P-type ATPase similar to the Menkes gene. Nat Genet 1993;5:327–337.
65. Tanzi RE, Petrukhin K, Chernove I, et al. The Wilson disease gene is a copper transporting ATPase with homology to the Menkes disease gene. Nat Genet 1993;5:344–350.
66. Gow PJ, Smallwood RA, Angus PW, Smith AL, Wall AJ, Sewell RB. Diagnosis of Wilson's disease: an experience over three decades. Gut 2000;46:415–419.
67. Arima M, Takeshita K, Yoshino K, Kitahara T, Suzuki Y. Prognosis of Wilson's disease in childhood. Eur J Pediatr 1977;126:147–154.
68. Menkes JH. Wilson disease. In: Pulst S-M, ed. Genetics of Movement Disorders. Amsterdam: Academic Press, 2003:341–352.
69. Wilson SAK. Progressive lenticular degeneration: a familial nervous disease associated with cirrhosis of the liver. Brain 1912;34:295–509.
70. Lingam S, Wilson J, Nazer H, Mowat AP. Neurological abnormalities in Wilson's disease are reversible. Neuropediatrics 1987;18:11–12.
71. Dooling EC, Schoene WC, Richardson EP Jr. Hallervorden–Spatz syndrome. Arch Neurol 1974;30:70–83.
72. Swaiman KF. Hallervorden–Spatz syndrome. Pediatr Neurol 2001;25:102–108.
73. Jankovic J, Kirkpatrick JB, Blomquist KA, Langlais PJ, Bird ED. Late-onset Hallervorden–Spatz disease presenting as familial parkinsonism. Neurology 1985;35:227–234.
74. Alberca R, Rafel E, Chinchon I, Vadillo J, Navarro A. Late onset parkinsonian syndrome in Hallervorden–Spatz disease. J Neurol Neurosurg Psychiatry 1987;50:1665–1668.
75. Taylor TD, Litt M, Kramer P, et al. Homozygosity mapping of Hallervorden–Spatz syndrome to chromosome 20p12.3-p13. Nat Genet 1996;14:479–481.
76. Zhou B, Westaway SK, Levinson B, Johnson MA, Gitschier J, Hayflick SJ. A novel pantothenate kinase gene (PANK2) is defective in Hallervorden–Spatz syndrome. Nat Genet 2001;28:345–349.
77. Hayflick SJ, Westaway SK, Levinson B, et al. Genetic, clinical, and radiographic delineation of Hallervorden–Spatz syndrome. N Engl J Med 2003;348:33–40.

78. Curtis AR, Fey C, Morris CM, et al. Mutation in the gene encoding ferritin light polypeptide causes dominant adult-onset basal ganglia disease. Nat Genet 2001;28:350–354.

79. Gitlin JD. Aceruloplasminemia. Pediatr Res 1998;44:271–276.

80. Hallervorden J, Spatz H. Eigenartige erkrankung im extrapyramidalen system mit besonderer beteiligung des globus pallidus und der substantia nigra. Z Gesamte Neurol Psychiatrie 1922:79:254–302.

81. Wakabayashi K, Yoshimoto M, Fukushima T, et al. Widespread occurrence of alpha-synuclein/NACP-immunoreactive neuronal inclusions in juvenile and adult-onset Hallervorden–Spatz disease with Lewy bodies. Neuropathol Appl Neurobiol 1999;25:363–368.

82. Wakabayashi K, Fukushima T, Koide R, et al. Juvenile-onset generalized neuroaxonal dystrophy (Hallervorden–Spatz disease) with diffuse neurofibrillary and Lewy body pathology. Acta Neuropathol (Berl) 2000;99:331–336.

83. Schapira AH, Cooper JM, Dexter D, Clark JB, Jenner P, Marsden CD. Mitochondrial complex I deficiency in Parkinson's disease. Neurochemistry 1990;54:823–827.

84. Swerdlow RH, Parks JK, Miller SW, et al. Origin and functional consequences of the complex I defect in Parkinson's disease. Ann Neurol 1996;40:663–671.

85. Gu M, Cooper JM, Taanman JW, Schapira AH. Mitochondrial DNA transmission of the mitochondrial defect in Parkinson's disease. Ann Neurol 1998;44:177–186.

86. Swerdlow RH, Parks JK, Davis JN II, et al. Matrilineal inheritance of complex I dysfunction in a multigenerational Parkinson's disease family. Ann Neurol 1998;44:873–881.

87. Simon DK, Pulst SM, Sutton JP, Browne SE, Beal MF, Johns DR. Familial multisystem degeneration with parkinsonism associated with the 11778 mitochondrial DNA mutation. Neurology 1999;53:1787–1793.

88. Gasser T, Bressman S, Dürr A, Higgins J, Klockgether T, Myers RH. Molecular diagnosis of inherited movement disorders: Movement Disorders Society Task Force on Molecular Diagnosis. Mov Disord 2003;18:3–18.

23

Clinical Diagnosis of Vascular Parkinsonism and Nondegenerative Atypical Parkinsonian Disorders

Madhavi Thomas and Joseph Jankovic

Idiopathic Parkinson's disease (PD) is the most common cause of parkinsonism, accounting for about 75% of all cases. Other causes of parkinsonism include multiple system atrophy (MSA), progressive supranuclear palsy (PSP), corticobasal degeneration (CBD), and a variety of other neurodegenerative disorders in which rest tremor, bradykinesia, rigidity, and other parkinsonian features are present. Since these disorders are often associated with other neurological deficits, such as dysautonomia (in MSA), vertical ophthalmoparesis (in PSP), and apraxia (in CBD), they are referred to as "parkinsonism plus syndromes." Whereas the above disorders are degenerative in nature, there are other forms of parkinsonism, which are secondary to a variety of etiologic factors including vascular parkinsonism (VP), hemiatrophy hemiparkinsonism, and toxic and metabolic causes.

It is important to review the cardinal features of PD that form the basis for diagnosis of parkinsonism. Cardinal motor features of PD are tremor, rigidity, bradykinesia, and postural instability. While these may occur in idiopathic PD, the atypical parkinsonian sydromes have a combination of these features in addition to the clinical features typical for each specific disorder. Proposed diagnostic criteria for PD include definite, probable, and possible PD and all of these require sustained response to levodopa (1). Although it is difficult to apply uniform diagnostic criteria to all the atypical parkinsonian syndromes, most of them share a common feature of poor or no response to levodopa. In this review we will discuss VP, and a variety of nondegenerative atypical parkinsonian syndromes (Table 1).

VASCULAR PARKINSONISM

VP, also known as arteriosclerotic parkinsonism, multi-infarct parkinsonism, and lower body parkinsonism, can result from lacunar infarctions, leukoaraiosis, and Binswanger's disease. In 1929, Critchley (2) described arteriosclerotic parkinsonism characterized by rigidity, pseudobulbar affect, dementia, incontinence, and short stepped gait in an elderly hypertensive individual with multiple ischemic insults in the basal ganglia. Zijlman et al. (3) in their report of clinico-pathological findings of VP showed the variability of clinical presentation of VP both clinically and pathologically. Based on the clinical evolution of symptoms in 17 patients in this clinico-pathological study, the following criteria for VP were proposed: parkinsonism in the presence of cerebrovascular disease, a relationship between the above two features, and (a) acute or delayed progressive onset with infarcts in or near areas that can increase basal ganglia output, or decrease the thalamocortical drive directly resulting in contralateral bradykinetic rigid syndrome termed Vpa, and (b) in the case of insiduous onset of parkinsonism with extensive subcortical white matter lesions, bilateral symptoms at onset, and the presence of early shuffling gait, or early cognitive dysfunction, termed Vpi (3). These patients with parkinsonism had atrophic gyri, ventricular dilatation, and major-artery atheroma on autopsy. There

From: *Current Clinical Neurology: Atypical Parkinsonian Disorders*
Edited by: I. Litvan © Humana Press Inc., Totowa, NJ

was extensive small vessel disease in the globus pallidus, caudate, putamen, and thalamus in the parkinsonian brains, and nigral cell loss was present in four patients. Microscopic pathology included gliosis, perivascular myelin pallor, hyaline thickening of arteriolar walls, and enlargement of perivascular spaces, along with macroscopically visible infarcts in the basal ganglia in those patients with VP. In all the 17 patients the pathologically examined frontal, temporal, parietal, occipital, and striatal areas were equally affected by the small-vessel disease pathology *(3)*. This study clearly demonstrates the pattern of pathology and variability of clinical findings in patients with VP. Clinical features are variable as shown in this study based on the onset of disease, resulting in a contralateral bradykinetic syndrome in the case of acute or delayed progressive onset, and a bilateral involvement in the case of insidious onset of VP. Three out of the 100 patients clinically diagnosed as PD had VP in the London Brain Bank study, showing that VP can very closely resemble PD *(4)*. Thompson and Marsden described parkinsonian features in a series of patients with Binswanger disease *(5)*. Binswanger's disease is a form of leukoencephalopathy that is mainly a result of hypoxic-ischemic lesions in the distal watershed periventricular areas, associated with aging, hyperviscocity, and increased fibrinogen levels, and has been reported to be associated with VP *(5–7)*. Based on a review of published series, VP can be defined as a syndrome resulting in short stepped gait, rigidity, with or without dementia, predominant lower body involvement in the absence of tremor, and poor levodopa responsiveness. Some patients also exhibit incontinence, pseudobulbar affect, and freezing of gait *(8–11)*.

VP can be clinically classified into three subgroups: (a) possible VP in patients who exhibit atypical parkinsonism and have a history of stroke and show vascular changes on their brain magnetic resonance imaging (MRI), (b) probable VP in patients with onset of parkinsonism within less than 1 mo after acute stroke supported by evidence of a multi-infarct state on brain MRI, and (c) definite VP, which is characterized clinically as possible or probable VP but at autopsy there is ischemic or hemorrhagic damage in the basal ganglia without any evidence of idiopathic PD, such the presence of Lewy bodies *(11)*. There are several clinical presentations of stroke-related parkinsonism, including a syndrome indistinguishable from idiopathic PD, vascular PSP with clinical features similar to those in idiopathic PSP *(12,13)*, lower body parkinsonism *(14)*, and parkinsonian gait disorders *(11,15–17)*.

As there were no previously established clinical criteria for VP, Winikates and Jankovic proposed a vascular rating scale for VP designed to establish diagnostic level of certainty *(11,13)*. Parkinsonism was defined as presence of at least two of the four cardinal signs of tremor at rest, bradykinesia, rigidity, and loss of postural reflexes. The vascular rating scale has scores ranging from 0 to 6 based on pathological, historical, and neuroimaging evidence of vascular disease. Two points were given for pathologically or angiographically proven diffuse vascular disease, one point for pathological evidence of both vascular and neurodegenerative changes, one point for onset of symptoms within 1 mo of a clinical stroke, a history of two or more strokes, a history of two or more risk factors for stroke, and neuroimaging evidence of diffuse vascular disease or vascular disease in two or more vascular territories. When a vascular score of 2 or higher was used as a designation of VP such patients could be clearly differentiated from idiopathic PD *(11,12)*. Zijlmans et al. *(3)* also proposed clinical criteria that include a differentiation between the unilateral and bilateral forms of VP.

Clinical features of patients with VP include older age at onset, male preponderance, higher frequency of dementia, and, as expected, vascular risk factors. About 25% of these patients may present with VP within a month after a stroke. Patients with VP typically present with gait difficulty and during the course have predominant lower body involvement, postural instability, history of falls, dementia, corticospinal findings, incontinence, pseudobulbar affect, and they are less likely to respond to levodopa *(8,10,11)*. Patients with severe subcortical ischemia (as evidenced by MRI) tend to have more gait difficulties *(4)*. In patients with lower body parkinsonism associated with VP, the upper body function is typically preserved. Some patients mainly have gait difficulties with and without freezing, mostly seen with multiple lacunar infarcts *(11,12)*. Quantitative gait analysis in 12 patients with PD, 12 with VP, and 10 controls showed that patients with VP had relatively well-preserved armswing, with anterior rotation of the shoulders *(17)*. Patients with VP were found to have more postural abnormalities on postural stability testing leading to balance problems on dynamic posturography testing *(18)*. Patients with VP have less flexion posture of the elbow, hip, knee, and trunk than patients with idiopathic PD. Larger studies using specific gait instruments, such as the Gait and Balance Scale (GABS) *(19)*, and other gait and balance analyses may help find other patterns of gait and balance abnormalities with high sensitivity and specificity for VP.

In addition to Binswanger's disease that has been associated with elevated fibrinogen levels, some VPs have been found to have high titers of anticardiolipin antibodies (ACLAs) *(20)*. In a study of 44 individuals with VP, 9 of the 22 tested (40.9%) patients had positive ACLA. Further studies are needed to document the exact incidence of ACLAs in patients with VP. Patients with cerebral autosomal dominant arteriopathy with subcortical infarcts and leukoencephalopathy (CADASIL) can sometimes present with parkinsonism. In the original descriptions patients had recurrent strokes, pseudobulbar palsy, and dementia. The abnormality on genetic linkage analysis was localized to chromosome 19q12, and the mutation in Notch-3 gene was subsequently identified *(21)*. In autopsied brains, patients with CADASIL have changes in the vessel wall similar to those seen in polyarteritis nodosa, manifested by eosinophilic granularity or fibrinoid necrosis of the tunica media coupled with basophilic granular degeneration of the media *(22)*.

Elevated homocysteine levels have been also associated with ischemic events resulting in VP, but this abnormality has been attributed to levodopa therapy *(23,24)*. In one study, patients treated with levodopa had a significant increase in plasma homocysteine levels compared to the levodopa-naive patients, and patients with homocysteine levels in the higher quartile had increased risk of coronary artery disease (relative risk 1.75) *(24)*. Although there is no evidence that stroke or coronary artery disease are any more frequent in PD patients than in individuals without PD, high homocysteine levels may increase the risk of dementia associated with PD.

Once VP is clinically suspected MRI scan of the brain must be performed to confirm the presences of subcortical ischemic changes on T1 and T2 images in the basal ganglia and white matter. As expected, in patients with VP the number and intensity of MRI lesions is greater *(10,25)*. Although some authors have not been able to correlate asymmetric lesions with the side of symptoms in patients with VP and PD *(16,26)*, Chang et al. *(27)* showed that most patients with VP had MRI correlates of ischemic changes. In their series of 11 patients they found common clinical features of akinesia, rigidity, shuffling gait, reduced armswing, hesitation while turning, very similar to PD, but these patients had more upright posture, more wide-based stance, and did not exhibit festination. They have identified three patterns of ischemia on computed tomography (CT) or MRI including frontal lobe, deep subcortical, and basal ganglia infarction associated with steady progression. They report that patients with specific basal ganglia lacunar infarcts had a better prognosis with resolution of PD symptoms, whereas those with frontal lobe infarction had a static course, and those with deep subcortical infarcts not specifically confined to the basal ganglia had a progressive course. Autopsy on one of their patients confirmed a multi-infarct state without any evidence of Lewy bodies *(27)*.

Using functional imaging, such as [123]I- β-CIT SPECT (single photon emission computed tomography) and TRODAT-1 scanning, may further enhance the diagnosis of VP *(28,29)*. TRODAT-1 is a cocaine analog that can bind to the presynaptic dopamine transporter and has been found to be useful in differentiating VP from PD. A significant reduction of the uptake was more pronounced in the contralateral putamen of patients idiopathic PD than that in patients with VP *(28)*. Proton MR spectroscopy shows preservation of dopaminergic neurons in VP *(30)*. Tohgi et al. *(31)* have shown narrowing of the width of SNc in patients who have both PD and vascular changes, but those with VP have normal width of SNc on the MRI brain. In a small study including 13 patients, EEG (electroencephelogram) slowing was less in those with VP compared to patients with PD *(32)*, but this observation needs to be confirmed in a larger group of patients.

A small proportion (up to 50%) of patients with VP respond to levodopa, the first line of therapy in this population *(5,14,16,33)*. Demikiran et al. *(16)* have also shown that 38% of patients with VP have a response to levodopa therapy. Depending on the identification of stroke risk factors patients should be started on antiplatelet therapy, or anticoagulation in those with atrial fibrillation and valvular heart disease with high risk of embolization. Occasionally, symptoms of VP may transiently improve with CSF (cerebrospinal fluid) drainage similar to that seen in Normal Pressure Hydrocephalus (NPH) *(34)*. This improvement, however, is rarely sustained and is not predictive of response to CSF shunting.

PARKINSONISM OWING TO TOXIN EXPOSURE

Several studies have explored the role of various environmental causes of parkinsonism, especially exposure to industrial toxins, organic solvents, pesticides, and other putative toxins *(35,36)*. Population studies have shown a link between risk of PD, and chronic (more than 20 yr) exposure to manganese, lead-copper combinations, and iron-copper *(37)*. Mercury exposure has also been linked to PD, but no firm evidence exists for mercury-induced parkinsonism. In the case-control study from Singapore, scalp hair mercury level has been shown to be a poor predictor of risk of PD *(38)*.

1-Methyl-4-Phenyl-1,2,3,6-Tetrahydropyridine

Exposure to 1-methyl-4-phenyl-1,2,3,6-tetrahydropyridine (MPTP) has been used as an experimental model of PD since the discovery in 1982 that this meperidine analog can cause parkinsonism in humans and certain animal species. MPTP after undergoing biotransformation to 1-methyl-4-phenylpyridium ion (MPP+) via monoamine-oxidase B, is taken up to the dopaminergic terminal by dopamine transporter where it inhibits complex I of the mitochondrial respiratory chain *(39–41)*. Individuals with MPTP-induced parkinsonism exhibited typical parkinsonian features including levodopa responsiveness and levodopa-induced dyskinesias, and at autopsy had moderate to severe depletion of pigmented neurons in the substantia nigra, gliosis, and microglial activation, but no convincing evidence of Lewy bodies. Another mitochondrial complex I inhibitor, rotenone, a lipophilic pesticide, has been described to cause parkinsonism in animals and has been used as a model for parkinsonism *(42)*. Unlike MPTP, rotenone is not selective for dopaminergic neurons, since it does not require the dopamine transporter to gain access to the neuronal interior. These findings show that the exposure to MPTP, and possibly other environmental toxins (such as paraquat and possibly other pesticides) can cause clinical, biochemical, and pathological changes similar to those seen in idiopathic PD.

Manganese

Manganese exposure has been known to cause parkinsonism in the form of progressive dystonia, parkinsonism, and psychiatric features for over 150 yr *(43)*. *Manganism* is a term used to describe neuropsychiatric symptoms in miners, smelters, and workers in the alloy industry. Clinical features of manganese induced parkinsonism, usually present in the late or established phase of this disease, include rigidiy, bradykinesia, and chiefly postural tremor. Patients also frequently exhibit dystonia, characteristic gait called "cock-walk," and postural instability with a tendency to fall backward, and poor response to levodopa. Characteristic MRI feature of manganese toxicity is T1 hyperintensity in the striatum and especially in the globus pallidus *(43)*. Pathologically manganese toxicity is associated with atrophy of globus pallidus, caudate nucleus, the putamen, and substantia nigra pars reticularis. Alzheimer's type II astrocytes are also seen in the basal ganglia, thought to represent the selective vulnerability of the basal ganglia *(44)*.

Welding fumes contain a variety of elements including manganese, which is argued to be the causative agent for parkinsonian symptoms in some welders. Racette et al. *(45)* performed a case-controlled study comparing clinical features of PD in 15 welders to that of a control group of PD patients. The welders had an earlier onset of PD, but otherwise the clinical features were identical to those of PD including levodopa responsiveness, motor fluctuations, and dyskinesias. 6-[^{18}F]fluoro-dopa PET (positron emission tomography), performed in only two of the welders, showed findings of decreased uptake in the posterior putamen similar to that seen in PD *(45)*.

Carbon Monoxide

Parkinsonism can develop immediately or several weeks (delayed onset) after exposure to carbon monoxide (CO) exposure. In a report of 242 patients who were exposed to CO, parkinsonism was diagnosed in 23 (9.5%) patients *(46)* The predominant features included "masked facies," short stepped gait, hypokinesia, rigidity, retropulsion, positive glabellar sign, grasp reflex, cognitive problems, and urinary and/or fecal incontinence; 43% patients had mutism. Intentional tremor and postural instability was described in 21% of the patients. Majority of patients had clinical correlation with abnormal CT scans with low-density lesions in the white matter, and in some low-density lesions were present in globus pallidus. There was no correlation between the CT findings and the location of the symptoms. Spontaneous recovery was noted in some patients, but most remained neurologically impaired without meaningful improvement with levodopa *(46,47)*. Lee and Marsden *(47)* described two forms of CO-induced parkinsonism: (a) progressive type and (b) delayed relapsing type (parkinsonian and akinetic mute form). Patients with the progressive form, although they usually recover from coma, have a poor prognosis. They remain in mute vegetative state with rigid, spastic state with little or no spontaneous movement. The delayed relapsing type presents with parkinsonism with variable symptoms including typical slow short stepped gait, with loss of armswing, retropulsion, rigidity and bradykinesia, and stooped posture; sometimes patients may have tremor. Some have dystonia of the hands and feet. In the akinetic mute patients the predominant features are apathy, mutism, along with incontinence, emotional lability, and rigidity. CT scan findings include white matter low-density lesions, and bilateral globus pallidus lesions that improve on subsequent scans in some cases *(47)*. In a study of 73 patients with CO poisoning, Parkinson et al. *(48)* found white matter changes in the centrum semiovale and the periventricular white matter, seen as T2 hyperintensities on MRI scans. Patients with lesions in the centrum semiovale were more likely to have cognitive deficits.

Cyanide Poisoning

Cyanide poisoning has been reported to cause parkinsonism in several case reports *(49–52)*. The observed deficits include progressive parkinsonism in association with dystonia, and apraxia of eyelid opening, with CT and MRI correlation of lesions in the basal ganglia, cerebellum, and cerebral cortex. T2 hyperintensities in the putamen are typical, but MRI changes may also include hemorrhagic necrosis in the cerebral cortex, especially in the sensorimotor cortex in addition to the changes in the basal ganglia *(52)*. These findings along with the temporal relationship to the onset of symptoms and the exposure to cyanide should help diagnose parkinsonism owing to cyanide poisoning *(53)*.

Solvent Exposure

Organic solvents have been long suspected to cause parkinsonism, including MSA *(35)*. Methanol has been reported to be associated with parkinsonism, especially after prolonged exposure. Patients present with metabolic acidosis, coma, and parkinsonian features, particularly rigidity and bradykinesia *(54,55)*. Other solvents such as toluene, methyl ethyl ketone, carbon disulfide, and *n*-hexane have all been linked to parkinsonism *(56)*. MRI of the brain in these cases shows white matter changes. [^{11}C] raclopride PET provided evidence of decreased dopamine receptor type 2 binding in a patient with methyl ethyl ketone exposure in addition to decreased F-dopa uptake on PET, identical to the changes seen in idiopathic PD *(56)*.

Ethanol

Alcohol-induced parkinsonism is a rare and poorly characterized disorder. Transient form of parkinsonism has been reported in alcoholics during withdrawal. This disorder is seen in chronic alcoholics of both sexes, usually older than 50 yr with no evidence of hepatic dysfunction *(57)*. The condition develops a few days after the consumption of the last drink; rarely during acute intoxication. The patients often show other features of alcohol withdrawal and alcoholism including postural tremor, ataxia, and confusion. Most of the patients have previous history of transient episodes of parkinsonism. CT and MRI studies do not show any specific changes. Some patients have moderate to severe brain atrophy resulting from alcoholism, and one patient had basal ganglia calcifications *(57)*. Levodopa has been tried in these patients with limited success. The condition is self-limited and all patients improve with abstinence. In some cases the duration of parkinsonism lasts up to weeks or months. None of the patients with these transient episodes have developed parkinsonism in a 10-yr follow-up study. The hypothesis is that patients susceptible to transient parkinsonism may have underlying nigral degeneration and develop parkinsonism owing to superimposed alcohol use *(57)*.

INFECTIOUS CAUSES OF PARKINSONISM

Human Immunodeficiency Virus

The association of human immunodeficiency virus (HIV) infection and movement disorders has been recognized since the first descriptions of neurological complications of HIV-associated AIDS *(58)*. Secondary parkinsonism has been reported by various authors as case reports, but Mattos et al. *(59)* have reported movement disorders in 28 HIV patients of whom 14 patients had parkinsonism. The mean age at onset of parkinsonism was 37.2 yr (range 25–63). They report mean Hoehn and Yahr scale of 2.5 (range of 1–5). The clinical features included tremor, and rapid progression of parkinsonian symptoms with time of onset to death being five mo in eight patients. Five patients were levodopa responsive. Imaging study with CT scans showed hydrocephalus ex-vacuo, and one patient had toxoplasmosis involving the basal ganglia. One patient with T1 enhancement on the MRI of the brain had ipsilateral ophthalmoplegia and contralateral parkinsonism. Only two of the patients with parkinsonism had other parkinsonian risk factors such as metaclopramide exposure and neurotoxoplasmosis *(59)*. Maggi et al. *(60)* described parkinsonism in a patient with AIDS and toxoplasmosis with abulia, VII cranial nerve impairment, hypomimia, speech impairment, difficulty arising from a chair, stooped posture, short stepped gait and freezing of gait, cogwheel rigidity, and bradykinesia in association with toxoplasma lesion in the bilateral lenticular nucleii and the right frontobasal region *(60)*. Presence of parkinsonism and tremor has been reported by other authors, and the management involves treatment of opportunistic infections, symptomatic treatment of parkinsonism, and antiretroviral therapy *(61)*. Bradykinesia, postural instability, gait disorder, and hypomimia are common features of HIV-related parkinsonism with dementia. Parkinsonian features have been reported in association with dopamine receptor antagonists, opportunistic infections such as toxoplasmosis, or HIV itself. Some patients with HIV have clinical features identical to idiopathic PD *(62)*. Dopaminergic medication has been thought to accelerate the course of HIV viral infection as shown in the study of levodopa and selegiline in the SIV-infected (Simian immunodeficiency virus) macaque model *(63)*.

Subacute Sclerosing Panencephalitis

Subacute sclerosing panencephalitis (SSPE), a slow viral disease caused by measles virus with a mutated M-protein, has been long recognized to cause parkinsonism, myoclonus, dystonia, chorea, athetosis, stereotypies, and a variety of other movement disorders. Sawaishi et al. *(64)* reported a case of SSPE with documented lesions in the substantia nigra as well as the putamen, globus pallidus, and caudate nuclei, seen on the MRI scans of the brain. Parkinsonian symptoms described in SSPE include bradykinesia and rigidity. Previous descriptions of MRI findings include lesions in the putamen and caudate, but sparing the globus pallidus and thalamus *(64)*. Treatment with levodopa and amantadine has been reported to provide some symptomatic relief *(65)*.

Other Infections

Mycoplasma pneumoniae has been reported to cause parkinsonism in a young boy with flulike symptoms, followed by parkinsonism with bradykinesia, hypomimia, hypophonia, and dystonia with MRI findings of increased signal (T1 or T2) in the basal ganglia *(66)*. The patient had elevated mycoplasma antibody levels and his symptoms and MRI abnormalities spontaneously resolved. Postencephalitic encephalitis has been associated with parkinsonism since the epidemic in early 1900s. Although the incidence of postencephalitic parkinsonism has markedly decreased, well-documented cases have been reported recently, including those caused by the West Nile virus *(67,68)*.

METABOLIC CAUSES OF PARKINSONISM

Important metabolic causes of parkinsonism include hypothyroidism and parathyroid dysfunction. Patients with hyperparathyroidism have clinical presentation identical to that of idiopathic PD, but the syndrome is levodopa resistant. The symptoms, however, may be relieved after resolution of the parathyroid dysfunction by surgical removal of the parathyroid adenoma. Hypoparathyroidism may also cause levodopa unresponsive parkinsonism *(69,70)*.

Bilateral striopallidodentate calcinosis, also known as Fahr's disease, is a rare disorder with calcium deposition in the subcortical nucleii and white matter bilaterally. Parkinsonism is reported in 57% of patients with this disorder; other movement disorders seen in Fahr's disease include chorea, tremor, dystonia, athetosis, and orofacial dyskinesias *(71)*. Additional neurological manifestations include cognitive impairment, cerebellar signs, speech disorder, gait disorder, pyramidal signs, sensory symptoms, and psychiatric features *(72)*. Patients have parkinsonism without evidence of parathyroid dysfunction in association with dementia and cerebellar signs. Lewy bodies may be found on autopsy. Response to levodopa is variable *(72)*. No gene has yet been identified although linkage to chromosome 14 has been suggested *(73)*.

POSTANOXIC PARKINSONISM

Parkinsonism can rarely result from hypoxic ischemic injury. Different movement disorders including chorea, tics, athetosis, dystonia, and myoclonus have been reported. Patients can develop parkinsonism with or without dystonia weeks to months after the ischemic event *(74)*. MRI findings include T1 hyper intensities in the basal ganglia bilaterally, indicative of ischemia or gliosis. In the case described by Li et al. *(74)*, the clinical findings included mainly an akinetic rigid syndrome with hypomimia, limitation of down gaze, dysarthria, rigidity, postural tremor, slow rapid alternating movements, shuffling gait, start hesitation, and freezing of gait occurring 3 wk after an anoxic injury owing to cardiac arrest. There was no improvement with dopaminergic drugs. The autopsy examination showed multiple old infarcts with the presence of macrophages indicative of old hemorrhagic infarct in the basal ganglia.

DRUG-INDUCED PARKINSONISM

A discussion of secondary parkinsonism would not be complete without at least a brief review of drug induced parkinsonism. Drug-induced parkinsonism, one of the most common causes of secondary parkinsonism, may coexist with tardive dyskinesia. In a study in patients in the hospital, 51% of the 95 patients had drug-induced parkinsonism *(75)*. The symptoms in drug induced parkinsonism are often bilateral at onset, whereas idiopathic PD is asymmetric at onset, but this clinical observation does not reliably differentiate between the two forms of parkinsonism. Tremor in drug-induced parkinsonism is generally high-frequency 7- to 8-Hz action tremor rather than a rest tremor as seen in idiopathic PD. Women tend to have drug-induced parkinsonism more frequently than men, the opposite of gender distribution in idiopathic PD. Most of the cases of drug-induced parkinsonism occur in patients over 40 yr of age. Parkinsonian symptoms occur generally 10–30 d after starting the drug. It is important to wait 3 months after withdrawal of medication before diagnosing drug-induced parkinsonism. The withdrawal of the suspected drug is usually followed 4–8 weeks later by the disappearance of clinical symptoms. In some cases, the parkinsonian symptoms, however, persist and these cases are suspected to have preclinical PD, in which the initial symptoms were triggered by the exposure to the dopamine receptor-blocking drug *(76)*. There are a variety of drugs including dopamine depletors, dopamine blockers, antihypertensives such as methyldopa and amiodarone, calcium channel blockers such as flunarizine and cinnarazine, and serotonine selective reuptake inhibitors such as fluoxetine, all of which can cause drug-induced parkinsonism. Drug-induced parkinsonism can be treated by withdrawal of the causative agent, but in some cases amantadine and levodopa have been useful *(77)*. Drug-induced parkinsonism is associated with other involuntary movements including bucco-lingulo-masticatory syndrome, focal dystonia, stereotypies, akathisia, and gait disturbance *(78)*. Recovery is noted in 60–70% patients in 7 weeks after drug withdrawal, but it may take about 15–18 months in some patients *(79)*. Hardie et al. *(78)* reported persistence of parkinsonian symptoms in 14 patients after drug withdrawal. Striatal dopamine transporter imaging is normal unlike that seen in idiopathic PD *(80)*.

PERIPHERALLY INDUCED TREMOR AND PARKINSONISM

There are several disorders that have been reported to result from trauma to the peripheral nervous system. These include tremor, dystonia, segmental myoclonus, hemifacial spasm, and in some cases parkinsonism. Among 146 patients with peripherally induced movement disorders, 28 had tremor with or without parkinsonism *(81)*. Eleven patients had tremor-dominant parkinsonism. Clinical features included rest and action tremor, and bradykinesia and rigidity in those with parkinsonism. Onset of movement disorder was temporally related to the injury, and was within 2–5 months after injury. Injuries varied from whiplash to sprain, dental procedure, fracture, overuse, or surgery. Patients had the injury in various areas including arm, neck, lumbar region, and teeth. A majority of patients had injuries in the arms. The condition seemed to spread to the other parts of the body beyond the initial site of injury, and it is unclear if any of them may have had predisposition to parkinsonism, and the trauma in some way has led to the earlier onset of parkinsonism *(81)*. F-Dopa PET scans showed a reduction in F-Dopa uptake suggesting that some patients with peripherally induced parkinsonism may be predisposed to develop the disorder because of a subclinical dopaminergic degeneration.

REVERSIBLE PARKINSONISM IN CHILDHOOD

Parkinsonism is uncommon in childhood and is often owing to a variety of genetic disorders such as parkin mutation, juvenile Huntington's disease, Wilson's disease, and pantothenate kinase-associated neurodegeneration *(82)*. Acquired causes of childhood onset parkinsonism include neuroleptic exposure, cytosine arabinoside, cyclophosphamide, amphotericin B, methotrexate, hypoxic ischemic encephalopathy, and hydrocephalus *(83,84)*.

DEVELOPMENTAL FORMS OF PARKINSONISM

Developmental forms of parkinsonism include syndromes induced by *in utero* or perinatal viral (or other) infection, such as maternal influenza during pregnancy or *in utero* or perinatal trauma or maternal stress. *In utero* influenza has been reported to be a cause of parkinsonism in a young child *(85)*. Parkinsonism was reported in children born to mothers with encephalitis lethargica *(85)*. Asphyxia during delivery, prenatal disturbances, premature birth, or early-childhood meningoencephalitis, often in combination with a complicated pregnancy, were all described to predispose to parkinsonian syndromes. The clinical symptoms included rigidity, hypokinesia, and in a small percentage, tremor. These children also had other neurological abnormalities including cognitive problems, behavioral difficulties, headaches, and strabismus. Treatment with levodopa was reported to be effective. Dyskinesia was noted to be a side effect 8–30 months after therapy, and by 3 years levodopa

Table 1
Secondary Causes of Parkinsonism

Vascular (includes parkinsonism and PSP): with vascular risk factors, hyperhomocystinemia, and CADASIL.

Toxin exposure: MPTP (1-methyl-4-phenyl-1,2,3,6- tetrahydropyridine), manganese, carbon monoxide, cyanide, ethanol, methanol, and other solvents.

Infectious: HIV (human immunodeficiency virus), SSPE (subacute sclerosing pan encephalitis), mycoplasma pneumoniae infection.

Metabolic: Hyperparathyroidism.

Post-anoxic

Drug-induced: Neuroleptic agents, dopamine depletors, amiodarone, calcium channel blockers.

Peripherally induced: parkinsonism owing to injury.

Reversible parkinsonism in childhood: Hypoxic ischemic injury, neuroleptics, cytosine arabinoside, cyclo-phosphamide, amphotericin B, methotrexate, encephalitis, pineal germinoma, neuroleptic malignant syndrome, stroke, head injury, hydrocephalus, kernicterus, and radiation necrosis.

Hemiatrophy-hemiparkinsonism

Structural lesions causing parkinsonism: Posterior fossa tumors, right temporal lobe hemorrhage, intrinsic brainstem tumors.

Other causes: Multiple sclerosis.

was withdrawn. This was a reversible syndrome with very slight progression, and was though to be a result of decreased metabolic activity. Overall, a minority of patients with pre- or perinatal infections or trauma present with parkinsonism with eventual resolution of symptoms and a favorable prognosis.

An important to recognize but poorly understood syndrome is that of cerebral palsy or static encephalopathy that later progresses and causes gradual neurological deterioration. In a study of delayed-onset progressive movement disorders after static brain lesions, about 15% had parkinsonism *(86)*. The precipitating insults included perinatal hypoxic ischemia, stroke, head injury, encephalitis, CO, kernicterus, and radiation necrosis.

HEMIPARKINSONISM-HEMIATROPHY

Hemiparkinsonism-hemiatrophy (HPHA) syndrome was first described by Klawans in 1981 *(87)*, who described four individuals with known hemiatrophy with narrow extremities on one side who developed delayed-onset hemiparkinsonism between ages 31 and 40 with tremor on the same side as the hemiatrophy along with rigidity, akinesia, and dystonia, but no evidence of hypomimia, or abnormal posture or lack of postural reflexes. Their symptoms remained unilateral between 5 and 35 yr after onset of illness. They did not respond well to levodopa. HPHA can be differentiated from idiopathic PD by the clinical features of hemiatrophy, asymmetric parkinsonism more prominent on the side of hemiatrophy, dystonia, early age at onset, history of birth injury, and slow progression of the disease. Mean age of onset of parkinsonism in HPHA is 43.7 yr (range 31–61), and mean duration of symptoms was 9.4 yr (range: 1–35 yr). The first symptom in majority of cases is tremor, followed by bradykinesia and dystonia. In some cases the tremor may become bilateral *(88–90)*. Greene et al. *(90)* have reported dopa-responsive dystonia in some patients with HPHA. In one case report of a 47-yr-old woman with HPHA, the patient developed unusual symptoms of exertional- induced weakness of the right ankle followed by prolonged inversion and dorsiflexion of her foot *(91)*. The symptoms later evolved into tremor, stiffness, and lack of dexterity of muscles on the right side. She had good

Table 2
Showing the Clinical Features of Nondegenerative Atypical Parkinsonian Disorders
that Help in Diagnosis

Parkinsonian Disorder	Distinguishing Clinical Features	Supportive MRI Findings
Vascular parkinsonism	Acute, delayed, or insidious onset with bradykinesia, rigidity, short stepped gait, with or without dementia, postural instability lower body involvement. Patients have freezing of gait, absence of tremor, poor levodopa responsiveness. Some patients have pseudobulbar affect. High index of suspicion in presence of vascular risk factors, and an older patient with atypical clinical presentation.	Subcortical ischemic changes on brain MRI
MPTP-induced parkinsonism	Features similar to idiopathic PD in presence of toxin exposure.	No specific changes
Manganese-induced parkinsonism	Parkinsonism with postural tremor, dystonia, cock-walk, postural instability in presence of exposure to manganese	T1 hyperintensity in the striatum and globus pallidus on brain MRI
Carbon monoxide-induced parkinsonism	Masked facies, short stepped gait, rigidity hypolinesia, cognitive impairment, mutism postural tremor, urinary or fecal incontinence, dystonia, emotional lability, postural instability	T2 hyperintensities in the white matter on brain MRI
Cyanide-induced parkinsonism	Parkinsonism, with dystonia, apraxia of eyelid opening, with temporal relation to the onset of symptoms and exposure to cyanide	T2 hyperintensities in the putamen hemorrhagic necrosis in the cerebral cortex, especially in the sensorimotor cortex
Methanol-induced parkinsonism	Metabolic acidosis, coma, parkinsonism, especially rigidity, and bradykinesia	Subcortical white matter changes
Ethanol-induced parkinsonism	Transient parkinsonism seen during alcohol withdrawal, developing a few days after consumption of the last drink. Most patients have previous transient episodes.	No specific changes
HIV-related parkinsonism	Rapid progression of parkinsonian symptoms tremor, in presence of HIV with or without related CNS infections such as toxoplasmosis	MRI abnormalities in case of CNS opportunistic infections such as toxoplasmosis, CMV (cytomegalovirus)
SSPE-related parkinsonism	Parkinsonism in presence of other abnormalities suggestive of SSPE	Lesions in caudate and putamen, but sparing the blobus pallidus and thalamus
Mycoplasma-related parkinsonism	Parkinsonism with flulike symptoms, and dystonia, with elevated mycoplasma antibody levels	Increased T1 and T2 signal in the basal ganglia
Bilateral striatopallidodentate calcinosis (Fahr's disease)	Parkinsonism, cognitive impairment, celebellar signs, speech abnormalities, pyramidal signs, psychiatric features and sensory abnormalities	MRI findings of calcium in the subcortical white matter and basal ganglia

Table 2 (Continued)

Parkinsonian Disorder	Distinguishing Clinical Features	Supportive MRI Findings
Post-anoxic parkinsonism	Parkinsonism with or without dystonia weeks to months after the ischemic event	T1 hyperintensities in the basal ganglia bilaterally
Drug-induced parkinsonism	Parkinsonism in association with other involuntary movements including bucco-lingulo-mastica-tory syndrome, dystonia, stereo-types, akathisia and gait disturbance with history of expo-sure todopamine receptor–blocking drug	No specific changes
Peripherally induced parkinsonism	Tremor-dominant parkinsonism following injury	No specific changes described
Developmental parkinsonism	Parkinsonism following some insult in utero, or immediate post-natal period in association with tremor, cognitive dysfuncion, behavioral abnormalities, head-aches, and strabismus	Abnormal in presence of clear ischemic event
Hemiatrophy-hemiparkinsonism	Hemiatrophy in association with hemiparkinsonism dystonia, but without postural instability Tends to remain unilateral for 5–35 yr after onset of parkinsonian symptoms; Early age at onset, history of birth injury, slow pro-gression of the disease are very typical features.	Hemiatrophy on MRI of the brain, may have associated skull asymmetry
Structural lesions causing parkin-sonism	Parkinsonism in presence of tumors, hemorrhage typically con-tralateral to the lesion and some-times ipsilateral to the lesion	MRI changes are usually consistent with the space occupying lesion.
Parkinsonism owing to multiple sclerosis	Parkinsonian features in presence of other symptoms of multiple sclerosis	MRI lesions in substantia nigra, and in the cervicomedullary junction

response of the dystonia parkinsonism to levodopa. Her MRI showed atrophy in the substantia nigra. The unusual constellation of exertional dystonia with parkinsonism and hemiatrophy demon-strates the wide range of clinical features seen in this syndrome. An unusual case of brain hemihypoplasia with contralateral hemiatrophy and hemiparkinsonism was described *(92)*. MRI of the brain showed skull and encephalic asymmetry and hypoplasia of the right side and the [99mTc] ECD SPECT showed global hypoperfusion of the right hemisphere.

STRUCTURAL LESIONS CAUSING PARKINSONISM

A variety of structural lesions can cause parkinsonism. Siderowf et al. *(93)* argue that the first described case of PSP in a patient with progressive opthalmoparesis and postural instability, and structural lesion with a tumor in the right cerebral peduncle is not idiopathic PSP. Brainstem astrocy-toma was reported to be the cause of unilateral parkinsonian symptoms; the symptoms resolved after resection of the tumor *(94)*. A frontal meningioma can sometimes present with rest tremor without other signs of parkinsonism *(95)*. Dopa-responsive parkinsonism has been reported resulting from a right temporal lobe hemorrhage *(96)*. Intrinsic brainstem tumors can cause parkinsonism. Posterior fossa tumors present with pyramidal tract signs, cerebellar signs, and hydrocephalus in addition to parkinsonism. The parkinsonian symptoms predominantly are seen contralateral to the lesion. In some cases ipsilateral symptoms have also been reported. The parkinsonism associated with mass lesions of the infratentorial compartment is usually on the contralateral side with other cranial nerve lesions or sensory symptoms depending on the location of the lesion. MRI of the brain is usually diagnostic. Pathophysiologic mechanisms include mechanical compression or distortion of the rostral midbrain and substantia nigra, infiltration and destruction of substantia nigra, impairment of the nigrostriatal pathways, and a combination of these mechanisms *(97)*.

OTHER UNUSUAL CAUSES OF SECONDARY PARKINSONISM

Parkinsonism was reported after a wasp sting resulting in a progressive syndrome of frequent freezing, rigidity, and bradykinesia, in addition to dystonia in the left arm *(98)*. The patient was reported to have had emotional lability and bilateral frontal release signs. The brain MRI showed marked destruction of the striatum and pallidum bilaterally, and enlargement of the lateral and third ventricles. There were circulating antibodies against the basal ganglia and cerebral cortex. The patient responded to immunosuppressive therapy with plasma exchange and intravenous immunoglobulin. Multiple sclerosis (MS) has also been reported to cause parkinsonism *(99)*. One patient presented mainly with gait difficulty, with slowness, short steps, and unsteadiness. She also developed rest tremor, hypomimia, and hypophonia. There were other features suggestive of multiple sclerosis in the form of diplopia, brisk reflexes, and sensory loss. The patient improved with steroids. So far in the literature nine cases including this case report of MS have been reported with findings of parkinsonism *(99)*. Three patients had hemiparkinsonism, and the rest of the patients had bilateral symptoms with rest tremor, hypomimia, rigidity, bradykinesia, and gait difficulties, very similar to idiopathic PD. Very limited information is available regarding levodopa responsiveness. MRI findings showed lesions in the periventricular area, pons, substantia nigra, and in corpus callosum in those with bilateral parkinsonism. In those with hemiparkinsonsim, lesions were in the left substantia nigra, periventricular area, and adjacent to the red nucleus *(99)*.

MAJOR RESEARCH ISSUES

As discussed above, there are several forms of nondegenerative parkinsonism with variable clinical features as shown in Table 2, VP being the most common. One of the mysteries of VP is what, besides the usual stroke risk factors, predisposes the affected individual to develop VP since not everyone with hypertension, diabetes, or other stroke risk factors develops VP. Further studies of the relationship between anticardiolipin antibodies and VP *(20)* are needed before routine screening of these patients for these antibodies can be recommended. It is not clear why some patients improve with dopaminergic drugs whereas others do not. CSF withdrawal may benefit some patients with VP, but this improvement is transient *(34)*. More studies are needed to determine whether CSF shunting would benefit some patients.

FUTURE DIRECTIONS

As discussed above, several of these non-degenerative forms of parkinsonism support the evidence for multiple etiologic factors leading to selective neuronal vulnerability.

Investigation of neuroprotective potential of specific agents such as CPI 1189 for HIV dementia has shown some improvement with motor function, but the study is not designed for efficacy *(100)*. Future studies in this area may help treat HIV-induced parkinsonism. Parkinsonism induced by toxic exposure or specific infectious etiology may provide a direct clue to the dysfunction in mitochondrial and other specific cellular mechanisms such as inflammation, and lysosomal dysfunction, which may help identify specific targets for therapy. Further research into the cellular mechanisms in various types of parkinsonism are needed in order to clarify the mode of insult an specific signal transduction pathways involved in disease mechanisms.

LEGEND TO VIDEOTAPE

Patient 1: Video segment shows a patient with a wide based gait, slightly decreased arm swing on the right side, with MRI findings of ischemic changes in the subcortical white matter. This patient with VP failed to respond to levodopa.

Patient 2: Patient shows freezing of gait with predominant gait difficulties in the absence of any upper body involvement typically observed in VP.

Patient 3: A patient with mild hypomimia, bradykinesia in the upper limbs, but disproportionate degree of gait difficulties showing broad-based gait, and freezing of gait while turning. The diagnosis of VP is supported by ischemic changes on MRI scan.

REFERENCES

1. Gelb DJ, Oliver E, Gilman S. Diagnostic criteria for Parkinson disease. Arch Neurol 1999;56:33–39.
2. Critchley M. Atherosclerotic parkinsonism. Brain 1929;52:23–83.
3. Zijlmans JCM, Daniel S, Hughes AJ, Revesz T, Lees AJ. A clinicopathological investigation of vascular parkinsonism (VP). Mov Disord published online March 16, 2004.
4. Daniel SE, Lees AJ. Parkinson's disease society brain bank, London: overview and research. J Neural Transm Suppl 1993;39:165–172.
5. Thompson PD, Marsden CD. Gait disorder of subcortical arteriosclerotic encephalopathy: Binswanger disease. Mov Disord 1987;2:1–8.
6. Roman GC. New insight into Binswanger disease. Arch Neurol 1999;56:1061–1106.
7. Mark MH, Sage JI, Walters AS, et al. Binswanger disease presenting as levodopa responsive parkinson's disease. Clinicopathological study of three cases. Mov Disord 1995;10:450–454.
8. Chang CM, Yu YL, Ng HK Leung SY, Fong KY. Vascular pseudoparkinsonism. Acta Neurol Scand 1992;86:588–592.
9. Yamanouchi H, Nagura H. Neurological signs and frontal white matter lesions in vascular parkinsonism—a clinico-pathological study. Stroke 1997;28:965–969.
10. Van Zagaten M, Lodder J, Kessels F. Gait disorder and parkinsonian signs in patients with stroke related to small deep infarcts and white matter lesions. Mov Disord 1998;13:89–95.
11. Winikates J, Jankovic J. Clinical correlates of vascular parkinsonism. Arch Neurol 1999;56:98–102 .
12. Dubinsky RM, Jankovic J. Progressive supranuclear palsy and a multi-infarct state. Neurology 1987;37:570–576.
13. Winikates J, Jankovic J. Vascular PSP. J Neural Transm Suppl 1994;42:189–201.
14. Fitzgerald P, Jankovic J. Lower body parkinsonism: evidence for vascular etiology. Mov Disord 1989;4:249–260.
15. Jankovic J, Nutt JG, Sudarsky L. Classification, diagnosis and etiology of gait disorders. In: Ruzicka E, Hallett M, Jankovic J, eds. Gait disorders. Advanced in Neurology, vol. 87, Philadelphia: Lippincott Williams & Wilkins, 2001:119–134.
16. Demikiran M, Bozdemir H, Sarica Y. Vascular parkinsonism, a distinct heterogeneous clinical entity. Acta Neurol Scand 2001;104:63–67.
17. Trenkwalder C, Paulus W, Keafeczyc S, et al. Postural stability differentiates "lower body" from idiopathic parkinsonism. Acta Neurol Scand 1995;91:444–452.
18. Zijlmans JCM, Poels PJE, Duysens J, et al. Quantitative gait analysis in patients with vascular parkinsonism. Mov Disord 1996;5:501–508.
19. Thomas M, Suteerawattanon M, Caroline KS, et al. Gait and Balance Scale: validation and utilization. J Neurol Sci 2004;217:89–99.
20. Huang Z, Jacewicz M, Pfeiffer RF. Anticardiolipin antibody in vascular parkinsonism. Mov Disord 2002;17:992–997.
21. Joutel A, Coprechot C, Ducros A, et al. Notch-3 mutation in CADASIL, a heriditary adult onset condition causing stroke and dementia. Nature 1997;383:707-710.
22. Rafalowska J, Fidzianska A, Dziewulska D, et al. CADASIL: new cases and new questions. Acta Neuropathol 2003;Sep 30 Epub ahead of print
23. Kuhn W, Roebroek R, Blom H, et al. Elevated plasma levels of homocysteine in Parkinson's disease. Eur Neurol 1998;40:225–227.
24. Rogers JD, Sanchez-Saffon A, Frol AB, Diaz-Arrstia R. Elevated plasma homocysteine levels in patients treated with levodopa. Association with vascular disease. Arch Neurol 2003;60:59–64.

25. Eadie MJ, Sutherland JM. Atherosclerosis in parkinsonism. J Neurol Neurosurg Psychiatry 1964;27:237–240.

26. Izelberg R, Bronstein NM, Reider I, Korczyn AD. Basal ganglia lacunes and parkinsonism. Neuroepidemiology 1994;13:108–112.

27. Chang CM, Yu Yl, Ng HK, Fong KY. Vascular pseudoparkinsonism. Acta Neurol Scand 1992;86:588–592.

28. Tzen KY, Lu CS, Yen TC, et al. Differential diagnosis of Parkinson's disease and vascular parkinsonism by ^{99m}Tc-TRODAT-I.J Nuclear Med 2001;42:408–413.

29. Bencsits G, Pirker W, Asenbaum, et al. Comparison of the ^{123}I beta-CIT snf SPECT in lower body parkinsonism and Parkinson's disease [Abstract]. Mov Disord 1998;13(Suppl):106.

30. Zijlmans JC, de Koster A, Van't Jof MA, et al. Proton magnetic resonance spectroscopy in suspected vascular parkinsonism. Acta Neurol Scand 1994;90:405–411.

31. Tohgi H, Takahashi S, Abe T, Utsugisawa K. Symptomatic characteristics of parkinsonism and the width of substantia nigra pars compacta on MRI according to the ischemic changes in the putamen and the cerebral white matter: implications for the diagnosis of vascular parkinsonism. Eur Neurol 2001;46:1–10.

32. Zijlmans JC, Pasman JW, Horstink MW, et al. EEG findings in patients with vascular parkinsonism. Acta Neurol Scand 1998;94:243–247.

33. Tolosa ES, Santamaria J. Parkinsonism and basal ganglia infarcts. Neurology 1984;34:1516–1518.

34. Ondo WG, Chan LL, Levy JK. Vascular parkinsonism: clinical correlates predicting motor improvement after lumbar puncture. Mov Disord 2002;17:91–97.

35. Hanna P, Jankovic J, Kilkpatrick J. Multiple system atrophy: the putative causative role of environmental toxins. Arch Neurol 1999;56:90–94;

36. Petrovitch H, Ross GW, Abbott RD, et al. Plantation work and risk of Parkinson disease in a population-based longitudinal study. Arch Neurol 2002;59:1787–1792.

37. Gorell JM, Johnson CC, Rybicki BA, et al. Occupational exposure to manganese, copper, lead, iron, mercury, and zinc and the risk of Parkinson's disease. Neurotoxicology 1999;20:239–247.

38. Ngim CH, Devathasan G. Epidemiologic study on association between body burden mercury level and idiopathic Parkinson's disease. Neuroepidemiology 1999;8:128–141.

39. Langston et al, 1999;Jenner P. The contribution of the MPTP-treated primate model to the development of new treatment strategies for Parkinson's disease. Parkinsonism Relat Disord 2003;9:131–137.

40. Langston JW, Ballard P, Tetrud J, Irwin I. Chronic parkinsonism in humans due to a product of meperidine analog synthesis. Science 1983;219:979–980.

41. Langston JW, Forno LS, Tetrud J, et al. Evidence of active nerve cell degeneration in the substantia nigra of humans years after 1-methyl-4-phenyl-1,2,3,6-tetrahydropyridine exposure. Ann Neurol 1999;46:598–605.

42. Gao HM, Liu B, Hong JS. Critical role for microglial NADPH oxidase in rotenone-induced degeneration of dopaminergic neurons. J Neurosci 2003;23:6181–6187.

43. Nelson K, Golnick J, Korn T, Angle C. Manganese encephalopathy: Utility of early magnetic resonance imaging. Br J Ind Med 1993;50:510–513.

44. Normadin L, Hazel AS. Manganese neurotoxicity: an update of pathophysiologic mechanisms. Met Brain Dis 2002;17:374–387.

45. Racette BA, McGee-Minnich L, Moerlein SM, et al. Welding-related parkinsonism clinical features and pathophysiology. Neurology 2001;56:8–13.

46. Choi IS. Parkinsonism after carbon monoxide poisoning. Eur Neurol 2002;48:30–33.

47. Lee MS, Marsden CD. Neurological sequelae following carbon monoxide poisoning: clinical course and outcome according to the clinical types and brain computed tomography scan findings. Mov Disord 1994;9:550–558.

48. Parkinson RB, Hopkins RO, Cleavinger HB et al.White matter hyperintensities and neuropsychological outcome following carbon monoxide poisoning. Neurology 2002;58:1525–1532.

49. Sohn YH, Jeong Y, Kim H, et al. The brain lesion responsible for parkinsonism after carbon monoxide poisoning. Arch Neurol 2000;57:1214–1218.

50. Carella F, Grassi MP, Savoiardo M, et al. Dystonic-parkinsonian syndrome after cyanide poisoning: clinical and MRI findings. J Neurol Neurosurg Psychiatry 1988;51:1345–1348.

51. Messing B. J Extrapyramidal disturbances after cyanide poisoning (first MRT-investigation of the brain). Neural Transm Suppl 1991;33:141-147.

52. Rachinger J, Fellner FA, Stieglbauer J, Trenler J. MR changes after acute cyanide intoxication. Am J Neuroradiol 2002;23:1398–1401.

53. Rosenow F, Herholz K, Lanfermann H, et al. Neurological sequelae of cyanide intoxication. The pattern of clinical, magnetic resonance imaging, and positron emission tomography findings. Ann Neurol 1995;38:825–828.

54. Ley CO, Gali FG. Parkinsonian syndrome after methanol intoxication. Eur Neurol 1983;22:405–409.

55. Finkelstein Y, Vardi J. Progressive parkinsonism in a young experimental physicist following long term exposure to methanol. Neurotoxicology 2002;23:521–525.

56. Hageman G, van Der Hock J, van Hout M, et al. Parkinsonism, pyramidal signs, polyneuropathy and cognitive decline after long term occupational solvent exposure. J Neurol 1999;246:198–206.

57. Neilman J, Lang AE, Fornazzari L, Carlen PL. Movement disorders in alcoholism: a review. Neurol 1990;40:741–746.

58. Nath A, Jankovic J, Pettigrew LC. Movement disorders and AIDS. Neurology 1987;37:36–41.

59. de Mattos JP, de Rosso ALZ, Correa RB, et al. Movement disorders in 28 HIV-infected patients. Arq. Neuro-psiquiatr. 2002;60:525–530.

60. Maggi P, de Mari M, Moramarco G, et al. Parkinsonism in a patient with AIDS and cerebral opportunistic granulomatous lesions. Neurol Sci 2000;21:173–176.

61. Cardoso F. HIV-related movement disorders: epidemiology, pathogenesis and management. CNS Drugs 2002;16: 663–668.

62. Kotsulieri E, Sopper S, Scheller C, et al. Parkinsonism in HIV dementia. J Neural Transm 2002;109:767–775.

63. Czub S, Koutsilleri E, Sopper S, et al. Enhancement of CNS pathology in early simian immunodeficiency virus infection by dopaminergic drugs. Acta Neuropathol 101:85–91.

64. Sawaishi Y, Yano T, Watanabe Y, Takada G. Migratory basal ganglia lesions in subacute sclerosing panencephalitis (SSPE): clinical implications of axonal spread. J Neurol Sci 1999;168:137–140.

65. Mossakowski MJ, Mathesian G. A parkinsonian syndrome in the course of subacute encephalitis. Neurology 1961;11:461–461.

66. Kim JS, Choi IS, Lee MC. Reversible parkinsonism and dystonia following probable mycoplasma infection. Mov Disord 1995;10:510–512.

67. Savant CS, Singhal BS, Jankovic J, Khan M, Virani A. Substantia nigra lesions in viral encephalitis. Mov Disord 2003;18:213–216.

68. Bosanko CM, Gilroy J, Wang A-M, et al. West Nile virus encephalitis involving the substantia nigra. Arch Neurol 2003;60:1448–1452.

69. Kovacs CS, Howse DC, Yendt HR. Reversible parkinsonism induced by hypercalcemia and primary hyperparathyroidism. Arch Intern Med 1993;153:1134–1136.

70. Hirooka Y, Yuasa K, Hibi K et al. Hyperparathyroidism associated with parkinsonism. Intern Med 1992;31:904–907.

71. Manyam BV, Walters AS, Nara KR. Bilateral striopallidodentate calcinosis: clinical characteristics of patients seen in a registry. Mov Disord 2001;16:258–264.

72. Manyam BV, Walters AS, Keller IA, Ghobrial M. Parkinsonism associated with autosomal dominant bilateral striopallidodentate necrosis. Parkinsonism Relat Disord 2001;7:289–295.

73. Brodaty H, Mitchell P, Luscombe G, Kwok JJ, et al. Familial idiopathic basal ganglia calcification (Fahr's disease) without neurological, cognitive and psychiatric symptoms is not linked to the IBGC1 locus on chromosome 14q. Hum Genet 2002;110:8–14.

74. Li JY, Lai PH, Chen CY, Wang JS, Lo YK. Post anoxic parkinsonism: clinical radiologic, and pathologic correlation. Neurology 2000;55:591–593.

75. Stephen PJ, Williamson J. Drug induced parkinsonism in the elderly. Lancet 1984;2:1082–1083.

76. Rajput A, Rozdilsky B, Hornykiewicz O, et al. Reversible drug-induced parkinsonism. Clinicopathologic study of two cases. Arch Neurol 1982;39:644–646.

77. Montastruc JL, Llau ME, Rascol O, Senard JM. Drug induced parkinsonism: a review. Fundam Clin Pharmacol 1994;8:293–306.

78. Hardie RJ, Lees AJ. Neuroleptic induced parkinson's syndrome: clinical features and results of treatment with levodopa. J Neurol Neurosurg Psych 1988;51:850–8554.

79. Consentino C, Torres L, Scortiati C et al. Movement disorders secondary to adulterated medication. Neurology 2000;55:598–599.

80. Tolosa E, Coelho M, Gallardo M. DAT imaging in drug-induced and psychogenic parkinsonism. Mov Disord 2003;18(Suppl 7):S28–S33.

81. Cardoso F, Jankovic J. Peripherally induced tremor and parkinsonism. Arch Neurol 1995;52:263–270.

82. Thomas M, Hayflick SJ, Jankovic J. Clinical heterogeneity of neurodegeneration with iron accumulation-1 (Hallervorden–Spatz syndrome) and pantothenate kinase associated neurodegeneration (PKAN). Mov Disord 2004;19:36–42.

83. Jankovic J, Newmark M, Peter P. Parkinsonism and acquired hydrocephalus. Mov Disord 1986;1:59–64.

84. Reiderer P, Foley P. Mini-review: multiple developmental forms of parkinsonism. The basis for further research as to the pathogenesis of parkinsonism. J Neural Transm 2002;109:1469–1475.

85. Pranzatelli M, Mott SH, Pavlakis SG, Conry JA, Tate ED. Clinical spectrum of secondary parkinsonism in childhood: a reversible disorder. Pediatr Neurol 1994;10:131–140.

86. Scott BL, Jankovic J. Delayed-onset progressive movement disorders after static brain lesions. Neurology 1996;46:68–74.

87. Klawans HL. Hemiparkinsonism as a late complication of hemiatrophy. Neurology 1981;31:625–628.

88. Buchman AS, Goetz C, Klawans HL. Hemiparkinsonism with hemiatrophy. Neurology 1988;38:527–530.

89. Jankovic J. Hemiparkinsonism and hemiatrophy. Neurology 1988;38:1815.

90. Greene PE, Bressman SB, Ford B, Hyland K. Parkinsonism, dystonia, hemiatrophy. Mov Disord 2000;15:537–541.

91. Lang AE. Hemiatrophy, Juvenile-onset exertional alternating leg paresis, hypotonia, and hemidystonia and adult-onset hemiparkinsonism: the spectrum of Hemiparkinsonism-Hemiatrophy syndrome. Mov Disord 1995;10:489–494.

92. Marchioni E, Soragna D, Versino M et al. Hemiparkinsonism-hemiatrophy with brain hemihypoplasia. Mov Disord 1999;14:359–363.

93. Siderowf AD, Galetta SL, Hurtig HI, Liu GT. Mov Disord 1998 ;13:170–174.

94. Cicarelli G, Pelecchia MT, Maiuri F, Barone P. Brain stem cystic astrocytoma presenting with pure parkinsonism. Mov Disord 1999;14:364–366.

95. Wenning GK, Luginger E, Sailer U, et al. Postoperative parkinsonian tremor in a patient with a frontal meningioma. Mov Disord 1999;14:366–368.

96. Ling M, Aggrawal A, Morris JGL. Dopa-responsive parkinsonism secondary to right temporal lobe hemorrhage Mov Disord 2002;17:402–403.

97. Pohle T, Krauss J. Parkinsonism in children resulting from mesencephalic tumors. Mov Disord 1999;14:842–846.

98. Leopold NA, Bara-Jimenez W, Hallett M. Parkinsonism after a wasp sting. Mov Disord 1999;14:122–127.

99. Folgar S, Gatto EM, Raina G, Micheli F. Parkinsonism as a manifestation of multiple sclerosis. Mov Disord 2003;18:108–113.

100. Clifford DB, McArthur JC, Schifitto G. A randomized clinical trial of CPI-1189 for HIV-associated cognitive-motor impairment. Neurology 2002;59:1568–1573.

Role of Electrophysiology in Diagnosis and Research in Atypical Parkinsonian Disorders

Josep Valls-Solé

INTRODUCTION

Correct clinical diagnosis of patients with parkinsonism is not always possible in spite of the continuous effort in defining diagnostic criteria *(1)*. Parkinsonism, defined as the combination of bradykinesia and rigidity *(2)*, may be a predominant clinical feature of several diseases, including idiopathic Parkinson's disease (IPD) and several other entities commonly known as "Parkinson-plus" syndromes or atypical parkinsonian disorders (APDs). In these entities, parkinsonism is accompanied by other clinical signs, or red flags *(3)*, that should warn the physician of the existence of a degenerative disorder. Even though rather specific clinical patterns have been described in patients with APDs, such as predominantly autonomic failure, cerebellar, or pyramidal dysfunction, in multiple system atrophy (MSA), axial rigidity, ocular motility disorders, and falls early in the course of the disease, in progressive supranuclear palsy (PSP), myoclonus and asymmetrical higher cortical limb dysfunction, in corticobasal degeneration (CBD), and fluctuating cognitive deficits, visual hallucinations, and REM sleep behavior disorder, in diffuse Lewy-body disease (LBD), these signs are not always evident or they may pass unrecognized by nonspecialized neurologists. In some conditions, such as for instance CBD, similar clinical expressions may be common to different pathologies *(4)*, and the same disease may encompass diverse clinical presentations *(5)*. In others, such as MSA with parkinsonian features (MSA-P), patients may behave like IPD until death *(6)*, making it almost impossible to establish a clinical separation between the two diseases. Nowadays, the definite clinical diagnosis still resides in the pathological postmortem examination *(1,7,8)*.

When in doubt, the clinician may seek help in laboratory exams. Unfortunately, however, there are not yet laboratory methods that can supply a diagnosis of certainty for APDs. Although single photon emission computer tomography (SPECT) and positron emission tomography (PET) have shown postsynaptic dopaminergic deficits in APDs *(9)*, these tests are not yet capable of differentiating between the various degenerative syndromes featuring parkinsonism. Though electrophysiological studies do not usually provide the diagnosis, they can be of great help in the recognition of pathophysiological mechanisms underlying the presentation of some symptoms and signs. In parkinsonism, pallidal hyperactivity might be responsible for reduced activation of thalamocortical projections, and for an abnormal control of brainstem circuits *(10–12)*. The situation might be slightly different in APDs, in which the basal ganglia pathology is accompanied by neuronal loss and atrophy in many nuclei of the brainstem and cerebellum, and dysfunctions might be present in various circuits. It is

From: *Current Clinical Neurology: Atypical Parkinsonian Disorders*
Edited by: I. Litvan © Humana Press Inc., Totowa, NJ

therefore logical that, although some clinical neurophysiological manifestations are common to both types of disorders, there are a few specific and distinctive features of each syndrome that may be clinically useful.

Neurophysiological studies are suited to demonstrate, document, and quantify clinical observations. They are not expensive, and mainly noninvasive. They may occasionally bring information on neurological functions that is not obtainable with other means. One such example is, for instance, the measure of excitability in neuronal structures or circuits. In this chapter, we describe the neurophysiological observations made in patients with the principal disorders grouped under the term APDs, and discuss how the results compare between different patient groups.

NEUROPHYSIOLOGICAL CORRELATE OF PARKINSONISM

Patients with APDs usually present with the main clinical signs characteristic of parkinsonism, i.e., bradykinesia and rigidity. Although clinicians identify bradykinesia and rigidity with no need for neurophysiological recordings, these are convenient for quantitation of the dysfunction. Bradykinesia and, specially, rigidity are present with varying degree and localization in patients with parkinsonism. They may not be observed at all in patients at early stages of the cerebellar variant of multiple system atrophy (MSA-C), though they will eventually appear during the course of the disease.

Hypokinesia and Bradykinesia

Hypokinesia and bradykinesia are abnormalities of movement, and the best way to quantify them is with the use of reaction time task paradigms. Akinesia is defined as a delay in movement initiation, whereas bradykinesia is defined as the slowness of movement execution *(13)*. There are many studies on reaction time in patients with IPD, but considerably less in APDs. Reaction time can be studied using different methods, ranging from the execution of a task *(14,15)*, the release of a switch or a lever *(16,17)*, the onset of limb displacement *(18,19)*, or the onset of electromyogram (EMG) activity *(20,21)*. In paradigms of simple reaction time (SRT), the subject knows all details about the requested motor performance before the imperative signal is delivered. In paradigms of choice reaction time (CRT), subjects have to process some of the information contained in the imperative signal itself. When measuring SRT as the onset of EMG activity in wrist extensors in patients with IPD, PSP, and MSA, Valldeoriola et al. *(22)* found a significantly larger delay of reaction time in patients with PSP in comparison to the other groups of patients (Fig. 1). This is in fitting with previously reported results of an investigation of reaction time to progressively complex tasks in PSP patients *(23)*. These authors found an increased central processing time in patients with PSP compared with both IPD and control subjects. PSP patients might have degraded cognition, with a delay in stimulus identification and categorization processes *(24)*.

The mechanisms underlying hypokinesia can be studied using EMG analysis of reaction time tasks. Hallett and Khoshbin *(10)* found that IPD patients were unable to appropriately scale the size of the first agonist burst to the requirements of a ballistic movement. They proposed that such defect represented a physiological mechanism of bradykinesia. It is likely that the increased pallidal inhibition of thalamocortical excitatory connections accounts for such an abnormal "energization" of the motor cortex. A proper study of the triphasic pattern in patients with APDs has not been done so far. However, in a small group of PSP patients, Molinuevo et al. *(25)* observed abnormalities of the triphasic pattern that were similar to those observed in IPD patients.

Rigidity

Rigidity in patients with parkinsonism manifests as a difficulty of complete muscle relaxation, with often permanent tonic background EMG activity *(11)*. Several neurophysiological tests have been used to assess rigidity, although direct clinico-neurophysiological correlations have proven more difficult than with bradykinesia. Rigidity has been considered to be the cause of some neurophysi-

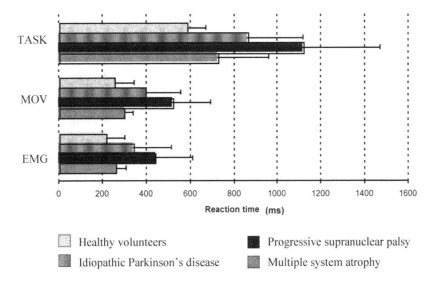

TASK

MOV

EMG

Reaction time (ms)

| ☐ Healthy volunteers | ■ Progressive supranuclear palsy |
| ▨ Idiopathic Parkinson's disease | ▨ Multiple system atrophy |

Fig. 1. Histograms of the mean and 1 standard deviation of simple reaction time values (expressed in ms) for EMG activity, onset of movement and task execution in healthy volunteers, and in patients with IPD, PSP, and MSA.

ological findings in IPD, such as an increased size of the F wave *(26)*, increased size of long loop reflex responses to stretch *(27)* or to electrical stimuli *(28–30)*, abnormalities in the silent period induced by transcranial magnetic stimulation *(31,32)*, reduced reciprocal inhibition *(33,34)*, and reduced autogenic (Ib) inhibition of the soleus H reflex *(35)*. However, none of those tests is specific for rigidity, which continues to be assessed by clinical evaluation of the resistance to passive movements.

Like with bradykinesia, most tests directed to the evaluation of rigidity have been proven in patients with IPD, and more scarcely in patients with APDs. However, it is not unreasonable to admit that when and where rigidity is present, patients with APDs would present similar abnormalities as those described for IPD. Direct surface electrophysiological recording of a muscle in rigid patients in resting conditions may be enough to notice that there is increased muscle activity with respect to normal subjects. Electrophysiological evidence for that can be found when testing the relaxation time after a sustained contraction *(36)*. The stretch reflex, which is the most paradigmatic electrophysiological test for limb rigidity, has not been properly tested in patients with APDs. In these patients, rigidity often predominates in axial muscles and is very mild in limb muscles, making it more difficult for neurophysiological evaluation. The shortening reaction *(37–40)* is a relatively poorly studied long latency reflex that occurs in the muscle shortened during a passive movement. Its frequent presence in patients with IPD could reflect the difficulties of these patients in modulating sensory signals generated by either joint afferents *(38)*, tendon organ afferents *(39)*, or both. Unfortunately, however, there have not been recent studies on such an interesting phenomenon.

The pathophysiology of rigidity may be related to abnormalities in propriospinal reflexes. In their study of IPD patients, Delwaide et al. *(35)* postulate that reduced autogenic inhibition mediated by Ib interneurons would be a neurophysiological correlate of rigidity. Interestingly, however, in the sole study published so far on spinal physiological mechanisms in APD patients, Fine et al. *(41)* reported increased Ib inhibition in patients with PSP. The observation of such an opposite behavior between IPD and PSP patients might be useful for differential diagnosis but points to the fact that neurophysiological observations might only be one manifestation of dysfunctional mechanisms. Further studies are required to find out the mechanisms by which the Ib interneurons are modulated in a different direction in PSP and IPD, and what is the exact role of this dysfunction in the generation of rigidity.

NEUROPHYSIOLOGICAL TESTS IN THE ASSESSMENT OF ATYPICAL PARKINSONIAN DISORDERS

Some neurophysiological features are specific or distinctive of patients with APDs. However, this does not mean that the electrophysiological findings hold the key for the diagnosis, since sensitivity and specificity of the tests has not been properly examined yet. The most relevant of these observations are described below, where they are grouped according to the neurophysiological method or technique in which the observation is based.

Brainstem Reflexes

The brainstem is a crucial structure for integration of reflexes and functions related to motor control. These structures receive modulatory inputs from more rostral centers, including the basal ganglia. There are many nuclei and circuits of interest in the brainstem for neurophysiological studies. However, it is still difficult to assign the results of some neurophysiological observations to specific brainstem centers or circuits. Therefore, most data gathered from the study of the brainstem in patients with APDs have the value of an empirical finding, and the exact anatomical/pathological correlation in humans is mainly based on hypothesis and theoretical knowledge from animal experiments.

Table 1 summarizes the observations made in patients with parkinsonism regarding facial movements and brainstem reflexes. Although many brainstem circuits are dysfunctional in patients with APDs, the examination of brainstem reflexes and functions yields more interesting results in patients with PSP than in any other form of parkinsonism.

Eye and Eyelid Movements

Some of the most striking features differentiating PSP from other disorders presenting with parkinsonism regard facial expression and gaze disturbances *(42)*. A list of abnormalities reported so far regarding eye or eyelid movements in these patients is shown in Table 2. The resting blink rate, of 24 per minute in normal controls, was found to be reduced in most patients with parkinsonism *(43)*, but significantly more so in patients with PSP, whose mean blinking frequency can be reduced to as little as 4 blinks per minute. Blinking rate may be an expression of the level of dopamine activity.

Clinical evidence of eye movement abnormalities is not always present in the initial phases of the disease *(42)*. If the possibility of PSP is suspected on the basis of some other clinical features, recording of eye movements by electro-oculography might be of some help. Surface electrodes are placed in the upper, lower, nasal, and temporal edges of the orbit and the subject is requested to make horizontal and vertical eye movements *(44)*. Electro-oculogram recordings may show characteristic abnormalities in patients with PSP *(45)*, including slowness of vertical eye movements, absent Bell's phenomenon, and square wave jerks (Fig. 2). In the study reported by Vidailhet and coworkers, 9 out of 10 patients with PSP had vertical-gaze paralysis with preserved reflex eye movements. Vidailhet et al. *(46)* also showed slowness of horizontal eye movement and microsaccades that would help in distinguishing patients with PSP from those with other parkinsonisms. Some eye movement abnormalities are already apparent at simple inspection. A PSP patient exhibiting slowness of saccades and limitation of vertical eye movement with preserved oculo-cephalic reflexes is shown in video segment 1.

Reflex Responses of the Orbicularis Oculi

In contrast to the reduced frequency of spontaneous blinking, reflex responses of the orbicularis oculi to trigeminal nerve inputs are of normal latency *(47)*. The normality of reflex responses to trigeminal nerve stimuli is in contrast to the absence or significant reduction of the responses to auditory inputs *(48)*. Whether the response of the orbicularis oculi to loud auditory stimulus is part of

Table 1
Characteristics of Some Brainstem Reflexes and Functions in Patients With Parkinsonism

Test	IPD	PSP	MSA	CBD
Spontaneous blinking frequency	Reduced	Extremely Reduced	Enhanced Normal Reduced	Normal
Excitability recovery curve (paired pulses)	Enhanced	Enhanced	Enhanced	Normal
Blinking to loud auditory stimuli	Normal	Reduced	Normal or Increased	Normal
Blinking to median nerve stimuli	Normal	Reduced or Absent	Normal	Normal
Auditory prepulse inhibition	Reduced	Reduced	?	?
Somatosensory prepulse inhibition	Normal	Reduced	?	?

IPD, idiopathic Parkinson's disease; PSP, progressive supranuclear palsy; MSA, multiple system atrophy (strionigral degeneration); CBD, corticobasal degeneration; ?, data unknown.

Table 2
Eye and Eyelid Movement Abnormalities Observed in Patients With PSP

Reduced spontaneous blinking *(43)*
Blepharospasm *(42)*
Supranuclear palsy of eyelid opening *(45)*
Supranuclear palsy of eyelid closing *(42)*
Reduced voluntary suppression of vestibular ocular reflex (VOR) *(42)*
Eyelid retraction (Cowper's sign) *(42)*
Square-wave jerks *(46)*
Absent eyelid responses to acoustic stimuli *(48)*
Absent eyelid responses to median nerve stimuli *(47)*

the generalized startle reaction or is an auditory blink reflex with separate physiological characteristics is still a matter of debate *(49,50)*. In any case, the reduction of orbicularis oculi responses to auditory stimuli is indeed an important observation of some clinical utility in the differential diagnosis of APDs.

The palmomental reflex is usually elicited by scratching the volar aspect of the thenar eminence or the thumb. This leads to a reflex movement of the chin that is considered abnormal when it shows reduced habituation *(51)*. Electromyographic recording of facial muscle responses during elicitation of the palmomental reflex permits the quantitation of the responses *(52)*. The facial reflex response is not limited to the mentalis muscle but is usually accompanied by an ipsilateral eyelid movement that can be apparent with simple inspection and readily demonstrated with surface electromyographic recording (Fig. 3A). Interestingly, in patients with PSP, contraction of eyelid muscles is not present even when the mentalis response is evident (see the second part of video segment 1 on accompanying DVD). In a protocolized study of facial reflexes in patients with parkinsonism, Valls-Solé et al. *(47)* analyzed the responses elicited simultaneously in the mentalis and orbicularis oculi muscles by median nerve electrical stimulation. The study included patients with IPD, PSP, MSA, CBD, and healthy volunteers. Responses in the mentalis muscle were found in most patients and in 2 out of 10 normal subjects. In all of them, whenever there were responses in the mentalis muscle, there were

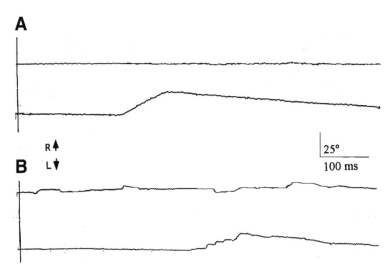

Fig. 2. Electro-oculogram in a healthy subject (**A**) and in a patient with PSP (**B**) during fixation to an object (upper traces) and voluntary saccades (lower traces). Note the presence of small eye movements during fixation, and of a slow and staircase eyeball displacement during the saccadic movement.

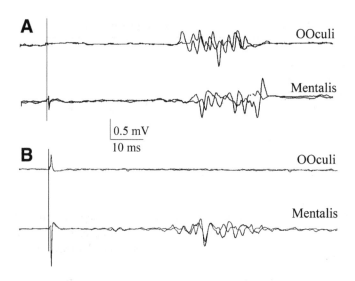

Fig. 3. Facial reflex responses to median nerve stimulation in a patient with IPD (**A**), and in a patient with PSP (**B**). Note the absence of orbicularis oculi response in the patient with PSP even though the mentalis muscle response (lower traces) is similar in both patients.

also responses in the orbicularis oculi muscle. The exception were the patients with PSP, who had no orbicularis oculi responses even if the responses of the mentalis muscle were not different from those observed in the other groups of patients (Fig. 3B). This abnormality probably reflects the activation of two different circuits by the median nerve afferent volley. The mentalis response could be conveyed through the cortico-nuclear tract, since this tract innervates predominantly lower facial motoneurons *(53)*, and a transcortical loop has been suggested because of the contiguity between thumb and chin areas in the brain sensorimotor region *(52,54)*. The selective damage of the pontine reticular formation in patients with PSP would be responsible for the absence of the orbicularis oculi response. Enhancement of mentalis response may occur because of disinhibition of thalamo-cortical connections from their striatal control *(54)*.

One of the earliest contributions of electromyography to the assessment of central nervous system (CNS) abnormalities in patients with parkinsonism was made by Kimura in 1973 *(55)*. Kimura demonstrated in these patients the existence of an abnormal decrease of habituation of the blink reflex to paired supraorbital nerve electrical stimuli. The fact that the abnormalities occurred in the R2 but not in the R1 component of the blink reflex suggested that the disturbance lies in the interneurons rather than in the motoneurons. Since then, many authors have studied the blink reflex excitability recovery curve to paired stimuli, by dividing the size of the response to the test stimulus by that of the response to the conditioning stimulus. This sign has been reported not only in parkinsonism, but in many other disorders as well *(56,57)*. It is therefore of little use for differential diagnosis between degenerative disorders. In clinical practice, the assessment of enhanced trigemino-facial reflex excitability may be of interest for documenting the existence of an abnormal function of brainstem interneurons in patients in whom clinical assessment is dubious or at early stages of their disease. We found similar interneuronal brainstem excitability enhancement in IPD, PSP, and MSA patients *(47)*. Figure 4 shows the proposed circuit of basal ganglia control of trigemino-facial reflex excitability, according to Basso and Evinger *(58)* and Basso et al. *(59)*, and the dysfunction likely occurring in parkinsonism.

Other Facial Reflexes

Neurophysiological abnormalities have been reported in other brainstem reflexes in parkinsonism, although they have not been investigated specifically in APDs *(60–62)*. It has been shown that the second inhibitory period of the masseteric exteroceptive inhibitory reflex has an enhanced excitability recovery cycle, similar to that of the blink reflex in patients with IPD. The same excitability recovery abnormalities have been reported in parkinsonism and dystonia *(60)*.

The Startle Reaction and the Startle-Induced Modulation of Reaction Time

The startle reaction in experimentation animals is known to be generated in the nucleus reticularis pontis caudalis (nRPC), which activates the reticulospinal tract inducing muscle responses in facial and spinal motoneurons *(63)*. In humans, the startle reaction is also thought to originate in corresponding nuclei of the brainstem, and spread caudally and rostrally to limb and facial muscles.

Abnormalities in the startle reaction can be related to enhancement or reduction of the response size. One example of abnormal startle response enhancement is hyperkeplexia *(64)*, whereas an abnormal startle response reduction takes place in patients with PSP *(48)*. The decrease of the startle reaction in PSP patients should not be surprising, since neuronal loss in these patients involves specifically the cholinergic neurons of the lower pontine reticular formation, where the startle reaction is generated. Neuronal loss has been reported in the pedunculo-pontine tegmental nucleus and the nucleus reticularis pontis caudalis *(65–67)*. In the study carried out by Vidailhet et al. *(48)*, the response was absent in three out of eight patients, and it was small and delayed in the other five patients. The same finding was later replicated by Valldeoriola et al. *(22)*, who carried out a comparative study of PSP and other APDs.

Whereas response enhancement is easy to identify because of reactions of larger size and decreased habituation, assessment of an abnormal reduction of the response may be more difficult because of the fact that the response habituates easily in healthy subjects *(49)*. For this reason, the observations made in experiments in which the startling stimulus was applied together with the imperative signal in the context of a reaction time task paradigm should be helpful for clinical purposes. Using such methods, Valls-Solé and coworkers *(68–70)* made a few interesting observations in healthy subjects:

1. The startling stimulus applied together with the imperative signal of a reaction time task induces a significant acceleration in the execution of the intended movement. The ballistic movement is executed without any distortion but at a significantly faster speed *(70)*.

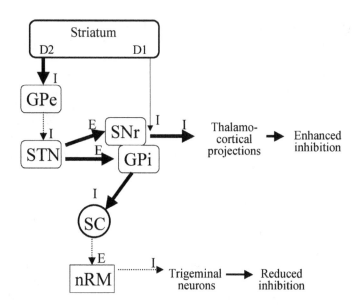

Fig. 4. Basal ganglia control of trigemino-facial reflex excitability. The basal ganglia modulate the excitability of the blink reflex through the output signals arising from the globus pallidus pars interna (GPi) and the substantia nigra pars reticulata (SNr). According to Basso et al. *(58)* and Basso and Evinger *(59)*, the GPi/SNr complex sends inhibitory inputs to the superior colliculus (SC), which is excitatory for the nucleus raphe magnus (nRM). This, in turn, inhibits the trigeminal neurons of the spinal nucleus. In PD, there is increased GPi/SNr inhibition of the SC which, as a consequence, reduces its excitatory inputs to the nRM. The less active nRM induces less inhibition of the spinal trigeminal nucleus, which becomes dis-inhibited (hyperexcitable). As with bradykinesia, it is difficult to know whether the same mechanisms apply to APDs. I, inhibitory; E, excitatory of stimulus.

2. The response to the startling stimulus is enhanced. The same startling stimulus that would give rise to a relatively small and inconsistent response when given alone induce a significantly larger response when is applied during motor preparation *(68)*.

3. Habituation of the response to the startling stimulus is significantly reduced. In a study in which auditory stimuli were applied at the same rate in different experimental conditions, Valls-Solé et al. *(69)* found that habituation of the response to the startling stimulus was reduced in facial and cervical muscles when subjects were engaged in preparation for a ballistic reaction.

Clinical application of the collision between a startle reaction and the voluntary activity in a reaction time task paradigm (the StartReact effect) was reported by Valldeoriola et al. *(22)*. These authors found that patients with PSP not only had absent startle reaction but they were also not able to accelerate their voluntary reaction when the startling stimulus was applied together with the imperative signal.

In contrast to patients with PSP, patients with MSA have normal auditory startle reaction in facial and cervical muscles *(71)*. Furthermore, when the responses of cranial and limb muscles are analyzed together, MSA patients had enhanced probability of a response, shortened onset latency, and enlarged response magnitude compared to normal controls *(72,73)*. In the only analysis of the startle response in patients with LBD, Kofler et al. *(73)* reported fewer and abnormally delayed ASR of low amplitude and short duration in extremity muscles in comparison to healthy controls. Two more details of the studies of Kofler and coworkers *(72,73)* are relevant for the discussion of the contribution of the startle reaction to the differential diagnosis of APD patients. One is the fact that three patients with MSA had no response to the startle reaction, indicating that absence of the startle reaction is not a feature exclusive to PSP patients *(48)*. A particularly high density of oligodendroglial cytoplasmatic inclusions in the brainstem area responsible for the generation of the reticulospinal tract was assumed to be the cause of absent startle response in those MSA patients. Another observation made by Kofler et al. *(72)* was the existence of subtle differences in the characteristics of the response between MSA-P and MSA-C patients. Whereas MSA-P patients had a higher startle probability and a larger area and shorter latency of the motor response, patients with MSA-C had less habituation. Differences between the two groups in the inhibitory effect of the cerebellum over the motor cortex may be responsible for such neurophysiological observation *(72)*.

Prepulse Inhibition

A weak stimulus preceding by about 100 ms the startling stimulus has an effect of inhibition upon the startle reaction (prepulse inhibition). The prepulse stimulus may be of the same or a different sensory modality as the stimulus inducing the startle *(50)*. In the blink reflex, an auditory prepulse causes enhancement of the R1 and depression of the R2 to electrical supraorbital nerve stimuli *(74)*. In a study of prepulse inhibition in patients with IPD, Nakashima et al. *(75)* found that auditory prepulse stimuli induced an abnormally reduced inhibition of the R2 response of the blink reflex, and Lozza et al. *(76)* reported an abnormally reduced blink reflex inhibition after index finger stimulation. However, some patients with IPD have an abnormal auditory prepulse inhibition and a normal somatosensory prepulse inhibition *(77)*. The different behavior of auditory and somatosensory prepulse stimuli in IPD patients could be owing to differences in the prepulse effectiveness of the same vs different sensory modality, differences in the arrival time of prepulse inputs to the brainstem centers, or to selective impairment of reticular formation neurons activated by auditory inputs. Patients with PSP have also absent or significantly reduced prepulse inhibition to both auditory and somatosensory prepulses (Fig. 5), revealing an even more striking dysfunction of the prepulse circuit in PSP compared to IPD. No data are available so far regarding prepulse inhibition in MSA patients.

Spinal Reflexes

A variety of tests determining the excitability of propriospinal interneurons *(78,79)* have been applied to patients with IPD, demonstrating reduced reciprocal *(33,34)* and autogenetic (Ib) inhibition *(35)*, possibly related to the clinical expression of rigidity. These exams have not been done in patients with APDs, except for a single study of autogenetic inhibition (Ib inhibition) in patients with PSP *(41)*. In such a study, the authors showed enhancement of the inhibition, the exact opposite of what was reported in patients with IPD. The explanation why opposite results have been found in these two groups of patients is, up to now, not clear.

Audiospinal facilitation is known as the effect of an auditory stimulus on spinal reflexes, specifically the soleus H reflex. The methods for audiospinal facilitation were developed by Rossignol and Jones *(80)* and Delwaide et al. *(81)*. The stimulus to the posterior tibial nerve to induce the H reflex is applied between 0 and 110 ms after a loud acoustic stimulus. Healthy subjects have H reflex facilitation beginning at intervals between 60 and 80 ms, and lasting until the intervals of 100 or 110 ms. However, audiospinal facilitation is abnormally reduced in patients with IPD *(12,81)*. Our own preliminary observations in patients with the clinical diagnosis of probable PSP is that they exhibit the same abnormality *(82)*.

Surface EMG Recording of Abnormal Movements

The recording of abnormal movements by means of surface EMG recording yields interesting information for the analysis of tremor, such as in patients with IPD *(82)*. Tremor has also been reported in up to 74% of MSA patients *(83)*. However, this figure included several types of tremor, with only a few patients exhibiting the resting tremor typical of IPD, and a large proportion of unclassifiable hands and finger "jerky" tremors, such as those shown in video segment 2. Electrophysiological studies of these latter movements have shown that their characteristics are closer to myoclonus than to tremor *(84)*. A piezoelectric accelerometer was used to record finger movements and analyze the

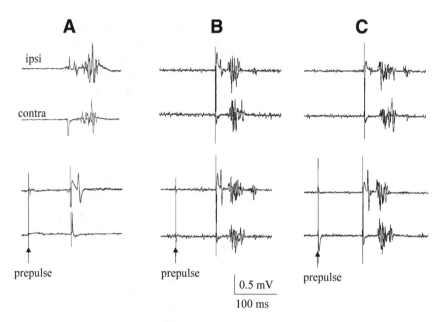

A   **B**   **C**

ipsi

contra

prepulse   prepulse   prepulse

0.5 mV

100 ms

Fig. 5. Prepulse inhibition of the blink reflex in a healthy volunteer and in a patient with PSP. The traces of the upper row show the responses to a stimulus to the supraorbital nerve applied at the vertical line. Ipsilateral recordings (ipsi) show R1 and R2 responses whereas contralateral recordings show only the R2. The traces of the lower row show the responses to the same stimulus when a prepulse is applied 100 ms before (*arrows*). (**A**) Normal auditory prepulse inhibition in a healthy volunteer; (**B**) Absent auditory prepulse inhibition in a patient with PSP. (**C**) Absent somatosensory prepulse inhibition in the same patient.

frequency spectrum of the signal through fast Fourier transformation. This procedure showed that movements of MSA patients were rather non-rhythmic in comparison to those of patients with other forms of tremor (Fig. 6). Salazar et al. *(84)* suggested the term minipolymyoclonus to be used to describe these small amplitude, irregular, jerklike abnormal movements. Other forms of myoclonus have been also reported in a few MSA patients *(30,85)*, which might have their origin in a reduced inhibition of the strio-palido-thalamo-cortical circuit *(86)*. Table 3 shows a list of disorders in which activity defined as minipolymyoclonus has been encountered, together with some of the most relevant neurophysiological findings.

Myoclonus is also an apparent feature in patients with CBD *(87)*, in whom they are thought to be of cortical origin in spite of lacking neurophysiological evidence. The expected findings of cortical myoclonus, such as giant somatosensory evoked potentials and jerk-locked EEG potentials, are inconsistent in CBD. The cortical response is occasionally absent, which is attributed to the marked frontoparietal cortical atrophy and neuronal degeneration characteristic of these patients *(88,89)*. Cortical atrophy of inhibitory neurons could lead to the enhanced (disinhibited) motor cortex excitability.

The "C" wave, or focal reflex myoclonus *(90)*, is a response seen in forearm muscles after electrical stimulation of ipsilateral cutaneous nerves of the hand. This response is thought to be mediated by fast-conducting afferent and efferent pathways and might have a latency as short as 43.1+/–3.2 ms *(87)*. In some patients, focal reflex myoclonus might be elicited by stimuli of an intensity below perception threshold, which suggests a direct connection from the thalamic nuclei to the motor cortex *(91)*. The "C" response should not be mistaken for the long latency excitatory response of the cutaneo-muscular reflexes *(92,93)*. The cutaneo-muscular reflex can be elicited during a sustained tonic voluntary contraction of the forearm muscles. The long latency excitatory component of the cutaneo-muscular reflex is abnormally enhanced in patients with IPD or MSA (30). However, the latency of such a response is longer than that of the "C" reflex.

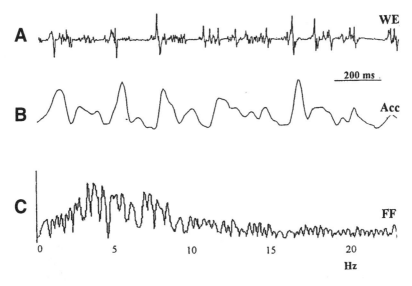

Fig. 6. Surface EMG recording from wrist extensors (**A**), accelerometric recording of finger movements (**B**), and FastFourier analysis of the movement recording (**C**) in a patient with MSA and minipolymyoclonus. See the absence of a dominant frequency peak.

Table 3
Disorders Featuring Minipolymyoclonus

Disorder	Dominant Clinical Sign	EMG Bursts	EEG	"C" wave
Motoneuron disease	Fasciculation atrophy	Asynchronous (1–20 Hz)	Not described	Not described
Polyneuropathy	Absent tendon jerks Severe sensory deficit	Slow and asynchronous	Not described	Not described
Alzheimer's disease	Dementia	Multifocal	Slow waves Epileptiform activity Negative frontal wave	Present
Myoclonic epilepsy	Seizures	Synchronized or irregular	Slow negative frontal wave	Present
Syringomyelia	Weakness. Spasticity Sensory deficit	Asynchronous and irregular	Not described	Not described
MSA-P	Rigid-akinetic syndrome	Synchronous (1–12 Hz)	Normal	Present

Autonomic Reflexes and Functions

Autonomic nervous system dysfunction is the key to the diagnosis in patients with MSA who present with parkinsonism or cerebellar syndromes *(3)*, and is presently a required criterion for the diagnosis of probable MSA *(94)*. Clinically relevant autonomic dysfunctions in these patients are orthostatic hypotension, urinary and fecal incontinence, erectile dysfunction in males, sudomotor disregulation, and abnormalities in respiratory control during sleep. Autonomic dysfunction, i.e., urinary incontinence (97%) and constipation (83%), has also been reported in patients with LBD *(95)*.

Orthostatic hypotension may result from the inability to increase sympathetic activity when standing. This can be shown as an abnormal regulation of baroreflex responses to different stimuli *(96)*. Using readily available electrophysiological equipment, it is also possible to monitor heartbeat frequency. Recording the R-R interval variation by means of the signal trigger and the delay line unit of an electromyograph shows graphically the reduced adaptation of the heart beat rate to a postural change or to the Valsalva maneuver *(77)*. The main drawback of this test is that patients with severe bradykinesia might be unable to perform adequately the maneuvers, and reduced R-R interval variation could actually be owing to insufficient stimulation. One of the possibilities to test R-R interval variation using methods that do not require the patient's cooperation is based on the fact that the startle response is normal in MSA patients *(71,72)*, and on the observation that a startle accelerates heartbeat frequency in normal subjects *(97)*. In a group of six MSA patients, a startling acoustic stimulus induced the normal motor component of the startle reaction but a significantly smaller change of the R-R interval in comparison to healthy volunteeers *(98)*.

The sympathetic sudomotor skin response, or SSR *(99)*, may reveal dysfunctions in the autonomic control of sudomotor reflexes. Loss of sympathetic neurons of the intermediolateral column might explain the finding of frequently abnormal SSRs in patients with MSA *(100)*. Other tests of sudomotor function, such as the evaluation of the amount of sweat production to direct gland stimulation with intradermal methacholine, have also demonstrated a decreased sweat response in patients with MSA *(101)*.

Sleep disorders are frequent in patients with MSA and in those with LBD. Some of these disorders might be related to autonomic dysfunction. In the study of Plazzi et al. *(102)*, 35 out of 39 patients with MSA had REM sleep behavior disorders. These preceded the diagnosis in 44% of the cases. Polysomnographic studies revealed subclinical obstructive sleep apnea in 6 patients, laryngeal stridor in 8 patients, and periodic leg movements during sleep in 10 patients. Laryngeal stridor, owing to vocal cord abductor paralysis during sleep, is probably caused by selective denervation atrophy of the cricoarytenoid muscle resulting from selective loss of neurons in the nucleus ambiguous *(103)*, and may lead to chocking and death in advanced stages of MSA. This can be prevented with tracheostomy *(104)* or with continuous positive air pressure *(105)*. REM sleep behavior disorder has also been considered a sign heralding LBD *(106)* and, in a more recent study, it is considered as a possible hallmark of a synucleinopathy in the setting of a cognitive dementia or parkinsonism *(107)*.

Needle EMG Recording of the Sphincter Muscles

In MSA patients, manifestations of autonomic dysfunctions such as erectile impotence are usually accompanied by increased urinary frequency and urgency, leading soon to incontinence, associated with large residual urine volumes *(108)*. The severity of urinary symptoms is one main red flag that should warn the neurologist of the possibility that the parkinsonian patient thought to have IPD is actually facing the diagnosis of probable MSA *(3)*. Urinary incontinence in MSA patients might be because of autonomic dysfunction, loss of pontine control of micturition, striatal sphincter denervation, or a combination of them all. Striatal sphincter denervation is attributed to the selective loss of motoneurons in the nucleus of Onuff at the S2-S3 medullary segments. Needle electromyography of the external anal sphincter, therefore, is considered an important neurophysiological test in the assessment of patients with parkinsonism, as most patients with MSA show denervation-reinnervation signs *(109,110)*. We and others have confirmed that anal sphincter denervation is prominent in patients with MSA, although similar types of abnormalities have been found in a large proportion of patients with PSP as well as in some patients with IPD *(111,112)*. Therefore, the utility of anal or vesical sphincter needle EMG in the diagnosis of MSA is still under debate *(113,114)*. Chronic constipation, local trauma related to delivery, and other pudendal nerve long-standing lesions may give rise also to sphincter denervation *(115,116)*, which may diminish the validity of the sign as a true marker of motoneuronal loss. In the consensus statement for the diagnosis of MSA *(94)*, sphincter EMG abnormalities are considered as a supportive laboratory finding.

Transcranial Magnetic Stimulation

There are not many studies published on the use of transcranial magnetic stimulation (TMS) in patients with APDs in comparison to the large body of literature published in patients with IPD. However, finding an abnormality in central conduction time in a patient with parkinsonism should be considered as a red flag to warn of the likely existence of a degenerative disorder different from IPD. Central motor conduction time has been found slightly delayed in a number of patients with MSA, in both the parkinsonian *(117)* and cerebellar variants *(118)*.

Many other cortical and subcortical functional measures can be determined with single-pulse TMS, including resting and active threshold, stimulus-response curves, silent period duration, or cortical maps, but only a few studies of this kind have been carried out in patients with APDs. Most of them have been performed in patients with CBD, a disorder featuring clinical signs of asymmetrical sensorimotor cortex involvement. Recording from muscles of the more affected side, Lu et al. *(119)* reported shortened TMS-induced silent period, and Strafella et al. *(120)* reported enhanced facilitation and reduced inhibition of MEPs modulated by digital nerve stimulation. These findings are likely reflecting motor cortical excitability enhancement.

Patients with CBD exhibit lack of voluntary control of limb movements (video segment 3), or "alien-hand" syndrome, which suggests a cortical dysfunction *(121,122)*. In normal subjects, unilateral TMS, applied with the figure of "8" coil, induces hand muscle responses restricted to the contralateral side. However, in 6 out of 10 patients with CBD, Valls-Solé et al. *(123)* found bilateral responses to focal, unilateral, TMS applied to the side contralateral to the alien hand (Fig. 7). Ipsilateral responses were delayed with respect to the contralateral ones by a mean of 7.7 ± 2.2 ms, a time allowing for conduction through the corpus callosum. Such abnormality was not found in any of 10 normal subjects, 8 patients with Alzheimer's disease, or 6 patients with IPD presenting with predominantly unilateral rigidity. This finding points again to an enhanced motor cortex excitability in the hemisphere contralateral to the alien hand, which may be unable to inhibit transcallosal excitatory inputs from the other hemisphere.

Paired-pulse TMS has been also used in the study of corticospinal tract functions in patients with APD. Intrahemispheric cortico-cortical inhibition was found abnormally reduced in patients with MSA-P, but not in patients with MSA-C *(124)*. It has also been abnormal in the study of patients with CBD *(125,126)*, suggesting the possibility of its clinical utility in the early phases of the disease *(126)*.

TMS is an important tool not only for the assessment of cortical motor function but also for the analysis of the modulatory effects that descending pathways might have on segmental reflexes. Using methods similar to those proposed by Delwaide and collaborators with auditory stimuli *(81)*, we examined the effects of TMS on the soleus H reflex in normal subjects and in patients with parkinsonism. In healthy volunteers, TMS induced early (5–30 ms) and late (60–100 ms) phases of significant facilitation of the soleus H reflex *(127)*. The second phase is absent or significantly reduced in about 50% of patients with IPD *(82)*, and in all eight patients with PSP examined so far (unpublished results).

Evoked Potentials

The early components of the somatosensory evoked potentials in patients with IPD are normal, except for the N30 recorded at the frontal lobe, which shows reduced amplitude *(128)*. According to Rossini and collaborators, the reduced amplitude of the N30 might be owing to an abnormal sensorimotor integration *(129)*. A different kind of abnormality has been reported in patients with PSP. In these patients, Kofler and collaborators *(130)* reported an enhancement of the amplitude of the early components of the somatosensory evoked potentials, which was considered to be the consequence of cortical disinhibition. More recently, Miwa and Mizuno *(131)* confirmed the finding and proposed that the observation of enlarged somatosensory evoked potentials can be useful in the differentiation of PSP patients from other patients with movement disorders.

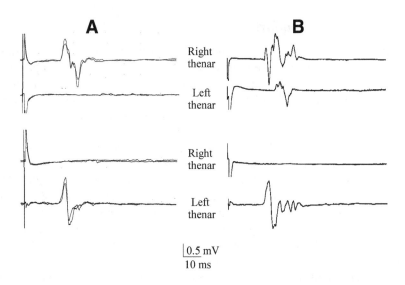

Fig. 7. Recordings from bilateral thenar muscles to focal, unilateral, transcranial magnetic stimulation (TMS) in a healthy control subject (*A*), and in a patient with CBD (*B*). Upper traces result from left-hemisphere TMS, and lower traces from right-hemisphere TMS. Note the presence of a delayed ipsilateral MEP in the patient.

The premotor evoked potentials are abnormal in patients with IPD, likely reflecting a disturbance in preparation of the motor act. Deecke et al. *(132)* showed that there was a delay and reduction of the bereitschaftpotential, and abnormalities in event-related potentials have been also published. However, there are no studies of the premotor potentials in patients with APDs.

NEUROPHYSIOLOGICAL TESTS MOST USEFUL
FOR DIFFERENTIAL DIAGNOSIS IN PATIENTS WITH APD

There is no single clinical neurophysiology test that can be used to distinguish with certitude between patients with APD at an individual level. This situation of clinical neurophysiology is common to many other conditions. In practicing clinical neurophysiology, the examiner is constantly looking for data that can bring more cues to confirm or refute an hypothesis made on the basis of clinical exam. The selection of tests useful for differential diagnosis in patients with APD can only be orientative or suggestive, but conclusive. One of the roles of those whose work is devoted to clinical neurophysiology should be to search for new methods and technical improvements to bring further understanding on pathophysiological mechanisms of the disease process.

From the author's point of view, the neurophysiological tests that better characterize parkinsonism and, specifically, the APDs, are listed in Table 4. Performance of ballistic movements within a reaction time task paradigm is useful to test the mechanisms of motor preparation and execution, even though very much should still be learned on the physiology of motor preparation for the test to provide its full potential of information. Brainstem and spinal reflexes have to be conveniently modulated by the descending motor commands for them to be integrated in the subject's normal motor behavior. Although many tests have given interesting information on the abnormal brainstem and spinal reflex modulation in patients with parkinsonism, a good clinical correlate of these abnormalities is still pending. The evaluation of autonomic reflexes and the sphincter EMG provides information on specific abnormalities that can be predominant in certain groups of patients. They reflect the involvement of specific groups of neurons, well correlated with pathologic findings. However, they are not useful for the diagnosis on an individual patient basis since similar abnormalities can be

Table 4

Selection of Neurophysiological Findings Allowing for Characterization of Specific Disorders Presenting With Parkinsonism

Disorder	Results of Neurophysiological Tests
IPD	Mild delay of reaction time in performance of ballistic movements
	Reduced prepulse inhibition of the blink reflex to auditory stimuli, with normal prepulse inhibition to somatosensory stimuli
	Regular alternating tremor at rest
PSP	Absent startle reaction to auditory stimuli
	Absent orbicularis oculi response to a median nerve electrical stimulus eliciting a response in the mentalis muscle
	Reduced prepulse inhibition of the blink reflex to both auditory and somatosensory stimuli
MSA	Signs of denervation-reinnervation in sphincter muscles
	Signs of autonomic dysfunction
	Minipolymyoclonus
CBD	Spontaneous and reflex myoclonus
	Asymmetry in cortical maps of representation of hand muscles
LBD	REM sleep behavior disorder

present in other groups of patients. TMS, short latency evoked potentials, and event-related potentials, are all offering many possibilities for the study of motor and sensory pathways as well as brain sensorimotor integration and high level processing of information. Although many studies have been carried out in patients with parkinsonism, very few reports on APDs have been published so far. A large amount of research is under way regarding the physiological mechanisms of TMS and event-related potentials. Many of them are already available for clinical application and more will be in the near future, allowing for better characterization of the abnormalities involving sensory and motor functions of patients with APDs.

FURTHER RESEARCH IN NEUROPHYSIOLOGY OF APD

There is a large amount of possibilities for research in neurophysiology of parkinsonism and of movement disorders in general. Neurophysiology offers the advantage of a good temporal resolution of events and should bring further understanding of what is wrong in the CNS that leads to motor dsyfunction. The research in clinical neurophysiology will probably continue until the pathophysiological mechanisms of the diseases are well understood. However, meaningful information can only be obtained if a careful neurological examination is followed by an imaginative albeit meticulous neurophysiological study. Undoubtedly, the most rewarding situation would be the one in which neurologists and clinical neurophysiologists join their efforts. Relevant and interesting information derived from neurophysiological studies should stir up the interest of clinicians, whereas challenging questions arising from clinical exams should stimulate the imagination of the clinical neurophysiologist in devising new techniques for more careful documentation of the signs.

Although the cooperation between clinical and neurophysiological experts is the first condition for the development of future lines of research, the second one is the development of better methods for clinical diagnosis of the diseases. Neurophysiology would be able to provide accurate information on the pathophysiology of movement disorders only if the diagnostic uncertainty is reduced to negligible levels. A thorough neurophysiological characterization of patients with APDs, appropriately classifed into well-differentiated groups, would certainly bring information that may be useful in the future to improve the diagnostic accuracy but, most of all, the pathophysiology of the diseases.

Suggestions for future research lines are listed in Table 5. Some of them are based on clinical features that should be the focuss of neurophysiological studies. However, some techniques may be

Table 5
Lines of Future Research in Neurophysiology of APD

Clinical Feature	Research Lines
Motor systems	Documentation of bradykinesia when performing natural tasks
	Methods for enhancing energization of the motor tract
	Readiness and premotor potentials
	Relationship between mental processes and motor actions
	Role of external cues and rhythms on movement performance
	Dysfunction of subcortical motor pathways
	Source of rest and action tremor oscillations
Sensory systems	Multilevel sensorimotor integration
	Long latency and event-related evoked potentials
	Intersensory facilitation vs collision between sensory stimuli
Spinal cord reflexes	Alpha motoneuronal excitability
	The role of propriospinal inhibitory circuits in rigidity
Brainstem physiology	Relationship between basal ganglia and brainstem nuclei
	Recording pedunculopontine tegmental nucleus functions
	Physiology of automatic movements
	Spontaneous and reflex blinks
Cortical stimulation	Modulation of cortical responses with sensory inputs
	Ipsilateral effects of TMS
	Repetitive transcranial magnetic stimulation

able to demonstrate features of the disease that point to the dysfunction of certain nervous system centers or structures. Among those techniques, TMS and event-related potentials are probably the most promising ones. Since their implantation, TMS and especially repetitive TMS (rTMS) have opened a large avenue of research in parkinsonism and other movement disorders. They will certainly bring more possibilities for neurophysiological interventions in the near future, including therapeutic actions. It has been demonstrated that the introduction of a variable amount of electrical current in brain tissues by applying rTMS of different intensities and frequencies induces excitability changes that can in turn be measured by conventional TMS or other methods *(133)*. Since 1994 *(134)*, rTMS has been used as a therapy in patients with IPD. Although there has been contradictory observations up to the most recently published papers *(135,136)*, researchers will certainly keep trying until the technique finds its position among the armamentarium of neurophysiological interventions in patients with APDs. Recording event-related brain potentials should provide information on structures that may be dysfunctional in parkinsonism. Cognitive negative variation has been reported to be improved after subthalamic nucleus stimulation *(137)*, indicating the sensitivity of the test to basal ganglia–cortical loop function. A variety of other neurophysiological techniques could be in the list of suggestions for future studies. The reader may find helpful information regarding many of those procedures in the specialized literature. However, apart from knowing technical details, the researcher interested in neurophysiology of parkinsonism should exercise imagination to find new ways to demonstrate specific features of the disease.

LEGENDS FOR THE VIDEO SEGMENTS

Video segment 1. Two patients with PSP featuring slow and limited voluntary eye movements. The second patient shows responses of the lower facial muscles, but not of the periocular muscles, to a scratch stimulus to the thenar eminence.

Video segment 2. Two patients with MSA-P showing minipolymyoclonus. Note the irregular movements, sometimes limited to one finger

Video segment 3. Two patients with corticobasal degeneration. The first patient shows some features of alien limb. The second patient had asymmetrical upper limb appraxia.

REFERENCES

1. Litvan I, Bhatia KP, Burn DJ, et al. SIC Task force appraisal of clinical diagnostic criteria for Parkinsonian disorders. Mov Disord 2003;18:467–486.
2. Jankovic J, Rajput AH, McDermott MP, Perl DP. The evolution of diagnosis in early Parkinson's disease. Arch Neurol 2000;57:369–372.
3. Quinn N. Multiple system atrophy—the nature of the beast. J Neurol Neursurg Psychiatry 1989;Suppl:78–89.
4. Boeve BF, Maraganore DM, Parisi JE, et al. Pathologic heterogeneity in clinically diagnosed corticobasal ganglionic degeneration. Neurology 1999;53:795–800.
5. Bergeron C, Pollanen MS, Weyer L, Black SE, Lang AE. Unusual clinical presentations of cortical basal ganglionic degeneration. Ann Neurol 1996;40:893–900.
6. Hughes AJ, Colosimo C, Kleedorfer B, Daniel SE, Lees AJ. The dopaminergic response in multiple system atrophy. J Neurol Neurosurg Psychiatry 1992;55:1009–1013.
7. Poewe W, Wenning G. The differential diagnosis of Parkinson's disease. Eur J Neurol 2002;9(Suppl 3):23–30.
8. Dickson DW, Bergeron C, Chin SS, et al. Office of rare diseases neuropathologic criteria for corticobasal degeneration. Exp Neurol 2002;61:935–946.
9. Brooks DJ, Ibáñez V, Sawle GV, et al. Striatal D2 receptor status in patients with parkinson's disease, striatonigral degeneration, and progressive supranuclear palsy, measured with IIC-raclopride and positron emission tomography. Ann Neurol 1992;31:184–192.
10. Hallett M, Khoshbin SA. A physiological mechanism of bradykinesia. Brain 1980;103:301–314.
11. Berardelli A, Sabra AF, Hallett M. Physiological mechanisms of rigidity in Parkinson's disease. J Neurol Neurosurg Psychiatry 1983;46:45–83.
12. Delwaide P, Pepin JL, DePasqua V, Maertens de Noordhout A. Projections from the basal ganglia to tegmentum: a subcortical route for explaining the pathophysiology of Parkinson's disease signs? J Neurol 2000;247(Suppl 2):75–81.
13. Hallett M. Clinical neurophysiology of akinesia. Rev Neurol 1990;146:585-590.
14. Rafal RD, Posner MI, Walker JA, Friedrich FJ. Cognition and the basal ganglia. Separating mental and motor components of performance in Parkinson's disease. Brain 1984;107:1083–1094.
15. Bloxham CA, Dick DJ, Moore M. Reaction times and attention in Parkinson's disease. J Neurol Neurosurg Psychiatry 1987;50:1178–1183.
16. Daum I, Quinn N. Reaction times and visuospatial processing in Parkinson's disease. J Clin Exp Neuropsychol 1991;13:972–982.
17. Godaux E, Koulischer D, Jacquy J. Parkinsonian bradykinesia is due to depression in the rate of rise of muscle activity. Ann Neurol 1992;31:93–100.
18. Evarts EV, Teravainen H, Calne DB. Reaction time in Parkinson's disease. Brain 1981;104:167–186.
19. Pullman SL, Watts RL, Juncos JL, Chase TN, Sanes JN. Dopaminergic effects on simple and choice reaction time performance in Parkinson's disease. Neurology 1988;38:249–254.
20. Berardelli A, Dick JPR, Rothwell JC, Day BL, Marsden CD. Scaling of the size of the first agonist EMG burst during rapid wrist movements in patients with Parkinson's disease. J Neurol Neurosurg Psychiatry 1986;49:1273–1279.
21. Pascual-Leone A, Valls-Solé J, Brasil-Neto JP, Cohen LG, Hallett M. Akinesia in Parkinson's disease. I. Shortening of simple reaction time with focal, single pulse transcranial magnetic stimulation. Neurology 1994;44:884–891.
22. Valldeoriola F, Valls-Solé J, Tolosa E, Ventura PJ, Nobbe FA, Martí MJ. The effects of a startling acoustic stimulus on reaction time in patients with different parkinsonian syndromes. Neurology 1998;51:1315–1320.
23. Dubois B, Pillon B, Legault F, Agid Y, Lhermitte F. Slowing of cognitive processing in progressive supranuclear palsy. A comparison with Parkinson's disease. Arch Neurol 1988;45:1194–1199.
24. Johnson R Jr, Litvan I, Grafman J. Progressive supranuclear palsy: altered sensory processing leads to degraded cognition. Neurology 1991;41:1257–1262.
25. Molinuevo JL, Valls-Solé J, Valldeoriola F. The effect of transcranial magnetic stimulation on reaction time in progressive supranuclear palsy. Clinical Neurophysiology 2000;111:2008–2013.
26. Abbruzzese G, Vische M, Ratto S, Abbruzzese M, Favale E. Assessment of motor neuron excitability in parkinsonian rigidity by the F wave. J Neurol 1985;232:246–249.
27. Rothwell JC, Obeso JA, Traub MM, Marsden CD. The behavior of the long latency stretch reflex in patients with Parkinson's disease. J Neurol Neurosurg Psychiatry 1983;46:35–44.
28. Deuschl G, Lucking CH. Physiology and clinical applications of hand muscle reflexes. Electroenceph Clin Neurophysiol 1990;Suppl 41:84–101.
29. Fuhr P, Zeffiro T, Hallett M. Cutaneous reflexes in Parkinson's disease. Muscle Nerve 1992;15:733–739.
30. Chen R, Ashby P, Lang AE. Stimulus-sensitive myoclonus in akinetic rigid syndromes. Brain 1992;115:1875–1888.

31. Cantello R, Gianelli M, Bettucci D, Civardi C, De Angelis MS, Mutani R. Parkinson's disease rigidity: magnetic MEPs in a small hand muscle. Neurology 1991;41:1449–1456.
32. Valls-Solé J, Pascual-Leone A, Brasil-Neto JP, McShane L, Hallett M. Abnormal facilitation of the response to transcranial magnetic stimulation in patients with Parkinson's disease. Neurology 1994;44:735–741.
33. Bathien N, Rondot P. Reciprocal continuous inhibition in rigidity of parkinsonism J Neurol Neurosurg Psychiatry 1977;40:20–24.
34. Lelli S, Panizza M, Hallett M. Spinal cord inhibitory mechanisms in Parkinson's disease. Neurology 1991;41:553–556
35. Delwaide P, Pepin JL, Maertens de Noordhout A. Short latency autogenic inhibition in patients with parkinsonian rigidity. Ann Neurol 1991;30:83–89.
36. Grasso M, Mazzini L, Schieppati M. Muscle relaxation in Parkinson's disease: a reaction time study. Mov Disord 1996;11:411–420.
37. Angel RW, Lewitt PA. Unloading and shortening reactions in Parkinson's disease. J Neurol Neurosurg Psych 1978;41:919–923.
38. Bathien N, Toma S, Rondot P. Étude de la réaction de raccourcissement présente chez l'homme dans diverses affections neurologiques. Electroenceph Clin Neurophys 1981;51:156–164.
39. Berardelli A, Hallett M. Shortening reaction of human tibialis anterior. Neurology 1984;34:242–246.
40. Diener C, Scholz E, Guschlbauer B, Dichgans J. Increased shortening reaction in Parkinson's disease reflects a difficulty in modulating long loop reflexes. Mov Disord 1987;2:31–36.
41. Fine EJ, Hallett M, Litvan I, Tresser N, Katz D. Dysfunction of Ib (autogenic) spinal inhibition in patients with progressive supranuclear palsy. Mov Disord 1998;13:668–672.
42. Golbe LI, Davis PH, Lepore FE. Eyelid movement abnormalities in progressive supranuclear palsy. Mov Disord 1989;4:297–302.
43. Karson CN, Burns S, LeWitt P, Foster NL, Newman RP. Blink rates and disorders of movement. Neurology 1984;34:677–678.
44. Heide W, Koenig E, Trillenberg P, Kömpf D, Zee DS. Electrooculography: technical standards and applications. Electroenceph Clin Neurophysiol 1999;(Suppl 52):223–240.
45. Chu FC, Reingold DB, Cogan DG, Williams AC. The eye movement disorders of progressive supranuclear palsy. Ophthalmology 1979;86:422–428.
46. Vidailhet M, Rivaud S, Gouider-Khouja N, et al. Eye movements in parkinsonian syndromes. Ann Neurol 1994;35: 420–426.
47. Valls-Solé J, Valldeoriola F, Tolosa E, Martí MJ. Distinctive abnormalities of facial reflexes in patients with progressive supranuclear palsy. Brain 1997;120:1877–1883.
48. Vidailhet M, Rothwell JC, Thompson PD, Lees AJ, Marsden CD. The auditory startle response in the Steele–Richardson–Olszewsky syndrome and Parkinson's disease. Brain 1991;115:1181–1192.
49. Brown P, Rothwell JC, Thompson PD, Day BL, Marsden CD. New observations on the normal auditory startle reflex in man. Brain 1991;114:1891–1902.
50. Valls-Solé J, Valldeoriola F, Molinuervo JL, Cossu G, Nobbe F. Prepulse modulation of the startle reaction and the blink reflex in normal human subjects. Exp Brain Res 1999;129:49–56.
51. Heilman KM. Exploring the enigmas of frontal lobe dysfunction. Geriatrics 1976;31:81–87.
52. Dehen H, Bathien N, Cambier J. The palmo-mental reflex. An electrophysiological study. Eur Neurol 1975;13:395–404.
53. Jenny AB, Saper CB. Organization of the facial nucleus and corticofacial projection in the monkey: a reconsideration of the upper motor neuron facial palsy. Neurology 1987;37:930–939.
54. Maertens de Noordhout A, Delwaide PJ. The palmomental reflex in Parkinson's disease. Comparisons with normal subjects and clinical relevance. Arch Neurol 1988;45:425–427.
55. Kimura J. Disorders of interneurons in parkinsonism. The orbicularis oculi reflex to paired stimuli. Brain 1973;96:87–96.
56. Smith SJ, Lees AJ. Abnormalities of the blink reflex in Gilles de la Tourette syndrome. J Neurol Neurosurg Psychiatry 1989;52:895–898.
57. Eekhof JL, Aramideh M, Bour LJ, Hilgevoord AA, Speelman HD, Ongerboer de Visser BW. Blink reflex recovery curves in blepharospasm, torticollis spasmodica, and hemifacial spasm. Muscle Nerve 1996;19:10–15
58. Basso MA, Powers AS, Evinger C. An explanation for reflex blink hyperexcitability in Parkinson's disease. I. Superior colliculus. J Neurosci 1996;16:7308–7317.
59. Basso MA, Evinger C. An explanation for reflex blink hyperexcitability in Parkinson's disease. II Nucleus raphe magnus. J Neurosci 1996;16:7318–7330.
60. Cruccu G, Pauletti G, Agostino R, Berardelli A, Manfredi M. Masseter inhibitory reflex in movement disorders. Huntington's chorea, Parkinson's disease, dystonia, and unilateral masticatory spasm. Electroenceph Clin Neurophysiol 1991;81:24–30.
61. Alfonsi E, Nappi G, Pacchetti C, et al. Changes in motoneuron excitability of masseter muscle following exteroceptive stimuli in Parkinson's disease. Electroencephalogr Clin Neurophysiol 1993;89:29–34
62. Deuschl G, Goddemeier C. Spontaneous and reflex activity of facial muscles in dystonia, Parkinson's disease, and in normal subjects. J Neurol Neurosurg Psychiatry 1998;64:320–324.

63. Davis M, Gendelman DS, Tischler MD, Gendelman PM. A primary acoustic startle circuit: lesion and stimulation studies. J Neurosci 1982;2:791–805.
64. Brown P, Rothwell JC, Thompson PD, Britton TC, Day BL, Marsden CD. The hyperekplexias and their relationship to the normal startle reflex. Brain 1991;114:1903–1928.
65. Zweig RM, Whitehouse PJ, Casanova MF, Walker LC, Jankel WR, Price DL. Loss of pedunculopontine neurons in progressive supranuclear palsy. Ann Neurol 1987;22:18–25.
66. Malessa S, Hirsch EC, Cervera P, et al. Progressive supranuclear palsy: loss of cholinergic acetyltransferase-like immunoreactive neurons in the pontine reticular formation. Neurology 1991;41:1593–1597.
67. Juncos JL, Hirsch EC, Malessa S, Duyckaerts C, Hersh LB, Agid Y. Mesencephalic cholinergic nuclei in progressive supranuclear palsy. Neurology 1991;41:25–30.
68. Valls-Solé J, Solé A, Valldeoriola F, Muñoz E, González LE, Tolosa ES. Reaction time and acoustic startle. Neurosci Lett 1995;195:97–100
69. Valls-Solé J, Valldeoriola F, Tolosa E, Nobbe F. Habituation of the startle reaction is reduced during preparation for execution of a motor task in normal human subjects. Brain Res 1997;751:155–159.
70. Valls-Solé J, Rothwell JC, Goulart F, Cossu G, Muñoz JE. Patterned ballistic movements triggered by a startle in healthy humans. J Physiol 1999;516:931–938.
71. Valldeoriola F, Valls-Solé J, Toloa E, Nobbe FA, Muñoz JE, Martí MJ. The acoustic startle response is normal in patients with multiple system atrophy. Mov Disord 1997;12:697–700.
72. Kofler M, Müller J, Seppi K, Wenning GK. Exaggerated auditory startle responses in multiple system atrophy: a comparative study of parkinson and cerebellar subtypes. Clin Neurophysiol 2003;114:541–547.
73. Kofler M, Müller J, Wenning G, et al. The auditory startle reaction in parkinsonian syndromes. Mov Disord 2001;16: 62–71.
74. Ison JR, Sanes JN, Foss JA, Pinckney LA. Facilitation and inhibition of the human startle blink reflexes by stimulus anticipation. Behav Neurosci 1990;104:418–429.
75. Nakashima K, Shimoyama R, Yokoyama Y, Takahashi K. Auditory effects on the electrically elicited blink reflex in patients with Parkinson's disease. Electroenceph Clin Neurophysiol 1993;89:108–112.
76. Lozza A, Pepin JL, Rapisarda G, Moglia A, Delwaide PJ. Functional changes of brainstem reflexes in Parkinson's disease. Conditioning of the blink reflex R2 component by paired and index finger stimulation. J Neural Transm 1997;104:679–687.
77. Valls-Solé J. Neurophysiological characterization of parkinsonian syndromes. Neurophysiol Clin 2000;30:352–367.
78. Pierrot-Deseilligny E, Mazières L. Circuits réflexes de la moelle epinière chez l'homme. Rev Neurol 1984;140(Part I):605–614
79. Pierrot-Deseilligny E, Mazières L. Circuits réflexes de la moelle epinière chez l'homme. Rev Neurol 1984;140(Part II):681–694.
80. Rossignol S, Jones GM. Audio-spinal influence in man studied by the H-reflex and its possible role on rhythmic movements synchronized to sound. Electroenceph Clin Neurophysiol 1976;41:83–92.
81. Delwaide P, Pepin JL, Maertens de Noordhout A. The audiospinal reaction in Parkinsonian patients reflects functional changes in reticular nuclei. Ann Neurol 1993;33:63–69
82. Valls-Solé J, Valldeoriola F. Neurophysiological correlate of clinical signs in Parkinson's disease. Clinical Neurophysiology 2002;113:792–805.
83. Wenning GK, Ben Shlomo Y, Magalhaes M, Daniel SE, Quinn NP. Clinical features and natural history of multiple system atrophy. An analysis of 100 cases. Brain 1994;117:835–845.
84. Salazar G, Valls-Solé J, Martí MJ, Chang H, Tolosa ES. Postural and action myoclonus in patients with parkinsonian type multiple system atrophy. Mov Disord 2000;15:77–83.
85. Gouider-Khouja N, Vidailhet M, Bonnet AM, Pichon J, Agid Y. "Pure" striatonigral degeneration and Parkinson's disease: a comparative clinical study. Mov Disord 1995;10:288–294.
86. Patel S, Slater P. Analysis of the brain regions involved in myoclonus produced by intracerebral picrotoxin. Neuroscience 1987;20:687–693.
87. Thompson PD, Day BL, Rothwell JC, Brown P, Britton TC, Marsden CD. The myoclonus in corticobasal degeneration. Evidence for two forms of cortical reflex myoclonus. Brain 1994;117:1197–1208.
88. Gibb WRG, Luthert PJ, Marsden CD. Corticobasal degeneration Brain 1989;112:1171–1192.
89. Brunt ERP, vanWeerden TW, Pruim J, Lakke JWPF. Unique myoclonic pattern in corticobasal degeneration. Mov Disord 1995;10:132–142.
90. Sutton GG, Mayer RF. Focal reflex myoclonus. J Neurol Neurosurg Psychiatry 1974;37:207–217.
91. Mauguière F, Desmedt JE, Courjon J. Astereognosis and dissociated loss of frontal or parietal components of somatosensory evoked potentials in hemispheric lesions: detailed correlations with clinical signs and computerized tomographic scanning. Brain 1983;106:271–311.
92. Caccia MR, McComas AJ, Upton ARM, Blogg T. Cutaneous reflexes in small muscles of the hand. J Neurol Neursurg Psychiatry 1973;36:960–977.

93. Jenner JR, Stephens JA. Cutaneous reflex responses and their central nervous pathways studied in man. J Physiol 1982;333:405-419.

94. Gilman S, Low PA, Quinn N, et al. Consensus statement on the diagnosis of multiple system atrophy. J Neurol Sci 1999;163:94–98.

95. Horimoto Y, Matsumoto M, Akatsu H, et al. Autonomic dysfunctions in dementia with Lewy bodies. J Neurol 2003;250:530–533.

96. Benarroch EE, Chang FLF. Central autonomic disorders. J Clin Neurophysiol 1993;10:39–50.

97. Holand S, Girard A, Laude D, Meyer-Bisch C, Elghozi JL. Effects of an auditory startle stimulus on blood pressure and heart rate in humans. J Hypertens 1999;17:1893–1897.

98. Valls-Solé J, Veciana M, León L, Valldeoriola F. Effects of a startle on heart rate in patients with multiple system atrophy. Mov Disord 2002;17:546–549.

99. Shahani BW, Halperin JJ, Boulu P, Cohen J. Sympathetic skin response: a method of assessing unmyelinated axon dysfunction in peripheral neuropathies. J Neurol Neurosurg Psychiatry 1984;47:536–542.

100. Bordet R, Benhadjali J, Destee A, Hurtevent JF, Bourriez JL, Guieu JD. Sympathetic skin response and R-R interval variability in multiple system atrophy and idiopathic Parkinson's disease. Mov Dis 1996;11:268–272.

101. Baser SM, Meer J, Polinsky RJ, Hallett M. Sudomotor function in autonomic failure. Neurology 1991;41:1564–1566.

102. Plazzi G, Corsini R, Provini F, et al. REM sleep behavior disorders in multiple system atrophy. Neurology 1997;48:1094–1097.

103. Bannister R, Gibson W, Michaels L, Oppenheimer DR. Laryngeal abductor paralsysis in multiple system atrophy. A report on three necropsied cases, with observation on the laryngeal muscles and the nuclei ambigui. Brain 1981;104:351–368.

104. Isozaki E, Naito A, Horiguchi S, Kawamura R, Hayashida T, Tanabe H. Early diagnosis and stage classification of vocal cord abductor paralysis in patients with multiple system atrophy. J Neurol Neurosurg Psychiatry 1996;60:399–402.

105. Iranzo A, Santamaría J, Tolosa E, et al. Continuous positive air pressure eliminates nocturnal stridor in multiple system atrophy. The Lancet 2000;356:1329–1330.

106. Turner RS. Idiopathic rapid eye movement sleep behavior disorder is a harbinger of dementia with Lewy bodies. J Geriatr Psychiatry Neurol 2002;15:195–199.

107. Boeve BF, Silber MH, Parisi JE, et al. Synucleinopathy pathology and REM sleep behavior disorder plus dementia or parkinsonism. Neurology 2003;61:40–45.

108. Kirby R, Fowler CJ, Gosling J, Bannister R. Urethro-vesical dysfunction in progressive autonomic failure with multiple system atrophy. J Neurol Neurosurg Psychiatry 1986;49:554–562.

109. Sakuta M, Nakanishi T, Toyokura Y. Anal muscle electromyograms differ in amyotrophic lateral sclerosis and Shy-Drager syndrome. Neurology 1978;28:1289–1293.

110. Eardley I, Quinn NP, Fowler CJ, et al. The value of urethral sphincter electromyography in the differential diagnosis of parkinsonism. Br J Urol 1989;64:360–362.

111. Valldeoriola F, Valls-Solé J, Tolosa ES, Martí MJ. Striated anal sphincter denervation in patients with progressive supranuclear palsy. Mov Disord 1995;10:550–555.

112. Giladi N, Simon ES, Korczyn AD, et al. Anal sphincter EMG does not distinguish between multiple system atrophy and Parkinson's disease. Muscle Nerve 2000;23:731–734.

113. Rodi Z, Denislic M, Vodusek DB. External anal sphincter electromyography in the differential diagnosis of parkinsonism. J Neurol Neurosurg Psychiatry 1996;60:460–461.

114. Libelius R, Johansson F. Quantitative electromyography of the external anal sphincter in Parkinson's disease and multiple system atrophy. Muscle Nerve 2000;23:1250–1256.

115. Kiff ES, Swash M. Slowed conduction in the pudendal nerves in idiopathic (neurogenic) faecal incontinence. Br J Surg 1984;71:614–616.

116. Podnar S, Vodusek DB. Standardization of anal sphincter electromyography: effect of chronic constipation. Muscle Nerve 2000;23:1748–1751.

117. Abbruzzese G, Marchese R, Trompetto C. Sensory and motor evoked potentials in multiple system atrophy: a comparative study with Parkinson's disease. Mov Disord 1997;12:315–321.

118. Cruz Martinez A, Arpa J, Alonso M, Palomo F, Villoslada C. Transcranial magnetic stimulation in multiple system and late onset cerebellar atrophies. Acta Neurol Scand 1995;92:218–224.

119. Lu CS, Ikeda A, Terada K, et al. Electrophysiological studies of early stage corticobasal degeneration. Mov Disord 1998;13:140–146.

120. Strafella A, Ashby P, Lang AE. Reflex myoclonus in cortical-basal ganglionic degeneration involves a transcortical pathway. Mov Disord 1997;12:360–369.

121. Goldberg G, Mayer NH, Toglia JU. Medial frontal cortex infarction and the alien hand sign. Arch Neurol 1981;38: 683–686.

122. Feinberg TE, Schindler RJ, Flanagan NG, Haber LD. Two alien hand syndromes. Neurology 1992;42:19–24.

123. Valls-Solé J, Tolosa E, Martí MJ, et al. Examination of motor output pathways in patients with corticobasal ganglionic degeneration using transcranial magnetic stimulation. Brain 2001;124:1131–1137.
124. Marchese R, Trompetto C, Buccolieri A, Abbruzzese G. Abnormalities of motor cortical excitability are not correlated with clinical features in atypical parkinsonism. Mov Disord 2000;15:1210–1214.
125. Hanajima R, Ugawa Y, Terao Y, Ogata K, Kanazawa I. Ipsilateral cortico-cortical inhibition of the motor cortex in various neurological disorders. J Neurol Sci 1996;140:109–116.
126. Frasson E, Bertolasi L, Bertasi V, et al. Paired transcranial magnetic stimulation for the early diagnosis of corticobasal ganglionic degeneration. Clin Neurophysiol 2003;114:272–278.
127. Goulart F, Valls-Solé J, Alvarez R. Posture-related modification of soleus H reflex excitability. Muscle Nerve 2000;23:925–932.
128. Rossini PM, Babiloni F, Bernardi G, et al. Abnormalities of short-latency somatosensory evoked potentials in parkinsonian patients. Electroenceph Clin Neurophysiol 1989;74:277–289.
129. Rossini PM, Filippi MM, Vernieri F. Neurophysiology of sensorimotor integration in Parkinson's disease. Clin Neurosci 1998;5:121–130.
130. Kofler M, Müller J, Reggiani L, Wenning GK. Somatosensory evoked potentials in progressive supranuclear palsy. J Neurol Sci 2000;179:85–91.
131. Miwa H, Mizuno Y. Enlargements of somatosensory-evoked potentials in progressive supranuclear palsy. Acta Neurol Scand 2002;106:209–212.
132. Deecke L, Englitz HG, Kornhuber HH, Schmitt G. Cerebral potential preceding voluntary movement in patients with bilateral or unilateral Parkinson akinesia. In: Desmedt JE, ed. Progress in Clinical Neurophysiology, vol. 1. Basel: Karger, 1977:151–163.
133. Rizzo V, Siebner HR, Modugno N, et al. Shaping the excitability of human motor cortex with premotor rTMS. J Physiol 2004;554:483–495.
134. Pascual-Leone A, Valls-Sole J, Brasil-Neto JP, Cammarota A, Grafman J, Hallett M. Akinesia in Parkinson's disease. II. Effects of subthreshold repetitive transcranial motor cortex stimulation. Neurology 1994;44:892–898.
135. Ikeguchi M, Touge T, Nishiyama Y, Takeuchi H, Kuriyama S, Ohkawa M. Effects of successive repetitive transcranial magnetic stimulation on motor performances and brain perfusion in idiopathic Parkinson's disease. J Neurol Sci 2003;209:41–46.
136. Okabe S, Ugawa Y, Kanazawa I. Effectiveness of rTMS on Parkinson's Disease Study Group. 0.2-Hz repetitive transcranial magnetic stimulation has no add-on effects as compared to a realistic sham stimulation in Parkinson's disease. Mov Disord 2003;18:382–388.
137. Gerschlager W, Alesch F, Cunnington R, et al. Bilateral subthalamic nucleus stimulation improves frontal cortex function in Parkinson's disease. An electrophysiological study of the contingent negative variation. Brain 1999;122:2365–2373.

25

Role of CT and MRI in Diagnosis and Research

Mario Savoiardo and Marina Grisoli

INTRODUCTION

In degenerative disorders, computed tomography (CT) is usually requested only to avoid a misdiagnosis or to exclude an unlikely tumor or another unexpected pathology. It is true, however, that CT can demonstrate atrophic changes that, in cases in which they are typically distributed, may contribute to the diagnosis.

In a few atypical parkinsonian disorders, such as progressive supranuclear palsy and olivopontocerebellar degeneration, CT was used up to the mid-1980s to support the clinical diagnosis. At present, however, its role is very limited. In this group of disorders, demonstration of atrophy or other structural changes of deep nuclei is not obtainable by CT and not even always by magnetic resonance imaging (MRI). There is no question, however, that, in atypical parkinsonian disorders, MRI is a very useful and easily available diagnostic tool. We shall, therefore, focus on the MRI findings that can be demonstrated in these diseases, and review what is now widely accepted and consolidated, what is strongly diagnostic if not pathognomonic of a specific disorder, what is less predictive or uncertain, and what should be studied in future investigations.

After a few comments on Parkinson's disease (PD), we shall discuss multiple system atrophy (MSA) of the parkinsonian type (MSA-P) and cerebellar type (MSA-C), progressive supranuclear palsy (PSP), corticobasal degeneration (CBD), dementia with Lewy bodies (DLB), and, briefly, vascular parkinsonism and toxic and metabolic conditions causing parkinsonism.

PARKINSON'S DISEASE

A few papers have described that, on MRI, atrophy of the pars compacta of the substantia nigra can be demonstrated in T2-weighted thin sections (1–3). Its isointense narrow band, delimited anteriorly by hypointensity of the medial part of the cerebral peduncle and the loss of signal intensity owing to iron deposits in the pars reticulata and, posteriorly, in the red nucleus, becomes progressively thinner. However, the smudging of the hypointensity, which should indicate atrophy of the pars compacta, can also be observed in an unknown proportion of cases in patients with atypical parkinsonian disorders (4,5). Other sequences and quantification of brain iron have been proposed (6,7). MRI observation of the substantia nigra is, therefore, not easy. It requires a dedicated examination that has not become a routine study in any center because of two other reasons. First, the neurologists do not need MRI to diagnose PD and, second, neuroradiologists and neurologists rely on other observations to support a differential diagnosis between PD and atypical parkinsonian disorders. Actually, in most of the papers dealing with MRI in PD and parkinsonisms, the substantia nigra is

From: *Current Clinical Neurology: Atypical Parkinsonian Disorders*
Edited by: I. Litvan © Humana Press Inc., Totowa, NJ

disregarded or ignored. The "normal" MRI features of patients with PD are used as a control for a series of other abnormalities affecting specific nuclei, structures, or areas that point to a specific parkinsonian disorder.

An important advancement in the MRI diagnosis of PD has been proposed by Hutchinson and Raff *(8,9)*. A ratio between the signals obtained with two different sequences suppressing the signal from white matter and gray matter, respectively, exquisitely demonstrated the substantia nigra to the point that serial studies could be expected to even predict the disease. So far, this technique has not been commonly used *(10)*, probably because of technical difficulties in obtaining the ratio.

The neuroradiological differential diagnosis of MSA, PSP, and CBD from PD, therefore relies upon the demonstration of lesions in the nuclei or areas that pathology shows to be characteristically affected in each specific disorder. In a few instances, the neuroradiologist has helped the pathologist to pinpoint subtle abnormalities that turned out to be useful for the diagnosis.

MULTIPLE SYSTEM ATROPHY

MSA has been separated into MSA-P and MSA-C according to the predominant parkinsonian or cerebellar features. The former corresponds to the old term *striatonigral degeneration* (SND), the latter to sporadic *olivopontocerebellar atrophy* (OPCA). The term *Shy–Drager syndrome* is no longer been considered useful by the Consensus Conference on MSA *(11)*, but a proposal to introduce the term MSA-A (autonomic features–predominant MSA) was recently made by Horimoto et al. *(12)* to indicate those MSA patients in whom autonomic dysfunction predominated over cerebellar or parkinsonian features.

For the purpose of identifying the MRI characteristic features or markers or pointers of the different atypical parkinsonian disorders, one should consider the pathology of the specific disorder *(13)*. There is no doubt that in MSA-P or SND the pathology is mostly in the putamen, whereas in MSA-C the changes are in the brainstem and cerebellum. In MSA-A, most of the abnormalities are in the spinal cord and may be, therefore, disregarded when considering MRI.

Multiple System Atrophy of the Parkinsonian Type

The MRI abnormalities observed in MSA-P have been described in several papers; they should be considered separately according to whether they are obtained at low- or high-field intensity MRI *(14–19)*.

Low-field intensity MRI (up to 0.5T) demonstrates increased signal intensity in proton density and T2-weighted images in the dorsolateral and posterior part of the putamen, where loss of neurons and gliosis in a loose tissue have been described *(20,21)*. These findings correspond to an increased amount of water in the tissue (Fig. 1). Atrophy of the putamen has been commonly observed *(22)* but only recently emphasized by Yekhlef et al. *(23)*.

High-field intensity MRI (usually 1.5T) shows a different feature, i.e., putaminal hypointensity in T2-weighted images that may completely or almost completely mask the hyperintensity described above *(16–19,24–26)*. The hypointensity is caused by a magnetic susceptibility effect mainly owing to deposits of iron in the same putaminal areas *(27)*; this effect is proportional to the square of the magnetic field intensity and is, therefore, usually evident only at high-field MRI. A lateral rim of hyperintensity, indicating a band devoid of iron right on the lateral margin of the posterior part of the putamen, may be recognizable *(25)*, particularly if we observe proton density and T2-weighted images together. In fact, the magnetic susceptibility effect is much less evident in proton density images. This "slit-like" lateral rim of hyperintensity has been briefly called the "putaminal slit" *(12)*. In conclusion, at 1.5 T MRI putaminal hypointensity in T2-weighted images more marked in the posterior part of this nucleus and the associated thin lateral rim of hyperintensity are the features of MSA-P *(17,25,26,28,29)* (Fig. 2).

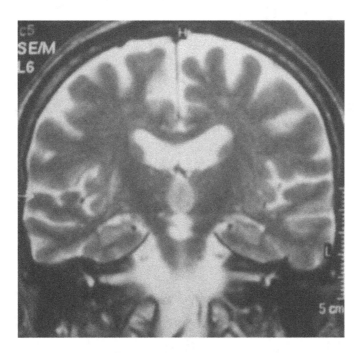

Fig.1. MSA-P. 0.5 T, coronal T2-weighted image shows increased signal intensity in the right putamen in a patient with parkinsonism prevalent on the left side.

A very thin line of milder hyperintensity along the entire lateral profile of the putamen, at the interface with the external capsule, may be confused with the "lateral hyperintense rim" or "putaminal slit." This very subtle line has been occasionally observed in atypical parkinsonian disorders *(30)*. In our experience, a very thin line that also borders the anterior part of the putamen, often without associated hypointensity, may be a nonsignificant finding since we have observed it, although rarely, mainly in normal subjects (Fig. 2B). As in the figure shown by Macia et al. *(30)*, it should be noted that the evidence of this line is mostly along the anterior part of the putamen, whereas the abnormalities documented by pathology in MSA-P and shown by MRI typically affect the posterior putamen *(21,27)*.

All these details are important when one is investigating sensitivity and specificity of MRI abnormalities in MSA-P. Specificity, sensitivity, and positive predictive value of the putaminal abnormalities have been investigated in a limited number of studies *(18,19,23)*. The specificity is high, but sensitivity has been considered low, generally not higher than 50–60% *(18,19)*. As most neuroradiologists know, conventional spin-echo (CSE) images are more sensitive than fast spin-echo (FSE) images to magnetic susceptibility effects owing to iron deposits in the tissue. In MSA-P, Righini et al. *(31)* have elegantly demonstrated that, by using CSE thin sections (3 mm) and comparison of proton density and T2-weighted images vs FSE 5 mm T2-weighted images, the sensitivity is increased from 45% to more than 83%.

Another trivial explanation of the difference in sensitivity between different series is the length of the disease at time of MRI examination. Only very few investigations have dealt with the MRI demonstration of the progression of MSA *(12,26)*. In the series reported by Watanabe et al. *(26)*, frequency of putaminal abnormalities went up from 38.5% in patients with 2 yr or less from motor impairment to 80% in patients with more than 4 yr from motor impairment.

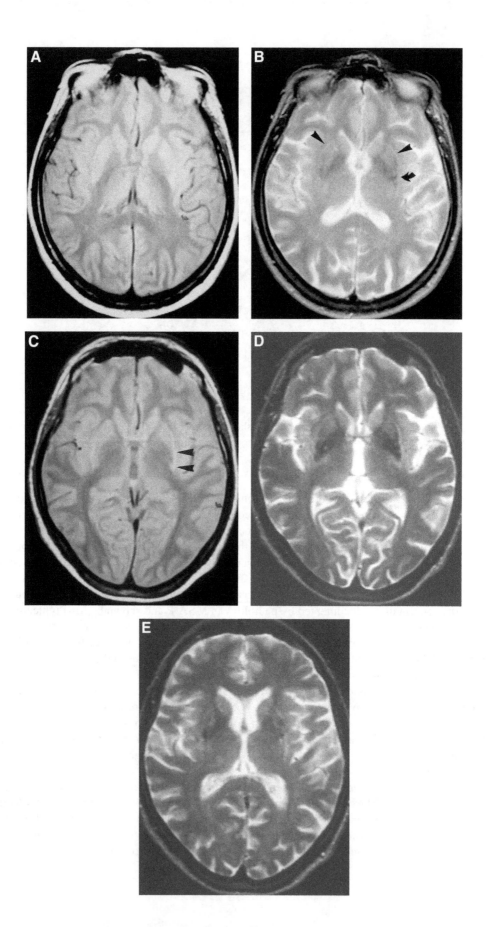

Of course, MRI abnormalities supporting the diagnosis of MSA-P have a greater importance if they are recognizable in the early stages of the disease, when the clinical diagnosis is still uncertain, rather than in its late stages. Detection of subtle abnormalities that may indicate the diagnosis of MSA-P rather than PD on the first MRI examination, performed at the time of the first visit by a neurologist, may occur, but such episodes are still anecdotical. How early the abnormalities appear is an aspect that needs to be clarified.

A few proton MR spectroscopy (MRS) studies have demonstrated that *N*-acetylaspartate (NAA) and choline (Cho) were reduced in the lentiform nucleus of MSA patients *(32,33)*. The NAA/creatine (Cr) ratio was particularly decreased in MSA-P patients, probably reflecting putaminal neuronal loss *(32)*. MRS, however, has not been widely used to help differentiate patients with MSA from patients with PD.

The use of diffusion-weighted imaging (DWI) has been recently proposed to help differentiating MSA-P from PD *(34)*. The Innsbruck group demonstrated that the patients with MSA-P presented an increased regional apparent diffusion coefficient (rADC) in the putamen compared with both patients with PD and normal subjects *(34)*. In another study, however, DWI failed to discriminate MSA-P and PSP *(35)*. The advantage of DWI is that one can obtain measurements and quantification. It is not clear, however, whether DWI studies of the basal ganglia in MSA-P patients will prove to have a greater sensitivity than the CSE sequences of MRI, as described by Righini et al. *(31)*.

Multiple System Atrophy of the Cerebellar Type

In MSA-C there are two types of abnormalities, atrophy and signal changes, which do not depend on magnetic field intensity *(36)*. Atrophy has a very characteristic distribution; it mainly involves the pons, middle cerebellar peduncles, and cerebellum. Therefore, the diagnosis can be suspected when one simply observes, in the MRI sagittal midline section, the decreased bulging of the pons compared to the midbrain and particularly the medulla oblongata. The flattening of the profile of the pons begins, in fact, in its caudal part (Fig. 3A). In addition to atrophy, signal changes may be recognized in proton density and T2-weighted images consisting of slight hyperintensity in the structures that degenerate or become gliotic *(36)*. They include: (a) the pontine nuclei and their fibers (the transverse pontine fibers) that run mostly on the anterior and posterior aspect of the basis pontis, cross the midline on the raphe, and reach the cerebellum through the middle cerebellar peduncles (Figs. 3B and C); and (b) the whole cerebellum, because of loss of Purkinje cells and degeneration of their fibers and consequent diffuse gliosis. To make the resulting MRI picture more characteristic, these signal abnormalities are combined with the signal preservation of the structures that do not degenerate *(17)*. They are mainly the superior cerebellar peduncles and the corticospinal tracts. The axial sections of the pons, therefore, present a typical aspect with a sort of cross recognized in the early papers *(36)*, later defined as the "hot cross bun sign" *(18,26)* or simply the "cross sign" *(12)* (Figs. 3B and C). Coronal sections are particularly useful to demonstrate the cerebellar hyperintensity when it is very slight, by allowing a comparison in the same image of the infratentorial and the supratentorial structures *(17,36)*. They also beautifully demonstrate the atrophy of the middle cerebellar peduncles *(36)*.

Fig. 2. (*opposite page*) MSA-P. 1.5 T, axial sections (**A–E**). First examination (**A,B**) performed when the patient, with a 2-yr history of dysautonomia, developed mild right-sided parkinsonism. The proton density image (A) is normal whereas the T2-weighted image (B) shows mildly decreased signal intensity in the posterior part of the left putamen (curved arrow), consistent with iron deposits. The very subtle bands of hyperintensity along the anterior part of the putamina (arrowheads) probably are a nonsignificant finding. On the follow-up examination performed 19 mo later, when the parkinsonian signs always prevalent on the right side had progressed, hyperintensity in proton density image (C) in the left posterior putamen has developed (arrowheads). In the T2-weighted sections (D and, adjacent cranial section, E), more marked hypointensity and a lateral rim of hyperintensity are visible.

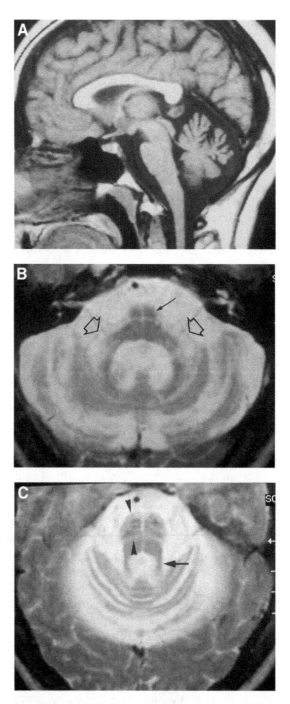

Fig. 3. MSA-C. T1-weighted midline sagittal section in an early case (**A**) shows flattening of the inferior part of the profile of the pons and cerebellar atrophy. In an advanced case, T2-weighted axial sections on the lower (**B**) and upper pons (**C**) show atrophy of the pons, middle cerebellar peduncles, and cerebellum with characteristic signal changes. The left corticospinal tract is indicated by an arrow; the margins of the hyperintense middle cerebellar peduncles (open arrows) are poorly defined with respect to the CSF (**B**). (**C**) Arrowheads point to the hyperintense anterior and posterior right transverse pontine fibers; an arrow indicates the left superior cerebellar peduncle. On the midline, the raphe is hyperintense.

Both specificity and sensitivity of MRI pontine and cerebellar signs in MSA-C are very high *(13,18,19)*. In the series reviewed by Schrag et al. *(19)*, 83% of MSA-C patients could be unequivocally classified based on the MRI findings. If the disease is advanced, sensitivity may be greater than 90% *(26)*. Specificity may decrease if we do not exclude patients with hereditary ataxias *(25)*. Patients with spinocerebellar ataxias (SCAs), particularly SCA1, SCA2, and SCA3, may share the same features both at MRI and histology *(37–39)*. A few of our cases of SCA2, which together with SCA1 is the most common inherited spinocerebellar ataxia in Italy, had an MRI scan that was indistinguishable from that of a patient with MSA-C except for the presence of some degree of cerebral atrophy.

As with MSA-P, one problem in MSA-C is to know how early the MRI signs of atrophy and signal changes develop in the course of the disease, i.e., how helpful can MRI be in the early stages of MSA-C. According to Horimoto et al. *(12)*, the initial changes of the "cross sign" were seen in all their cases of MSA-C within the first 2 or 3 yr after onset of symptoms. As expected, patients with MSA-C normally present pontine and cerebellar changes earlier, with greater severity and more rapid progression than other signs of MSA such as putaminal changes, which usually appear later and have a slower progression. Reciprocally, patients with MSA-P have earlier and more severe putaminal involvement, though posterior fossa changes in these patients may appear later and remain milder. It is, therefore, somewhat misleading to consider indifferently the putaminal and the posterior fossa abnormalities as indicators of MSA and to verify their specificity and sensitivity. In our opinion, one must always consider the clinical presentation (MSA-P or MSA-C or perhaps MSA-A) and should then investigate whether the appropriate MRI signs, i.e., those fitting with the diagnosis, are present *(13,17,19,23,26)*. Occasionally, however, the "inappropriate" MRI sign had an earlier progression than the clinically appropriate one *(12)*. Of course, both putaminal and brainstem-cerebellar signs should be present in a "full-blown" MSA.

Large multicentric studies including hundreds of patients from different countries will probably answer all the questions regarding specificity, sensitivity, positive predictive values, time of appearance, and progression of the MRI signs in MSA-P, MSA-C, and PSP *(40)*.

In the attempt to find measurable data, Kanazawa et al. *(41)* investigated brainstem and cerebellar involvement in patients with MSA-C using DWI. They found significant differences in the apparent diffusion coefficient (ADC) values of the pons, middle cerebellar peduncles, cerebellar white matter, and putamen between MSA-C patients and controls. The ADC values also correlated with the duration of the disease. ADC values of MSA-C patients in the pons, middle cerebellar peduncles, and cerebellar white matter were also higher than those obtained in a few patients with SCA3 and SCA6.

Measurable data can also be obtained by MRS. Mascalchi et al. demonstrated decreased NAA/Cr and Cho/Cr ratios in the pons and cerebellum of MSA-C patients vs controls *(42)*. MRS, however, is a complex and time-consuming examination that is performed in only a few specialized centers. To obtain measurable data, it is easier to obtain DWI sequences that require a very short acquisition time and calculate the ADC maps *(35)*.

Measurable data are required when dealing with large number of patients in research studies. They are also necessary in longitudinal studies to quantify the progression of the disease. They are hardly needed in the everyday examinations of patients with atypical parkinsonian disorders in whom a diagnosis or a support to a specific diagnosis is required by the clinician. Specificity and sensitivity of MRI findings in these disorders are not yet fully established; much more time will be needed to evaluate sensitivity and specificity in diffusion or spectroscopy studies.

PROGRESSIVE SUPRANUCLEAR PALSY

With regard to MRI diagnosis of PSP, all the attention has been given to atrophy of the midbrain where pathologic changes are known to occur *(43)*. Signal changes in this region have also been noted. Less attention has been paid to basal ganglia abnormalities and cerebral atrophy, which are more variable and less useful for the diagnosis.

MRI simply confirmed what pneumoencephalography first, and later CT *(44,45)* have shown: demonstration of midbrain atrophy is the cardinal neuroradiologic feature of PSP diagnosis. This demonstration can be achieved by observing the midbrain size either in axial sections or in the midline sagittal section *(17,23,25)*. The latter has the advantage of showing a direct comparison between the size of the midbrain and that of the pons, not only in the sagittal diameter, but also in "height," or vertical or caudo-cranial diameter. The midbrain size is, in fact, reduced in all the directions. The upper profile of the normal midbrain in sagittal section is characterized by a slight superior convexity with the highest point approximately midway between the aqueduct and the mamillary bodies. In PSP, this profile flattens and may even become concave in its posterior part, because of atrophy and reduced height of the midbrain tegmentum associated with enlargement of the third ventricle. Thinning of the tectum particularly in its superior part may also be observed in sagittal sections *(25)* (Fig. 4A). Atrophy of the midbrain is found in 75–89% of the clinically diagnosed PSP patients *(19,23,46)*.

Simple linear measurements of the midbrain have been suggested in axial and sagittal sections *(47)*. No overlap was found between the measures obtained in PSP patients (range of midbrain diameter: 11–15 mm) vs PD patients and normal subjects (range 17–19 and 17–20 mm, respectively), whereas some overlapping occurred between PSP and MSA-P patients (range 14–19 mm, mean 16.7).

As mentioned above, disproportionate dilatation of the third ventricle, compared to the lateral ones, may be caused by diencephalic extension of atrophy. This finding was evident in about one-fourth of our cases.

One absolutely marginal feature that is sometimes seen in PSP patients in sagittal MR images is hyperextension of the head. This feature, however, may be a clue for the diagnosis. The hyperextended position may be assumed during the examination by patients who were correctly positioned by the MRI technician at the beginning of the examination. The neuroradiologist who recognizes the unusual hyperextension of the head should immediately observe the midbrain, looking for atrophy and signal changes that may confirm the suspicion of PSP *(17,25)*.

Signal changes in the midbrain are the second aspect that one should look for in suspected PSP patients. When present, they consist of mild hyperintensity in proton density and T2-weighted images, mainly in the tegmentum and periaqueductal region where gliosis and tau-positive lesions are found in pathological sections *(48,49)* (Fig. 4B). These abnormalities may extend caudally to the pontine tegmentum *(49)*. Signal changes in the midbrain are recognizable in about 60% of the PSP patients *(46)*.

Mild to moderate cerebral atrophy may be observed in most of the patients, sometimes more marked in the frontal and temporal lobes *(19)*, but without the focal and asymmetric distribution found in CBD *(46)* (*see* the following section).

Occasional abnormalities in the basal ganglia (atrophy of the lenticular nucleus with pallidal hyperintensity) have sometimes been reported *(19)*, but the typical combination of T2 putaminal hypointensity with lateral hyperintense rim seen in 1.5 T studies of MSA-P patients are absent *(25,28)*.

DWI has only rarely been used to study PSP. In one study, regional ADCs (rADCs) were increased in the basal ganglia of PSP patients; the values allowed discrimination from patients with PD but did not discriminate PSP and MSA-P *(35)*. No results of the MRI observations were given so that it remains undefined whether DWI performs better, equally, or worse than MRI in discriminating PSP, MSA-P, and PD. In another study on only five PSP patients, ADCs in the prefrontal and precentral white matter were higher than in controls *(50)*.

MRS reports on PSP are also rare. NAA deficit in the lentiform nucleus, consistent with neuronal loss, was found in PSP and in MSA patients, whereas patients with PD did not differ from controls *(33)*. Tedeschi et al. *(51)* examined patients with PD, PSP, and CBD. Compared with the control subjects, PSP patients presented reduced NAA/Cr or NAA/Cho in the brainstem, centrum semiovale, frontal and precentral cortex, and lentiform nucleus. These data demonstrate that, in addition to brainstem and basal ganglia involvement, the frontal association and motor cortex are also affected; abnormalities in the centrum semiovale suggest involvement of the axons connecting the basal gan-

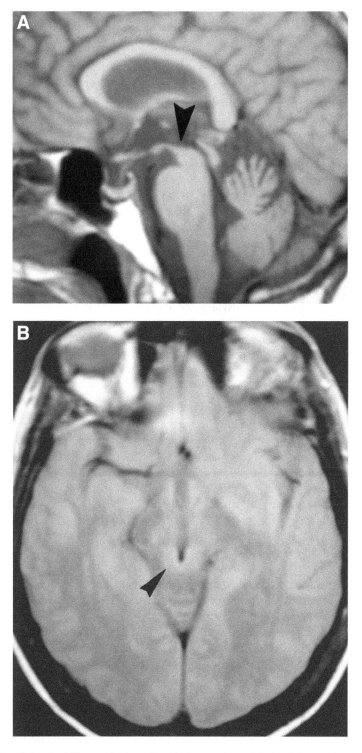

Fig. 4. PSP. T1-weighted midline sagittal section (**A**) in a patient with 5-yr history of disease. The midbrain is atrophic. The superior profile is concave (arrowhead); the tectum is thin in its cranial part; the antero-posterior diameter is 14 mm. Compare with the normal midbrain of Fig. 3A. The tectal and periaqueductal areas show a mild or questionable hyperintensity (arrowhead) in the proton density image (**B**).

glia to the cortex *(51)*. In another PSP series, in which a decrease of NAA in the lentiform nucleus was found, the authors reported that three of their nine PSP patients presented the "eye of the tiger" sign in the pallida *(52)*. A similar observation was made by other authors in a case of CBD *(53)*, suggesting that the "eye of the tiger" sign described by Sethi et al. *(54)* is not specific of Hallervorden–Spatz disease (HSD). In 1.5 T T2-weighted images, the pallidum is normally hypointense in adults or old patients because of normal accumulation of iron. Any hyperintense area within the pallidum, because of lacunar infarct or dilatation of Virchow–Robin spaces or rarefaction of fibers and gliosis that probably accompany calcium deposits, may justify the appearance of the "eye of the tiger." In fact, contrary to what we expected, we have observed some hyperintensity in T2-weighted images in a few cases in which CT demonstrated calcifications in the pallidum, a nearly physiologic finding in old age. What is striking in children or adolescents with HSD, is that the hypointensity owing to iron deposits is extraordinarily marked for their age. Even if HSD may present in adulthood, the age of the patient should be considered when one sees an anteromedial hyperintensity in a hypointense pallidum. In other words, the hypointensity should be evaluated considering the patient's age.

HSD was recently found to be related to mutations in the gene encoding pantothenate kinase 2 (PANK2), and the specific MRI pattern described *(54,55)* has been found to distinguish patients with PANK2 mutations *(56)*. The same MRI findings may be seen in HARP syndrome (hypoprebeta-lipoproteinemia, acanthocytosis, retinitis pigmentosa, and pallidal degeneration) which is, however, part of the pantothenate kinase–associated neurodegeneration *(57)*. It will, therefore, be very interesting to carefully rule out any possible misinterpretation (i.e., lacunar infarcts or dilated perivascular spaces) and eventually obtain the appropriate genetic tests in the patients with PSP or other disorders presenting the "eye of the tiger" sign or similar signal abnormalities.

CORTICOBASAL DEGENERATION

MRI diagnosis of CBD has been examined in only a few papers *(19,23,46,58–61)*. The essential aspect that should be sought to support the clinical diagnosis of CBD is asymmetrical posterior frontal and parietal atrophy; atrophy occurs in the hemisphere contralateral to the side of the clinical manifestations. The unilateral atrophy is manifested by dilatation of the ipsilateral cortical sulci and lateral ventricle, with concomitant loss of bulk of the white matter (Fig. 5). The cortical atrophy may be marked, with sometimes a "knife edge" thinning of the postcentral gyrus (Fig. 5F). Occasionally, slightly increased signal intensity in proton density and T2-weighted images may be seen in the atrophic cortex and subjacent white matter. Proton density or FLAIR images are more reliable than T2-weighted images in showing the cortical hyperintensity (Figs. 5C,D,F); in T2-weighted images, the hyperintensity of the cortex may be masked by the higher signal intensity of the adjacent cerebrospinal fluid.

One interesting aspect is that the asymmetric atrophy is usually not mentioned in MRI reports, unless the neuroradiologist is aware of the possibility of a specific diagnosis based on the asymmetry. We did not mention asymmetry in our first reports of CBD cases. When the neurologist called our attention to this aspect, we easily recognized the site of predominant atrophy (always contralateral to the side of prevalent clinical involvement, unknown to us) in all the six cases that had been studied.

Fig. 5. *(opposite page)* CBD. In a 66-yr-old male with clinical manifestations prevalent on the left side (**A–E**), the T1-weighted sagittal sections on the left (A) and right (B) hemispheres show more marked right atrophy, prevalent in the parietal area. FLAIR coronal sections on the anterior and posterior parietal areas (C and D) confirm the asymmetry of atrophy. The right ventricle is slightly larger and minimal hyperintensity is present in the white matter of the right parietal lobe. Marked hyperintensity around the occipital horns is present bilaterally (D). In the same patient, right parietal atrophy is also evident on CT scan (E). In a different patient, a 72-yr-old woman with clinical manifestations on the left side, axial proton density image (**F**) shows hyperintense cortex in the atrophic postcentral gyrus (arrowheads).

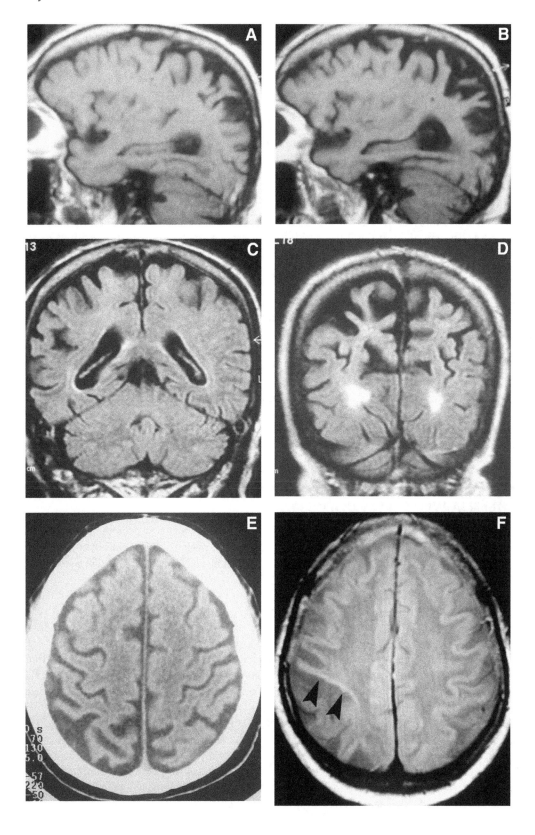

Atrophy, of course, can be recognized in the axial sections of the brain on MRI, but coronal sections are particularly helpful to demonstrate the asymmetry, which is the cardinal feature for diagnosis of CBD. Coronal sections, however, are not routinely obtained in many institutions: this is perhaps the reason for the relatively scarce sensitivity of a few reported MRI studies in diagnosing CBD *(19)*. Three-dimensional volume-rendered images may beautifully demonstrate the extent and distribution of the cortical involvement *(61)* but a surface display of MR-generated images is not part of a standard examination of the brain and is very rarely performed.

In spite of the known pathologic involvement of the basal ganglia and substantia nigra, in these areas signal abnormalities such as pallidal hyperintensity or putaminal hypointensity are rarely observed on MRI *(19,60)*. Putaminal hypointensity associated with the hyperintense posterolateral rim was never observed in our 25 patients. However, Yekhlef et al. reported a constant presence of putaminal atrophy in their series of 26 cases. They also reported midbrain atrophy in 75% of their patients, whereas this feature was very rare (1 of 16 cases, or 6.3%) in our series *(46)*, so that it could be used for differentiation of CBD from PSP. Our last review *(60)* confirms the rarity of midbrain atrophy in patients with CBD (2 of 25 cases, or 8%).

As we have seen, there are very marked discrepancies between the various series; further observations are needed to assess the value of MRI in the diagnosis of CBD. The basic bias is owing to the fact that asymmetry is considered the hallmark of CBD, whereas from pathology we know that cases with symmetric involvement are indeed present and also a few MRI series report cases with clinical diagnosis of CBD without cortical asymmetries *(46,58)*. Undoubtedly, if asymmetry is considered crucial for the neuroradiological diagnosis, occurrence of CBD will be underestimated.

Regarding DWI, it has been suggested that patients with CBD may present white matter abnormalities more severe on the side with predominant cortical atrophy, even when no abnormalities are detected by T2-weighted and FLAIR images *(62)*. To our knowledge, however, no series with a significant number of cases of CBD has been studied with DWI.

Nine CBD patients were studied with MRS by Tedeschi et al. *(51)*. Reduced NAA/Cho or NAA/Cr were found in the lentiform nucleus, parietal cortex, and centrum semiovale. Significant asymmetries were present in the parietal areas with more marked abnormalities in the parietal cortex contralateral to the clinically most affected side.

DEMENTIA WITH LEWY BODIES

MRI studies on DLB are rather rare, probably because they do not show peculiar signal changes or localized atrophy that may support the diagnosis. Except for a report by Hashimoto et al. *(63)*, most MRI studies have been published by the group of Barber et al. in Newcastle upon Tyne *(64–67)*. The few studies we performed in our patients with DLB concur with the published data.

The essential findings of a series of volumetric studies indicate that patients with dementia, either vascular or owing to Alzheimer's disease (AD) or DLB, present brain atrophy compared with control subjects. Atrophy in DLB is less marked than in patients with AD, with particular preservation of mesial temporal structures including amigdala, hippocampus, subiculum, and parahippocampal and dentate gyri. Preservation of these structures may, therefore, help to differentiate DLB from AD *(63,65)*. Total brain volume is not significantly different in patients with DLB and vascular dementia *(66)*, but white matter and basal ganglia hyperintensities in T2-weighted images are more frequent and extensive in patients with vascular dementia than in patients with AD and DLB *(64)*.

Occipital hypoperfusion has been demonstrated in DLB *(68,69)*. Because the visual hallucinations of DLB might also be related to structural changes in the occipital lobes, volumetric MRI measurements have been performed *(70,71)*. The results are conflicting: in one series, occipital lobe volumes in DLB were not significantly different from those of AD and control groups *(70)*; in the other series *(71)*, occipital lobe atrophy was found in DLB but also in AD patients. Therefore, on the basis of these volumetric studies, discrimination of these two types of dementia was not possible.

VASCULAR PARKINSONISM

Although the concept of vascular parkinsonism, proposed by Critchley in 1929, was almost abandoned for many years, it has once more come to the fore. The prevalence and incidence of vascular parkinsonism is variable in different series. Diagnosis of vascular parkinsonism is usually suggested by acute onset or other signs of cerebrovascular disease, but needs to be confirmed by imaging studies *(72)*. This is the form of parkinsonism that frequently can be diagnosed by CT, without requiring MRI to demonstrate the lesions.

The lesions usually are lacunar or small infarcts in the basal ganglia, mostly in the putamina (Fig. 6). A single lesion in one putamen may sometimes justify the contralateral parkinsonism. Parkinsonism may also be associated with multiple infarcts or white matter lesions in the subcortical arteriosclerotic encephalopathy *(72)*, which is more accurately shown by MRI. In this disease, precise clinicoradiological correlations are difficult to obtain. Parkinsonian symptoms and signs may be associated with lesions in the basal ganglia or in the white matter of the cerebral hemispheres probably because of involvement of the striato-thalamic connections with the frontal cortex.

TOXIC AND METABOLIC PARKINSONISM

A long series of toxic and metabolic disorders, acquired or inherited, may cause parkinsonian symptoms and signs *(72)*. Many times the diagnosis is straightforward, known from the medical history, but the support of imaging studies may be useful in defining at least the extent of damage. This is the case of post-anoxic encephalopathy or carbon monoxide intoxication, in which the lesions involve the white matter and the basal ganglia where they are prevalent in the pallida *(73,74)*. The same prevalent pallidal location is seen in cyanide intoxication *(75)*. In other conditions, such as the unusual parkinsonian presentation of Wilson's disease, the correct diagnosis may be unsuspected and MRI, by demonstrating putaminal and lateral thalamic abnormalities or more extensive basal ganglia and brainstem involvement *(25)*, may orient the diagnostic work-up to a rapid conclusion.

One condition in which MRI may suggest the correct diagnosis is manganese intoxication. This is manifested by hyperintensity in T1-weighted images in the pallida, sometimes extending caudally to the substantia nigra. Manganese accumulates in the pallida in many conditions, including liver cirrhosis with portacaval shunt and hepatic encephalopathy *(76,77)*, long-term parenteral nutrition *(78)*, environmental exposure in miners or industrial workers *(79)*, or in other less clear conditions *(80)*. Therefore, demonstration of pallidal hyperintensities in T1-weighted images should prompt investigations of blood manganese concentrations (Fig. 7).

PROSPECTS FOR FUTURE RESEARCH

In research on atypical parkinsonian disorders, MR investigations can be expanded in at least two main directions.

One implies the collection of large series in multicentric studies, particularly regarding the less common disorders such as CBD or DLB, so that the sensitivity and specificity of the MRI findings can be reliably established. However, in order to make them widely and reliably applicable, the study protocols should be carefully planned, taking into account the existing knowledge of the sensitivity of different sequences and the total time required for an examination. Longitudinal studies are also needed. Comparison of sensitivity and specificity of MRI findings in a certain disease observed in different series may be meaningless if the series are not comparable because of different disease duration. Up to now, longitudinal studies have only been performed very rarely and in very few diseases. By observing the evolution of the various imaging findings, the neuroradiologist will be able to recognize the earliest findings of a given disorder and thus anticipate the diagnosis.

The other direction of MR investigations regards the advanced MR techniques, such as MRS, diffusion studies, and volumetric and functional studies. The latter are discussed in another chapter.

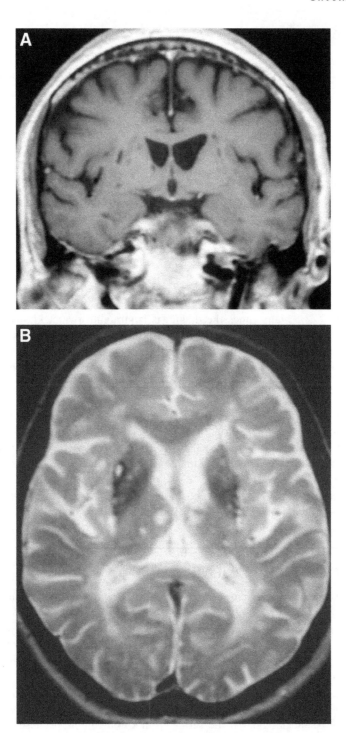

Fig. 6. Vascular parkinsonism. In this 66-yr-old patient with pseudobulbar signs and progressive parkin-sonism with shuffling gait, coronal T1- (**A**) and axial T2-weighted sections (**B**) show multiple lacunes or small infarcts in the basal ganglia and thalami. Hyper- and hypointensity consistent with an old, small hemorrhagic lesion is present in the right putamen (**B**).

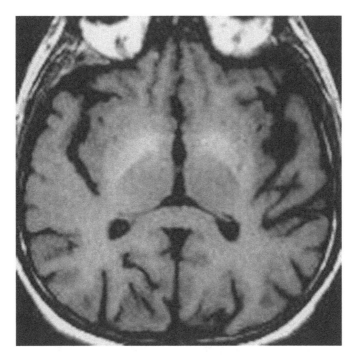

Fig. 7. Parkinsonism in chronic manganese intoxication. Pallidal hyperintensity in T1-weighted axial section prompted investigations on possible manganese intoxication. Improvement following chelating treatment was obtained (courtesy of Dr. M. C. Valentini, Turin).

As for MRS and diffusion imaging, we tried to give an overview of what is now available. The number of studies dealing with these techniques, however, is rather limited. First of all, these techniques should be applied in a greater number of cases and the results should be compared with the MRI results in the same patients in order to understand their relative diagnostic value and to establish if they offer some advantage in terms of diagnosis. They can, of course, bring additional knowledge and offer quantitative data; quantification is necessary when dealing with large series of patients and in longitudinal studies.

In MRS, most studies have focused on changes in NAA, a neuronal marker that is expected to decrease in degenerative disorders, and on choline and creatine, which are considered indicators of cell membranes turnover and energy supply in the tissue, respectively. Since gliosis is often prominent in various degenerative disorders, short TE techniques (such as STEAM with TE = 34 ms) should be used more widely in order to evaluate myoinositol, a putative marker of gliosis.

Diffusion-tensor MR imaging characterizes the diffusion of water molecules in the tissue and makes measurements of the damage to the brain tissue at microscopic level possible. In a few atypical parkinsonisms, regional ADC values in the appropriate areas have been examined. From the tensor, it is possible to calculate the degree of anisotropy of the tissue. Fractional anisotropy, which is an index that measures the anisotropy of the tissue, could also be applied in investigations on fiber tract damage in degenerative disorders such as MSA-C in which fiber tract abnormalities are a characteristic MRI feature.

Correlating all these in vivo measurements with the corresponding pathologic findings will be necessary to assess the value of these new techniques and gain further insights in the pathogenesis of the disorders in which they are applied.

Table 1
Distribution of Characteristic MR Abnormalities in Atypical Parkinsonian Disorders

	MSA-P	MSA-C	PSP	CBD
MRI Atrophy	Putamen	Pons, middle cerebellar peduncles, cerebellum	Midbrain and diencephalon	Parieto-frontal regions, asymmetrical
MRI signal abnormalities	1.5T: hypointensity in T2-w.i. in posterior lateral putamen with lateral rim of hyperintensity 0.5T: usually only hyper-intensity in PD and T2-w.i. in posterior lateral putamen	Hyperintensity in PD and T2-w.i. in transverse pontine fibers ("cross sign"), middle cerebellar peduncles, cerebellum	Slight hyperintensity in PD and T2-w.i. in periaqueductal area	Rare, slight hyperintensity in PD and T2-w.i. in atrophic cortex and subcortical white matter
DWI	↑ ADC in putamen	↑ ADC in pons, middle cerebellar peduncles, cerebellum	↑ ADC in basal ganglia and frontal white matter	Asymmetrical white matter abnormalities reported in atrophic regions
MRS	↓ NAA and Cho in lentiform nucleus	↓ NAA and Cho in pons and cerebellum	↓ NAA in brainstem, lentiform nucleus, frontal and motor cortex, centrum semiovale	↓ NAA in lentiform nucleus, parietal cortex and centrum semiovale

---

PROSPECTS FOR FUTURE MR RESEARCH

MRI
- large series in multicentric studies to evaluate its sensitivity and specificity in different atypical parkinsonian disorders
- longitudinal studies to assess the course of the disease

MRS
- for early detection and quantification of metabolic abnormalities

DWI and diffusion tensor imaging (DTI)
- for early detection and quantification of changes of diffusivity in different brain areas

MRS, DWI, and DTI: are they better than MRI in early diagnosis?

ACKNOWLEDGMENTS

We are indebted to Dr. Floriano Girotti for his helpful discussions and comments.

REFERENCES

1. Duguid JR, De La Paz R, De Groot J. Magnetic resonance imaging of the midbrain in Parkinson's disease. Ann Neurol 1986;20:744–747.
2. Rutledge JN, Hilal SK, Silver AJ, Defendini R, Fahn S. Study of movement disorders and brain iron by MR. AJNR Am J Neuroradiol 1987;8:397–411.
3. Braffman BH, Grossman RI, Goldberg HI, et al. MR imaging of Parkinson disease with spin-echo and gradient-echo sequences. AJNR Am J Neuroradiol 1988;9:1093–1099.
4. Stern MB, Braffman BH, Skolnick BE, Hurtig HI, Grossman RI. Magnetic resonance imaging in Parkinson's disease and parkinsonian syndromes. Neurology 1989;39:1524–1526.
5. Gorell JM, Ordidge RJ, Brown GG, Deniau J-C, Buderer NM, Helpern JA. Increased iron-related MRI contrast in the substantia nigra in Parkinson's disease. Neurology 1995;45:1138–1143.
6. Oikawa H, Sasaki M, Tamakawa Y, Ehara S, Tohyama K. The substantia nigra in Parkinson disease: proton density-weighted spin-echo and fast short inversion time inversion-recovery MR findings. AJNR Am J Neuroradiol 2002;23:1747–1756.
7. Vymazal J, Righini A, Brooks RA, et al. T1 and T2 in the brain of healthy subjects, patients with Parkinson disease, and patients with multiple system atrophy: relation to iron content. Radiology 1999;211:489–495.
8. Hutchinson M, Raff U. Parkinson's disease: a novel MRI method for determining structural changes in the substantia nigra. J Neurol Neurosurg Psychiatry 1999;67:815–818.
9. Hutchinson M, Raff U. Structural changes of the substantia nigra in Parkinson's disease as revealed by MR imaging. AJNR Am J Neuroradiol 2000;21:697–701.
10. Hu MTM, White SJ, Herlihy AH, Chaudhuri KR, Hajnal JV, Brooks DJ. A comparison of ^{18}F-dopa PET and inversion recovery MRI in the diagnosis of Parkinson's disease. Neurology 2001;56:1195–1200
11. Gilman S, Low PA, Quinn N, et al. Consensus statement on the diagnosis of multiple system atrophy. J Auton Nerv Syst 1998;74:189–192.
12. Horimoto Y, Aiba I, Yasuda T, et al. Longitudinal MRI study of multiple system atrophy - when do the findings appear, or what is the course? J Neurol 2002;249:847–854.
13. Testa D, Savoiardo M, Fetoni V, et al. Multiple system atrophy: clinical and MR observations on 42 cases. Ital J Neurol Sci 1993;14:221–216.
14. Drayer BP, Olanow W, Burger P, Johnson GA, Herfkens R, Riederer S. Parkinson plus syndrome: diagnosis using high field MR imaging of brain iron. Radiology 1986;159:493–498.
15. Pastakia B, Polinsky R, Di Chiro G, Simmons JT, Brown R, Wener L. Multiple system atrophy (Shy–Drager syndrome): MR imaging. Radiology 1986;159:499–502.
16. Savoiardo M, Strada L, Girotti F, et al. MR imaging in progressive supranuclear palsy and Shy–Drager syndrome. J Comput Assist Tomogr 1989;13:555–560.
17. Savoiardo M, Girotti F, Strada L, Ciceri E. Magnetic resonance imaging in progressive supranuclear palsy and other parkinsonian disorders. J Neural Transm 1994;42(Suppl):93–110.
18. Schrag A, Kingsley D, Phatouros C, et al. Clinical usefulness of magnetic resonance imaging in multiple system atrophy. J Neurol Neurosurg Psychiatry 1998;65:65–71.
19. Schrag A, Good CD, Miszkiel K, et al. Differentiation of atypical parkinsonian syndromes with routine MRI. Neurology 2000;54:697–702.
20. Fearnley JM, Lees AJ. Striatonigral degeneration. A clinicopathological study. Brain 1990;113:1823–1842.
21. Goto S, Matsumoto S, Ushio Y, Hirano A. Subregional loss of putaminal efferents to the basal ganglia output nuclei may cause parkinsonism in striatonigral degeneration. Neurology 1996;47:1032–1036.

22. Konagaya M, Konagaya Y, Iida M. Clinical and magnetic resonance imaging study of extrapyramidal symptoms in multiple system atrophy. J Neurol Neurosurg Psychiatry 1994;57:1528–1531.
23. Yekhlef F, Ballan G, Macia F, Delmer O, Sourgen C, Tison F. Routine MRI for the differential diagnosis of Parkinson's disease, MSA, PSP, and CBD. J Neural Transm 2003;110:151–169.
24. Lang AE, Curran T, Provias J, Bergeron C. Striatonigral degeneration: iron deposition in putamen correlates with the slit-like void signal of magnetic resonance imaging. Can J Neurol Sci 1994;21:311–318.
25. Savoiardo M, Grisoli M. Magnetic resonance imaging of movement disorders. In: Jankovic JJ, Tolosa E, eds. Parkinson's Disease and Movement Disorders, 4th ed. Philadelphia: Lippincott Williams & Wilkins, 2002:596–609.
26. Watanabe H, Saito Y, Terao S, et al. Progression and prognosis in multiple system atrophy. An analysis of 230 Japanese patients. Brain 2002;125:1070–1083.
27. Borit A, Rubinstein LJ, Urich H. The striatonigral degenerations: putaminal pigments and nosology. Brain 1975;98: 101–112.
28. Kraft E, Schwarz J, Trenkwalder C, Vogl T, Pfluger T, Oertel WH. The combination of hypointense and hyperintense signal changes on T2-weighted magnetic resonance imaging sequences. A specific marker of multiple system atrophy? Arch Neurol 1999;56:225–228.
29. Bhattacharya K, Saadia D, Eisenkraft B, et al. Brain magnetic resonance imaging in multiple-system atrophy and Parkinson disease. A diagnostic algorithm. Arch Neurol 2002;59:835–842.
30. Macia F, Yekhlef F, Ballan G, Delmer O, Tison F. T2-hyperintense lateral rim and hypointense putamen are typical but not exclusive of multiple system atrophy. Arch Neurol 2001;58:1024–1026.
31. Righini A, Antonini A, Ferrarini M, et al. Thin section MR study of the basal ganglia in the differential diagnosis between striatonigral degeneration and Parkinson disease. J Comput Assist Tomogr 2002;26:266–271.
32. Davie CA, Wenning GK, Barker GJ, et al. Differentiation of multiple system atrophy from idiopathic Parkinson's disease using proton magnetic resonance spectroscopy. Ann Neurol 1995;37:204–210.
33. Federico F, Simone IL, Lucivero V, et al. Proton magnetic resonance spectroscopy in Parkinson's disease and atypical parkinsonian disorders. Mov Disord 1997;12:903–909.
34. Schocke MFH, Seppi K, Esterhammer R, et al. Diffusion-weighted MRI differentiates the Parkinson variant of multiple system atrophy from PD. Neurology 2002;58:575–580.
35. Seppi K, Schocke MFH, Esterhammer R, et al. Diffusion-weighted imaging discriminates progressive supranuclear palsy from PD, but not from the parkinson variant of multiple system atrophy. Neurology 2003;60:922–927.
36. Savoiardo M, Strada L, Girotti F, et al. Olivopontocerebellar atrophy: MR diagnosis and relationship to multisystem atrophy. Radiology 1990;174:693–696.
37. Bürk K, Abele M, Fetter M, et al. Autosomal dominant cerebellar ataxia type I. Clinical features and MRI in families with SCA 1, SCA 2, and SCA 3. Brain 1996;119:1497–1505.
38. Murata Y, Yamaguchi S, Kawakami H, et al. Characteristic magnetic resonance imaging findings in Machado–Joseph disease. Arch Neurol 1998;55:33–37.
39. Di Donato S. The complex clinical and genetic classification of inherited ataxias. I. Dominant ataxias. Ital J Neurol Sci 1998;19:335–343.
40. Verin M, Rolland Y, Defebvre L, Delmaire C, Payan C, the NNIPPS Study Group. Neuroprotection and natural hystory in Parkinson plus syndrome (NNIPPS): preliminary results of the magnetic resonance imaging (MRI) study in progressive supranuclear palsy (PSP) and multiple system atrophy (MSA). Neurology 2003;60(Suppl 1):A293–A294.
41. Kanazawa M, Shimohata T, Tanaka K, Onodera O, Tsuji S, Okamoto K. Evaluation of brainstem involvement of multiple system atrophy by diffusion-weighted MRI. Neurology 2003;60(Suppl 1):A210.
42. Mascalchi M, Cosottini M, Lolli F, et al. Proton MR spectroscopy of the cerebellum and pons in patients with degenerative ataxia. Radiology 2002;223:371–378.
43. Steele JC, Richardson JC, Olszewski J. Progressive supranuclear palsy. Arch Neurol 1964;10:333–359.
44. Masucci EF, Borts FT, Smirniotopoulos JG, Kurtzke JF, Schellinger D. Thin-section CT of midbrain abnormalities in progressive supranuclear palsy. AJNR Am J Neuroradiol 1985;6:767–772.
45. Schonfeld SM, Golbe LI, Sage JI, Safer JN, Duvoisin RC. Computed tomographic findings in progressive supranuclear palsy: correlation with clinical grade. Mov Disord 1987;2:263–278.
46. Soliveri P, Monza D, Paridi D, et al. Cognitive and magnetic resonance imaging aspects of corticobasal degeneration and progressive supranuclear palsy. Neurology 1999;53:502–507.
47. Warmuth-Metz M, Naumann M, Csoti I, Solymosi L. Measurement of the midbrain diameter on routine magnetic resonance imaging. A simple and accurate method of differentiating between Parkinson disease and progressive supranuclear palsy. Arch Neurol 2001;58:1076–1079.
48. Aiba I, Hashizume Y, Yoshida M, Okuda S, Marakani N, Ujihira N. Relationship between brainstem MRI and pathological findings in progressive supranuclear palsy—study in autopsy cases. J Neurol Sci 1997;152:210–217.
49. Yagishita A, Oda M. Progressive supranuclear palsy: MRI and pathological findings. Neuroradiology 1996;38(Suppl):S60–S66.

50. Ohshita T, Oka M, Imon Y, Yamaguchi S, Mimori Y, Nakamura S. Apparent diffusion coefficient measurements in progressive supranuclear palsy. Neuroradiology 2000;42:643–647.

51. Tedeschi G, Litvan I, Bonavita S, et al. Proton magnetic resonance spectroscopic imaging in progressive supranuclear palsy, Parkinson's disease and corticobasal degeneration. Brain 1997;120:1541–1552.

52. Davie CA, Barker GJ, Machado C, Miller DH, Lees AJ. Proton magnetic resonance spectroscopy in Steele–Richardson–Olszewski syndrome. Mov Disord 1997;12:767–771.

53. Molinuevo JL, Muñoz E, Valldeoriola F, Tolosa E. The eye of the tiger sign in cortical-basal ganglionic degeneration. Mov Disord 1999;14:169–171.

54. Sethi KD, Adams RJ, Loring DW, el Gammal T. Hallervorden–Spatz syndrome: clinical and magnetic resonance imaging correlations. Ann Neurol 1988;24:692–694.

55. Savoiardo M, Halliday WC, Nardocci N, et al. Hallervorden–Spatz disease: MR and pathologic findings. AJNR Am J Neuroradiol 1993;14:155–162.

56. Hayflick SJ, Westaway SK, Levinson B, et al. Genetic, clinical, and radiographic delineation of Hallervorden–Spatz syndrome. N Engl J Med 2003;348:33–40.

57. Ching KHL, Westaway SK, Gitschier J, Higgins JJ, Hayflick SJ. HARP syndrome is allelic with pantothenate kinase-associated neurodegeneration. Neurology 2002;58:1673–1674.

58. Giménez-Roldán S, Mateo D, Benito C, Grandas F, Pérez-Gilabert Y. Progressive supranuclear palsy and corticobasal ganglionic degeneration: differentiation by clinical features and neuroimaging techniques. J Neural Transm 1994;42(Suppl):79–90.

59. Grisoli M, Fetoni V, Savoiardo M, Girotti F, Bruzzone MG. MRI in corticobasal degeneration. Eur J Neurol 1995;2:547–552.

60. Savoiardo M, Grisoli M, Girotti F. Magnetic resonance imaging in CBD, related atypical parkinsonian disorders, and dementias. In: Litvan I, Goetz CG, Lang AE, eds. Corticobasal Degeneration and Related Disorders. Advances in Neurology, vol. 82. Philadelphia: Lippincott Williams & Wilkins, 2000:197–208.

61. Kitagaki H, Hirono N, Ishii K, Mori E. Corticobasal degeneration: evaluation of cortical atrophy by means of hemispheric surface display generated with MR images. Radiology 2000;216:31–38.

62. Ikeda K, Iwasaki Y, Ichikawa Y. Cortical and MRI aspects of corticobasal degeneration and progressive supranuclear palsy [Letter]. Neurology 2000;54:1878.

63. Hashimoto M, Kitagaki H, Imamura T, et al. Medial temporal and whole-brain atrophy in dementia with Lewy bodies: a volumetric MRI study. Neurology 1998;51:357–362.

64. Barber R, Scheltens P, Gholkar A, et al. White matter lesions on magnetic resonance imaging in dementia with Lewy bodies, Alzheimer's disease, vascular dementia, and normal aging. J Neurol Neurosurg Psychiatry 1999;67:66–72.

65. Barber R, Gholkar A, Scheltens P, Ballard C, McKeith IG, O'Brien JT. Medial temporal lobe atrophy on MRI in dementia with Lewy bodies. Neurology 1999;52:1153–1158.

66. Barber R, Ballard C, McKeith IG, Gholkar A, O'Brien JT. MRI volumetric study of dementia with Lewy bodies. A comparison with AD and vascular dementia. Neurology 2000;54:1304–1309.

67. Barber R, McKeith IG, Ballard C, Gholkar A, O'Brien JT. A comparison of medial and lateral temporal lobe atrophy in dementia with Lewy bodies and Alzheimer's disease: magnetic resonance imaging volumetric study. Dement Geriatr Cogn Disord 2001;12:198–205.

68. Ishii K, Yamaji S, Kitagaki H, Imamura T, Hirono N, Mori E. Regional cerebral blood flow difference between dementia with Lewy bodies and AD. Neurology 1999;53:413–416.

69. Lobotesis K, Fenwick JD, Phipps A, et al. Occipital hypoperfusion on SPECT in dementia with Lewy bodies but not AD. Neurology 2001;56:643–649.

70. Middelkoop HAM, van der Flier WM, Burton EJ, et al. Dementia with Lewy bodies and AD are not associated with occipital lobe atrophy on MRI. Neurology 2001;57:2117–2120.

71. Gerlach M, Stadler K, Aichner F, Ransmayr G. Dementia with Lewy bodies and AD are not associated with occipital lobe atrophy on MRI [Letter]. Neurology 2002;59:1476.

72. Riley DE. Secondary parkinsonism. In: Jankovic JJ, Tolosa E, eds. Parkinson's Disease and Movement Disorders, 4th ed. Philadelphia: Lippincott Williams & Wilkins, 2002:199–211.

73. Chang KH, Han MH, Kim HS, Wie BA, Han MC. Delayed encephalopathy after acute carbon monoxide intoxication: MR imaging features and distribution of cerebral white matter lesions. Radiology 1992;184:117–122.

74. Sohn YH, Jeong Y, Kim HS, Im JH, Kim JS. The brain lesions responsible for parkinsonism after carbon monoxide poisoning. Arch Neurol 2000;57:1214–1218.

75. Rosenow F, Herholz K, Lanfermann H, et al. Neurological sequelae of cyanide intoxication—the patterns of clinical, magnetic resonance imaging, and positron emission tomography findings. Ann Neurol 1995;38:825–828.

76. Spahr L, Butterworth RF, Fontaine S, et al. Increased blood manganese in cirrhotic patients: relationship to pallidal magnetic resonance signal hyperintensity and neurological symptoms. Hepatology 1996;24:1116–1120.

77. Hauser RA, Zesiewicz TA, Martinez C, Rosemurgy AS, Olanow CW. Blood manganese correlates with brain magnetic resonance imaging changes in patients with liver disease. Can J Neurol Sci 1996;23:95–98.

78. Fell JM, Reynolds AP, Meadows N, et al. Manganese toxicity in children receiving long-term parenteral nutrition. Lancet 1996;347(9010):1218–1221.

79. Kim Y, Kim KS, Yang JS, et al. Increase in signal intensities on T1-weighted magnetic resonance images in asymptomatic manganese-exposed workers. Neurotoxicology 1999;20:901–907.

80. Hernandez EH, Valentini MC, Discalzi G. T1-weighted hyperintensity in basal ganglia at brain magnetic resonance imaging: are different pathologies sharing a common mechanism? Neurotoxicology 2002;23:669–674.

26

Role of Functional Magnetic Neuroimaging in Diagnosis and Research

Hartwig Roman Siebner and Günther Deuschl

INTRODUCTION

Recent advances in magnetic resonance imaging (MRI) have opened up new possibilities to map distinct aspects of human brain function in vivo. Functional magnetic resonance imaging (fMRI) is widely used to assess changes in regional neuronal activity at high spatial and temporal resolution *(1,2)*. Magnetic resonance spectroscopy (MRS) provides a means to probe distinct aspects of brain metabolism at a regional level *(3,4)*. Water diffusion magnetic resonance imaging (dMRI) can be used to study the integrity of white matter tracks in the brain *(5)*. MRI has already been successfully applied to study the pathophysiology of movement disorders such as Parkinson's disease (PD) *(6,7)*. The aim of this chapter is to summarize how these innovative MRI methods may be useful for diagnosis and research of atypical parkinsonian disorders.

FUNCTIONAL MAGNETIC RESONANCE IMAGING

Neuroimaging techniques, such as single photon emission tomography (SPECT), positron emission tomography (PET), and fMRI, provide a means of mapping regional neuronal activity in vivo in the intact human brain. Blood oxygen level-dependent (BOLD) fMRI uses echo-planar imaging (EPI) to detect changes in the oxygenation state of the blood *(8)*. Recent studies of the monkey brain combined BOLD-sensitive fMRI with electrophysiological measurements to demonstrate that the BOLD signal primarily measures the input and processing of neuronal information within a brain region *(2)*.

Since the BOLD signal is an intrinsic signal, BOLD-sensitive fMRI does not require the injection of a contrast agent. Compared to PET and SPECT, BOLD-sensitive fMRI does not involve exposure to radiation, is widely available, and offers a higher spatial and temporal resolution. Moreover, event-related fMRI protocols allow studies to investigate changes in the BOLD signal related to a single movement, whereas SPECT and PET can only map the averaged regional cerebral blood flow (rCBF) changes caused by multiple trials. Because of these methodological advantages, BOLD-sensitive fMRI has largely replaced PET and SPECT of rCBF as a tool to study the functional architecture of the human brain.

In recent years, BOLD-sensitive fMRI has been extensively used as a research tool to study the functional consequences of nigrostriatal dopamine loss in idiopathic PD. So far, most studies have investigated changes in BOLD signal related to volitional hand movements *(9–12)*. These studies have disclosed a movement-related dysfunction in basal ganglia-thalamocortical loops that are

From: *Current Clinical Neurology: Atypical Parkinsonian Disorders*
Edited by: I. Litvan © Humana Press Inc., Totowa, NJ

involved in manual motor control. However, the pattern of abnormal movement-related activity in frontal motor areas has been variable across studies *(9–12)*. Since these studies used motor tasks that differed in terms of movement parameters and cognitive load, the implication is that, in PD, functional impairment of the various basal ganglia-thalamocortical motor loops is highly dependent on the motor context. In addition to motor activation studies, BOLD-sensitive fMRI has also successfully been employed to assess nonmotor functions such as attention to action and working memory in PD *(12,13)*. Repeated fMRI measurements have also been used to image the acute effects of a therapeutic intervention. For instance, pharmacological fMRI studies have consistently demonstrated a partial normalization of movement-related activation in frontal motor areas after oral administration of levodopa *(9–11)*.

At present, there are no fMRI studies investigating atypical parkinsonian disorders. However, the experience with fMRI gathered in PD indicates that fMRI can successfully be applied in atypical parkinsonian disorders. The main potential of fMRI lies in its ability to assess the functional consequences of the underlying neurodegenerative process. Activation studies with fMRI can not only reveal regional abnormalities in task-related activity but also disclose abnomal functional integration among brain regions that form a functional network *(12)*. The pathology of atypical parkinsonian disorders affects brain regions that are not subject to neurodegeneration in PD *(14)*. Therefore, fMRI studies may be particularly revealing if the behavioral paradigm activates a functional system that is specifically affected by the suspected atypical parkinsonian syndrome. For instance, in patients with progressive supranuclear palsy (PSP), fMRI studies that explore distinct aspects of voluntary control of eye movements such as smooth pursuit and saccade generation may reveal specific functional abnormalities in regions involved in ocular motor control. Therefore, fMRI may provide a better understanding of the pathophysiology and help to establish a specific profile of abnormal brain activation for the various atypical parkinsonian disorders.

In contrast to PET activation studies, fMRI activation studies allow to acquire many hundreds of brain volumes during a single session. Therefore, single-subject fMRI provides sufficient statistical power to analyze individual activation patterns. This is of relevance in atypical parkinsonian disorders since it may be difficult to recruit a sufficient number of well-characterized patients to ensure sufficient statistical power for between-group comparisons.

Pharmacological fMRI provides a means to objectively measure the functional effects of therapeutic agents on neuronal activity. Serial fMRI measurements of the functional response to levodopa can be used to address the question why a subgroup of patients with multiple system atrophy (MSA) shows a sustained levodopa response during the course of the disease. In conjunction with structural MRI, long-term fMRI studies might be of value to monitor disease progression in patients with atypical parkinsonian disorders.

MAGNETIC RESONANCE SPECTROSCOPY

MRS provides chemical information on tissue metabolites *(3,4)*. The molecules that can be studied by MRS in human brain tissue are hydrogen 1 (^{1}H) and phosphorus 31 (^{31}P). Magnetic resonance sensitivity is far greater for protons than it is for phosphorus *(3)*. Therefore, most commercial MR scanners are capable of only proton MRS. Spectra are usually obtained from localized brain regions. The brain region is defined on a single slice by placing a small voxel, on the order of 1 or 2 cm^2, in the area of interest. The compounds that can be observed in proton spectra are primarily identified by their frequency (i.e., their position in the spectrum), expressed as the shift in frequency in pars per million (ppm) relative to a standard. A normal spectrum shows peaks from *N*-acetyl groups, especially *N*-acetylaspartate (NAA) at 2.0 ppm, creatine (Cr), and phosphocreatine at 3.0 ppm, and choline-containing phospholipids (Ch) at 3.2 ppm *(3)*. An additional peak at 1.3 ppm arises from the methyl resonance of lactate and is normally barely visible above the baseline noise *(3)*. Pathologic conditions that involve regional neuronal loss lead to region-specific decreases in the relative NAA concentrations *(3,4)*. Since NAA is a marker of neuronal integrity, proton MRS provides a noninvasive means of quantifying neuronal loss or damage in vivo. Ch and other lipids are markers of altered neuronal membrane synthesis. Cr is a possible marker of defective energy metabolism. Typically, individual metabolic ratios obtained from peak areas of the spectrum are used as input to the statistical analysis. Because total Cr concentration is relatively resistant to change, Cr is often used as an internal standard to which the concentrations of other metabolites are normalized.

Proton MRS has been used by several groups to study brain metabolism in nondemented PD yielding conflicting results *(15–27)*. In general, the majority of these studies have failed to detect consistent abnormalities for NAA, Ch, or Cr in the basal ganglia *(15–19,21,24,25*; but *see* refs. *20,26,27)* or the cerebral cortex *(19,21,25*; but *see* refs. *22,23)*. A multicenter study that included 151 patients with PD and 97 age-matched controls found no overall differences in the striatal proton spectra between groups *(16)*. However, there was a decrease in the NAA/Cho ratio in a subgroup of elderly patients (aged 51–70 yr) and patients that were not treated with levodopa *(16)*. These findings suggest that proton MRS may reveal subtle metabolic abnormalities in patients with PD depending on age and medication. Therefore, heterogeneities of clinical features across patient groups may at least in part account for discrepancies across studies *(15–27)*.

Three out of four proton MRS studies have reported abnormal proton spectra in patients with atypical parkinsonian disorders *(15,18,19*; but *see* ref. *26)*. Davie et al. *(15)* performed proton MRS of the lentiform nucleus in seven patients with MSA-P (predominantly striatonigral variant) and five patients with MSA-C (olivocerebellar variant). Compared with healthy controls, the NAA/Cr ratio was significantly decreased in patients with MSA *(15)*. Tedeschi et al. *(19)* found a reduced NAA/Cre ratio in the brainstem, centrum semiovale, and frontal and precentral cortex, and a reduced NAA/Ch ratio in the lentiform nucleus in 12 patients with PSP compared with healthy controls (Fig. 1). The same study also included nine patients with corticobasal degeneration (CBD). CBD patients also showed an abnormal metabolic pattern with a reduced NAA/Cre ratio in the centrum semiovale and a reduced NAA/Ch ratio in the lentiform nucleus and the parietal cortex contralateral to the most affected side (Fig. 1). A reduction in NAA/Ch and NAA/Cr ratios in the lentiform nucleus was also observed by Federico et al. *(18)* in seven patients with MSA and seven patients with PSP. All three studies additionally examined the proton spectra in a group of PD patients and found no abnormalities in the selected region of interest *(15,18,19)*. It should be noted, however, that Clarke et al. failed to find any abnormality for NAA, Ch, and Cr in six patients with probable MSA *(26)*.

In summary, the published data suggest that proton MRS may be of potential diagnostic value in atypical parkinsonian disorders. However, the demonstration of significant group differences in patients with well-defined clinical features does not imply that proton MRS can reliably discriminate between PD and atypical parkinsonian disorders in individual patients. A recent study by Alexon et al. used pattern recognition techniques (i.e., neural network and related data analyses) to analyze proton spectra in 15 patients with probable PD, 11 patients with possible PD, 5 patients with atypical PD, and 14 healthy age-matched controls *(27)*. In contrast to conventional analyses, all information within the proton spectrum can be entered in the statistical analysis simultaneously. The neuronal networks approach allowed them to distinguish between the four groups with considerable accuracy; approximately 88% of the predictions were correct. By contrast, conventional analysis revealed no significant differences in metabolite ratios among groups.

Proton MRS of the basal ganglia in conjunction with statistical analyses that take into account the pattern of the entire proton spectrum may help to distinguish PD from atypical parkinsonian disorders at initial presentation. Discriminative power may be further increased by using a multimodal imaging approach that combines MRS with other imaging techniques such as structural MRI or ^{18}F-6-fluorodopa PET.

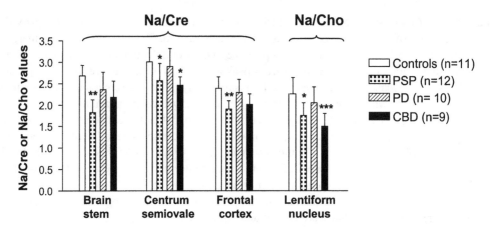

Fig 1. H-MRS findings in control subjects and patients with parkinsonian disorders.PSP, progressive supra-nuclear palsy; PD, Parkinson's disease; CBD, corticobasal degeneration. Columns and error bars present means ± SD. Asterisks indicate significant differences between controls and PSP patients and between controls and CBD ($^*p = 0.05$, $^{**}p < 0.01$, $^{***}p < 0.001$). The data were taken from Table 2 published in ref. *19*.

Phosphorus MRS provides information on levels of cerebral phospholipids and high-energy phosphates. The cerebral phosphorus spectra contains at least seven resonances that can be attributed to phosphomonoesters (PME), inorganic phosphate (Pi), phosphodiesters (PDE), phosphocreatine (PCr), and adenosine triphosphate (ATP). So far, only one group has used MRS to investigate the phosphorus spectra in 13 patients with PD and 15 patients with MSA *(28)*. Assuming a constant cytosolic concentration of ATP, Barbiroli et al. measured PCr and Pi and calculated cytosolic pH and free Mg^{2+} *(28)*. Compared with an age-matched control group, patients with PD showed a significant increase in Pi and a decrease in cytosolic free Mg^{2+}, whereas PCr was reduced and Pi was increased in patients with MSA. In the MSA group, there was no difference in the phosphorus spectra between the MSA-P and the MSA-C variants of MSA. A discriminant analysis that considered only the concentrations of PCr and Mg^{2+} provided a correct classification of MSA and PD patients in 93% of the cases. These preliminary data suggest that, in addition to proton MRS, phosphorus MRS may be useful to probe cerebral phosphate metabolism and ion contents in patients with atypical parkinsonian disorders.

DIFFUSION-WEIGHTED MAGNETIC RESONANCE IMAGING

Water diffusion-weighted MRI produces quantitative maps of microscopic displacement of water molecules that occur as part of the physical diffusion process. This is achieved by sensitizing the magnetic resonance signal to the random motion of water molecules by using strong magnetic field gradients. By varying the magnetic field gradient, one can obtain different degrees of diffusion-weighted images and calculate an apparent diffusion coefficient (ADC) for each voxel *(5)*.

Since diffusion of water molecules is highly sensitive to microstructural changes in the cerebral tissue, diffusion-weighted MRI has become a firmly established method to probe the functional integrity of brain tissue, especially in acute cerebral ischemia *(29)*. Diffusion-weighted MRI has a high sensitivity to detect structural abnormalities. However, it is important to bear in mind that diffusion-weighted MRI has a low specificity in terms of underlying pathophysiology since various mechanisms (e.g., edema, neurotoxicity, Wallerian degeneration) can affect the diffusion process in the cerebral tissue.

Three studies have characterized water diffusion in patients with atypical parkinsonian disorders. Patients with PSP showed an increase in ADCs in the prefrontal and precentral white matter *(30)* and the basal ganglia *(31,32)*. An increase in ADCs was also found in patients with the MSA-P variant of MSA *(32)*, but not in patients with PD *(31,32)*. These data indicate that diffusion-weighted imaging may help to distinguish between PD and atypical parkinsonian disorders, but fails to discriminate between PSP and MSA.

The microstructure of the brain tissue imposes directional constraints to the diffusion of water molecules in the brain (referred to as anisotropy). Diffusion is particularly anisotropic in white matter tracts because water preferentially diffuses along the direction of white matter fibres. Anisotropic diffusion is more adequately characterized by a diffusion tensor. A diffusion tensor is an array of nine coefficients that fully characterizes the directional properties of water diffusion in space.

Diffusion tensor-encoded MRI (DT-MRI) uses different gradient orientations to characterize the diffusion tensor in each voxel of the brain *(5)*. The diffusion tensor is often displayed as an elipsoid *(5)*. The average size of the ellipsoid represents the overall displacement of the water molecules in a given voxel (mean diffusivity). The eccentricity of the ellipsoid characterizes the degree of anisotropy. A sphere indicates isotropic diffusion whereas an elongated (cigar-shaped) or flat (pancake-shaped) ellipsoid indicates anisotropic diffusion. The main axis of the ellipsoid corresponds to the preferential direction of diffusion.

In the white matter, the main axis of the diffusion tensor is thought to represent the prevailing orientation of white matter bundles in each voxel. DT-MRI allows one to track white matter fibers by connecting neighboring voxels on the basis of their main direction of the diffusion tensor (i.e., main fiber orientation) *(33)*. Anisotropy measurements can be used to identify subtle abnormalities in the organization of white matter tracks that are not evident with plain, anatomical MRI *(34)*. However, it is worth bearing in mind that currently available DT-MRI techniques can only visualize white matter bundles that consist of a large number of axons, limiting fiber tracking to the white matter. Furthermore, DT-MRI can not probe the directional and functional status of the information flow along the white matter tracts. DT-MRI also has a considerable potential for functional mapping of subcortical gray matter. A recent study employed DT-MRI to differentiate the nuclei in the thalamus and to map their connectivity *(35)*.

Because DT-MRI provides a unique approach to tracking anatomical connectivity in vivo, DT-MRI can provide important new insights into the neuroanatomical basis of atypical parkinsonian disorders linking clinical symptoms with impaired anatomical connectivity. Though no DT-MRI study has been published on atypical parkinsonian disorders at this stage, it is safe to state that DT-MRI provides a promising tool to pinpoint characteristic patterns of abnormal connectivity, especially in CBD and MSA. This may be used to separate atypical parkinsonian disorders from PD.

MRI-BASED MORPHOMETRY

MRI-based volumetry of structural MR images can reveal the pattern of atrophic changes in patients with atypical parkinsonian syndromes. Using a region-of-interest (ROI) analysis, it has been shown that the patterns of atrophy in predefined regions of interest allow the separation PD from MSA and PSP *(36)* as well as PSP from CBD *(37)*. For instance, a recent study by Gröschel and colleagues demonstrated that the volumes of midbrain, parietal white matter, temporal gray matter, brainstem, frontal white matter, and pons separate best between patients with PSP or CBD *(37)*. A stepwise linear discriminant analysis resulted in two canonical discriminant functions, which allowed for the correct prediction of the diagnosis in 95% of healthy control subjects as well as in 76% of all PSP and 83% of all CBD patients *(37)*. The discriminant functions revealed similar results in patients with definite PSP/CBD and in patients with possible and probable PSP/CBD *(37)*. Prospective studies are now needed to show whether MRI-based volumetry will have clinical applicability.

In recent years, voxel-based morphometry (VBM) of structural MRI data has been introduced as a simple and objective approach for characterizing small-scale differences in white and gray matter *(36)*. VBM refers to a voxel-wise statistical comparison of the local concentration of gray (or white) matter between two groups of subjects. The procedure involves spatial normalization of high-resolution MR images into the same stereotactic space followed by segmentation of the gray (or white) matter. The smoothed gray matter segments are then compared using parametric statistical tests and the theory of Gaussian random fields *(38)*. Other voxel-based morphometric approaches, such as deformation-based or tensor-based morphometry, allow the study of regional differences in brain shapes between groups of subjects *(38)*. In contrast to conventional ROI analyses, VBM and related approaches provide whole-brain coverage and are highly sensitive to subtle structural changes within a single brain region. Since VBM is an automated procedure, the analysis is highly observer independent. Finally, VBM is not affected by partial volume effects. VBM cannot only be applied to high-resolution structural MRI, but VBM can also be used to investigate between-group differences of ADC maps or fractional anisotropy maps. This allows to screen for regional changes in neuronal integrity (i.e., VBM of ADC maps) or regional changes in fiber orientation (i.e., VBM of DT-weighted MRI).

FUTURE DIRECTIONS

Apart from proton MRS, none of the MRI approaches described in this chapter have yet been used to study the pathophysiology of atypical parkinsonian disorders. Therefore, the potential of these techniques for the diagnosis and research of atypical parkinsonian disorders remains to be defined. Based on the MRI experience gathered with other neuropsychiatric disorders, we anticipate that fMRI, MRS, and water diffusion MRI will significantly contribute to early diagnosis and advance our understanding of pathophysiological evolution of the different atypical parkinsonian disorders. Future advances in MR technology and new MR techniques (e.g., magnetization transfer technique) will further increase the diagnostic and research potential of MRI in parkinsonian disorders *(39)*.

It is important to bear in mind that these MRI techniques can readily be combined with each other and with high-resolution structural MRI. Indeed, multimodal MRI studies that combine structural and functional MR techniques represent the most promising approach to exploit MRI as a research tool. Since VBM of structural MRI images maps the pattern of structural abnormalities, VBM provides complementary anatomic information for the interpretation of altered neuronal activity as revealed by fMRI. The same applies for DT-MRI which, in combination with fMRI, might provide important clues to altered functional connectivity in patients with atypical parkinsonism. On an individual basis, interfacing fMRI with structural MRI and DT-MRI may considerably enhance diagnostic accuracy of MRI in the differential diagnosis of the atypical parkinsonian disorders.

ROLE OF FUNCTIONAL MAGNETIC RESONANCE IMAGING IN DIAGNOSIS AND RESEARCH OF ATYPICAL PARKINSONIAN SYNDROMES

A. Functional magnetic resonance imaging (fMRI)

Mapping the functional consequences of neurodegeneration
Assessing the effect of therapeutic interventions
Monitoring disease progression

B. Magnetic resonance spectroscopy (MRS)

Noninvasive characterization of regional abnormalities in tissue metabolism
Discrimination between PD and atypical parkinsonian syndromes

C. Diffusion-weighted magnetic resonance imaging (dMRI)

Probing for microstructural changes in the cerebral tissue (ADC-maps)
Mapping abnormalities in the organization of white matter tracts (DT-imaging)
PD, Parkinson's disease; ADC, apparent diffusion coefficient; DT, diffusion tensor.

REFERENCES

1. Turner R, Howseman A, Rees GE, Josephs O, Friston K. Functional magnetic resonance imaging of the human brain: data acquisition and analysis. Exp Brain Res 1998;123:5–12.
2. Logothetis NK. The neural basis of the blood-oxygen-level-dependent functional magnetic resonance imaging signal. Phil Trans R Soc Lond B 2002;357:1003–1037.
3. Rudkin TM, Arnold DL. Proton magnetic resonance spectroscopy for the diagnosos and management of cerebral disorders. Arch Neurol 1999;56:919–926.
4. Ross B, Bluml S. Magnetic resonance spectroscopy of the human brain. Anat Rec 2001;265:54–84.
5. Le Bihan D. Looking into the functional architecture of the brain with diffusion MRI. Nature Rev Neurosci 2003;4: 469–480.
6. Brooks DJ. Morphological and functional imaging studies on the diagnosis and progression of Parkinson´s disease. J Neurol 2000;247(Suppl 2):11–18.
7. Ceballos-Baumann AO. Functional imaging in Parkinson´s disease: activation studies with PET, fMRI and SPECT. J Neurol 2003;250(Suppl 1):15–23.
8. Ogawa S, Lee TM, Nayak As, Glynn P. Oxygenation-sensitive contrast in magnetic reonance image of rodent brain at high magnetic fields. Magn Resonance Med 1990;14:68–78.
9. Sabatini U, Boulanouar K, Fabre N, Martin F, Carel C, Colonnese C, et al. Cortical motor reorganization in akinetic patients with Parkinson's disease: a functional MRI study. Brain 2000;123:394–403.
10. Haslinger B, Erhard P, Kampfe N, Boecker H, Rummeny E, Schwaiger M, et al. Event-related functional magnetic resonance imaging in Parkinson's disease before and after levodopa. Brain 2001;124:558–570.
11. Buhmann C, Glauche V, Sturenburg HJ, Oechsner M, Weiller C, Buchel C. Pharmacologically modulated fMRI: cortical responsiveness to levodopa in drug-naive hemiparkinsonian patients. Brain 2003;126:451–461.
12. Rowe J, Stephan KE, Friston K, Frackowiak R, Lees A, Passingham R. Attention to action in Parkinson's disease: impaired effective connectivity among frontal cortical regions. Brain 2002;125:276–289.
13. Mattay VS, Tessitore A, Callicott JH, Bertolino A, Goldberg TE, Chase TN, et al. Dopaminergic modulation of cortical function in patients with Parkinson's disease. Ann Neurol 2002;51:156–164.
14. Brooks D. Diagnosis and management of atypical parkinsonian syndromes. J Neurol Neurosurg Psychiatry 2002;72(Suppl.1):i10–i16.
15. Davie CA, Wenning GK, Barker GJ, Tofts PS, Kendall BE, Quinn N, et al. Differentiation of multiple system atrophy from idiopathic Parkinson's disease using proton magnetic resonance spectroscopy. Ann Neurol 1995;37:204–210.
16. Holshouser BA, Komu M, Moller HE, Zijlmans J, Kolem H, Hinshaw DB Jr, et al. Localized proton NMR spectroscopy in the striatum of patients with idiopathic Parkinson's disease: a multicenter pilot study. Magn Reson Med. 1995;33:589–594.
17. Clarke CE, Lowry M, Horsamn A. Unchanged basal ganglia N-acetylaspartate and glutamate in idiopathic Parkinson´s disease as measured by proton magnetic resonance spectroscopy. Mov Dis 1997;12:297–301.
18. Federico F, Simone IL, Lucivero V, De Mari M, Giannini P, Iliceto G, et al. Proton magnetic resonance spectroscopy in Parkinson's disease and progressive supranuclear palsy. J Neurol Neurosurg Psychiatry. 1997;62:239–242.
19. Tedeschi G, Litvan I, Bonavita S, Bertolino A, Lundbom N, Patronas N J, et al. Proton magnetic resonance spectroscopic imaging in progressive supranuclear palsy, Parkinson's disease and corticobasal degeneration. Brain 1997;120:1541–1552.
20. Choe BY, Park JW, Lee KS, Son BC, Kim MC, Kim BS, et al. Neuronal laterality in Parkinson's disease with unilateral symptom by in vivo 1H magnetic resonance spectroscopy. Invest Radiol. 1998;33:450–455.
21. Hoang TQ, Bluml S, Dubowitz DJ, Moats R, Kopyov O, Jacques D, et al. Quantitative proton-decoupled 31P MRS and 1H MRS in the evaluation of Huntington's and Parkinson's diseases. Neurology 1998;50:1033–1040.
22. Hu MT, Taylor-Robinson SD, Chaudhuri KR, Bell JD, Morris RG, Clough C, et al. Evidence for cortical dysfunction in clinically non-demented patients with Parkinson's disease: a proton MR spectroscopy study. J Neurol Neurosurg Psychiatry 1999;67:20–26.
23. Lucetti C, Del Dotto P, Gambaccini G, Bernardini S, Bianchi MC, Tosetti M, et al. Proton magnetic resonance spectroscopy (1H-MRS) of motor cortex and basal ganglia in *de novo* Parkinson's disease patients. Neurol Sci 2001;22:69–70.
24. O'Neill J, Schuff N, Marks WJ Jr, Feiwell R, Aminoff MJ, Weiner MW. Quantitative 1H magnetic resonance spectroscopy and MRI of Parkinson's disease. Mov Disord 2002;17:917–927.
25. Summerfield C, Gomez-Anson B, Tolosa E, Mercader JM, Marti MJ, Pastor P, et al. Dementia in Parkinson disease: a proton magnetic resonance spectroscopy study. Arch Neurol. 2002;59:1415–1420.
26. Clarke CE, Lowry M. Basal ganglia metabolite concentrations in idiopathic Parkinson's disease and multiple system atrophy measured by proton magnetic resonance spectroscopy. Eur J Neurol 2000;7:661–665.
27. Axelson D, Bakken IJ, Susann Gribbestad I, Ehrnholm B, Nilsen G, Aasly J. Applications of neural network analyses to in vivo 1H magnetic resonance spectroscopy of Parkinson disease patients. J Magn Reson Imaging. 2002;16:13–20.
28. Barbiroli B, Martinelli P, Patuelli A, Lodi R, Iotti S, Cortelli P, et al. Phosphorus magnetic resonance spectroscopy in multiple system atrophy and Parkinson's disease. Mov Disord 1999;14:430–435.

29. Moseley ME, Kucharczyk J, Mintorovitch J, Cohen Y, Kurhanewicz J, Derugin N, et al. Diffusion-weighted MR-imaging of acute stroke.: correlation with T2-weighted an magnetic susceptibility-enhanced imaging in cats. Am L Neuroradiol 1990;11;423–429.
30. Oshiata T, Oka M, Imon Y, Yamaguchi S, Mimori Y, Nakamura S. Apparent diffusion coefficient measurements in progressive nuclear palsy. Neuroradiology 2000;42:643–647.
31. Schocke MF, Seppi K, Esterhammer R, Kremser C, Jaschke W, Poewe W, et al. Diffusion-weighted MRI differentiates the Parkinson variant of multiple system atrophy from PD. Neurology 2002;58:575–580.
32. Seppi K, Schocke MF, Esterhammer R, Kremser C, Brenneis C, Mueller J, et al. Diffusion-weighted imaging discriminates progressive supranuclear palsy from PD, but not from the parkinson variant of multiple system atrophy. Neurology 2003;60:922–927.
33. Conturo TE, Lori NF, Cull TS, Akbudak E, Snyder AZ, Shimony JS, et al. Tracking neuronal fibre pathways in the living human brain. Proc Natl Acad Sci USA 1999;96:10422–10427.
34. Sommer M, Koch MA, Paulus W, Weiller C, Buechel C. Disconnection of speech-relevant brain areas in persistent developmental stuttering. Lancet 2002;360:380–383.
35. Behrens TE, Johansen-berg H, Woolrich MW, Smith SM, Wheeler-Kingshott CA, Boulby PA, et al. Non-invasive mapping of connections between human thalamus and cortex using diffusion imaging. Nat Neurosci 2003;6:750–757.
36. Schulz JB, Skalej M, Wedekind D, Luft AR, Abele M, Voigt K, et al. Magnetic resonance imaging-based volumetry differentiates idiopathic Parkinson´s syndrome from multiple system atrophy and progressive supranuclear palsy. Ann Neurol 1999;45:65–74.
37. Gröschel K, Hauser TK, Luft A, Patronas N, Dichgans J, Litvan I, et al. Magnetic resonance imaging-based volumetry differentiates progressive supranuclear palsy from corticobasal degeneration. Neuroimage 2004;21:714–724.
38. Ashburner J, Friston K. Voxel-based morphometry—the methods. Neuroimage 2000;11:805–821.
39. Hanyu H, Asano T, Sakurai H, takasaki M, Shindo H, Abe K. Magnetisation transfer measurements of the subcortical grey and white matter in Parkinson´s disease with and without dementia in progressive nuclear palsy. Neuroradiology 2001;43:542–546.

27

PET and SPECT Imaging in Atypical Parkinsonian Disorders

Alexander Gerhard and David J. Brooks

In this chapter we discuss the roles of positron emission tomography (PET) and (single photon emission computed tomography (SPECT) in the diagnosis and pathological understanding of atypical parkinsonian disorders. We will concentrate on multiple system atrophy (MSA), progressive supranuclear palsy (PSP), and corticobasal degeneration (CBD), but also consider dementia with Lewy bodies (DLB).

INTRODUCTION

PET and SPECT are both imaging modalities using radioactively labeled tracers to image receptor binding, metabolic pathways or blood flow in the brain. PET relies on short-lived [11]C- and ^{18}F-based tracers prepared on site with the aid of a cyclotron and its resolution is usually better (~4–5 mm) than that of conventional SPECT cameras (~7–8 mm) but SPECT is cheaper and more widely available as it uses [123]I- and ^{99m}Tc-based tracers with longer half-lives that can be produced centrally.

Some PET and SPECT tracers in routine use and the parameters that they measure when used in the investigation of atypical parkinsonian disorders are listed in Table 1.

These relatively noninvasive techniques are unique in their ability to monitor the function of biological pathways in vivo. This is especially true for PET as positron-emitting radiotracers can usually be prepared without altering the chemical properties of the molecule—carbon and hydrogen atoms are ubiquitous in organic molecules and can be substituted by the positron emitting isotopes ^{11}C and [18]F—for a review, *see* ref. *1*.

PET and SPECT biomarkers allow us to image variations in receptor binding, activity of metabolic pathways, and perfusion in typical and atypical parkinsonian disorders and so characterize and diagnose these disorders. These imaging techniques are also well suited for longitudinal measurements.

A general caveat when defining the functional imaging characteristics of parkinsonian disorders is the fact that these disorders can be classified with a degree of certainty during life only based on consensus clinical criteria. It is well known that this clinical diagnosis may subsequently prove erroneous when compared retrospectively with autopsy findings (*see* Chapter 4).

The pathology of each disorder will briefly be described to the extent that is necessary to understand the principle of the PET and SPECT techniques with reference to the relevant chapters in this book.

From: *Current Clinical Neurology: Atypical Parkinsonian Disorders*
Edited by: I. Litvan © Humana Press Inc., Totowa, NJ

Table 1
Commonly Used PET and SPECT Tracers With the Receptors/Processes They Label In Vivo

PET

    ^{18}FDG—glucose metabolism

    $H_2^{15}O$—blood flow

    [^{18}F]dopa—marker of the ability (of the putamen and caudate) to decarboxylate exogenous levodopa
       and store the resultant dopamine

    [^{11}C]SCH23390—D1-type receptor binding

    [^{11}C]raclopride and [^{11}C]methylspiperone—D2-type receptor binding

    [^{11}C]diprenorphine—nonselective opioid binding

    [^{11}C] PK11195—marker of microglial activation

    [^{11}C]NM4PA and ^{11}C-physostigmine acetylcholinesterase levels

SPECT

    [^{123}I]β-CIT and [^{123}I]FP-CIT—dopamine transporter density

    [^{123}I]IBZM and [^{123}I]epidipride—D2 receptors

MULTIPLE SYSTEM ATROPHY

MSA is a sporadic neurodegenerative disease characterized by a progressive akinetic-rigid syndrome, cerebellar dysfunction, and autonomic insufficiency *(2)*. Typical histopathological changes consist of neuronal loss in the nigrostriatal and olivopontocerebellar pathways with α-synuclein positive, argyrophilic staining, glial cytoplasmic inclusions *(3)* associated with reactive astrocytes, and activated microglia *(4)*.

PET and SPECT have been used to assess the following aspects of the underlying pathology: metabolic changes, dopaminergic dysfunction, opioid dysfunction, and microglial activation.

In this chapter we use the terminology recommended by the most recent consensus statement *(2)* designating patients as MSA-P if parkinsonian features predominate and MSA-C if cerebellar features predominate. The consensus criteria have only been stringently applied in more recent papers; previously the less well-defined terms striatonigral degeneration (SND) and sporadic olivopontocerebellar atrophy (sOPCA) have been used to describe these forms of MSA.

Metabolic Changes

^{18}FDG PET measures regional cerebral glucose metabolism (rCMRGlc), reflecting primarily the function of nerve terminal synaptic vesicles. The metabolic rate in a given region, therefore, reflects the activity of afferent projections to and interneurons in a region rather than that of its efferent projections. It is currently not possible to decide whether increases in rCMRGlc detected with PET represent excitatory or inhibitory activity *(5)*.

A number of ^{18}FDG PET studies have investigated the changes in rCMRGlc in MSA. In patients with the parkinsonian type of MSA, decreases of rCMRGlc in the lentiform nuclei and brainstem have been described *(6–9)*. This contrasts with idiopathic Parkinson's disease (PD) where lentiform glucose metabolism is normal or slightly elevated *(10,11)*. On the basis of these reports ^{18}FDG PET seems to be able to discriminate 80–100% of MSA-P and idiopathic PD cases by comparing striatal rCMRGglc (Fig. 1).

MSA patients with cerebellar features show decreases in cerebellar rCMRGglc *(8,12)*, in some cases even without obvious cerebellar atrophy on MRI *(13)*. Glucose hypometabolism in frontal regions *(6)*—possibly owing to the degeneration of fiber systems connecting the cortex and basal ganglia—is apparent in more advanced patients but usually absent in early cases *(12,14)*.

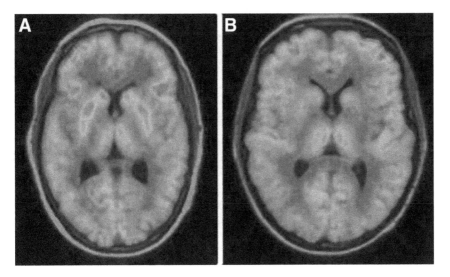

Fig. 1. Integrated images of ^{18}FDG uptake of (**A**) a healthy control person (**B**) a patient with probable MSA-P coregistered to the individual MRI (horizontal section); ^{18}FDG uptake is markedly reduced in the caudate and putamen of the MSA patient.

Dopaminergic Dysfunction

[^{18}F]-dopa is the most commonly used PET radiotracer for the study of striatal dopaminergic nerve terminal function in parkinsonism. [^{18}F]-dopa PET measures the rate of decarboxylation of [^{18}F]fluorodopa to [^{18}F]fluorodopamine by the enzyme dopa-decarboxylase and its subsequent storage in the striatal dopaminergic nerve terminals (presynaptic marker) *(15)*. [^{11}C]nomifensine is a marker of striatal monaminergic reuptake sites. Widely used presynaptic SPECT markers that bind to the striatal dopamine transporter (DAT) are the tropane derivatives [^{123}I]β-CIT and [^{123}I]FP-CIT.

The postsynaptic dopaminergic system has been studied with [^{11}C]SCH23390 (a PET D1 receptor ligand) and [^{11}C]raclopride and [^{123}I]IBZM (PET and SPECT D2 receptor ligands, respectively).

In patients with MSA-P, the function of both the pre- and postsynaptic dopamine system is impaired. Mean putaminal uptake of [^{18}F]-dopa , [^{11}C]nomifensine, and [^{123}I]β-CIT are reduced to ~50% of normal values *(16–18)* and individual levels of putaminal [^{18}F]-dopa uptake correlate with locomotor function (Fig. 2) *(16,19)*.

Pathological studies suggest that the substantia nigra is more uniformly affected in MSA than in PD where ventrolateral areas are targeted *(20,21)*. A number of studies using markers of presynaptic dopaminergic function have reported similar putamen reductions in MSA-P and PD but a greater reduction of uptake in the caudate nucleus in the former, a "relative sparing of caudate function" being observed in PD *(9,16,18)*. Other groups have not replicated this greater involvement of caudate dopaminergic function in MSA compared with PD and reported that caudate [^{18}F]-dopa Ki values are of limited value for discriminating between these disorders *(11,19)*.

Using formal discriminant analysis, Burn and coworkers were able to distinguish MSA-P from PD correctly in about 70% of cases with ^{18}F-dopa PET *(22)*, suggesting it is a less sensitive tool than FDG PET for the differential diagnosis of these disorders.

Studies on postsynaptic D2 receptor binding with [^{11}C]raclopride PET have found varying degrees of overlap between normals, PD, and MSA patients. Brooks and colleagues found a lesser decline of striatal [^{11}C]raclopride binding in L-dopa-resistant striatonigral degeneration than in chronically L-dopa-treated PD patients *(23)*. In other studies, patients with probable MSA-P have been more readily

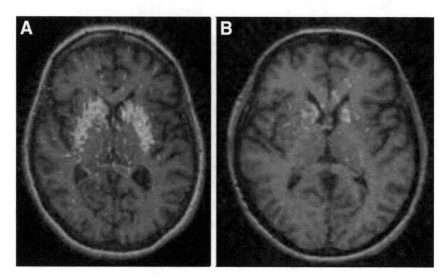

Fig. 2. Parametric Ki maps of [^{18}F]-dopa PET scans of (**A**) a healthy control person (**B**) a patient with probable MSA-P coregistered to the individual MRI (horizontal section) showing almost completely reduced Ki values in the caudate and putamen of the MSA patient.

discriminated from PD patients and normal controls showing reduced striatal *(19)* or putaminal *(11)* D2 binding. MSA putaminal D2 binding correlated with locomotor scores in one study *(19)*.

Similar results have been obtained with the D2 receptor marker [^{123}I]IBZM and SPECT, which correctly distinguished five out of seven patients with probable MSA from normals and PD patients on the basis of their decreased striatal D2-binding potential *(24)*. IBZM SPECT correctly predicts the response to dopaminergic medication in 70% of parkinsonian patients, those subjects having normal striatal IBZM uptake usually showing a good response. On follow up after 24–56 mo, the diagnosis of MSA-P and PD remained unaltered in the majority of these subjects *(25,26)*.

[^{123}I]β-CIT SPECT is a marker of dopamine transporter function and sensitively visualizes the presynaptic dopaminergic lesion in MSA-P patients, revealing a mean 50% reduction in striatal binding. However, a similar reduction is seen in PD and so [^{123}I]β-CIT SPECT is of limited value for distinguishing these disorders *(27)*. As expected, the differentiation of the disorders improves markedly when [^{123}I]β-CIT SPECT is combined with the marker of D2 receptors [^{123}I]iodobenzfuran SPECT *(24)*.

Opioid Dysfunction

Striatal projections to the external pallidum contain the opioid peptide enkephalin whereas those to the internal pallidum express dynorphin. The basal ganglia are rich in μ, κ, and δ opioid receptor subtypes.

[^{11}C]diprenorphine is a nonspecific opioid antagonist that binds with similar affinity to all three receptor subtypes. From autopsy studies it is known that metenkephalin levels in the striatum are reduced in MSA-P whereas they are preserved in PD *(28)*. Burn and colleagues were able to demonstrate in a small series that putaminal uptake of [^{11}C]diprenorphine was reduced in 50% of MSA-P patients but normal in nondyskinetic PD patients *(29)*.

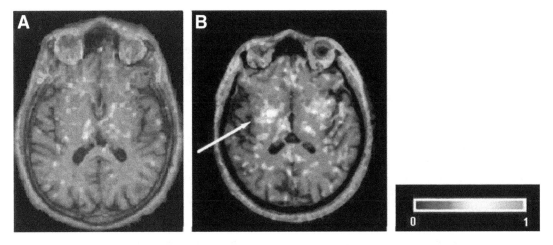

Fig. 3. Binding potential map for a patient with probable MSA-P (**B**) coregistered to the individual MRI. Increased [^{11}C]^{47}-PK11195 binding can be seen in the putamen and pallidum (indicated by the arrow). The color scale is callibrated for binding potential values from 0 to 1. White indicates values >1. Extracerebral binding has been masked. (**A**) Illustrates the typical distribution of binding in a 59-yr-old healthy volunteer in transverse view (BP map coregistered to the MRI).

Microglial Activation

In MSA, microglial activation has been described as part of the neuropathological process *(4)*. Microglia constitute 20% of glial cells and are ontogenetically related to cells of mononuclear-phagocyte lineage. They respond to brain injury by swelling and expressing cytokines and other immunologically relevant molecules and have been used as an early marker of active brain disease *(30)*. The mitochondria of activated microglia express *peripheral benzodiazepine binding sites* (PBBSs). PK11195 [1-(2-chlorophenyl)-*N*-methyl-*N*-(1-methylpropyl)-3-isoquinoline carboxamide] is a selective ligand for PBBSs *(31)* and, when labeled with [^{11}C], can be used as a PET tracer. In lesions without invading blood-borne cells, activated microglia are the primary source of PBBS expression *(32)*.

In five patients with probable MSA, we were recently able to detect increased [^{11}C]-PK11195 signal in the dorsolateral prefrontal cortex, caudate, putamen, pallidum, thalamus, pons, and substantia nigra (Fig. 3) *(33)*.

This pattern accords well with the known neuropathological distribution of microglial activation in MSA and provides information about the location of *active* disease. [^{11}C]-PK11195 PET seems to be a valuable tool to characterize the inflammatory component of the pathological process in MSA.

PROGRESSIVE SUPRANUCLEAR PALSY

Metabolic Studies

Neuropathological criteria for PSP include the accumulation of intraneuronal globose neurofibrillary tangles in and often atrophy of the following structures: pallidum and subthalamic nucleus, substantia nigra, pontine tegmentum, oculomotor and pontine nuclei, striatum, and prefrontal and precentral cortices *(34)*. These pathological findings have been reflected by changes in function observed in a number of PET and SPECT studies using ^{18}FDG or blood flow markers *(35–41)*. The studies reported ~25% decreases of regional cerebral metabolism in the frontal cortex, striatum, and thalamus.

Two more recent studies localized the metabolic changes in PSP using SPM (statistical parametric mapping) *(42)*, which explores focal changes in brain metabolism without having to make *a priori* hypotheses. This confirmed the earlier studies using region of interest analysis but highlighted the involvement of the frontal eye fields in premotor cortex *(43,44)*.

The decreases in frontal metabolism (hypofrontality) may reflect primary frontal cortical pathology but are more likely to arise because of pallidal degeneration since internal pallidal neurons project via the ventrolateral thalamus to premotor and prefrontal areas *(45)*.

Dopaminergic System

In PSP the nigrostriatal dopaminergic projections are uniformly affected and caudate and putamen dopamine content is equivalently reduced to 10–25 % of normal levels *(46,47)*.

The uniform degeneration of nigrostriatal dopaminergic projections is reflected by findings from PET and SPECT studies of the presynaptic dopaminergic system in PSP. The first [^{18}F]dopa PET study in PSP found a decrease in striatal dopamine formation and storage that correlated with disease severity but was unable to clearly separate caudate and putamen signals owing to the low 1.5-cm resolution of the PET camera *(36)*. Using higher-resolution cameras it became possible to show that, in contrast to PD, the Ki values in the PSP group were uniformly reduced in putamen and caudate to ~40% of normal values *(48)*. Applying discriminant analysis the differential involvement of the caudate [^{18}F]dopa uptake has allowed 90% of clinically probable PSP patients to be seperated from PD *(22)*. A similar difference in the degree of caudate involvement between PSP and PD was found using the PET dopamine transporter marker [^{11}C]-WIN 35,428 *(49)*. Another interesting application of [^{18}F]dopa PET has been the demonstration of reduced striatal [^{18}F]dopa uptake in 5 out of 15 asymptomatic members of a PSP kindred; one of these subjects developed clinical PSP 2 yr after the scan, thus indicating that [^{18}F]dopa PET has the ability to detect familial PSP preclinically *(43)*.

[^{123}I]β-CIT and FP-CIT SPECT have also been used in PSP to demonstrate presynaptic degeneration of dopamine terminals. Although it has been possible to demonstrate the "relative caudate sparing" in PD compared to PSP, especially in relatively early cases *(50,51)*, other groups have found these approaches of limited value in discriminating PSP from PD *(27)*.

D2 receptor binding in PSP patients has been examined as early as 1986 using the D2 antagonist [^{76}Br]bromospiperone *(52)*. A mean fall of 24% in equilibrium striatum/cerebellar uptake ratios was observed, but 50% of their PSP cases had striatal D2 binding within the normal range.

Brooks and colleagues studied nine PSP patients with [^{11}C]raclopride PET *(53)*; the PSP group showed 24% and 9% significant reductions of tracer caudate and putamen:cerebellar uptake ratios, and again only 50% of patients had individually reduced uptake ratios. In a larger series of 32 patients with probable PSP, 20 of these subjects showed reduced basal ganglia/frontal cortex [^{123}I-IBZM signal ratios, indicating a reduction of D2 receptors in approx two-thirds of PSP patients *(54)*. A smaller number of patients with probable PSP (*n* = 6) were scanned with the D2 marker [^{123}I]iodobenzfuran (IBF SPECT); 8% and 21% reductions of binding potential in the posterior putamen and caudate were found, which failed to reach statistical significance *(24)*.

These PET and SPECT findings of moderate reductions of striatal D2 receptor binding in PSP are in agreement with neuropatholgical findings reporting ~30% reductions in D2 density in the caudate and putamen of these patients *(55)*.

Cholinergic, Opioid, and Benzodiazepine Binding

Burn and colleagues examined striatal opioid binding in PSP *(29)*. [^{11}C]diprenorphine binding was reduced in all six PSP patients. Interestingly, caudate and putamen were equally affected, whereas in MSA-P patients caudate binding remained normal.

When using *N*-methyl-4-[^{11}C]piperidyl and PET to measure acetylcholinesterase (AChE) activity in 12 patients with PSP, Shinotoh and coworkers found a prominent reduction (–38%) of thalamic

AChE activity whereas the cortical activity was only slightly reduced *(56)*. Using ^{11}C-physostigmine PET, Pappata and colleagues have also reported reduced striatal AChE levels in PSP, which correlated with disability *(57)*.

A recent autoradiographic study in PSP *(58)* found degeneration of striatal cholinergic and dopaminergic terminals, whereas central benzodiazepine receptor binding remained unaffected. Since basal ganglia cholinergic terminals seem to degenerate in a selective manner in PSP, striatal VAChT (acetylcholine vesicular transporter) reduction may provide a unique neurochemical imaging marker for distinction of PSP from other types of basal ganglia neurodegeneration.

PET and [^{11}C]flumazenil (FMZ), a nonselective central benzodiazepine receptor antagonist, can be used to examine the density of benzodiazepine/$GABA_A$ receptors. Since probably all cortical neurons express $GABA_A$ receptors, the density of these receptors provides a measure of the integrity of intrinsic cerebral cortical neurons. In a group of 12 PSP patients, a slight reduction of [^{11}C]flumazenil was detected in the anterior cingulate gyrus but no other abnormalities were found *(59)*.

Although it is known from autoradiographic postmortem studies that benzodiazepine binding is reduced in the pallidum and preserved in the striatum of PSP patients *(58)*, the low expression of these receptors in the pallidum and proximity of the putamen probably make current functional imaging techniques too insensitive to detect these changes *(60)*.

CORTICOBASAL DEGENERATION

Metabolic Studies

In CBD there is a characteristic asymmetrical distribution of swollen ubiquitin- and tau-positive achromatic neurons in the posterior frontal, inferior parietal, and superior temporal cortical areas as well as in the thalamus, striatum, and substantia nigra *(61)*.

Over the last 12 yr a number of groups have examined regional cerebral oxygen metabolism (rCMRO2) *(62)* and rCMRGlc *(63–66)* in patients with clinically probable CBD. All these studies, which examined between five and eight patients each, found strikingly asymmetrical reductions in resting levels of brain function, with the hypometabolism being most evident in the brain hemisphere contralateral to the more affected limbs. Particularly targeted were the posterior frontal, inferior parietal, and superior temporal regions along with thalamus and striatum. Whereas these studies used a region of interest approach, Hosaka and colleagues recently performed a voxel-based comparison of rCMRGlc with statistical parametric mapping and essentially found a similar pattern of hypometabolism in their group of CBD patients *(44)*.

The pattern of decreased metabolic activity in frontal and parietal cortex and basal ganglia has also been shown with SPECT and the perfusion marker [99]Technetiumhexamethylpropylenamine (HMPAO) *(67)*. These changes were not only found in the hemisphere contralateral to the more affected body side but also ipsilaterally suggesting that the disease process is bilateral even at a stage when the clinical manifestations are unilateral.

Dopaminergic System

In CBD the substantia nigra is uniformly involved, which results in similar levels of dopamine loss in both caudate and putamen *(68)*.

Sawle and coworkers *(62)* found striatal ^{18}F-6-fluorodopa uptake was reduced in an asymmetric pattern, caudate and putamen being similarly involved in all six cases examined with the reduction being most pronounced contralateral to the clinically more affected limbs. Uptake into mesial frontal cortex was also halved, indicating that not only the nigrostratal but also the mesofrontal dopaminergic projections are impaired in this condition.

A subsequent report using [^{18}F]dopa PET confirmed Sawle's findings *(65)*, whereas Laureys and colleagues noted relatively minor caudate involvement in their early CBD cases *(69)*.

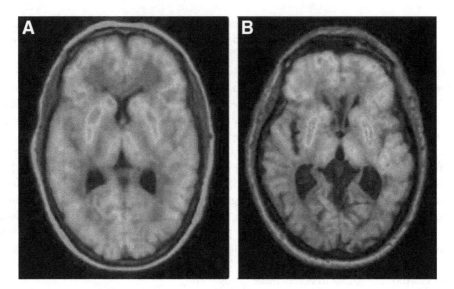

Fig. 4. Integrated images of [18]FDG uptake of (**A**) a healthy control person (**B**) a patient with dementia with Lewy bodies co-registered to the individual MRI (horizontal section); [18]FDG uptake is markedly reduced in the occipital lobe of the DLB patient.

Investigation of D2 receptor density with [^{123}I]IBZM and SPECT suggests a reduction in the striatum of CBD patients but has been restricted to a single case so far *(70)*.

DEMENTIA WITH LEWY BODIES

Metabolic Studies

DLB has not been examined as extensively with PET and SPECT as other atypical parkinsonian disorders. Albin and colleagues have reported the [18]FDG PET findings of six demented individuals with pathologically verified diffuse Lewy body disease *(71)*, three of whom had had pure DLB and three combined DLB and Alzheimer's disease (DLB-AD) pathology. These patients showed hypometabolism in association cortices with relative sparing of subcortical structures and primary somatomotor cortex, a pattern reported previously in AD. The main difference in comparison to patients with AD was the more pronounced hypometabolism in the occipital association cortex and primary visual cortex, indicating the presence of diffuse cortical abnormalities in DLB and suggesting that FDG-PET may possibly be useful in discriminating DLB from AD antemortem (Fig. 4).

This finding has been confirmed in larger series of 13 patients with DLB and 53 patients with AD *(72)*. Similar differences in brain perfusion patterns between DLB and AD have been found using [99m]Technetium labeled perfusion markers and SPECT *(73)*.

A direct metabolic comparison of patients with PD and DLB has not been performed to date to our knowledge; since occipital decreases in occipital metabolic activity has been described in PD *(74)* as well, it would be very interesting to determine whether occipital hypometabolism discriminates not only between DLB and AD but also between DLB and PD.

Dopaminergic System

The presynaptic system has been characterized in DLB using both PET and SPECT. Using [^{18}F]dopa PET, Hu and colleagues *(75)* described a reduction of striatal dopamine uptake in 6 patients with DLB whereas the values in the 10 AD patients were not significantly different from normal.

Table 2

Synopsis of the Characteristic PET and SPECT Findings in Different Parkinsonian Disorders

Imaging Modality and Measured Parameter	MSA-P	PSP	CBD	DLB	PD
FDG-PET (glucose metabolism in afferent projections and interneurons)	decreased in lentiform nucleus and frontal regions	decreased in striatum, thalamus, and frontal areas	decreased in striatum, thalamus, inferior parietal, and posterior frontal cortex; often asymmetric	decreased in occipital cortex	normal or slightly elevated in lentiform nucleus
F-dopa-PET (presynaptic dopa metabolism)	reduced in putamen ± caudate	reduced in putamen and caudate	reduced in caudate and putamen	reduced in caudate and putamen	reduced in putamen ± caudate
Raclopride-PET and IBZM SPECT (postsynaptic putaminal D2 receptor density)	low or normal	low or normal	low in striatum	?	normal or raised
Diprenorphine PET (opioid receptor density)	reduced in putamen	reduced in caudate and putamen	?	?	reduced in striatum of dyskinetic patients

Walker and coworkers have recently evaluated the integrity of the the nigrostriatal metabolism using the presynaptic marker ^{123}I-labeled 2'-carbomethoxy-3'-(4-iodophenyl)-N-(3-fluoropropyl)nortropane (FP-CIT), and SPECT in 27 patients with DLB, 17 with AD, 19 drug-naive PD patients, and 16 controls. There was a good seperation of the DLB and PD patients from AD patients and normals on the basis of the reduced striatal uptake ratios in these two groups whereas it was not possible to distinguish DLB and PD patients *(76)*. As the DLB cases were all rigid, however, and the AD cases were not, the FP-CIT SPECT may simply have been discriminating the parkinsonism rather than the type of dementia.

CONCLUSIONS

A general problem when examining parkinsonian disorders remains the fact that clinical criteria only allows one to diagnose these disorders with limited certainty. Only a few PET or SPECT series have later been compared with neuropathology, but clearly this is necessary to determine how sensitive and specific imaging modalities are when used for the purposes of differential diagnosis. Nevertheless, PET has been shown to be helpful in distinguishing around 80% of atypical parkinsonian disorders from idiopathic PD and, to a lesser extent, from each other by demonstrating different degrees and patterns of metabolic and dopaminergic impairment.

Table 2 gives a synopsis of the characteristic PET and SPECT findings in different parkinsonian disorders.

Since PET and SPECT have the unique ability to measure physiological and pathological parameters of brain metabolism and receptors, they are invaluable research tools given that they are relatively noninvasive and allow longitudinal examinations. The possibility of longitudinal measurements has been explored in atypical PD in only one β-CIT SPECT study so far *(77)*, demonstrating a more rapid degeneration of the nigrostriatal dopaminergic system in atypical parkinsonian disorders than in idiopathic PD.

For example, we are currently undertaking a longitudinal study comparing findings with serial [^{11}C][47]-PK11195 and ^{18}F-dopa PET in MSA and PD hoping to clarify the still largely hypothetical role of "neuroinflammatory" glial responses in neurodegenerative diseases. PET studies like this have the potential to elucidate the neuropathological processes in atypical parkinsonian disorders and will hopefully ultimately lead to better treatment options.

SUMMARY/ OUTLOOK

- PET and SPECT are unique imaging tools that allow to investigate physiological and pathological aspects of Parkinsonian disorders in vivo and longitudinally.
- Especially FDG PET is helpful in distinguishing atypical Parkinsonian disorders from idiopathic PD and from each other.
- Future research should be aimed at correlating different imaging modalities to each other and where possible to postmortem findings.
- The use of new PET markers for microglial activation and amyloid deposits for "in vivo pathology" will aid the development and evaluation of new therapies (e.g., of minocyline in MSA to suppress microglial activation).

REFERENCES

1. Cherry SR, Phelps ME. Imaging brain function with positron emission tomography. In: Toga AW, Mazziotta JC, eds. Brain Mapping: The Methods. San Diego: Academic, 1996:191–222.
2. Gilman S, Low PA, Quinn N, et al. Consensus statement on the diagnosis of multiple system atrophy. J Auton Nerv Syst 1998;74:189–192.
3. Lantos PL, Papp MI. Cellular pathology of multiple system atrophy: a review [Editorial]. J Neurol Neurosurg Psychiatry 1994;57:129–133.
4. Schwarz SC, Seufferlein T, Liptay S, et al. Microglial activation in multiple system atrophy: a potential role for NF-kappaB/rel proteins. Neuroreport 1998;9:3029–3032.
5. Jueptner M, Weiller C. Review: does measurement of regional cerebral blood flow reflect synaptic activity? Implications for PET and fMRI. Neuroimage 1995;2:148–156.
6. De Volder AG, Francart J, Laterre C, et al. Decreased glucose utilization in the striatum and frontal lobe in probable striatonigral degeneration. Ann Neurol 1989;26:239–247.
7. Eidelberg D, Takikawa S, Moeller JR, et al. Striatal hypometabolism distinguishes striatonigral degeneration from Parkinson's disease. Ann Neurol 1993;33:518–527.
8. Gilman S, Koeppe RA, Junck L, Kluin KJ, Lohman M, St Laurent RT. Patterns of cerebral glucose metabolism detected with positron emission tomography differ in multiple system atrophy and olivopontocerebellar atrophy. Ann Neurol 1994;36:166–175.
9. Otsuka M, Ichiya Y, Hosokawa S, et al. Striatal blood flow, glucose metabolism and 18F-dopa uptake: difference in Parkinson's disease and atypical parkinsonism. J Neurol Neurosurg Psychiatry 1991;54:898–904.
10. Antonini A, Vontobel P, Psylla M, et al. Complementary positron emission tomographic studies of the striatal dopaminergic system in Parkinson's disease. Arch Neurol 1995;52:1183–1190.
11. Ghaemi M, Hilker R, Rudolf J, Sobesky J, Heiss WD. Differentiating multiple system atrophy from Parkinson's disease: contribution of striatal and midbrain MRI volumetry and multi-tracer PET imaging. J Neurol Neurosurg Psychiatry 2002;73:517–523.
12. Perani D, Bressi S, Testa D, et al. Clinical/metabolic correlations in multiple system atrophy. A fludeoxyglucose F 18 positron emission tomographic study. Arch Neurol 1995;52:179–185.
13. Otsuka M, Ichiya Y, Kuwabara Y, et al. Glucose metabolism in the cortical and subcortical brain structures in multiple system atrophy and Parkinson's disease: a positron emission tomographic study. J Neurol Sci 1996;144:77–83.
14. Taniwaki T, Nakagawa M, Yamada T, et al. Cerebral metabolic changes in early multiple system atrophy: a PET study. J Neurol Sci 2002;200:79–84.
15. Firnau G, Sood S, Chirakal R, Nahmias C, Garnett ES. Cerebral metabolism of 6-[18F]fluoro-L-3,4-dihydroxyphenylalanine in the primate. J Neurochem 1987;48:1077–1082.
16. Brooks DJ, Salmon EP, Mathias CJ, et al. The relationship between locomotor disability, autonomic dysfunction, and the integrity of the striatal dopaminergic system in patients with multiple system atrophy, pure autonomic failure, and Parkinson's disease, studied with PET. Brain 1990;113:1539–1552.
17. Salmon E, Brooks DJ, Leenders KL, et al. A two-compartment description and kinetic procedure for measuring regional cerebral [11C]nomifensine uptake using positron emission tomography. J Cereb Blood Flow Metab 1990;10:307–316.

18. Brucke T, Asenbaum S, Pirker W, et al. Measurement of the dopaminergic degeneration in Parkinson's disease with [123I] beta-CIT and SPECT. Correlation with clinical findings and comparison with multiple system atrophy and progressive supranuclear palsy. J Neural Transm Suppl 1997;50:9–24.

19. Antonini A, Leenders KL, Vontobel P, et al. Complementary PET studies of striatal neuronal function in the differential diagnosis between multiple system atrophy and Parkinson's disease. Brain 1997;120:2187–2195.

20. Goto S, Hirano A, Matsumoto S. Subdivisional involvement of nigrostriatal loop in idiopathic Parkinson's disease and striatonigral degeneration. Ann Neurol 1989;26:766–770.

21. Fearnley JM, Lees AJ. Striatonigral degeneration. A clinicopathological study. Brain 1990;113:1823–1842.

22. Burn DJ, Sawle GV, Brooks DJ. Differential diagnosis of Parkinson's disease, multiple system atrophy, and Steele–Richardson–Olszewski syndrome: discriminant analysis of striatal 18F-dopa PET data. J Neurol Neurosurg Psychiatry 1994;57:278–284.

23. Brooks DJ, Ibanez V, Sawle GV, et al. Striatal D2 receptor status in patients with Parkinson's disease, striatonigral degeneration, and progressive supranuclear palsy, measured with 11C-raclopride and positron emission tomography. Ann Neurol 1992;31:184–192.

24. Kim YJ, Ichise M, Ballinger JR, et al. Combination of dopamine transporter and D2 receptor SPECT in the diagnostic evaluation of PD, MSA, and PSP. Mov Disord 2002;17:303–312.

25. Schwarz J, Tatsch K, Arnold G, et al. 123I-iodobenzamide-SPECT predicts dopaminergic responsiveness in patients with de novo parkinsonism. Neurology 1992;42:556–561.

26. Schwarz J, Tatsch K, Gasser T, et al. 123I-IBZM binding compared with long-term clinical follow up in patients with de novo parkinsonism. Mov Disord 1998;13:16–19.

27. Pirker W, Asenbaum S, Bencsits G, et al. [123I]beta-CIT SPECT in multiple system atrophy, progressive supranuclear palsy, and corticobasal degeneration. Mov Disord 2000;15:1158–1167.

28. Goto S, Hirano A, Matsumoto S. Met-enkephalin immunoreactivity in the basal ganglia in Parkinson's disease and striatonigral degeneration. Neurology 1990;40:1051–1056.

29. Burn DJ, Rinne JO, Quinn NP, Lees AJ, Marsden CD, Brooks DJ. Striatal opioid receptor binding in Parkinson's disease, striatonigral degeneration and Steele–Richardson–Olszewski syndrome, A [11C]diprenorphine PET study. Brain 1995;118:951–958.

30. Kreutzberg GW. Microglia: a sensor for pathological events in the CNS. Trends Neurosci 1996;19:312–318.

31. Banati RB, Newcombe J, Gunn RN, et al. The peripheral benzodiazepine binding site in the brain in multiple sclerosis: Quantitative in vivo imaging of microglia as a measure of disease activity. Brain 2000;123:2321–2337.

32. Banati RB, Myers R, Kreutzberg GW. PK ("peripheral benzodiazepine")—binding sites in the CNS indicate early and discrete brain lesions: microautoradiographic detection of [3H]PK11195 binding to activated microglia. J Neurocytol 1997;26:77–82.

33. Gerhard A, Banati RB, Goerres GB, et al. [11C](R)-PK11195 PET imaging of microglial activation in multiple system atrophy. Neurology 2003;61:686–689.

34. Hauw JJ, Daniel SE, Dickson D, et al. Preliminary NINDS neuropathologic criteria for Steele–Richardson–Olszewski syndrome (progressive supranuclear palsy). Neurology 1994;44:2015–2019.

35. D'Antona R, Baron JC, Samson Y, et al. Subcortical dementia. Frontal cortex hypometabolism detected by positron tomography in patients with progressive supranuclear palsy. Brain 1985;108:785–799.

36. Leenders KL, Frackowiak RS, Lees AJ. Steele–Richardson–Olszewski syndrome. Brain energy metabolism, blood flow and fluorodopa uptake measured by positron emission tomography. Brain 1988;111:615–630.

37. Johnson KA, Sperling RA, Holman BL, Nagel JS, Growdon JH. Cerebral perfusion in progressive supranuclear palsy. J Nucl Med 1992;33:704–709.

38. Otsuka M, Ichiya Y, Kuwabara Y, et al. Cerebral blood flow, oxygen and glucose metabolism with PET in progressive supranuclear palsy. Ann Nucl Med 1989;3:111–118.

39. Karbe H, Grond M, Huber M, Herholz K, Kessler J, Heiss WD. Subcortical damage and cortical dysfunction in progressive supranuclear palsy demonstrated by positron emission tomography. J Neurol 1992;239:98–102.

40. Goffinet AM, De Volder AG, Gillain C, et al. Positron tomography demonstrates frontal lobe hypometabolism in progressive supranuclear palsy. Ann Neurol 1989;25:131–9.

41. Foster NL, Gilman S, Berent S, Morin EM, Brown MB, Koeppe RA. Cerebral hypometabolism in progressive supranuclear palsy studied with positron emission tomography. Ann Neurol 1988;24:399–406.

42. Friston K, Holmes AP, Worsley KJ, Poline JP, Frith CD, Frackowiak R. Statistical parametric maps in functional imaging: a general linear approach. Hum Brain Mapp 1995;2:189–210.

43. Piccini P, de Yebenez J, Lees AJ, et al. Familial progressive supranuclear palsy: detection of subclinical cases using 18F-dopa and 18fluorodeoxyglucose positron emission tomography. Arch Neurol 2001;58:1846–1851.

44. Hosaka K, Ishii K, Sakamoto S, et al. Voxel-based comparison of regional cerebral glucose metabolism between PSP and corticobasal degeneration. J Neurol Sci 2002;199:67–71.

45. Alexander GE, DeLong MR, Strick PL. Parallel organization of functionally segregated circuits linking basal ganglia and cortex. Annu Rev Neurosci 1986;9:357–381.
46. Kish SJ, Chang LJ, Mirchandani L, Shannak K, Hornykiewicz O. Progressive supranuclear palsy: relationship between extrapyramidal disturbances, dementia, and brain neurotransmitter markers. Ann Neurol 1985;18:530–536.
47. Ruberg M, Javoy-Agid F, Hirsch E, et al. Dopaminergic and cholinergic lesions in progressive supranuclear palsy. Ann Neurol 1985;18:523–529.
48. Brooks DJ, Ibanez V, Sawle GV, et al. Differing patterns of striatal 18F-dopa uptake in Parkinson's disease, multiple system atrophy, and progressive supranuclear palsy. Ann Neurol 1990;28:547–555.
49. Ilgin N, Zubieta J, Reich SG, Dannals RF, Ravert HT, Frost JJ. PET imaging of the dopamine transporter in progressive supranuclear palsy and Parkinson's disease. Neurology 1999;52:1221–1226.
50. Messa C, Volonte MA, Fazio F, et al. Differential distribution of striatal [123I]beta-CIT in Parkinson's disease and progressive supranuclear palsy, evaluated with single-photon emission tomography. Eur J Nucl Med 1998;25:1270–1276.
51. Antonini A, Benti R, De Notaris R, et al. 123I-Ioflupane/SPECT binding to striatal dopamine transporter (DAT) uptake in patients with Parkinson's disease, multiple system atrophy, and progressive supranuclear palsy. Neurol Sci 2003;24: 149–150.
52. Baron JC, Maziere B, Loc'h C, et al. Loss of striatal [76Br]bromospiperone binding sites demonstrated by positron tomography in progressive supranuclear palsy. J Cereb Blood Flow Metab 1986;6:131–136.
53. Brooks DJ, Playford ED, Ibanez V, et al. Isolated tremor and disruption of the nigrostriatal dopaminergic system: an 18F-dopa PET study. Neurology 1992;42:1554–1560.
54. Arnold G, Schwarz J, Tatsch K, et al. Steele-Richardson-Olszewski-syndrome: the relation of dopamine D2 receptor binding and subcortical lesions in MRI. J Neural Transm 2002;109:503–512.
55. Pierot L, Desnos C, Blin J, et al. D1 and D2-type dopamine receptors in patients with Parkinson's disease and progressive supranuclear palsy. J Neurol Sci 1988;86:291–306.
56. Shinotoh H, Namba H, Yamaguchi M, et al. Positron emission tomographic measurement of acetylcholinesterase activity reveals differential loss of ascending cholinergic systems in Parkinson's disease and progressive supranuclear palsy. Ann Neurol 1999;46:62–69.
57. Pappata S, Traykov L, Tavitian B, et al. Striatal reduction of acetycholinesterase in patients with progressive supranuclear palsy (PSP) as measured in vivo by PET and ^{11}C-physiostigmine (^{11}C-PHY). J Cereb Blood Flow Metab 1997;17:687.
58. Suzuki M, Desmond TJ, Albin RL, Frey KA. Cholinergic vesicular transporters in progressive supranuclear palsy. Neurology 2002;58:1013–1018.
59. Foster NL, Minoshima S, Johanns J, et al. PET measures of benzodiazepine receptors in progressive supranuclear palsy. Neurology 2000;54:1768–1773.
60. Eidelberg D, Dhawan V. Can imaging distinguish PSP from other neurodegenerative disorders? Neurology 2002;58:997–998.
61. Gibb WR, Luthert PJ, Marsden CD. Corticobasal degeneration. Brain 1989;112:1171–1192.
62. Sawle GV, Brooks DJ, Marsden CD, Frackowiak RS. Corticobasal degeneration. A unique pattern of regional cortical oxygen hypometabolism and striatal fluorodopa uptake demonstrated by positron emission tomography. Brain 1991;114:541–556.
63. Eidelberg D, Dhawan V, Moeller JR, et al. The metabolic landscape of cortico-basal ganglionic degeneration: regional asymmetries studied with positron emission tomography. J Neurol Neurosurg Psychiatry 1991;54:856–862.
64. Blin J, Vidailhet MJ, Pillon B, Dubois B, Feve JR, Agid Y. Corticobasal degeneration: decreased and asymmetrical glucose consumption as studied with PET. Mov Disord 1992;7:348–354.
65. Nagasawa H, Tanji H, Nomura H, et al. PET study of cerebral glucose metabolism and fluorodopa uptake in patients with corticobasal degeneration. J Neurol Sci 1996;139:210–217.
66. Nagahama Y, Fukuyama H, Turjanski N, et al. Cerebral glucose metabolism in corticobasal degeneration: comparison with progressive supranuclear palsy and normal controls. Mov Disord 1997;12:691–696.
67. Markus HS, Lees AJ, Lennox G, Marsden CD, Costa DC. Patterns of regional cerebral blood flow in corticobasal degeneration studied using HMPAO SPECT; comparison with Parkinson's disease and normal controls [see comments]. Mov Disord 1995;10:179–187.
68. Riley DE, Lang AE, Lewis A, et al. Cortical-basal ganglionic degeneration. Neurology 1990;40:1203–1212.
69. Laureys S, Salmon E, Garraux G, et al. Fluorodopa uptake and glucose metabolism in early stages of corticobasal degeneration. J Neurol 1999;246:1151–1158.
70. Frisoni GB, Pizzolato G, Zanetti O, Bianchetti A, Chierichetti F, Trabucchi M. Corticobasal degeneration: neuropsychological assessment and dopamine D2 receptor SPECT analysis. Eur Neurol 1995;35:50–54.
71. Albin RL, Minoshima S, D'Amato CJ, Frey KA, Kuhl DA, Sima AA. Fluoro-deoxyglucose positron emission tomography in diffuse Lewy body disease. Neurology 1996;47:462–466.
72. Minoshima S, Foster NL, Sima AA, Frey KA, Albin RL, Kuhl DE. Alzheimer's disease versus dementia with Lewy bodies: cerebral metabolic distinction with autopsy confirmation. Ann Neurol 2001;50:358–365.

73. Donnemiller E, Heilmann J, Wenning GK, et al. Brain perfusion scintigraphy with 99mTc-HMPAO or 99mTc-ECD and 123I-beta-CIT single-photon emission tomography in dementia of the Alzheimer-type and diffuse Lewy body disease. Eur J Nucl Med 1997;24:320–325.

74. Hu MT, Taylor-Robinson SD, Chaudhuri KR, et al. Cortical dysfunction in non-demented Parkinson's disease patients: a combined (31)P-MRS and (18)FDG-PET study. Brain 2000;123:340–352.

75. Hu XS, Okamura N, Arai H, et al. 18F-fluorodopa PET study of striatal dopamine uptake in the diagnosis of dementia with Lewy bodies. Neurology 2000;55:1575–1577.

76. Walker Z, Costa DC, Walker RW, et al. Differentiation of dementia with Lewy bodies from Alzheimer's disease using a dopaminergic presynaptic ligand. J Neurol Neurosurg Psychiatry 2002;73:134–140.

77. Pirker W, Djamshidian S, Asenbaum S, et al. Progression of dopaminergic degeneration in Parkinson's disease and atypical parkinsonism: a longitudinal beta-CIT SPECT study. Mov Disord 2002;17:45–53.

28

Current and Future Therapeutic Approaches

Elmyra V. Encarnacion and Thomas N. Chase

INTRODUCTION

Approaches to the pharmacotherapy of the "atypical" parkinsonian or "Parkinson plus" disorders have, as yet, met with little success. Drugs attempting to replace or mimic specific neurotransmitters are relatively ineffective, as evidenced, for example, by the inconsistent response rates to dopamine (DA) replacement by the administration of levodopa. This variable and modest efficacy contrasts with the predictable and significant benefit obtained with dopaminomimetics in Parkinson's disease (PD); in this case, core symptoms arise from the loss of a single transmitter system. By contrast, clinical disability in the atypical parkinsonian disorders reflects more diffuse neuronal damage and multiple neurotransmitter involvement. Nigral dopaminergic neurons degenerate, but so do serotonergic, noradrenergic, and cholinergic neurons. Replacing DA thus can improve parkinsonian rigidity and bradykinesia, but the overall benefit is poor and generally disappears with disease progression. Studies of drugs targeting cholinergic and other monoaminergic systems have usually reported disappointing results. On the other hand, there is a paucity of well-controlled trials of single transmitter replacement strategies, and clinical studies that systematically address multiple system deficiencies are virtually unknown. Indeed, whether a transmitter replacement strategy can be effective in the symptomatic treatment of the Parkinson plus disorders remains uncertain. However, current neurosciences research is providing rapidly increasing insight into the pathogenesis of PD and atypical parkinsonian disorders. With this new understanding comes the possibility of discovering interventions that will slow or stop disease progression. Progress in the search for radiologic and biochemical surrogate markers promises not only earlier and more definitive diagnosis but also efficient and more reliable therapeutic trials.

For the purpose of this review, the atypical parkinsonian disorders have been categorized as follows: (a) multiple system atrophy (MSA), further grouped into MSA-C, previously called olivopontocerebellar atrophy, OPCA; MSA-A, previously called Shy–Drager, SD; MSA-P, previously called striatonigral degeneration SND; (b) progressive supranuclear palsy (PSP); (c) corticobasal degeneration (CBD); and (d) dementia with lewy bodies (DLB). An initial analysis of current therapeutic approaches, based on clinical trial results published since 1980 and organized by the major neurotransmitter system targeted, will be followed by consideration of possible directions for future therapeutic research.

From: *Current Clinical Neurology: Atypical Parkinsonian Disorders*
Edited by: I. Litvan © Humana Press Inc., Totowa, NJ

PARKINSONISM AND MOVEMENT DISORDERS

Dopaminergic

Since degeneration of the nigrostriatal system occurs in all parkinsonian disorders, drugs targeting the principal transmitter deficiency, DA, remain the treatment of choice for associated motor dysfunction, especially rigidity and bradykinesia. Positron emission tomography (PET) studies have shown decreased striatal 18flourodopa uptake and decreased striatal regional blood flow indicative of the loss of nigral dopaminergic neurons (1,2). Moreover, a preferential loss of postsynaptic DA-D2 receptors in the posterior putamen occurs in relation to levodopa resistance, suggesting the additional degeneration of striatal spiny neurons (3,4). Similarly, 123I-iodobenzamide (IBZM) single photon emission computed tomography (SPECT) studies indicate lower mean striatal DA-D2 receptor binding in patients with atypical parkinsonian disorders than in those with PD (5). A comparison using [123I]β-CIT SPECT reveals a reduction of striatal DA transporter density in parkinsonian disorders, including PD (6–8), but long-term studies have shown a more rapid decline in the atypical disorders; in MSA and PSP putamen-caudate nucleus ratios are reduced and in CBD there is an increase in binding asymmetry (9).

In MSA, analyses of 203 pathologically proven cases indicated that although the overall response to levodopa was poor, some patients might initially respond well (10). Indeed, response rates reported for levodopa range from 33% up to 68% (11,12). As striatal degeneration occurs, receptor sites for the postsynaptic activity of DA produced by levodopa treatment declines, and thus clinical efficacy consequently fades, leaving only supportive measures for later-stage patients. Those enjoying good response may develop levodopa-induced axial, orofacial, and limb dyskinesias of the dystonic or choreiform type (10,13). In general, DA agonists are no more effective than levodopa, although an open-label evaluation on apomorphine, the most potent dopamine agonist, suggested some motor benefit in patients with MSA (14). Uncontrolled studies of bromocriptine (10–80 mg) also noted benefit (15), whereas evaluations of pergolide yielded inconsistent results (16). A controlled trial of lisurude (up to 2.4 mg per day) observed improvement in one (who was also levodopa responsive) out of seven patients (17).

In PSP, local cerebral blood flow (LCBF) using xenon-enhanced computed tomography reveal lower striatal baseline values and no increase following the intravenous administration of levodopa compared to PD (18). Extensive degeneration of downstream basal ganglia structures may account for levodopa-unresponsive motor dysfunction (19). Thus, a review of 12 pathologically proven cases of PSP indicated that one-third of the patients had modest, but nonsustained, improvement while receiving levodopa with a peripheral decarboxylase inhibitor (20). Similarly, a retrospective review of clinically diagnosed cases showed that 54% had mild to moderate improvement with levodopa (21). Reports on dopamine agonists appear to be even more negative. Pramipexole (4.5 mg daily) for 2 mo was not effective (22), and lisuride (mean daily dose of 2.5 mg) provided no overall benefit when used alone and in combination with levodopa (23). Dyskinesias and other side effects are rare, with only isolated cases of levodopa-induced oromandibular dystonia, dyskinesia, and apraxia of eyelid opening (24–26).

A review of 14 pathologically proven CBD cases found that virtually all developed asymmetric or unilateral akinetic-rigid parkinsonism and gait disorder, and that none had a dramatic response to levodopa therapy (27). A chart review of 147 clinically diagnosed CBD patients from eight major movement disorders centers noted that 92% received some kind of dopaminergic medication, specifically levodopa with a peripheral decarboxylase inhibitor (87%), bromocriptine or pergolide (25%), and selegiline (20%) (28). Overall, clinical improvement occurred in 24% receiving any of these dopaminergic agents, with levodopa being the most effective drug given at a median dose of 300 mg and ranging from 100 to 2000 mg. Dopamine agonists (pergolide and bromocriptine) and selegiline were less successful, producing 6% and 10% benefit, respectively. Parkinsonian signs improved the most, and dyskinesias were not observed even with high-dose levodopa. Side effects included drug-associated worsening of parkinsonism, dystonia, myoclonus, and gait dysfunction, whereas nonmotor side effects included gastrointestinal complaints, confusion, somnolence, dizziness, and hallucinations. A relative failure or lack of efficacy of dopaminergic therapy in a parkinsonian patient with cortical dysfunction should raise the suspicion of CBD.

Cholinergic

Cholinergic neuronal depletion *(29,30)* as well as reductions in such enzymatic markers as cholineacetyltransferase *(31–33)* and acetylcholinesterase *(33)* occur in the atypical parkinsonian disorders, although with differences in the degree and distribution of affected neurons. For example, several cholinergic nuclei undergo degeneration in PSP *(32,34,35)*, whereas immunohistochemical analyses of autopsy material indicate that in CBD the forebrain cholinergic system is more vulnerable than the midbrain *(36)*. The generalized loss of striatal cholinergic interneurons accounts for observed reduction in DA-D2 receptors *(37)* and thus the ineffectiveness of dopaminergic drugs in PSP. Unfortunately, cholinergic replacement therapy alone has been no more effective in palliating symptoms, secondary to the severity of cholinergic deficits and the more widespread impairment of monoaminergic systems in PSP *(38)*.

In patients with PSP, cholinergic stimulation by intravenous physostigmine had no significant motor or neurobehavioral effects at any dose, whereas cholinergic blockade by intravenous scopolamine, in low and medium doses, impaired memory performance in PSP patients as well as normal individuals and exacerbated gait disability in some patients *(39)*. Similarly, controlled trials of orally administered physostigmine failed to benefit any of the motor functions tested *(40,41)*. An open study of the acetylcholinesterase inhibitor, donepezil, lasting 3 mo also did not appear to improve cognitive dysfunction or activities of daily living *(38)*. A controlled trial of donepezil in 21 PSP patients did, however, suggest modest benefit in some cognitive measures but worsened mobility scores *(42)*. The effect of donepezil on motor dysfunction ranges from none *(38)* to deleterious *(42)*. Similarly, the direct cholinergic agonist RS-86 did not improve motor function, eye movements, or psychometric performance in a controlled trial in 10 PSP patients *(43)*.

In clinically diagnosed CBD cases, 27% received anticholinergics, which briefly benefited some individuals but were often poorly tolerated *(28)*.

Adrenergic, Serotoninergic, GABAergic, Glutamatergic

Neurotransmitter systems downstream from the degenerating nigrostriatal dopaminergic pathway have also been targeted therapeutically. The rationale for these pharmacological interventions parallels that for DA replacement, i.e., the restoration of transmitter function, lost as a consequence of the degenerative process.

Adrenergic system dysfunction occurs in atypical parkinsonian disorders and could contribute to clinical disability. For example, there is degeneration of the locus ceruleus in PSP, where quantitative autoradiographic analysis of tissue sections shows a dramatic reduction in α-2 adrenoceptor density compared to controls *(44)*. Nevertheless, a randomized blinded study revealed that the α-2 adrenergic antagonist idazoxan improved balance and manual dexterity in about half of PSP patients *(45)*, whereas a similarly designed evaluation of efaroxan, another potent α-2 antagonist, did not significantly alter any of the assessed measures of motor function *(46)*.

The effect of serotoninergic drugs in the atypicals has not been extensively studied. Open-label evaluations suggested methysergide, a serotonin 5HT2 receptor antagonist that blocks the facilitatory effects of raphe stimulation on bulbospinal neurons, affords relief to some PSP patients when used alone or in combination with antiparkinsonian agents *(47,48)*; marked improvement was reported in patients with severe dysphagia *(48)*. These studies, however, have not been replicated, and methysergide is no longer being used owing to its clear side effects (e.g., retroperitoneal fibrosis).

γ-Aminobutyric acid (GABA) system function has been assessed in the atypical parkinsonian disorders using PET with [^{11}C]flumazenil. GABA-type A/benzodiazepine receptor binding appears to be decreased in the brainstem and cerebellum of MSA patients with MSA-C, but not in MSA-A syndrome; however, binding still remains largely preserved in the cerebral hemispheres, basal ganglia, thalamus, and brainstem as well as cerebellum in both MSA groups compared to normal controls *(49)*. Results from a randomized blinded study of vigabatrin, an irreversible inhibitor of GABA-transaminase, given to patients with MSA-C at a daily oral dose of 2–4 g for 4 mo, indicate that agents that increase central GABA concentrations are unlikely to confer symptomatic benefit *(50)*.

In PSP, PET studies revealed a 13% global reduction in [^{11}C]flumazenil binding, particularly in the anterior cingulate gyrus *(51)*, and a reduced density of GABA neurons was seen in the caudate nucleus, ventral striatum, and internal and external pallidum *(52)*. A controlled study of zolpidem, a hypnotic with putative GABA-A receptor agonist activity, at doses of 5–10 mg, found improvement in parkinsonian signs (>20% improvement), dysarthria, and eye movements, although sedation appeared at the highest dose *(53)*. In clinically diagnosed CBD, benzodiazepines, primarily clonazepam, reportedly improves myoclonus (23%) and dystonia (9%) *(28)*, whereas clinical experience suggests that baclofen and tizanidine can have a modest beneficial effect on rigidity and tremor *(54)*.

Possible involvement of glutamatergic systems in the atypical parkinsonian syndromes has been little explored, although some studies have addressed the therapeutic efficacy of drugs purporting to inhibit glutamate receptors of the *N*-methyl-D-aspartate (NMDA) type. For example, an uncontrolled study of the NMDA antagonist, amantadine, in eight patients with MSA-C lasting on average for over 40 mo suggested improved performance on measures of reaction and movement time *(55)*. On the other hand, a short-term pilot study of amantadine at relatively high doses (400–600 mg/d) failed to find consistent benefit *(56)*. Nevertheless, a salutatory response was observed in a blinded and controlled study involving 30 MSA-C patients that used lower doses of amantadine (200 mg/d) for 3–4 mo *(57)*. Amantadine is neither much used nor very effective in patients with CBD *(28)*.

Others

Tricyclics

A blinded trial of amitriptyline, a norepinephrine and serotonin reuptake blocker, beginning at 25 mg at bedtime and increasing to 50 mg in a week or two as needed, showed modest benefit in gait *(58)*.

Botulinum Toxin

Dystonia can be a disabling feature in at least a third of CBD cases *(28,59)* as well as in other atypical parkinsonian disorders. Open-label studies of botulinum toxin (BTx)-A injections suggest that the treatment of limb dystonia depends on the severity of the deformity and degree of contractures *(60)*, temporarily improving hand and arm function in early disease, while reducing pain, facilitating hygiene, and preventing secondary contractures in more advanced stages *(61)*. BTx-A also reportedly improved orofacial dystonia using clinical and electromyogram (EMG) examinations as outcome measures *(61)*, and can be particularly effective in the relief of blepharospasm and PSP-associated retrocollis *(61)*, and apraxia of eyelid opening *(62)*. Adverse effects are generally mild and transient, although severe dysphagia has been reported, with onset a few days after treatment and persisting for several months *(63)*.

Neurosurgical Approaches

Stereotactic procedures, such as pallidotomy or pallidal/subthalamic nucleus (STN) stimulation, have had limited success in the atypical parkinsonian disorders *(64)*, and are not generally recommended. On the other hand, bilateral STN stimulation reportedly benefited rigidity and akinesia in four MSA patients *(65)*. Neural transplantation approaches are currently being explored in the atypicals, although beset by the same methodological and ethical issues associated with these procedures in PD. A placebo-controlled study is under way to assess the safety, tolerability, and efficacy of glial cell-derived neurotrophic factor (GDNF) continuously infused directly into striatum on motor dysfunction in PSP patients.

Electroconvulsive Therapy (ECT)

ECT appeared to improved motor signs in five PSP patients after nine treatments, although treatment-induced confusion and prolonged hospitalization limit the usefulness of this technique *(66)*.

AUTONOMIC DYSFUNCTION

Most studies of autonomic dysfunction in atypical parkinsonian disorders focus on MSA, where this feature is far more common than in CBD, PSP, or DLB. Neuropathological studies reveal neuronal loss in central adrenergic pathways, especially catecholaminergic neuron depletion in the rostral ventrolateral medulla, but not in the sympathetic ganglia *(67,68)*. Asymptomatic orthostatic hypotension generally does not require treatment in MSA, since autoregulation seems preserved down to a systolic blood pressure of 60 mmHg, a value well below the 80 mmHg at which autoregulation fails in normal subjects *(69)*.

For symptomatic orthostatic hypotension, fludrocortisone, acting through expanding plasma volume and reducing natriuresis, and midodrine, an α-1 adrenoreceptor agonist, generally appear to be the treatments of choice. A large, randomized, controlled trial showed that midodrine reduced orthostatic hypotension by increasing peripheral resistance *(70)*. Midodrine can be initiated at 2.5 mg three times a day, increased up to 10 mg three times a day, if needed, whereas fludrocortisone, which has never been studied formally, is usually started at .1 mg daily, and increased to a maximum of four tablets per day in two or three divided doses *(62)*. A placebo-controlled trial in 35 patients comparing the pressor effects of phenylpropanolamine (12.5 mg and 25 mg), yohimbine (5.4 mg), indomethacin (50 mg), ibuprofen (600 mg), caffeine (250 mg), and methylphenidate (5 mg) on seated systolic blood pressure showed a significant pressor response with phenylpropanolamine, yohimbine, and indomethacin; comparison of phenylpropanolamine (12.5 mg) and midodrine (5mg) in a subgroup of patients elicited similar effects *(71)*.

In an uncontrolled, dose-ranging study of L-threo-dihydroxyphenylserine, 100, 200, and 300 mg twice daily were well tolerated, and the 300-mg dose seemed to offer the most effective control of symptomatic orthostatic hypotension (72). Similar results were observed when 60° head-up-tilt was performed after the daily oral administration of 300 mg L-threo-dihydroxyphenylserine for 2 wk *(73)*. A small, open evaluation of chronic subcutaneous octreotide at 100 µg three times a day also suggested functional improvement *(74)*. Furthermore, isolated cases include treatment with vasopressin in refractory hypotension *(75)* and erythropoietin in those with anemia *(76)*.

Urinary problems also commonly afflict those with atypical parkinsonian syndromes. α1-adrenergic receptors are present in the proximal urethra where impaired relaxation may be responsible for difficulty voiding and increased residual urine. An uncontrolled study showed that α1-adrenergic antagonists, prazosin (nonselective) and moxisylyte (selective), reduced residual urine volume, although side effects related to orthostatic hypotension were common in those with postural hypotension of more than −30 mmHg *(77)*. An open study suggested that desmopressin at night may reverse nocturia *(78)*. For incontinence, peripherally acting anticholinergics, such as tolterodine, oxybutynin, and propiverene, are used, albeit at the expense of causing retention *(79)*. Although no formal studies have been done on these drugs, recommended doses are tolterodine 2–4 mg at bedtime or twice daily, oxybutinin 5–10 mg at bedtime, or propantheline 15–30 mg at bedtime if the pathophysiology involves detrusor hyperreflexia *(62)*.

Other common autonomic disturbances include erectile dysfunction and constipation. A randomized controlled study showed that sildenafil citrate (50 mg) is efficacious in the treatment of impotence, but may unmask or exacerbate preexisting hypotension *(80)*; measurement of orthostastic blood pressure is thus recommended prior to the administration of this drug. General recommendations for constipation are a high-fiber diet, and over-the-counter laxatives or lactulose. In an open evaluation, macrogol 3350 was found to diminish constipation *(81)*. Open-label studies have also suggested that subcutaneous bethanechol chloride, a muscarinic receptor agonist, improves tearing, salivation, sweating, gastrointestinal, and bladder functions *(82)*, whereas sublingual atropine benefits sialorrhea, although with such side effects as delirium and hallucinations *(83)*. Anticholinergics also risk exacerbating confusion and constipation as well as preexisting prostatism and glaucoma.

COGNITIVE DYSFUNCTION

Cholinergic

Drugs enhancing central cholinergic function provide a rational approach to the treatment of cognitive dysfunction associated with the Parkinson plus disorders. In PSP, however, a controlled trial of physostigmine showed only borderline changes in long-term memory *(41)*, although improved visual attention has been reported *(92)*. An open study of donepezil did not appear to ameliorate cognitive dysfunction *(38)*, whereas a controlled trial suggested modest benefit in some cognitive measures but worsened mobility scores *(42)*. A controlled trial on the direct cholinergic agonist RS-86 revealed comparable unsatisfactory results *(43)*.

DLB is attended by brain cholinergic deficits such as an early loss of cholinacetyltransferase activity *(93)* as well reductions in hippocampal muscarinic and nicotinic receptors *(94)*. An uncontrolled assessment of the cholinesterase inhibitor, rivastigmine, suggested improvement after 24 wk of treatment in cognition, activities of daily living, and behavioral and psychiatric symptoms measured by the Neuropsychiatric Inventory *(95)*. A subsequent placebo-controlled study observed similarly benefits with rivastigmine (6–12 mg daily) on behavior and cognition, with most parameters of cognitive performance returning to pretreatment levels after 3 wk of drug discontinuation *(96)*. Prospective studies on donepezil, another cholinesterase inhibitor, also found improvement in cognitive and noncognitive symptoms, without a worsening of motor function *(97,98)*. Cholinergic replacement therapy should thus be considered in DLB patients.

On the other hand, the use of drugs that possess anticholinergic activity, such as tricyclic antidepressants, risk worsening confusion *(28)*.

BEHAVIORAL DYSFUNCTION

Dopaminergic and Serotoninergic

Classical antipsychotic drugs that potently block dopaminergic receptors can ameliorate psychotic symptoms but worsen parkinsonism, at times seriously enough to require levodopa *(84)*. Better results in treating psychosis have been obtained with the atypical neuroleptics, possibly owing to their predominant antiserotoninergic rather than antidopaminergic activity. An extensive chart review revealed that 90% of DLB patients had partial to complete resolution of psychosis using long-term quetiapine, although in 27% motor worsening was noted at some point during treatment *(85)*. A large, randomized blinded trial found that olanzapine (5 or 10 mg) reduces psychosis without exacerbating parkinsonism *(86)*. Relatively small doses of clozapine have also been used successfully for the relief of paranoid delusions, psychosis, and agitation, albeit at the risk of agranulocytosis *(84)*. Indeed, caution is generally warranted in using neuroleptics, since sedation, confusion, immobility, postural instability, and other serious side effects are hardly uncommon *(87,88)*. Neuroleptic malignant syndrome (NMS) is a rare but fatal adverse effect more common with typical neuroleptics, such as haloperidol, owing to potent dopaminergic blockade *(84,85)*. Dopaminomimetic agents (DA agonists more so than levodopa) are more likely to worsen than improve cognitive and affective function associated with the atypical parkinsonian disorders. The management of psychosis should thus first involve lowering the dose of anti-parkinsonian medication in this order: anticholinergics, amantadine, selegiline, DA agonists, and then levodopa; only if the improvement is inadequate, should a cautious trial of antipsychotic medication be considered *(87)*. There are isolated reports of improvement in depression with levodopa *(89)*, or with levodopa combined with L-threodihydroxyphenylserine and thyroid-releasing hormone *(90)*. The successful use of clozapine in treatment-resistant psy-

Table 1
Most Commonly Recommended Drugs for Each Dysfunction

Motor	Levodopa, variable response but best drug
	Other dopaminergic agents, less beneficial
Autonomic	Orthostatic hypotension—fludrocortisone, midodrine
	Urinary incontinence—tolterodine, oxybutinin, propantheline
	Erectile dysfunction—sildenafil citrate
Cognitive	Cholinesterase inhibitors (donepezil, rivastigmine)
Behavioral	Psychosis—atypical neuroleptics (quetiapine, clozapine)
	Depression—SSRI

chotic depression without aggravating neurological disabilities has also been observed *(91)*. In the absence of formal trials of antidepressants in patients with atypical parkinsonism, serotonin reuptake inhibitors, such as those used for PD, are generally prescribed.

Others

ECT has been effective in the treatment of depression in the atypical parkinsonian disorders, but produces inconsistent benefits on motor or cognitive dysfunction *(99–101)*.

FUTURE

The atypical parkinsonian disorders present clinically with a myriad of symptoms owing to the diffuse nature of the underlying neuronal involvement. Current palliative pharmacotherapies, largely seeking to normalize resultant transmitter system abnormalities, are largely unsuccessful because of poor efficacy, prominent adverse effects, or both. A variety of factors contribute to this unfortunate situation. The number of patients afflicted by these disorders is small, insufficient to stimulate specific pharmaceutical development efforts. Attempts to rigorously assess possible extensions of existing drugs to the treatment of the atypical parkinsonian syndromes have been uncommon. There are no reliable means for early and accurate diagnosis, although the National Institutes of Health–Progressive Supranuclear Palsy (NINDS–PSP) criteria is specific. There is also a need for validated animal models, but studies are under way *(102–105)*. Finally, most clinical trials have been so limited and poorly designed as to preclude reliable interpretation. In this setting, physicians have largely been left to make their own best therapeutic judgments. Treatment remains symptomatic and largely supportive (Table 1) while awaiting the emergence of neuroprotective strategies to slow or stop disease progression. Palliative therapies include ambulatory aids and rehabilitation, which are discussed in another chapter.

Neuroprotection

Notwithstanding the rapid advances in basic neurosciences research, the causes of neurodegenerative disease remain obscure. Without more detailed etiologic information, the probability of discovering an effective protective therapy is small. Current research implicates a complex combination of genetic predispositions and endogenous and/or environmental factors. Oxidative stress, excitotoxicity, mitochondrial deficiency, microglial activation, apoptotic triggering, and protein-processing abnormalities have all been suggested as possibly contributory (Table 2). Recently, the proteins α-synuclein, which interfere with membrane protein function, and tau, a microtubular-associated protein, which plays an important role in neuronal transport, have received increasing investigative attention. The discovery of these proteins has prompted classification of the atypical parkinsonian disorders into α-synucleopathies, specifically MSA *(106,107)* and DLB *(108)*,

**Table 2
Possible Disease Etiologies and Areas to Explore for Neuroprotection**

Oxidative stress
Excitotoxicity
Mitochondrial deficiency
Microglial activation
Apoptotic triggering
Protein processing abnormalities (i.e., accumulation of α-synuclein, tau)

and tauopathies, specifically PSP and CBD *(109,110)*. Pathological overlap exists, however, and colocalization of α-synuclein and tau does occur *(111–114)*. A possible role for these proteins in pathogenesis could also provide a basis for developing surrogate spinal fluid outcome measures to assist in the clinical evaluation of therapeutic candidates. Stimulation of axonal regeneration through glial cell-derived neurotrophic factor (GDNF) has already received attention. Neuroradiologic advances also promise to provide clearer insight into such matters as local cerebral blood flow, transmitter system function, and intracellular metabolic abnormalities, needed to identify the cause of the selective neurodegenerative processes and to discover successful therapeutic interventions.

REFERENCES

1. Brooks DJ, Ibanez V, Sawle GV, Quinn N, Lees AJ, Mathias CJ, et al. Differing patterns of striatal 18F-dopa uptake in Parkinson's disease, multiple system atrophy, and progressive supranuclear palsy. Ann Neurol 1990;28(4):547–555.
2. Leenders KL, Frackowiak RSJ, Lees AJ. Steele–Richardson–Olszewski syndrome. Brain energy metabolism, blood flow and fluorodopa uptake measured by positron emission tomography. Brain 1988;111(Pt 3):615–630.
3. Antonini A, Leenders KL, Vontobel P. Complementary PET studies of striatal neuronal function in the differential diagnosis between multiple system atrophy and Parkinson's disease. Brain 1997;120(Pt 12):2187–2195.
4. Churchyard A, Donnan GA, Hughes A. Dopa resistance in multiple-system atrophy: loss of postsynaptic D2 receptors. Ann Neurol 1993;34(2):219–226.
5. Hierholzer J, Cordes M, Venz S, Schelosky L, Harisch C, Richter W, et al. Loss of dopamine-D2 receptor binding sites in Parkinsonian plus syndromes. J Nucl Med 1998;39(6):954–960.
6. Pirker W, Asenbaum S, Bencsits G, Prayer D, Gerschlager W, Deecke L, et al. [123I]beta-CIT SPECT in multiple system atrophy, progressive supranuclear palsy, and corticobasal degeneration. Mov Disord 2000;15(6):1158–1167.
7. Ransmayrl G, Seppi K, Donnemiller E, Luginger E, Marksteiner J, Riccabona G, et al. Striatal dopamine transporter function in dementia with Lewy bodies and Parkinson's disease. Eur J Nucl Med 2001;28(10):1523–1528.
8. Varrone A, Marek KL, Jennings D, Innis RB, Seibyl JP. [(123)I]beta-CIT SPECT imaging demonstrates reduced density of striatal dopamine transporters in Parkinson's disease and multiple system atrophy. Mov Disord 2001;16(6):1023–1032.
9. Pirker W, Djamshidian S, Asenbaum S, Gerschlager W, Tribl G, Hoffmann M, et al. Progression of dopaminergic degeneration in Parkinson's disease and atypical parkinsonism: a longitudinal beta-CIT SPECT study. Mov Disord 2002;17(1):45–53.
10. Wenning GK, Tison F, Ben-Shlomo Y, Daniel SE, Quinn NP. Multiple system atrophy: a review of 203 pathologically proven cases. Mov Disord 1997;12(2):133–147.
11. Rajput AH, Rozdilsky B, Rajput A, Ang L. Levodopa efficacy and pathological basis of Parkinson syndrome. Clin Neuropharmacol 1990;13(6):553–558.
12. Colosimo C, Albanese A, Hughes A, de Brun VM, Lees AJ. Some specific clinical features differentiate multiple system atrophy (stritaonigral variety) from Parkinson's disease. Arch Neurol 1995;52:248–294.
13. Boesch SM, Wenning GK, Ransmayr G, Poewe W. Dystonia in multiple system atrophy. J Neurol Neurosurg Psychiatry 2002;72(3):300–303.
14. Rossi P, Colosimo C, Moro E, Tonali P, Albanese A. Acute challenge with apomorphine and levodopa in parkinsonism. Eur Neurol 2000;43(2):95–101.
15. Goetz CG, Tanner CM, Klawans HL. The pharmacology of olivopontocerebellar atrophy. Adv Neurol 1984;41:143–148.
16. Kurlan R, Miller C, Levy R, Macik B, Hamill R, Shoulson I. Long-term experience with pergolide therapy of advanced parkinsonism. Neurology 1985;35(5):738–742.
17. Lees A, Bannister R. The use of lisuride in the treatment of multiple system atrophy with autonomic failure (Shy–Drager syndrome). J Neurol Neurosurg Psychiatry 1981;44(4):347–351.

18. Kobari M, Fukuuchi Y, Shinohara T, Nogawa S, Takahashi K. Local cerebral blood flow and its response to intravenous levodopa in progressive supranuclear palsy. Comparison with Parkinson's disease. Arch Neurol 1992;49(7):725–730.

19. Henderson JM, Carpenter K, Cartwright H, Halliday GM. Loss of thalamic intralaminar nuclei in progressive supranuclear palsy and Parkinson's disease: clinical and therapeutic implications. Brain 2000;123(Pt 7):1410–1421.

20. Kompoliti K, Goetz CG, Litvan I, Jellinger K, Veiny M. Pharmacological therapy in progressive supranuclear palsy. Arch Neurol 1998; 55(8):1099–1102.

21. Nieforth KA, Golbe LI. Retrospective study of drug response in 87 patients with progressive supranuclear palsy. Clin Neuropharmacol 1993;16(4):338–346.

22. Weiner W J, Minagar A, Shulman LM. Pramipexole in progressive supranuclear palsy. Neurology 1999;52(4):873–874.

23. Neophytides A, Lieberman AN, Goldstein M, Gopinathan G, Leibowitz M, Bock J, Walker R. The use of lisuride, a potent dopamine and serotonin agonist, in the treatment of progressive supranuclear palsy. J Neurol Neurosurg Psychiatry 1982;45(3):261–263.

24. Defazio G, De Mari M, De Salvia R, Lamberti P, Giorelli M, Livrea P. "Apraxia of eyelid opening" induced by levodopa therapy and apomorphine in atypical parkinsonism (possible progressive supranuclear palsy): a case report. Clin Neuropharmacol 1999;22(5):292–294.

25. Kim JM, Lee KH, Choi YL, Choe GY, Jeon BS. Levodopa-induced dyskinesia in an autopsy-proven case of progressive supranuclear palsy. Mov Disord 2002;17(5):1089–1090.

26. Tan EK, Chan LL, Wong MC. Levodopa-induced oromandibular dystonia in progressive supranuclear palsy. Clin Neurol Neurosurg 2003;105(2):132–134.

27. Wenning GK, Litvan I, Jankovic J, Granata R, Mangone CA, McKee A, et al. Natural history and survival of 14 patients with corticobasal degeneration confirmed at postmortem examination. J Neurol Neurosurg Psychiatry 1998; 64(2):184–189.

28. Kompoliti K, Goetz CG, Boeve BF, Maraganore DM, Ahlskog JE, Marsden CD, et al. Clinical presentation and pharmacological therapy in corticobasal degeneration. Arch Neurol 1998;55(7):957–961.

29. Benarroch EE, Schmeichel AM, Padsi JE. Depletion of mesopontine cholinergic and sparing of raphe neurons in multiple system atrophy. Neurology 2002;59(6):944–946.

30. Benarroch EE, Schmeichel AM, Padsi JE. Preservation of branchimotor neurons of the nucleus ambiguus in multiple system atrophy. Neurology 2003;60(1):115–117.

31. Kish SJ, Robitaille Y, el-Awar M, Deck JH, Simmons J, Schut L, et al. Non-Alzheimer-type pattern of brain cholineacetyltransferase reduction in dominantly inherited olivopontocerebellar atrophy. Ann Neurol 1989; 26(3):362–367.

32. Ruberg M, Javoy-Agid F, Hirsch E, Scatton B, LHeureux R, Hauw JJ, et al. Dopaminergic and cholinergic lesions in progressive supranuclear palsy. Ann Neurol 1985;18(5):523–529.

33. Kish SJ, Chang LJ, Mirchandani L, Shannak K, Hornykiewicz O. Progressive supranuclear palsy: relationship between extrapyramidal disturbances, dementia, and brain neurotransmitter markers. Ann Neurol 1985;18(5):530–536.

34. Hirsch EC, Graybiel AM, Duyckaerts C, Javoy-Agid F. Neuronal loss in the pedunculopontine tegmental nucleus in Parkinson disease and in progressive supranuclear palsy. Proc Natl Acad Sci USA 1987;84(16):5976–5980.

35. Juncos JL, Hirsch EC, Malessa S, Duyckaerts C, Hersh LB, Agid Y. Mesencephalic cholinergic nuclei in progressive supranuclear palsy. Neurology 1991;41(1):25–30.

36. Kasashima S, Oda Y. Cholinergic neuronal loss in the basal forebrain and mesopontine tegmentum of progressive supranuclear palsy and corticobasal degeneration. Acta Neuropathol (Berl) 2003;105(2):117–124.

37. Javoy-Agid F. Cholinergic and peptidergic systems in PSP. J Neural Transm Suppl 1994;42:205–218.

38. Fabbrini G, Barbanti P, Bonifati V, Colosimo C, Gasparini M, Vanacore N, et al. Donepezil in the treatment of progressive supranuclear palsy. Acta Neurol Scand. 2001;103(2):123–125.

39. Litvan I, Blesa R, Clark K, Nichelli P, Atack JR, Mouradian MM, et al. Pharmacological evaluation of the cholinergic system in progressive supranuclear palsy. Ann Neurol 1994;36(1):55–61.

40. Frattali CM, Sonies BC, Chi-Fishman G, Litvan I. Effects of physostigmine on swallowing and oral motor functions in patients with progressive supranuclear palsy: a pilot study. Dysphagia 1999;14(3):165–168.

41. Litvan I, Gomez C, Atack JR, Gillespie M, Kask AM, Mouradian MM, et al. Physostigmine treatment of progressive supranuclear palsy. Ann Neurol 1989;26(3):404–407.

42. Litvan I, Phipps M, Pharr VL, Hallett M, Grafman J, Salazar A. Randomized placebo-controlled trial of donepezil in patients with progressive supranuclear palsy. Neurology 2001;57(3):467–473.

43. Foster NL, Aldrich MS, Bluemlein L, White RF, Berent S. Failure of cholinergic agonist RS-86 to improve cognition and movement in PSP despite effects on sleep. Neurology 1989;39(2 Pt 1):257–261.

44. Pascual J, Berciano J, Gonzalez AM, Grijalba B, Figols J, Pazos A. Autoradiographic demonstration of loss of alpha 2-adrenoceptors in progressive supranuclear palsy: preliminary report. J Neurol Sci 1993;114(2):165–169.

45. Cole DG, Growdon JH. Therapy for progressive supranuclear palsy: past and future. J Neural Transm Suppl 1994;42:283–290.

46. Rascol O, Sieradzan K, Peyro-Saint-Paul H, Thalamas C, Brefel-Courbon C, Senard JM, et al. Efaroxan, an alpha-2 antagonist, in the treatment of progressive supranuclear palsy. Mov Disord 1998;13(4):673–676.

47. Di Trapani G, Stampatore P, La Cara A, Azzoni A, Vaccario ML. Treatment of progressive supranuclear palsy with methysergide. A clinical study. Ital J Neurol Sci 1991;12(2):157–161.
48. Rafal RD, Grimm RJ. Progressive supranuclear palsy: functional analysis of the response to methysergide and antiparkinsonian agents. Neurology 1981;31(12):1507–1518.
49. Gilman S, Koeppe RA, Junck L, Kluin KJ, Lohman M, St Laurent RT. Benzodiazepine receptor binding in cerebellar degenerations studied with positron emission tomography. Ann Neurol 1995;38(2):176–185.
50. Bonnet AM, Esteguy M, Tell G, Schechter PJ, Hardenberg J, Agid Y. A controlled study of oral vigabatrin (gamma-vinyl GABA) in patients with cerebellar ataxia. Can J Neurol Sci 1986;13(4):331–333.
51. Foster NL, Minoshima S, Johanns J, Little R, Heumann ML, Kuhl DE, et al. PET measures of benzodiazepine receptors in progressive supranuclear palsy. Neurology 2000;54(9):1768–1773.
52. Levy R, Ruberg M, Herrero MT, Villares J, Javoy-Agid F, Agid Y, et al. Alterations of GABAergic neurons in the basal ganglia of patients with progressive supranuclear palsy: an in situ hybridization study of GAD67 messenger RNA. Neurology. 1995;45(1):127–134.
53. Daniele A, Moro E, Bentivoglio AR. Zolpidem in progressive supranuclear palsy. N Engl J Med 1999;341(7):543–544.
54. Stover NP, Watts RL. Corticobasal degeneration. Semin Neurol 2001;21(2):49–58.
55. Botez MI, Botez-Marquard T, Elie R, Le Marec N, Pedraza OL, Lalonde R. Amantadine hydrochloride treatment in olivopontocerebellar atrophy: a long-term follow-up study. Eur Neurol 1999;41(4):212–215.
56. Colosimo C, Merello M, Pontieri FE . Amantadine in parkinsonian patients unresponsive to levodopa: a pilot study. J Neurol 1996;243(5):422–425.
57. Botez MI, Botez-Marquard T, Elie R, Pedraza OL, Goyette K, Lalonde R. Amantadine hydrochloride treatment in heredodegenerative ataxias: a double blind study. J Neurol Neurosurg Psychiatry 1996;61(3):259–264.
58. Newman GC. Treatment of progressive supranuclear palsy with tricyclic antidepressants. Neurology 1985;35(8):1189–1193.
59. Vanek ZF, Jankovic J. Dystonia in corticobasal degeneration. Mov Disord. 2001;16(2):252–257.
60. Cordivari C, Misra VP, Catania S, Lees AJ. Treatment of dystonic clenched fist with botulinum toxin. Mov Disord 2001;16(5):907–913.
61. Muller J, Wenning GK, Wissel J, Seppi K, Poewe W. Botulinum toxin treatment in atypical parkinsonian disorders associated with disabling focal dystonia. J Neurol 2002;249(3):300–304.
62. Mark MH. Lumping and splitting the Parkinson plus syndromes: dementia with Lewy bodies, multiple system atrophy, progressive supranuclear palsy, and cortical-basal ganglionic degeneration. Neurol Clin 2001;19(3):607–627.
63. Thobois S, Broussolle E, Toureille L, Vial C. Severe dysphagia after botulinum toxin injection for cervical dystonia in multiple system atrophy. Mov Disord 2001;16(4):764–765.
64. Lang AE, Lozano Am. Parkinson's disease. Second of two parts. N Engl J Med 1998;339(16):1130–1143.
65. Visser-Vandewalle V, Temel Y, Colle H, van der Linden C. Bilateral high-frequency stimulation of the subthalamic nucleus in patients with multiple system atrophy—parkinsonism. Report of four cases. J Neurosurg 2003;98(4):882–887.
66. Barclay CL, Duff J, Sandor P, Lang AE. Limited usefulness of electroconvulsive therapy in progressive supranuclear palsy. Neurology 1996;46(5):1284–1286.
67. Benarroch EE, Smithson IL, Low PA, Parisi JE. Depletion of catecholaminergic neurons of the rostral ventrolateral medulla in multiple systems atrophy with autonomic failure. Ann Neurol 1998;43(2):156–163.
68. Mathias CJ. Autonomic disorders and their recognition. N Engl J Med 1997;336(10):721–724.
69. Thomas DJ, Bannister R. Preservation of autoregulation of cerebral blood flow in autonomic failure. J Neurol Sci 1980; 44(2–3):205–212.
70. Wright R, Kaufman HC, Perera R, Opker-Gehring TL, McElligot MA, Cheng KN. A double-blind, dose response study on midodrine in neurogenic orthostatic hypotension. Neurology 1998;51(1):120–124.
71. Jordan J, Shannon JR, Biaggioni I, Norman R, Black BK, Robertson D. Contrasting actions of pressor agents in severe autonomic failure. Am J Med 1998;105(2):116–124.
72. Mathias CJ, Senard JM, Braune S, Watson L, Aragishi A, Keeling JE, et al. L-threo-dihydroxyphenylserine (L-threo-DOPS; droxidopa) in the management of neurogenic orthostatic hypotension: a multi-national, multi-center, dose-ranging study in multiple system atrophy and pure autonomic failure. Clin Auton Res 2001;11(4):235–242.
73. Yoshozawa T, Fuhita T, Mizusawa H, Shoji S. L-threo-3,4-dihydroxyphenylserine enhances the orthostatic responses of plasma renin activity and angiotensin II in multiple system atrophy. J Neuro 1999;246(3):193–197.
74. Bordet R, Benhadjali J, Destee A, Belabbas A, Libersa C. Octreotide in the management of orthostatic hypotension in multiple system atrophy: pilot trial of chronic administration. Clin Neuropharmacol 1994;17(4):380–383.
75. Vallejo R, DeSouza G, Lee J. Shy–Drager syndrome and severe unexplained intraoperative hypotension responsive to vasopressin. Anesth Analg 2002;95(1):50–52.
76. Perrera R, Isola L, Kaufman H. Effect of recombinant erythropoietin on anemia and orthostatic hypotension in primary autonomic failure. Clin Auton Res 1995;5(4):211–213.
77. Sakakibara R, Hattori T, Uchiyama T, Suenaga T, Takahashi H, Yamanishi T, et al. Are alpha-blockers involved in lower urinary tract dysfunction in multiple system atrophy? A comparison of prazosin and moxisylyte. J Auton Nerv Syst 2000;79(2–3):191–195.

78. Sakakibara R, Matsuda S, Uchiyama T, Yoshiyama M, Yamanishi T, Hattori T. The effect of intranasal desmopressin on nocturnal waking in urination in multiple system atrophy patients with nocturnal polyuria. Clin Auton Res 2003;13(2):106–108.

79. Colosimo C, Pezzella FR. The symptomatic treatment of multiple system atrophy. Eur J Neurol 2002;9(3):195–199.

80. Hussain IF, Brady CM, Swinn MJ, Mathias CJ, Fowler CJ. Treatment of erectile dysfunction with sildenafil citrate (Viagra) in parkinsonism due to Parkinson's disease or multiple system atrophy with observations on orthostatic hypotension. J Neurol Neurosurg Psychiatry 2001;71(3):371–374.

81. Eichhorn TE, Oertel WH. Macrogol 3350/electrolyte improves constipation in Parkinson's disease and multiple system atrophy. Mov Disord 2001;16(6):1176–1177.

82. Khurana RK. Cholinergic dysfunction in Shy–Drager syndrome: effect of the parasympathomimetic agent, bethanechol. Clin Auton Res 1994;4(1–2):5–13.

83. Hyson HC, Johnson AM, Jog MS. Sublingual atropine for sialorrhea secondary to parkinsonism: a pilot study. Mov Disord 2002;17(6):1318–1320.

84. Geroldi C, Frisoni GB, Bianchetti A, Trabucchi M. Drug treatment in Lewy body dementia. Dement Geriatr Cogn Disord 1997;8(3):188–197.

85. Fernandez HH, Trieschmann ME, Burke MA, Friedman JH. Quetiapine for psychosis in Parkinson's disease versus dementia with Lewy bodies. J Clin Psychiatry 2002;63(6):513–515.

86. Cummings JL, Street J, Masterman D, Clark WS. Efficacy of olanzapine in the treatment of psychosis in dementia with lewy bodies. Dement Geriatr Cogn Disord 2002;13(2):67–73.

87. Barber R, Panikkar A, McKeith IG. Dementia with Lewy bodies: diagnosis and management. Int J Geriatr Psychiatry 2001;16(Suppl 1):S12–S18.

88. McKeith I, Fairbairn A, Perry R, Thompson P, Perry E. Neuroleptic sensitivity in patients with senile dementia of Lewy body type. BMJ 1992;305(6855):673–678.

89. Fetoni V, Soliveri P, Monza D, Testa D, Girotti F. Affective symptoms in multiple system atrophy and Parkinson's disease: response to levodopa therapy. J Neurol Neurosurg Psychiatry 1999;66(4):541–544.

90. Goto K, Ueki A, Shimode H, Shinjo H, Miwa C, Morita Y. Depression in multiple system atrophy: a case report. Psychiatry Clin Neurosci 2000;54(4):507–511.

91. Parsa MA, Simon M, Dubrow C, Ramirez LF, Meltzer HY. Psychiatric manifestations of olivo-ponto-cerebellar atrophy and treatment with clozapine. Int J Psychiatry Med 1993;23(2):149–156.

92. Kertzman C, Robinson DL, Litvan I. Effects of physostigmine on spatial attention in patients with progressive supranuclear palsy. Arch Neurol 1990;47(12):1346–1350.

93. Shiozaki K, Iseki E, Hino H, Kosaka K. Distribution of m1 muscarinic acetylcholine receptors in the hippocampus of patients with Alzheimer's disease and dementia with Lewy bodies-an immunohistochemical study. J Neurol Sci 2001;193(1):23–28.

94. Martin-Ruiz C, Court J, Lee M, Piggott M, Johnson M, Ballard C, et al. Nicotinic receptors in dementia of Alzheimer, Lewy body and vascular types. Nicotinic receptors in dementia of Alzheimer, Lewy body and vascular types. Acta Neurol Scand Suppl 2000;176:34–41.

95. Grace J, Daniel S, Stevens T, Shankar KK, Walker Z, Byrne EJ, et al. Long-Term use of rivastigmine in patients with dementia with Lewy bodies: an open-label trial. Int Psychogeriatr 2001;13(2):199–205.

96. Wesnes KA, McKeith IG, Ferrara R, Emre M, Del Ser T, Spano PF, et al. Effects of rivastigmine on cognitive function in dementia with lewy bodies: a randomised placebo-controlled international study using the cognitive drug research computerised assessment system. Dement Geriatr Cogn Disord 2002;13(3):183–92.

97. Samuel W, Caligiuri M, Galasko D, Lacro J, Marini M, McClure FS, et al. Better cognitive and psychopathologic response to donepezil in patients prospectively diagnosed as dementia with Lewy bodies: a preliminary study. Int J Geriatr Psychiatry 2000;15(9):794–802.

98. Shea C, MacKnight C, Rockwood K. Donepezil for treatment of dementia with Lewy bodies: a case series of nine patients. Int Psychogeriatr 1998;10(3):229–238.

99. Hooten WM, Melin G, Richardson JW. Response of the parkinsonian symptoms of multiple system atrophy to ECT. Am J Psychiatry 1998;155(11):1628.

100. Roane DM, Rogers JD, Helew L, Zarate J. Electroconvulsive therapy for elderly patients with multiple system atrophy: a case series. Am J Geriatr Psychiatry 2000;8(2):171–174.

101. Ruxin RJ, Ruedrich S. ECT in combined multiple system atrophy and major depression. Convuls Ther 1994;10(4):298–300.

102. Feany MB, Bender WW. A Drosophila model of Parkinson's disease. Nature 2000;404(6776):394–398.

103. Sahara N, Lewis J, DeTure M, McGowan E, Dickson DW, Hutton M, et al. Assembly of tau in transgenic animals expressing P301L tau: alteration of phosphorylation and solubility. J Neurochem 2002;83(6):1498–1508.

104. Giasson BI, Duda JE, Quinn SM, Zhang B, Tojanowksi JQ, Lee VM-Y. Neuronal a-synucleinopathy with severe movement disorder in mice expressing A53T human a-synuclein. Neuron 2002; 34(4):521–533.

105. Neumann M, Kahle PJ, Giasson BI, Ozmen L, Borroni E, Spooren W, et al. Misfolded proteinase K-resistant hyperphosphorylated a-synuclein in aged transgenic mice with locomotor deterioration and in human a-synucleinopathies. J Clin Invest 2002;110(10):1429–1439.

106. Gai WP, Pountney DL, Power JH, Li QX, Culvenor JG, McLean CA, et al. Alpha-Synuclein fibrils constitute the central core of oligodendroglial inclusion filaments in multiple system atrophy. Exp Neurol 2003;181(1):68–78.

107. Duda JE, Giasson BI, Gur TL, Montine TJ, Robertson D, Biaggioni I, et al. Immunohistochemical and biochemical studies demonstrate a distinct profile of alpha-synuclein permutations in multiple system atrophy. J Neuropathol Exp Neurol 2000;59(9):830-41.

108. Marui W, Iseki E, Nakai T, Miura S, Kato M, Ueda K, et al. Progression and staging of Lewy pathology in brains from patients with dementia with Lewy bodies. J Neurol Sci 2002;195(2):153–159.

109. Arai T, Ikeda K, Akiyama H, Tsuchiya K, Iritani S, Ishiguro K, et al. Different immunoreactivities of the microtubule-binding region of tau and its molecular basis in brains from patients with Alzheimer's disease, Pick's disease, progressive supranuclear palsy and corticobasal degeneration. Acta Neuropathol (Berl) 2003;105(5):489–498.

110. Houlden H, Crook R, Dolan RJ, McLaughlin J, Revesz T, Hardy J. A novel presenilin mutation (M233V) causing very early onset Alzheimer's disease with Lewy bodies. Neurosci Lett 2001;313(1–2):93–95.

111. Piao YS, Hayashi S, Wakabayashi K, Kakita A, Aida I, Yamada M, et al. Cerebellar cortical tau pathology in progressive supranuclear palsy and corticobasal degeneration. Acta Neuropathol (Berl) 2002;103(5):469–474.

112. Ishizawa T, Mattila P, Davies P, Wang D, Dickson DW. Colocalization of tau and alpha-synuclein epitopes in Lewy bodies. J Neuropathol Exp Neurol 2003;62(4):389–397.

113. Iseki E, Togo T, Suzuki K, Katsuse O, Marui W, de Silva R, et al. Dementia with Lewy bodies from the perspective of tauopathy. Acta Neuropathol (Berl) 2003;105(3):265–270.

114. Takanashi M, Ohta S, Matsuoka S, Mori H, Mizuno Y. Mixed multiple system atrophy and progressive supranuclear palsy: a clinical and pathological report of one case. Acta Neuropathol 2002;103(1):82–87.

29

Rehabilitation of Patients With Atypical Parkinsonian Disorders

Daniel K. White, Douglas I. Katz, Terry Ellis, Laura Buyan-Dent, and Marie H. Saint-Hilaire

INTRODUCTION

Atypical parkinsonism encompasses several disorders that may have disease-specific or individual-specific characteristics, however common features include akinesia, rigidity, gait difficulties, and cognitive decline with gradual worsening of the symptoms. These features result in a variety of deficits that affect the patient's ability to function in their usual capacity at home, on the job, and within their community. As in other neurodegenerative disorders, patients with atypical parkinsonian disorders (APDs) become increasingly disabled and have a decline in their quality of life. The rehabilitation team's goal is to improve the patient's functional ability and quality of life. Use of a disablement model provides a conceptual framework helpful in delineating the level at which intervention is best applied. The team must appreciate the impact of intervention at the pathology, impairment, functional, and disability levels in order to choose the appropriate treatment direction. The evidence supporting rehabilitation in idiopathic Parkinson's disease (PD) can be useful in gaining an appreciation of the impact of treatment across the different levels in order to help guide rehabilitation direction in patient's with APDs. Treatment direction may encompass both restorative and compensatory strategies to improve function and quality of life and should be considered to supplement pharmacologic and other medical interventions.

A CONCEPTUAL FRAMEWORK

Rehabilitation teams often use a model of disablement to describe the relationship from disease to disability and to clearly identify the effects of disease on an individual. A disablement model is useful in providing a conceptual framework to help focus rehabilitation efforts in an appropriate direction. A model is also helpful in establishing clear communication among the members of the rehabilitation team. The Nagi Disablement model, developed by the sociologist, Saad Nagi, is one such model often adopted by rehabilitation teams. It contains four levels of dysfunction, which include the pathology, impairment, functional limitation, and disability (1). APDs are examples of pathologies, which encompass the disease state at the organ level. Impairments refer to the anatomical, physiological, mental, or emotional abnormalities or losses related to structure or function. It is helpful to distinguish between direct and indirect impairments. Direct impairments are those that arise as a direct result of the pathology. In APDs, direct impairments may include rigidity, bradykinesia, and tremor. Indirect impairments may arise from the direct impairments or from adopting a more seden-

From: *Current Clinical Neurology: Atypical Parkinsonian Disorders*
Edited by: I. Litvan © Humana Press Inc., Totowa, NJ

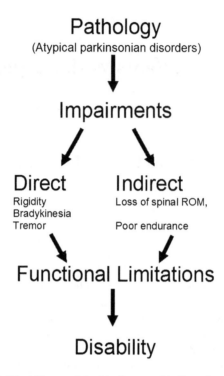

Fig 1. Disability model with direct and indirect impairment.

tary lifestyle over time. For example, in APDs, the presence of axial rigidity often leads to indirect impairments such as loss of range of motion into spinal rotation and extension. Indirect impairments such as poor endurance may evolve because of a decline in activity level as the disease progresses. Functional limitations include limitations in performance at the level of the whole person such as walking, moving in bed, rising from a chair, and handwriting. Disability refers to limitations in performance of socially defined roles and tasks including work, travel, and other leisure or recreational activities. (*See* Fig. 1.)

The role of the rehabilitation team is to choose and administer the appropriate therapeutic interventions with the goal of maximizing function and minimizing disability ultimately leading to improving quality of life. In order to choose the most appropriate interventions, the level of impact must be defined. The neurologist typically intervenes with pharmacological intervention aimed at the pathology level. A myriad of medications to optimize availability of dopamine or to replace dopamine are administered with the goal of reducing severity of impairments such as rigidity, which may lead to improvements in mobility at the functional level. However, in patients with APDs, medication effectiveness is less than optimal and often leads to only modest changes at the impairment and functional levels. Given the limited effect of pharmacological intervention, rehabilitation may play an even more important role in maximizing function in patients with APDs than idiopathic PD.

EFFICACY OF REHABILITATION

The efficacy of rehabilitation in patients with APDs is largely unknown, however a number of studies have investigated the efficacy of physical therapy in addition to medication therapy in individuals with PD. Most studies reveal positive effects of physical therapy in patients with PD. De Goede and colleagues conducted a meta-analysis of 12 studies investigating the effects of physical therapy in addition to medications in individuals with PD *(2)*. All studies included in the analysis were classified as true or quasi-experiments. The physical therapy interventions varied across studies and included gait training with external cues, behavioral training to improve activities of daily living (ADL), exercises to improve mobility, stretching, strengthening, karate, skills training, and education. A statistically significant summary effect size was found with regard to ADL (0.40), stride length (0.46), and walking speed (0.49). The summary effect size with regard to neurological signs (0.22) was not significant. The authors concluded that individuals with PD benefit from physical therapy (PT) added to their standard medication. Murphy and Tickle-Degnen conducted a meta-analysis of 16 studies investigating the effects of occupational therapy (OT)-related treatments for individuals with PD *(3)*. Studies included contained a variety of experimental designs including randomized controlled trials (RCTs), cohort, pretest–posttest, and case-control studies. A statistically significant summary effect size was found for outcomes classified at the capabilities and abilities level (0.50), the activities and tasks level (0.54), and on overall outcomes (0.54). The results of this meta-analysis suggest small to moderate positive effects of OT-related interventions in individuals with PD. Deane and coauthors concluded in two systematic reviews that there was not enough evidence to reject or to support the efficacy of PT for patients with PD, however a meta-analytic review was not conducted *(4,5)*.

A randomized control trial (RCT) (*n* = 68) investigating the efficacy of PT in patients with PD revealed significant improvements at the disability level regarding quality of life as it relates to physical mobility. The most robust findings occurred at the functional level with respect to walking speed and ADL *(6)*. No significant improvements were found at the impairment level with regard to neurological signs. Several other investigations support these findings. Formisano et al. investigated the benefits of a PT program in comparison to a control group and found greater improvements regarding ADL and a 10-m walking test in the group who had received PT *(7)*. Patti and coauthors investigated the effects of a multidisciplinary rehabilitation program in an RCT on individuals with idiopathic PD and found significant increases in walking speed and stride length compared to a nonintervention control condition *(8)*. In a nonrandomized study, Szekely and coauthors reported significant improvements in step length and walking speed for a small group of individuals with PD who participated in a group exercise program *(9)*. Scandalis and colleagues reported significant gains in strength, stride length, and walking velocity compared to pretreatment values in 14 individuals with PD who participated an 8-wk course of resistance training *(10)*. Muller et al. randomly assigned 29 patients with PD to either a control group receiving nonspecific psychological treatment or a behavioral treatment group focusing on strategies to improve initiation and coordination of walking and ADL. The behavior treatment group showed faster onset of gait initiation and improvements in the Unified PD Rating Scale (UPDRS) ADL section compared to the control group *(11)*. Thaut et al. investigated the use of rhythmic auditory stimulation (RAS) as a pacemaker in a 3-wk home-based gait-training program for individuals with PD. In comparison to a control group, the patients who trained with RAS significantly improved gait velocity by 25% and stride length by 12% *(12)*. These studies all provide evidence supporting the functional gains that occur following PT intervention in the PD population. These interventions were focused at the functional level targeting walking, balance, and transitional movements supporting the importance of task-specific training at the functional level.

The impact of rehabilitation on direct impairments stemming from PD appears minimal. The meta-analysis by deGoede and colleagues and the RCT by Ellis and coauthors revealed no significant changes in neurological signs *(2,6)*. However, in a randomized crossover study, Comella et al. found significant improvements in the UPDRS motor scores following participation in a rehabilitation program, suggesting a potential impact on neurological signs *(13)*. The impact of rehabilitation on indirect impairments appears stronger. In an RCT, Schenkman and colleagues demonstrated improved axial mobility and flexibility in individuals with PD who participated in a 10-wk exercise program *(14)*. Scandalis and coauthors reported strength gains after participation in a resisted strengthening program in individuals with PD *(10)*. Bridgewater and coauthors reported gains in cardiorespiratory fitness and habitual activity levels following participation in a 12-wk aerobic-exercise program *(15)*.

DIRECTING REHABILITATION APPROACHES

Therapists may choose from a variety of treatment approaches and strategy. These include treatments that target problems at the impairment or functional level, and interventions that aim to *restore* to a previous level of functioning or *compensate* for loss of previous healthy functioning. Although the literature on rehabilitation with patients with PD is not yet adequate to establish comprehensive evidenced-based guidelines, the growing body of evidence supports the efficacy of rehabilitation and suggests approaches that rehabilitation teams may use in patients with idiopathic PD and APDs. Consistent themes that arise from the research in idiopathic PD include improvements in walking ability and ADL status following rehabilitation targeting these functional areas. Task-specific training at the functional level appears to be a critical ingredient. Studies of other neurologic disorders support the notion that performance of tasks improves in relation to direct task practice *(16,17)*. Furthermore, Lin and colleagues suggest the adult neurological population is more likely to put effort into purposeful everyday tasks, as opposed to tasks perceived as nonpurposeful or less meaningful *(18)*.

The lack of effect of rehabilitation at the impairment level in patients with PD suggests that rehabilitation programs aimed at reducing rigidity, tremor, and other PD impairments are less likely to lead to changes in functional status. However, indirect impairments such as flexibility, range of motion, strength and cardiorespiratory status may benefit. Interventions targeting these indirect impairments yield improvements in function and quality of life.

The choice of restorative vs compensatory strategies can vary among individuals, for different treatment goals and at different times in the progression of the disease. The success of restorative approaches is in part linked to improvement at the indirect impairment level. For example, as axial mobility of the spine improves with treatment aimed at increasing range of motion, the patient's ability to get out of bed in a way that resembles premorbid performance of the task also improves. If underlying impairments do not improve significantly enough to allow successful use of previous movement patterns in the functional task, a compensatory approach may be required to improve function. For example, if axial mobility remains limited, a new strategy relying less on spinal mobility may be introduced to compensate for a loss of mobility. In this case, successful completion of the task can still occur by adopting this new strategy. In idiopathic PD, a combination of restorative and compensatory strategies is often implemented to improve function and quality of life. In early PD, when medications are most effective in treating direct impairments and indirect impairments are most amenable to change with rehabilitation, a restorative approach is often successful. As the disease progresses, fewer changes at the impairment level are expected and a greater emphasis on compensatory strategies to improve function should be adopted. In APDs, the impact of intervention on impairments is usually less than that expected in idiopathic PD. The effect of medication on the reduction in direct impairments, such as rigidity, and indirect impairments, such as spinal mobility, are often less than what is expected in idiopathic PD. In order to improve function in those with APDs, a compensatory approach at the functional level is usually necessary. For example, if a patient with an APD is having difficulty rising from a chair, adopting a strategy using momentum or counting may improve ability to perform the task. In addition, changing the environmental conditions such as raising the height of the chair or using a chair with arm rests is often a successful compensatory strategy.

In summary, indirect impairments have the potential to be modified but greater changes would be expected to occur in the idiopathic PD population compared to the APD population. Frequent reassessment to evaluate the degree of change is necessary to help steer or adjust treatment direction. Several studies support the effectiveness of task specific practice at the functional level to yield improvements in functional status in patients with PD. A restorative approach may be successful when underlying impairments are amenable to improvement; otherwise compensatory approaches in strategy and environmental constraints may yield the greatest changes in functional status and quality of life.

OVERVIEW OF A MOVEMENT DISORDERS REHABILITATION PROGRAM

Our institution has developed a specialized inpatient movement disorders program that focuses on patients with atypical and idiopathic PD and their unique cognitive, motor, and medication-related issues. The program consists of a team of neurologists, nurses, physical, occupational, and speech therapists specializing in movement disorders. Upon admission, the initial goals of the team are to record a patient's movement performance and cognitive function throughout the day. This information is used to identify particular problems specific to that individual, and establish a working diagnosis of the movement disorder to guide treatment decisions. The next goal is to make appropriate medication adjustments to minimize impairments and optimize functional mobility throughout the day. During this process patients participate in individual- and group-therapy sessions where team members treat and monitor movement and cognitive behavior.

Physical and occupational therapists evaluate patient's functional status daily with a battery of short timed tests. Impairment-level assessments are made twice weekly by neurologists examining tremor, bradykinesia, rigidity, and other impairment-level elements of the UPDRS. Once data are collected and evaluations are complete, patient cases are discussed at weekly movement disorders rounds attended by the patient's therapy team and the movement disorders team. A brief summary of any medication side effects or fluctuations of motor or cognitive status is presented to the movement disorders neurologists, who then direct appropriate medication adjustments. The patient's motor and cognitive function continues to be tracked and presented at the next round to determine the effectiveness of any medication changes.

A neurologist specializing in movement disorders can play a key role on a rehabilitative team by assisting in the identification and potential treatment of atypical syndromes. Movement disorder specialists serve as a resource for new developments, diagnostic criteria, and novel treatments. The input of the specialist can be particularly valuable since the diagnosis of APD is not straightforward. Frequently, the response or lack of response to dopaminergic medications is key to the diagnosis. The coordinated efforts of the movement disorders specialist and the rehabilitation team provides a unique and desirable setting to diagnose APDs and the response to medication.

Rehabilitation team members are able to spend a significant amount of time evaluating and interacting with patients, and if knowledgeable regarding extrapyramidal disorders, can detect subtleties that may not be available to a neurologist evaluating a patient in the usual clinical setting. For example, in the typical outpatient office visit, determining the response to medication throughout the day is largely done by anecdotal information provided by the patient and family. In a medically supervised setting such as a rehabilitation center, the potential exists for close observation and documentation by staff specially trained and guided by movement disorders specialists to determine more precisely what is actually occurring in a patient over time. Acquisition of this kind of information can greatly improve diagnosis and treatment, which is often a formidable challenge in patients with atypical PD.

Monitoring of Side Effects and Timing of Medication

In addition to carrying out daily motor and cognitive assessments, therapists and nursing staff are knowledgeable of the indications and potential side effects of the dopaminergic medications used in the treatment of extrapyramidal movement disorders. Issues regarding administration of these medications with respect to meals and activities are emphasized. The nursing staff is focused on keeping to dosage schedules, often challenging in patients with frequent dosing of multiple medications. The staff recognizes the importance of accurate documentation of actual times medications are received so there is reliable information to guide further medication adjustments.

The rehabilitation team monitors medication effects and side effects. Educational inservices are given to assure correct identification of parkinsonian signs and side effects including tremor, freezing, wearing-off phenomena, dyskinesias, hallucinations, and orthostasis. Clinical responses are documented and tracked in relation to medication dosing. These observations are key for medication adjustment decisions.

Cognitive Performance Measures

The primary measure used to track cognitive performance is the Mini Mental Status Exam (MMSE) *(19)*. The MMSE is an 11-item test examining five areas of cognitive function including orientation, registration, attention, calculation, language, and recall. This is performed at least once during admission to obtain baseline information or may be used for comparison in future admissions. Scores may be used to monitor cognitive decline after medication changes. If cognitive difficulty is a significant problem, neuropsychology may provide further assessment. Behavioral problems are managed using the combined expertise of the rehabilitation team, with input from psychology, neuropsychology, and neurology.

Motor Performance Measures

The therapy staff records motor performance measures to objectively track a patient's response to a medication regimen. When selecting a test, therapists attend to the particular areas of functional mobility that fluctuate throughout the day and choose a physical measure that incorporates this particular motor task, such as turning, ambulating, or transitioning from sitting to standing. The motor test should be administered around the patient's medication schedule accounting for peak ("on") and trough ("off") times. Subsequent retests should be carried out at similar times to help distinguish random fluctuations in motor behavior from those related to medication dosing. Again, strict timing of administration of medications is emphasized to ensure motor performance can be related to a possible medication effect.

Physical-performance measures that have been found to be valid and reliable in idiopathic PD population include the 2-min walk, the timed up and go (TUG), and the timed supine to stand and stand to supine *(20,21)*. The results of these tests is documented in the chart for team members to track changes over time and in relation to medication interventions.

The 2-Min Walk

The 2-min walk involves measuring the distance a patient can ambulate at a comfortable pace in 2 min. The test should be carried on a flat level surface with two cones or markers delineating the repeated walking path. The distance between the markers should be kept consistent between tests to improve reliability. The patient can use an assistive device during the test if necessary. This test has been shown to identify the loss of walking endurance in those with idiopathic PD compared to healthy controls *(20)*. The 2-min walk is more appropriate than a 6- or 12-min walk test in patients with APDs. The test requires two practice walks followed by one recorded walk to control for learning effects. An example of how to administer this test is included on the CD-ROM.

The Timed Up and Go

The TUG is a simple test that can be quickly administered. The TUG records the time it takes to stand up from a chair with armrests, walk 3 m, turn, return to the chair, and sit down. The patient can use an assistive device such as a walker or cane during the test. The TUG has been shown to have excellent interrater reliability (ICC = 0.99) and intrarater reliability (ICC = 0.99) *(22)*. The test also has been found to correlate moderately with gait speed, balance, and functional capacity *(22)*. The TUG has been shown to be responsive to changes in motor performance in individuals with idiopathic PD. The test is performed twice with a practice first trial and a recorded second trial. An example of how to administer this test is included on the CD-ROM.

The Timed Supine to Stand and Stand to Supine

This test records the amount of time it takes for a patient to transfer from a supine to standing position and separately records time to transfer from standing to supine. The timed supine to stand and stand to supine test has been found to be a stable measure with good test–retest reliability (ICC = 0.77 for supine to stand, and 0.80 for stand to supine) *(21)*. As with the TUG, this test incorporates functional elements that patients with APDs usually have difficulty with. In the clinic, the test can be modified to a sitting position instead of a standing position for those patients unable to stand unassisted, however the patient must be able to transfer unassisted. Patients perform one practice trial and the average of two subsequent test trials yields the time that is recorded. An example of how to administer this test is included on the CD-ROM.

Intervention Approaches

Both *restorative* and *compensatory* approaches are implemented in the inpatient movement disorders program at our institution. Whereas most patients demonstrate some potential for change of indirect impairments, the majority respond best to interventions aimed at functional-level tasks. Sometimes both strategies are combined through the collaborative efforts of physical or occupational therapy.

For example, axial rigidity, a common direct impairment, results in the indirect impairment of limited range of motion in spinal rotation and extension. To address these indirect impairments, a physical therapist can have patients pass a therapy ball laterally from side to side in a seated or standing position. Patients can achieve more axial extension through increasing the height at which the therapy ball is passed. Increased axial rotation can be achieved through seating the patients more perpendicular to one another.

Both of these indirect impairments can be further treated within a functional context using meaningful tasks, such as meal preparation, upper- or lower-body dressing, or grooming. PT and OT can employ these activities in constructing tasks to address loss of axial range of motion (ROM). For instance, placing canned goods in overhead cabinets during meal preparation activities improves spinal ROM. Patients can reach for food items positioned laterally to facilitate spinal rotation and place the items in an overhead cabinet facilitate spinal extension. For most patients, compensatory techniques will be appropriate to accomplish this task in the home environment, and can be introduced through educating patients to place items on lower shelves to compensate for limited axial extension. Patients can then actively practice utilizing this compensatory strategy in the functional kitchen environment.

A video illustrating an example of one approach aimed at the indirect impairment level followed by the functional level can be found on the CD-ROM.

CASE STUDY

The following case study illustrates some of the essential components of our movement disorders program at our institution for a patient with an APD.

MG is an 89-yr-old male who reported progressive worsening of gait and increased frequency of falls. He was started on L-dopa/carbidopa several months prior to admission by his primary neurologist, who suspected the patient had idiopathic PD. It was not clear that medication produced an improvement in function. His past medical history was significant for hypertension, coronary artery disease, chronic anemia, and a coronary artery bypass graft. Upon admission MG had no frank rigidity, but mild cogwheeling (left greater than right), and a mild to moderate symmetric bilateral action tremor. Functionally, the patient was able to walk with a minimal amount of assistance for distances of 100 ft with a rolling walker. His gait was characterized by an overall slow cadence, short step length, and a decreased base of support. On admission the patient was receiving one and a half tabs of L-dopa/carbidopa 25/100 three times a day. Given the patient's questionable response to L-dopa/carbidopa and his cardiovascular risk factors, the initial working diagnosis of the movement disorders team was APD.

Since MG was able to ambulate with a minimal amount of assistance, the patient was appropriate for functional testing using the TUG and 2-min walk. The supine to stand test was not appropriate since MG required assistance with bed mobility upon admission. After baseline measures were col-

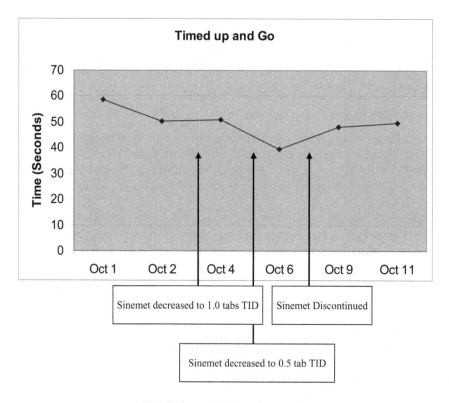

Fig. 2. Case study: timed up and go.

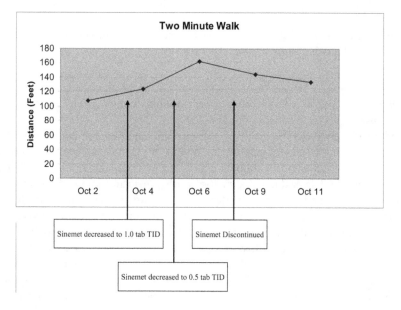

Fig. 3. Case study: 2-min walk.

lected, L-dopa/carbidopa was tapered and discontinued because of the lack of evidence that it provided clear benefit. To ensure the patient had no negative effects from the medication taper, functional measures were collected after each medication change. Figures 2 and 3 describe performance on functional measures regarding medication changes.

At discharge the patient's functional measures were improved, about 10 s faster with the TUG and 26 ft farther with the 2-min walk from initial measures. The improvement in functional measures despite tapering L-dopa/carbidopa suggested that the improvement was the result of rehabilitation interventions. At discharge, the patient returned to assistive living.

This case illustrates several important contributions a movement disorders rehabilitation team can provide patients with atypical PD. Aside from the benefits of rehabilitation interventions, the team provided systematic objective measures of function to accurately conclude that MG did not benefit from pharmacological intervention.

CONCLUSION

Patients with atypical PD present numerous unique challenges to the health care team and their families. Rehabilitation can play an important role in improving function and quality of life especially for treatment of this patient population since current medical and surgical therapies are limited for treating this patient population. Although the efficacy of rehabilitation in patients with APD has not been adequately studied, themes emerge from the rehabilitation literature in idiopathic PD, which may be helpful in the treatment of individuals with APD. Rehabilitation may focus at an impairment or functional level and may employ restorative or compensatory strategies. Research evidence is strongest for rehabilitative treatment at a functional level but some combination of strategies, employing a variety of activities and the combined efforts of multiple disciplines may be most effective. Rehabilitation efforts need to be closely coordinated with medication adjustments. A multidisciplinary team with expertise in the treatment of patient with movement disorders can facilitate such a coordinated effort using standardized protocols to track progress, response to medication, and side effects.

FUTURE RESEARCH DIRECTIONS FOR REHABILITATION OF PATIENTS WITH APDS

- Additional randomized control trials are needed to determine the efficacy of rehabilitation across the short and long term.
- An investigation of the relationship between functional gains and the impact on quality of life is needed.
- The relationship between impairment-level gains and change in function needs to be examined.
- The critical aspects of treatment that lead to improved function and quality of life need to be identified.
- Guidelines are needed to categorize which patients are "responders" or "non-responders" to rehabilitation and which patients benefit from a *compensatory* vs a *restorative* approach.

VIDEO LEGENDS

Functional Tests

- Timed Up and Go

   Demonstration of the Timed up and Go with a patient with PD.

- 2-Min Walk

   Demonstration of the 2-Min walk test with a patient with PD.

- Timed Supine to Stand and Stand to Supine

  Demonstration of the Timed Supine to Stand and Stand to Supine with a patient with PD.

MD Program Treatment

- Movement Disorders Program Axial Rotation

  Demonstration of intervention directed at the indirect impairment level for two patients with PD.

- Movement Disorders Program Kitchen Activity

  The first section is of a higher-level patient performing a kitchen activity to improve axial rotation and extension. The second section is of a lower-level patient performing the same task, but modified for his level of function.

REFERENCES

1. Verbrugge LM, Jette AM. The disablement process. Soc Sci Med 1994;38(1):1–14.
2. de Goede CJ, Keus SH, Kwakkel G, Wagenaar RC. The effects of physical therapy in Parkinson's disease: A research synthesis. Arch Phys Med Rehabil 2001;82:509–515.
3. Murphy S, Tickle-Degnen L. The effectiveness of occupational therapy-related treatments for persons with Parkinson's disease: a meta-analytic review. Am J Occup Ther 2001;55(4):385–392.
4. Deane KH, Ellis-Hill C, Jones D, Whurr R, Ben-Shlomo Y, Playford ED, et al. Systematic review of paramedical therapies for Parkinson's disease. Mov Disord 2002;17(5):984–991.
5. Deane KH, Jones D, Ellis-Hill C, Clarke CE, Playford ED, Ben-Shlomo Y. Physiotherapy for Parkinson's disease: a comparison of techniques (Cochrane Review). In: The Cochrane library, Issue 3, 2002. Oxford: Update Software.
6. Ellis T, deGoede CJT, Feldman RG, Wolters ECH, Kwakkel G, Wagenaar RC. Efficacy of a physical therapy program in patients with Parkinson's disease: a randomized controlled trial. Arch Phys Med Rehab 2004. In press.
7. Formisano R, Pratesi L, Modarelli FT, Bonifati V, Meco G. Rehabilitation and Parkinson's disease. Scand J Rehabil Med 1992;24(3):157–160.
8. Patti F, Reggio A, Nicoletti F, Sellaroli T, Deinite G, Nicoletti Fr. Effects of rehabilitation therapy on Parkinsonian's disability and functional independence. J Neurol Rehabil 1996;10:223–231.
9. Szekely BC, Kosanovich NN, Sheppard W. Adjunctive treatment in Parkinson's disease: physical therapy and comprehensive group therapy. Rehabil Lit 1982;43(3-4):72–76.
10. Scandalis TA, Bosak A, Berliner JC, Helman LL, Wells MR. Resistance training and gait function in patients with Parkinson's disease. Am J Phys Med Rehabil 2001;80(1):38–43; quiz 44–46.
11. Muller V, Mohr B, Rosin R, Pulvermuller F, Muller F, Birbaumer N. Short-term effects of behavioral treatment on movement initiation and postural control in Parkinson's disease: a controlled clinical study. Mov Disord 1997;12(3):306–314.
12. Thaut MH, McIntosh GC, Rice RR, Miller RA, Rathbun J, Brault JM, Rhythmic auditory stimulation in gait training for Parkinson's disease patients. Mov Disord 1996;11(2):193–200.
13. Comella CL, Stebbins GT, Brown-Toms N, Goetz CG. Physical therapy and Parkinson's disease: a controlled clinical trial. Neurology 1994;44(3 Pt 1):376–378.
14. Schenkman M, Cutson TM, Kuchibhatla M, Chandler J, Pieper CF, Ray L, et al. Exercise to improve spinal flexibility and function for people with Parkinson's disease: a randomized, controlled trial. J Am Geriatr Soc 1998;46(10):1207–1216.
15. Bridgewater KJ, Sharpe MH. Trunk muscle performance in early Parkinson's disease. Phys Ther 1998;78(6):566–576.
16. Wagenaar RC. Effects of stroke rehabilitation. In: Kaufman T, ed. Rehabilitation of the Geriatric Patient. New York: Churchill Livingstone, 2000:130–134.
17. Richards CL, Malouin F, Wood-Dauphinee S, Williams JI, Bouchard JP, Brunet D. Task-specific physical therapy for optimization of gait recovery in acute stroke patients. Arch Phys Med Rehabil 1993;74(6):612–620.
18. Lin K, Wu C, Tickle-Degnen L, Coster W. Enhancing occupational performance through occupationally embedded exercise: A meta-analytic review. Occupational Therapy Journal of Research 1997;12:25–47.
19. Folstein M, Folstein SE, McHugh PR. "Mini-mental state." A practical method for grading the cognitive state of patients for the clinician. J Psychiatr Res 1975;12(3):189–198.
20. Light K, Behrman A, Thigpen M, Triggs M. The 2-minute walk test: A tool for evaluating walking endurance in clients with Parkinson's disease. Neurol Rep 1997;21(4):136–139.
21. Schenkman M, Cutson TM, Kuchibhatla M, Chandler J, Pieper C. Reliability of impairment and physical performance measures for persons with Parkinson's disease. Phys Ther 1997;77(1):19–27.
22. Podsiadlo D, Richardson S. The timed "Up & Go": A test of basic functional mobility for frail elderly persons. J Am Geriatr Soc 1991;39(2):142–148.

30
Overview and Future Research

Andrew Lees

Diagnosis is a system of more or less accurate guessing in which the end point achieved is a name. These names applied to disease come to assume the importance of specific entities, whereas they are for the most part no more than insecure and temporary conceptions.
—Sir Thomas Lewis (1931)

Despite its imprecision, *atypical parkinsonism* is a useful clinical term. It unites a group of disorders linked by the predominant presence of bradykinesia, but where additional clinical features exclude Parkinson's disease (PD; hence the analogous but currently less-favored term *Parkinson's plus*). In most cases, disease progression is rapid and relentless and the response to dopaminergic drugs minimal or temporary. Multiple system atrophy (MSA) is the most common example among the primary neurodegenerations, but a substantial number of cases are found at autopsy to have neurofibrillary tangle degeneration, or a combination of neocortical and subcortical Lewy bodies. Extensive subcortical cerebrovascular disease without additional neurodegenerative pathological change is another relatively common cause, but one that presents considerable diagnostic difficulties in clinical practice. Because so many of these pathologies carry a grim and hopeless prognosis, the delicate nuance of uncertainty implicit within the term atypical parkinsonism may be preferable to a more precise alternative clinical label. Nonetheless, names given to neurological disorders assume great importance, both within the medical profession and for those individuals who acquire them: "giving a name to the enemy," however baleful, is often greeted, at least initially, with a sense of relief— "better the devil you know!"

Division into more precise nosological entities is also essential for research. MSA is a synucleinopathy whereas progressive supranuclear palsy (PSP) and corticobasal degeneration (CBD) are four-repeat primary tauopathies. Erroneous inclusion of cases of vascular Parkinson's syndrome could invalidate a genetic study on MSA or an epidemiological study of PSP.

Recent clinico-pathological studies of Parkinson's syndromes have led to an increased awareness among neurologists of MSA of the parkinsonism type (MSA-P, striatonigral degeneration, Shy–Drager syndrome), vascular Parkinson's syndrome, and a motley collection of conditions united by the abnormal accumulation of hyperphosphorylated tau protein in the brain and subcortical neurofibrillary degeneration. The best-recognized conditions in this group are PSP, CBD, and frontotemporal dementia with parkinsonism (FTDP). Much rarer, but of great contemporary interest, are the inherited heavy-metal storage disorders including Hallervorden–Spatz disease and HARP syndrome (recessively inherited and caused by mutations in pantothenate kinase 2 [PANK 2] on chromosome 20), neuroferritinopathy (dominantly inherited and caused by a light ferritin chain mutation on

From: *Current Clinical Neurology: Atypical Parkinsonian Disorders*
Edited by: I. Litvan © Humana Press Inc., Totowa, NJ

chromosome 19),Wilson's disease (recessively inherited and caused by mutations of copper-transporting P-type ATPase on chromosome 13), and acaeruloplasminaemia (recessively inherited and caused by mutations of the caeruloplasmin gene on chromosome 3).

As concepts of what constitutes the clinical picture of PD continue to evolve, our definition of atypical Parkinsonism will also be modified. For example, early autonomic failure, early severe dementia, a negative response to 1000 mg per day of L-dopa for at least 6 wk, and more than one affected first-degree relative have been considered "red flags" for atypical parkinsonism, and yet all of these have been linked with Lewy body pathology in clinico-pathological studies (1). On the other hand, "minimal change" MSA with an excellent sustained response to L-dopa may be indistinguishable from PD throughout the whole course of the illness (2).

A 4–6 Hz "pill-rolling rest tremor" remains the single best clinical marker for PD (3) but a few patients never notice one; in others it may be slight and unobtrusive, and some lose their rest tremor completely as the clinical picture evolves (4) Greater attention to olfaction in the clinical examination may become important as preliminary data indicate that the majority of patients with PD and dementia with Lewy bodies (DLB) have hyposmia, whereas olfactory discrimination in vascular Parkinson's, PSP, CBD, and parkin mutations is usually normal (5). Formed visual hallucinations, which occur commonly in PD and DLB, are extremely rare in MSA, PSP, and CBD and may be another rather neglected red flag for PD especially in the absence of any associated dementia.

PSP (Steele–Richardson–Olszewski disease) is usually included as an important cause of atypical parkinsonism, but Richardson in his seminal descriptions emphasized the marked clinical differences between PSP and PD, although he later conceded that the phenomenology of PSP was likely to broaden with greater clinical awareness and further pathological study (6). L-Dopa-unresponsive symmetrical bradykinesia with prominent axial involvement, preserved downgaze, and extensive subcortical neurofibrillary tangle formation is now recognized as one of the more common causes of atypical parkinsonism, but it is questionable whether this should be included as a clinical variant of Steele–Richardson–Olszewski disease (7,8). CBD, a much rarer clinico-pathological entity, is also included in the list of neurodegenerative disorders presenting with parkinsonism. Despite this, a presentation with predominant parkinsonism must be extraordinarily rare as unilateral myoclonus, jerky tremor, rigidity, cortical sensory loss, dyspraxia, and dystonia usually dominate the clinical picture.

Much interest is at present focused on the parkinsonian signs seen in DLB. This clinical syndrome first described by Kosaka and other Japanese colleagues presents with prominent cognitive decline, delirium, and visual hallucinations, usually in the seventh and eighth decades of life, but the histopathological findings cannot be reliably distinguished in an individual case from those found in PD. Many of these cases also have extensive additional neocortical neurofibrillary tangles, hence the alternative name "Lewy body variant of Alzheimer's disease." However, there is a very interesting group of young patients with pure diffuse cortical and subcortical Lewy body pathology who present with rapidly progressive dementia, behavioral disturbance, and atypical parkinsonism (9). Parkinsonism is seen at some stage in most cases of DLB and it has been reported that the therapeutic response to L-dopa is poorer and rest tremor less frequent and intrusive than in PD (10). However, it is my clinical impression that the L-dopa response is also less striking in many elderly PD patients—especially when there is associated cognitive impairment (11)—and it is now accepted that rest tremor may disappear in the later stages of PD. It seems justified on clinical grounds to distinguish PD and DLB, but from a molecular biological perspective both are likely to share very similar if not identical pathological processes.

In comparison with PD the atypical Parkinson's syndromes are all uncommon, at least in Caucasians. There are some very preliminary data to suggest that atypical features, including a poorer response to L-dopa, may be more common in Africans and Indians with presumed PD, and that an increased frequency of comorbid cerebrovascular disease or associated diabetes mellitus does not account for this difference (12,13). In one South London movement disorder clinic survey, the percentage of atypical parkinsonism was found to be 22% in black African and African/Caribbean patients and 20% in South Asian patients compared to 7% in whites *(14)* This raises the interesting possibility that the phenotype of PD may vary somewhat from race to race, but pathological diagnosis is needed to take this interesting possibility further. A higher incidence of atypical parkinsonism has also been reported among the Chamorros of the Mariana Islands (bodig) *(15)*, the Afro-Caribbean population of the French Antilles *(16)* and the indigenous population of New Caledonia. For example in Guadeloupe, of 220 consecutive patients examined at the CHU Pointe a Pitre, 26.5% fulfilled National Institute of Neurological Disorders and Stroke (NINDS) criteria for PSP and 43.8% were unclassifiable using available published clinical criteria for the recognized parkinsonian syndromes *(17)*. The possibility that cycad or annonacae toxicity may explain these geographic clusters of atypical parkinsonism has been proposed: however, genetic factors may also be important and it is now recognized that spinocerebellar ataxia (SCA) 2 and SCA 3 may present with atypical parkinsonism particularly in Afro-Caribbean and Oriental populations *(18–20)*.

Huntington's disease is another autosomal dominantly inherited disorder that occasionally presents with atypical parkinsonism in middle age *(21)*.

Neuroleptic-provoked Parkinson's syndrome, which is often clinically indistinguishable from PD in the elderly, remains a much more common condition than MSA, PSP, or DLB, although it seems likely that more judicious use of the older antipsychotic drugs and employment of the newer drugs with reputedly fewer extrapyramidal side effects may have reduced its frequency a little. There is a poor or negligible response to L-dopa *(22)*, so if the history of neuroleptic intake is overlooked these cases may be misdiagnosed as MSA or PSP *(23)*. A proportion of elderly-onset cases do not improve even a year after neuroleptic withdrawal, indicating that the drug has probably unmasked latent PD.

The clinical diagnosis of vascular Parkinson's syndrome remains at best an insecure one. Most neurologists now recognize the syndrome of "lower half parkinsonism" with a broad-based, shuffling gait and freezing, with only minimal hand bradykinesia, hypomimia, and often normal speech. Diffuse cerebrovascular disease, especially if there is a history of hypertension, is the most common pathological finding. Striatal cerebrovascular disease is, however, a relatively common associated pathological finding in the elderly parkinsonian patient *(1)* and it is probable that in some patients this modifies the clinical picture. Parkinsonism following a stroke is less well accepted, but there are a number of reported cases in the literature with supportive neuroimaging or pathological confirmation *(24,25)*.

In the absence of specific biological or genetic markers for any of the neurodegenerative processes associated with atypical Parkinson's syndromes, their diagnosis and differentiation depend primarily on scrupulous history taking and a full clinical examination. Diagnosis of the established classical presentation of MSA or PSP is straightforward but "overlap syndromes," "atypical presentations," and early incomplete clinical pictures are frequent, and pose formidable challenges. A recent cross-sectional survey in two tertiary university hospital referral centers for movement disorders in Western Europe revealed that at any one time there were about 5% of atypical parkinsonian patients who could not be more precisely categorized using currently available clinical diagnostic criteria *(26)*. A clinico-pathological study of the first 100 patients diagnosed as PD by UK neurologists 20 yr ago coming to autopsy at the Queen Square Brain Bank for Neurological Disorders (QSBB) in London revealed that 24% did not have severe nigral and locus coeruleus neuronal loss with Lewy bodies in surviving neurones. However, retrospective application of the QSBB criteria for the clinical diagnosis of PD by a movement disorder specialist blinded to the pathological diagnosis improved the accuracy of clinical diagnosis retrospectively to 86%. The most common pathology in the misdiagnosed cases was extensive subcortical neurofibrillary tangles *(27)*. Conversely 12% of 100 cases fulfilling operational criteria for the pathological diagnosis of PD were found to have clinical signs that would have excluded a diagnosis of PD using QSBB operational criteria *(1)*. Ten years later, using identical ascertainment and methodology, diagnostic accuracy had risen to 90% and did not improve further with retrospective application of the QSBB criteria; on this second review MSA-P had taken over as the commonest cause for misdiagnosis. This improvement is likely to reflect a greater clinical awareness among UK neurologists of the wide spectrum of atypical parkinsonian disorders and the publication of sets of consensus criteria to aid clinical diagnosis *(28)*.

A recent review of 60 cases diagnosed clinically with PSP who came to autopsy at the QSBB showed that the clinical diagnosis was accurate in 47 (78%). Sources of diagnostic error included DLB, MSA, tauopathies, and motor neuron disease (MND)-ubiquitin inclusion dementia. Retrospective application of the NINDS and Society for PSP Consensus criteria marginally improved the accuracy of initial clinical diagnosis, but none of the existing diagnostic criteria for PSP could significantly improve accuracy of the final clinical diagnosis *(29)*. A similar methodological study with MSA revealed that 51 of 59 clinically suspected cases were confirmed pathologically in the QSBB, with PD as the most common false positive; this study showed a high diagnostic accuracy for the clinical diagnosis of MSA. Retrospective application of either the Quinn or Consensus criteria for MSA further improved clinical diagnosis in the early stages, but not at the time of the last hospital visit before death *(30)*. In an earlier study from the QSBB, Wenning et al. found that one-third of pathologically confirmed cases carried an alternative clinical diagnosis at death—usually PD *(31)*. Litvan and colleagues *(32)* using material derived from a number of brain banks, found that only 50% of cases with pathologically proven MSA had been accurately diagnosed by their primary neurologist, whereas retrospective analysis by movement disorder specialists improved the accuracy to around 70%. Several studies have compared the clinical features of pathologically proven MSA with idiopathic PD and developed scoring systems weighted for different clinical features *(33)*. These have produced sensitivities of 90%. However, application of these scoring systems in prospective clinical series is likely to be less impressive, as they are internally derived and may overestimate their true performance.

In an attempt to see whether greater accuracy of clinical diagnosis could be achieved by movement disorder specialists working in a university hospital setting, the detailed case notes of 143 pathological cases of parkinsonism thoroughly investigated at the National Hospital for Neurology, Queen Square, by at least one staff movement disorder expert between 1990 and 1999 were scrutinized. The positive predictive value of a clinical diagnosis of MSA was 85.7 (30 out of 35), and the sensitivity was 88.2% (30 out of 34). For PSP, comparable figures were positive predictive value 80% (16 out of 20) and sensitivity 84.2% (16 out of 19). The positive predictive value for PD in this study was extremely high at 98.6% (72 out of 73) with a sensitivity of 91.1%, owing to seven false-negative cases. This suggests that neurologists with special training in movement disorders can expect to achieve around a 90% overall diagnostic accuracy rate for Parkinson's syndromes in the late stages of disease *(34)*.

For more than a century the semiology of the Parkinson's syndromes has been based on a combination of the clinical picture and the neuropathological findings. Even with this traditional two-dimensional classification, new nosological entities continue to be described. Recent advances in genetics and molecular pathology have led to reappraisal of what constitutes a disease: disorders with very different clinical features are linked through identical histopathological changes and patients carrying the same genetic mutation may have very different physical signs. Further confusion stems from the finding that patients fulfilling operational clinical diagnostic criteria for a particular Parkinson's syndrome are sometimes found to have incompatible pathological lesions, and that dual or even multiple pathologies are commonly found at postmortem examination of the elderly. Our conception of PD has been under modification ever since James Parkinson's seminal description of the shaking palsy: his original description was embellished by the 19th-century neurologists, particularly Charcot and Gowers, and the pathological discoveries of Lewy and Tretiakoff provided substance for the notion that it was a distinct entity. However, not long after, following the pandemic of von Economo's disease and the realization that syphilis, head trauma, and cerebrovascular disease could additionally produce parkinsonism, the very existence of the shaking palsy (PD) was called into question. In the 1960s a cluster of previously unrecognized clinico-pathological entities with bradykinesia as a prominent feature were delineated and neuroleptic drugs started to replace postencephalitic parkinsonism as the most common cause of secondary parkinsonism. Attempts to distinguish these atypical cases from PD have led to the development of operational exclusion criteria and supportive red flags to aid diagnostic accuracy of brainstem Lewy body PD.

It has always been recognized that PD is protean in its clinical manifestations and natural history which has led to proposals for tremulous, akinetic-rigid, young-onset, senile, and benign and malignant subtypes. Widespread acknowledgement of the malady's clinical heterogeneity has also led to calls for abolition of the term PD in favor of *idiopathic Parkinsonism*. The cloning of at least four gene mutations in familial Parkinson's syndrome—in which the clinical picture closely resembles classical sporadic PD—has further led to a reconsideration of clinical terminology. Some molecular pathologists link PD, DLB, and MSA because all three are associated with the abnormal misfolding and aggregation of alpha-synuclein. PSP, corticobasal ganglionic degeneration, and some rare familial cases of frontotemporal degeneration, on the other hand, have been embraced under the rubric of primary tauopathy.

The paradigm for treatment of neurodegenerative disease has largely hinged on the success of L-dopa in PD and the clinico-biochemical/pathological correlate linking bradykinesia with dopaminergic lesions in the pars compacta of the substantia nigra. However, the success of this approach has served to hide its shortcomings: as neurologists record the constellation of symptoms and signs in a patient with atypical parkinsonism and speculate on why specific brain regions appear selectively vulnerable at postmortem examination, they should not forget Sir Thomas Lewis's cautionary words to his cardiological colleagues 70 yr ago, that what were then considered discrete entities would in time prove to be no more than ephemeral conceptions. In fact what we often perceive as entities are really processes, each made up of a finite number of specific events.

Neurodegeneration results from a limited number of pathological events each of which engenders biochemical consequences at cellular level. These are modified by genetic and environmental factors and may result in nerve cell death by apoptosis or necrosis. What determines—in an atypical parkinson's case—why a particular neurone takes the tau/tangle or synuclein/Lewy body/glial cytoplasmic inclusion route to cell death may depend on many factors, including the particular chemistry of that neuron, the timing of the event, and the influence of supporting glia. Greater understanding of the mechanisms that cause these destructive biochemical cascades will shed light on the causes of the atypical Parkinson syndromes and, with luck, lead to effective new disease-modifying treatments. The words of L'Hermitte and Cornil from 1921 remain as relevant today as then:

> We must either admit that there exists in addition to multiple Parkinsonian syndromes, an authentic Parkinson's disease with particular lesions and a characteristic evolution and symptomatology or we must say that there is no Parkinson's disease just as there is no hemiplegic disease or pseudobulbar disease.

As we evolve from the traditional clinico-pathological concept of disease entities to a more dynamic consideration of pathological processes, it may be more useful for neurologists in future to describe patients who fulfill a definition of parkinsonism (bradykinesia plus rigidity and/or rest tremor) in terms of their associated physical signs (e.g., dementia, autonomic failure, supranuclear downgaze palsy), functional and physical disability (as quantified by rating scales), disease duration, response to dopaminergic therapy, and genetic profile, rather than attempting to guess the associated histopathological findings on the basis of pattern recognition. In the meantime, however, we must use the crumbs of knowledge we have gathered by clinical observation and research about these brutal clinical syndromes to inform and relieve suffering in our patients.

REFERENCES

1. Hughes AJ, Daniel SE, Blankson S, Lees AJ. A clinicopathologic study of 100 cases of Parkinson's disease. Arch Neurol 1993;50(2):140–148.

2. Wenning GK, Quinn N, Magalhaes M, Mathias C, Daniel SE. "Minimal change" multiple system atrophy. Mov Disord 1994;9(2):161–166.
3. Stadlan EM, Yahr MD. The pathology of parkinsonism. Proceedings of the 5th International Congress of Neuropathology 1965;100:569–571.
4. Winogrodzka A, Wagenaar RC, Bergmans P, et al. Rigidity decreases resting tremor intensity in Parkinson's disease: a (123)beta-CIT SPECT study in early, non-medicated patients. Mov Disord 2001;16:1033–1040.
5. Hawkes C. Olfaction in neurodegenerative disorder. Mov Disord 2003;18(4):364–372.
6. Steele J, Richardson J, Olszewski J. Progressive supranuclear palsy. Arch Neurol 1964;10:333–359.
7. Daniel SE, de Bruin VM, Lees AJ. The clinical and pathological spectrum of Steele–Richardson–Olszewski syndrome (progressive supranuclear palsy): a reappraisal. Brain 1995;118(Pt 3):759–770.
8. Morris HR, Gibb G, Katzenschlager R, et al. Pathological, clinical and genetic heterogeneity in progressive supranuclear palsy. Brain 2002;125(Pt 5):969–975.
9. Gibb WR, Esiri MM, Lees AJ. Clinical and pathological features of diffuse cortical Lewy body disease (Lewy body dementia). Brain 1987;110(Pt 5):1131–1153.
10. Levy G, Tang MX, Cote LJ, et al. Motor impairment in PD: relationship to incident dementia and age. Neurology 2000;55(4):539–544.
11. Burn DJ, Rowan EN, Minett T, et al. Extrapyramidal features in Parkinson's disease with and without dementia and dementia with Lewy bodies: A cross-sectional comparative study. Mov Disord 2003;18(8):884–889.
12. Chaudhuri KR, Hu MT, Brooks DJ. Atypical parkinsonism in Afro-Caribbean and Indian origin immigrants to the UK. Mov Disord 2000;15(1):18–23.
13. Schrag A, Bhatt M, Soonawala N, Quinn NP, Bhatia KP. Occurrence of atypical parkinsonism in Indians and Caucasians. Acta Neurol Scand 2004;109(2):155–156.
14. Hu M. Cortical and Striatal Function in a Cross-Racial Parkinson's Disease Population. London: Guys, Kings and St. Thomas's School of Medicine, 2000. PhD thesis, University of London.
15. Hirano A, Kurland L, Krooth R, Lessell S. Parkinsonism-dementia complex, an endemic disease on the island of Guam. 1. Clinical Features. Brain 1961;84:642–661.
16. Caparros-Lefebvre D, Elbaz A. Possible relation of atypical parkinsonism in the French West Indies with consumption of tropical plants: a case-control study. Caribbean Parkinsonism Study Group. Lancet 1999;354(9175):281–286.
17. Caparros-Lefebvre D, Sergeant N, Lees A, et al. Guadeloupean parkinsonism: a cluster of progressive supranuclear palsy–like tauopathy. Brain 2002;125(Pt 4):801–811.
18. Subramony SH, Hernandez D, Adam A, et al. Ethnic differences in the expression of neurodegenerative disease: Machado–Joseph disease in Africans and Caucasians. Mov Disord 2002;17(5):1068–1071.
19. Furtado S, Farrer M, Tsuboi Y, et al. SCA-2 presenting as parkinsonism in an Alberta family: clinical, genetic, and PET findings. Neurology 2002;59(10):1625–1627.
20. Payami H, Nutt J, Gancher S, et al. SCA2 may present as levodopa-responsive parkinsonism. Mov Disord 2003;18(4):425–429.
21. Reuter I, Hu MT, Andrews TC, Brooks DJ, Clough C, Chaudhuri KR. Late onset levodopa responsive Huntington's disease with minimal chorea masquerading as Parkinson plus syndrome. J Neurol Neurosurg Psychiatry 2000;68(2):238–241.
22. Hardie RJ, Lees AJ. Neuroleptic-induced Parkinson's syndrome: clinical features and results of treatment with levodopa. J Neurol Neurosurg Psychiatry 1988;51(6):850–854.
23. Tolosa E, Coelho M, Gallardo M. DAT imaging in drug-induced and psychogenic parkinsonism. Mov Disord 2003;18(Suppl 7):S28–S33.
24. Tolosa ES, Santamaria J. Parkinsonism and basal ganglia infarcts. Neurology 1984;34(11):1516–1518.
25. Ziljmans J, Daniel SE, Hughes AJ, Revesz T, Lees AJ. Clinico-Pathological Investigation of Vascular Parkinsonism(VP) Including Clinical Criteria for the Diagnosis of VP. Mov Disord, published online, March 16, 2004.
26. Katzenschlager R, Cardoso A, Tolosa E, Lees A. Unclassifiable parkinsonism in two European tertiary referral centres for movement disorders. Mov Disord 2003;18:1123–1131.
27. Hughes AJ, Daniel SE, Kilford L, Lees AJ. Accuracy of clinical diagnosis of idiopathic Parkinson's disease: a clinico-pathological study of 100 cases. J Neurol Neurosurg Psychiatry 1992;55(3):181–184.
28. Hughes AJ, Daniel SE, Lees AJ. Improved accuracy of clinical diagnosis of Lewy body Parkinson's disease. Neurology 2001;57(8):1497–1499.
29. Osaki Y, Ben-Shlomo Y, Lees AJ, et al. Accuracy of Clinical Diagnosis of Progressive Supranuclear Palsy. Mov Disord 2004;19:181–189.
30. Osaki Y, Wenning GK, Daniel SE, et al. Do published criteria improve clinical diagnostic accuracy in multiple system atrophy? Neurology 2002;59(10):1486–1491.
31. Wenning GK, Ben-Shlomo Y, Magalhaes M, Daniel SE, Quinn NP. Clinicopathological study of 35 cases of multiple system atrophy. J Neurol Neurosurg Psychiatry 1995;58(2):160–166.
32. Litvan I, Goetz CG, Jankovic J, et al. What is the accuracy of the clinical diagnosis of multiple system atrophy? A clinicopathologic study. Arch Neurol 1997;54(8):937–944.

33. Colosimo C, Albanese A, Hughes AJ, de Bruin VM, and Lees AJ. Some specific clinical features differentiate multiple system atrophy (striatonigral variety) from Parkinson's disease. Arch Neurol 1995;52(3):294–298.
34. Hughes AJ, Daniel SE, Ben-Shlomo Y, Lees AJ. The accuracy of diagnosis of parkinsonian syndromes in a specialist movement disorder service. Brain 2002;125(Pt 4):861–870.

Index

A

AD, see Alzheimer's disease
Agitation, definition and identification, 162
α (alpha)-Synuclein, see Synucleins
ALS, see Amyotrophic lateral sclerosis
Alzheimer's disease (AD)
    coexistence with Dementia with Lewy
        bodies, 140, 141
    Lewy bodies, 116, 117
    neuropathology, 47
    tau pathology, 124
Amyotrophic lateral sclerosis (ALS), par-
    kinsonism dementia complex of
    Guam, 47
Anxiety, definition and identification, 162
Apathy, definition and identification, 162,
    185
Aphasia, see Speech and language distur-
    bances
ApoE4, dementia with Lewy bodies risks,
    141, 142
Apraxia, see also Speech and language
    disturbances
    comparison in parkinsonian disorders,
        205
    computer modeling of abnormal kine-
        matics during pointing movement
        and errors in praxis
        bread-slicing gesture simulations, 104
        cortical networks, 101
        finger-to-nose test simulations, 102,
            103
        tasks, 99
    corticobasal degeneration, 202–204
    definition, 195
    eyelid opening, 202
    face apraxia, 202
    limb apraxia
        assessment, 196, 197
        diseases, 195
        error patterns, 197, 198
        ideational apraxia, 199
        ideomotor apraxia, 199–201

        limb-kinetic apraxia, 201, 202
        prospects for study, 206
    Parkinson's disease, 204, 205
    progressive supranuclear palsy, 204
    whole body apraxia, 202
Argyrophilic grain disease, neuropathol-
    ogy, 119, 123
Ataxia telangiectasia, eye movements, 245
Autonomic reflexes
    assessment, 419, 420
    dysautonomia clinical evaluation, 157
    dysfunction management, 349–351, 477,
        478
    multiple system atrophy function testing
        bladder function, 341, 342
        cardiovascular function, 341

B

Botulinum toxin, dystonia management,
    476
Bradykinesia, clinical evaluation, 154, 410
Brainstem reflexes, see Eye movements;
    Neurophysiological assessment
Brain tumors, parkinsonism induction, 403,
    404

C

Carbon monoxide, parkinsonism induc-
    tion, 397
CBD, see Corticobasal degeneration
Charcot, Jean-Martin, Parkinson's disease
    research contributions, 11–13
Childhood onset parkinsonism, causes, 400
Cholinesterase inhibitors, dementia with
    Lewy bodies management, 368, 369
Computed tomography (CT)
    progressive supranuclear palsy, 298, 440
    vascular parkinsonism, 443
Computer modeling, basal ganglia disor-
    ders
    abnormal kinematics during pointing
        movement and errors in praxis
        bread-slicing gesture simulations, 104
        cortical networks, 101

CPSIA information can be obtained
at www.ICGtesting.com
Printed in the USA
LVHW062136201222
735671LV00004B/36

9 781588 293312